E. Klipp, R. Herwig, A. Kowald,
C. Wierling, H. Lehrach
Systems Biology in Practice

Further Titles of Interest

C. Sensen (Ed.)

Handbook of Genome Research

**Genomics, Proteomics, Metabolomics,
Bioinformatics, Ethics & Legal Issues**

2005
ISBN 3-527-31348-6

C. Sensen (Ed.)

**Essentials of Genomics and
Bioinformatics**

2002
ISBN 3-527-30541-6

R. D. Schmid, R. Hammelehle

**Pocket Guide to Biotechnology
and Genetic Engineering**

2003
ISBN 3-527-30895-4

M. Schena, S. Knudsen

**Guide to Analysis of DNA
Microarray Data. 2nd Edition**
and Microarray Analysis Set

2004
ISBN 0-471-67853-8

O. Kayser, R. H. Müller (Eds.)

Pharmaceutical Biotechnology

Drug Discovery and Clinical Applications

2004
ISBN 3-527-30554-8

S. C. Gad (Ed.)

Drug Discovery Handbook

2005
ISBN 0-471-21384-5

C. M. Niemeyer, C. A. Mirkin (Eds.)

Nanobiotechnology

Concepts, Applications and Perspectives

2004
ISBN 3-527-30658-7

G. Gellissen (Ed.)

Production of Recombinant Proteins

**Novel Microbial and Eukaryotic Expression
Systems**

2005
ISBN 3-527-31036-3

E. Klipp, R. Herwig, A. Kowald, C. Wierling, H. Lehrach

Systems Biology in Practice

Concepts, Implementation and Application

WILEY-VCH

WILEY-VCH Verlag GmbH & Co. KGaA

Dr. Edda Klipp
Dr. Ralf Herwig
Dr. Axel Kowald
Christoph Wierling
Prof. Dr. Hans Lehrach
MPI für Molekulare Genetik
Ihnestraße 73
14195 Berlin
Germany

1st Edition 2005
  1st Reprint 2006

Library of Congress Card No. applied for

British Library Cataloguing-in-Publication Data: A catalogue record for this book is available from the British Library.

Die Deutsche Bibliothek –
CIP Cataloguing-in-Publication Data:
Die Deutsche Bibliothek lists this publication in the Deutsche Nationalbibliografie; detailed bibliographic data is available in the Internet at http://dnb.ddb.de

Printed in the Federal Republic of Germany
Printed on acid-free paper

Composition   ProSatz Unger, Weinheim
Printing   betz-druck GmbH, Darmstadt
Bookbinding   Litges & Dopf Buchbinderei GmbH, Heppenheim

ISBN-13:   978-3-527-31078-4
ISBN-10:   3-527-31078-9

Preface

Systems biology is the coordinated study of biological systems by (1) investigating the components of cellular networks and their interactions, (2) applying experimental high-throughput and whole-genome techniques, and (3) integrating computational methods with experimental efforts. In this book we attempt to give a survey of this rapidly developing field. The systematic approach to biology is not new, but it has recently gained new attraction due to emerging experimental and computational methods. This book is intended as an introduction for students of biology, biophysics, and bioinformatics and for advanced researchers approaching systems biology from a different discipline.

We see the origin and the methodological foundations for systems biology (1) in the accumulation of detailed biological knowledge with the prospect of utilization in biotechnology and health care, (2) in the emergence of new experimental techniques in genomics and proteomics, (3) in the tradition of mathematical modeling of biological processes, (4) in the developing computer power as a prerequisite for databases and for the calculation of large systems, and (5) in the Internet as *the* medium for quick and comprehensive exchange of information.

Recently, researchers working in different fields of biology have expressed the need for systematic approaches. They have frequently demanded the establishment of computer models of biochemical and signaling networks in order to arrive at testable quantitative predictions despite the complexity of these networks. For example, Hartwell and colleagues (1999) argue that "[t]he best test of our understanding of cells will be to make quantitative predictions about their behavior and test them. This will require detailed simulations of the biochemical processes taking place within [cells]. ... We need to develop simplifying, higher-level models and find general principles that will allow us to grasp and manipulate the functions of [biochemical networks]." Fraser and Harland (2000) state, "As the sophistication of the data collection improves, so does the challenge of fully harvesting the fruits of these efforts. The results to date show a dizzying array of signaling systems acting within and between cells. ... In such settings, intuition can be inadequate, often giving incomplete or incorrect predictions. ... In the face of such complexity, computational tools must be employed as a tool for understanding." Noble laureate Nurse (2000) writes, "Perhaps a proper understanding of the complex regulatory networks making up cellular systems like the cell cycle will require a ... shift from

Systems Biology in Practice. Concepts, Implementation and Application.
E. Klipp, R. Herwig, A. Kowald, C. Wierling, H. Lehrach
Copyright © 2005 WILEY-VCH Verlag GmbH & Co. KGaA, Weinheim
ISBN: 3-527-31078-9

common sense thinking. We might need to move into a strange more abstract world, more readily analyzable in terms of mathematics." And Kitano (2002 a) emphasizes that "computational biology, through pragmatic modeling and theoretical exploration, provides a powerful foundation from which to address critical scientific questions head-on."

The requirement to merge experimental techniques and theoretical concepts in the investigation of biological objects has been acknowledged, for example, by Kitano (2002 a): "To understand complex biological systems requires the integration of experimental and computational research – in other words a systems biology approach." Levchenko (2003) recommends "the systems biology approach, relying on computational modeling coupled with various experimental techniques and methodologies, ... combining the dynamical view of rapidly evolving responses and the structural view arising from high-throughput analyses of the interacting species." Ideker and colleagues (2001) state, "Systems biology studies biological systems by systematically perturbing them (biologically, genetically, or chemically); monitoring the gene, protein, and informational pathway responses; integrating these data; and ultimately, formulating mathematical models that describe the structure of the system and its response to individual perturbations."

Aebersold and colleagues (2000) see the fundamental experimental contribution in large-scale facilities for genome-wide analyses, including DNA sequencing, gene expression measurements, and proteomics, while Hood (2003) explains his path to systems biology in the following way: "Our view and how we practice biology have been profoundly changed by the Human Genome Project."

Importantly, it has been discovered that cellular regulation is organized into complex networks and that the various interactions of network elements in time and space must be studied. Kitano (2002 b) stresses that "[t]o understand biology at the system level, we must examine the structure and dynamics of cellular and organismal function, rather than the characteristics of isolated parts of a cell or organism. Properties of systems, such as robustness, emerge as central issues, and understanding these properties may have an impact on the future of medicine." Kholodenko and colleagues want to "untangle the wires" and "trace the functional interactions in signaling and gene networks." Levchenko (2003) sees advantages in understanding signaling: "A new view of signaling networks as systems consisting of multiple complex elements interacting in a multifarious fashion is emerging, a view that conflicts with the single-gene or protein-centric approach common in biological research. The postgenomic era has brought about a different, network-centric methodology of analysis, suddenly forcing researchers toward the opposite extreme of complexity, where the networks being explored are, to a certain extent, intractable and uninterpretable."

There are many fields of application besides the understanding of cellular regulation. With respect to modeling of the heart as whole organ, Noble (2002) discusses that "[s]uccessful physiological analysis requires an understanding of the functional interactions between the key components of cells, organs, and systems, as well as how these interactions change in disease states. This information resides neither in the genome nor even in the individual proteins that genes code for. It lies at the level of protein interactions within the context of subcellular, cellular, tissue, organ, and system structures." Kirkwood and colleagues (2003) observe a need to apply "e-biology" on aging in order to integrate theory and data.

There is no need to add another definition of systems biology. More important than such a definition is the operational meaning and the *modus vivendi*. However, we would like to emphasize the view that although the *new* property of systems biology is the computational aspect, the trinity of experimentation, data handling, and mathematical modeling is crucial for further successful development of biological science.

Although deciphering of the DNA sequences of many organisms including man has been acknowledged as an important step towards the exact representation of biology, it is currently not possible to calculate the phenotype of an organism from genotype or to simulate a living cell using only the information encoded in these sequences. We will show in the following chapters what can be achieved at present. An old proverb states, "What you expect is what you will get." Knowledge of different concepts, methodologies, and sources of information will support researchers in interpreting their data in a broader context.

This book is divided into three parts. The first part gives an introduction to three main foundations of systems biology – cell biology, mathematics, and experimental techniques. This will be very basic for advanced readers but will prove helpful for those approaching systems biology from a different scientific discipline.

The second part of the book presents current strategies of computational modeling and data mining. It covers in detail various cellular processes such as metabolism, signaling, the cell cycle, and gene expression, as well as the interactions between them. We introduce different concepts of modeling and discuss how the different models can be used to tackle a number of frequent problems, including such questions as how regulation is organized, how data can be interpreted, or which model to apply under specific settings.

The third part gives an overview on currently available help and resources from the Internet. We represent modeling tools that we frequently use ourselves. We also give an overview on databases that are indispensable for information exchange and therefore constitute an essential support for systems biology.

The ideas presented in this book rely on the work of many colleagues currently or formerly active in the field. Our contribution to systems biology has been influenced by many other scientists and our teachers, whom we wish to acknowledge.

We also thank a number of people who helped us in finishing this book. We are especially grateful to Bente Kofahl, Dr. Wolfram Liebermeister, and Dr. Damini Tapadar for reading and commenting on the manuscript. Hendrik Hache and Mario Drungowski contributed with data analysis. Parts of the experimental data used throughout the book were generated in collaboration with Dr. Marie-Laure Yaspo, Dr. James Adjaye and Dr. Pia Aanstad. We thank Monica Shevack for the artistic preparation of many figures.

E.K. wishes to thank her family for support, especially her sons for patience and hot dinners. R.H. thanks his family for supporting him throughout the course of writing. Funding from the following sources is appreciated: E.K. and A.K. are supported by the German Federal Ministry for Education and Research and by the Berlin Center of Genome Based Bioinformatics. C.W. is financed by the EU FP6 grant (LSHG-CT-2003–503269) and R.H. and H.L. by the Max Planck Society.

References

AEBERSOLD, R., HOOD, L.E. and WATTS, J.D. Equipping scientists for the new biology (2000) Nat. Biotechnol. *18*, 359

FRASER, S.E. and HARLAND, R.M. The molecular metamorphosis of experimental embryology (2000) Cell *100*, 41–55

HARTWELL, L.H., HOPFIELD, J.J., LEIBLER, S. and MURRAY, A.W. From molecular to modular cell biology (1999) Nature *402*, C47–52

HOOD, L. Systems biology: integrating technology, biology, and computation (2003) Mech. Ageing Dev. *124*, 9–16

IDEKER, T., GALITSKI, T. and HOOD, L. A new approach to decoding life: systems biology (2001) Annu. Rev. Genomics Hum. Genet. *2*, 343–72

KIRKWOOD, T.B., BOYS, R.J., GILLESPIE, C.S., PROCTOR, C.J., SHANLEY, D.P. and WILKINSON, D.J. Towards an e-biology of ageing: integrating theory and data (2003) Nat. Rev. Mol. Cell. Biol. *4*, 243–9

KITANO, H. Computational systems biology (2002 a) Nature *420*, 206–10

KITANO, H. Systems biology: a brief overview (2002 b) Science *295*, 1662–4

LEVCHENKO, A. Dynamical and integrative cell signaling: challenges for the new biology (2003) Biotechnol. Bioeng. *84*, 773–82

NOBLE, D. Modeling the heart–from genes to cells to the whole organ (2002) Science *295*, 1678–82

NURSE, P. A long twentieth century of the cell cycle and beyond (2000) Cell *100*, 71–8

Foreword

Systems biology is an emergent discipline that is gaining increased attention. A desire to understand systems of living organisms is not a new one. It can be traced back a few decades. Walter Cannon's homeostasis, Norbert Wiener's cybernetics, and Ludwig von Bertalanffy's general systems theory all points to essentially the same direction – system-level understanding of biological systems. Since the discovery of double helix structure of DNA and a series of efforts that gave birth to molecular biology, astonishing progress has been made on our understanding on living forms as molecular machinery. The climax came as completion of human genome sequencing.

With accumulating knowledge of genes and proteins, the next natural question to ask is how they are working together? What are principles that govern at the system-level? With the progress of molecular biology, genomics, computer science, and control theory, the old question is now being revisited with new concepts and methodologies.

A system is not just an assembly of components. There are principles that govern at the system-level. Unlike genes and proteins that are rather tangible objects, a system is no tangible. The essence of the system lies in dynamics that is not tangible. This makes the game of systems biology complicated, and may sound alien to many molecular biologists who are accustomed to a molecular-oriented view of the world. Needless to say system-level understanding has to be grounded onto molecular-level so that a continuous spectrum of knowledge can be established.

The enterprise of systems biology research requires both breadth and depth of understanding for various aspects of biological, computational, mathematical, and even engineering issues. So far, there has not been a coherent textbook in the field that covers broad aspects of systems biology. (I wrote a textbook in 2001 perhaps the first textbook in systems biology, but it was only in Japanese.) In this textbook, the authors have successfully covered sufficiently broad aspects of biology and computation that is essential in getting started in systems biology research. It is essential that both computational and experimental aspects of biology are described consistently and seamlessly. The students who learned through this textbook will make no barrier between computation and experiments. They would use advanced computational tools just like using PCR. I am expecting to see a new generation of systems biologists who get the first touch of the field from this book.
Bon voyage
Tokyo, Japan, September 26 2004

Hiroaki Kitano

Systems Biology in Practice. Concepts, Implementation and Application.
E. Klipp, R. Herwig, A. Kowald, C. Wierling, H. Lehrach
Copyright © 2005 WILEY-VCH Verlag GmbH & Co. KGaA, Weinheim
ISBN: 3-527-31078-9

Contents

Systems Biology in Practice. Concepts, Implementation and Application.
E. Klipp, R. Herwig, A. Kowald, C. Wierling, H. Lehrach
Copyright © 2005 WILEY-VCH Verlag GmbH & Co. KGaA, Weinheim
ISBN: 3-527-31078-9

Part I
General Introduction

Systems Biology in Practice. Concepts, Implementation and Application.
E. Klipp, R. Herwig, A. Kowald, C. Wierling, H. Lehrach
Copyright © 2005 WILEY-VCH Verlag GmbH & Co. KGaA, Weinheim
ISBN: 3-527-31078-9

1
Basic Principles

1.1
Systems Biology is Biology!

Life is one of the most complex phenomena in the universe. It has been studied by using systematic approaches in botany, zoology, and ecology as well as by investigating the composition and molecular biology of single cells. For a long time biologists have thoroughly investigated how parts of the cell work: they have studied the biochemistry of small and large molecules, the structure of proteins, the structure of DNA and RNA, and the principles of DNA replication as well as transcription and translation and the structure and function of membranes. In addition, theoretical concepts about the interaction of elements in different types of networks have been developed. The next step in this line of research is further effort towards a systematic investigation of cells, organs, and organisms and of (mainly) cellular processes such as cellular communication, cell division, homeostasis, and adaptation. This approach has been termed systems biology.

Now the time has come to integrate different fields of biology and natural science in order to better understand how cells work, how cellular processes are regulated, and how cells react to environmental perturbations or even anticipate those changes. The development of a more systematic view of biological processes is accompanied by and based on a revolution of experimental techniques and methodologies. New high-throughput methods allow measurement of the expression levels of all genes of a cell at the same time and with reasonable temporal resolution, although this is still very expensive. Fluorescence labeling and sophisticated microscopic techniques allow tracing individual molecules within a single cell. A fine-grained study of cell components and cell processes in time and in space is an important prerequisite for the further elucidation of cellular regulation.

Systems biology is driven partly by the curiosity of scientists, but even more so by the high potential of its applications. Biotechnological production requires tools with high predictive power to design cells with desired properties cheaply and reliably. There are many promises for health care: models of regulatory networks are necessary to understand their alterations in the case of disease and to develop methods to cure the disease. Furthermore, since there is an observable trend in health care towards individualized and predictive medicine (Weston and Hood 2004), there will be

Systems Biology in Practice. Concepts, Implementation and Application.
E. Klipp, R. Herwig, A. Kowald, C. Wierling, H. Lehrach
Copyright © 2005 WILEY-VCH Verlag GmbH & Co. KGaA, Weinheim
ISBN: 3-527-31078-9

an increasing need for the exact formulation of cellular networks and the prediction of systems behavior in the areas of drug development, drug validation, diagnostics, and therapy monitoring. For example, it has been shown that the epidermal growth factor receptor, which is targeted by a new generation of cancer drugs, belongs to a family of at least four related receptors. These receptors can be turned on by more than 30 different molecules. Thus, such a complex setup makes it necessary to derive the wiring diagram to understand how each component plays its role in responding to various stimuli and causing disease. Once a detailed model has been constructed, all effects of possible perturbations can be predicted fairly cheaply *in silico*. Furthermore, models gained by systems biology approaches can be used for prediction of the behavior of the biological system even under conditions that are not easily accessible with experiments.

Systems biology approaches offer the chance to predict the outcome of complex processes, e. g., the effect of different possible courses of cancer treatment on the tumor (how effectively the treatment eliminates the tumor as well as possible metastatic cells) and the patient (what the cancer treatment does to other rapidly growing tissues, how bad the predicted side effects of a specific treatment in a specific patient are).

These and many other problems that could have enormous effects on our survival, our health, our food supplies, and many other issues that are essential to our existence and our well being might very well be almost impossible to approach without the tools of systems biology that are currently being developed. E. g., to optimize the treatment of an individual cancer patient, we have to be able to accurately predict the outcome of the possible courses of treatment. This would be easy if we were able to understand the complex processes (drug effects, drug side effects, drug metabolism, etc.) the way that we understand some processes in physics (e. g., the famous equation $E = mc^2$ describing the dependence of mass and energy) or even some of the basic processes in biology (the genetic code). This is very unlikely for the complex, highly connected systems we are faced with in many real-world problems in biology. It is not even clear whether our current approach of studying such systems – analyzing small segments (often one or a few genes at a time) – will ever give us enough insight to be able to make useful prediction, as, at least in mathematics, many systems cannot be subdivided in that form. The only option we have might therefore very well be to generate as much information as possible on the system, using the tools of functional genomics, and to model the entire process in as much detail as necessary to allow quantitative predictions of the parameters we are interested in.

Systems biology relies on the integration of experimentation, data processing, and modeling. Ideally, this is an iterative process. Experimentally obtained knowledge about the system under study together with open questions lead to an initial model. The initial model allows predictions that can be verified or falsified in new experiments. Disagreements stimulate the next step of model development, which again results in experimentally testable predictions. This iteration continues until a good agreement is achieved between the data obtained in the experiment and the model predictions.

A major topic of current systems biology is the analysis of networks: gene networks, protein interaction networks, metabolic networks, signaling networks, etc. Initially, investigation of abstract networks was fashionable. However, it has become clear that it is necessary to study more realistic and detailed networks in order to un-cover the peculiarities of biological regulation. Different theoretical attempts have been made to study the different types of networks. For example, gene regulatory networks are sometimes described by Boolean logic assigning to genes one of two states, on or off; protein relations are mainly characterized by a static view of putative interactions measured by yeast two-hybrid methods, and metabolic networks are determined by the set of catalyzing enzymes and the possible metabolic fluxes and intrinsic modes of regulation.

A unified view of a cellular network is currently emerging in the sense that each action of a cell involves different levels of cellular organization, including genes, proteins, metabolism, or signaling pathways. Therefore, the current description of the individual networks must be integrated into a larger framework.

Systems biology also employs theoretical concepts that are only rough representations of their biological counterparts. For example, the representation of gene regulatory networks by Boolean networks, the description of complex enzyme kinetics by simple mass action laws, or the simplification of multifarious reaction schemes by black boxes proved to be helpful understatements. Although being a simplification, these models elucidate possible network properties and help to check the reliability of basic assumptions and to discover possible design principles in nature. Simplified models can be used to test mathematically formulated hypothesis about system dynamics. And simplifying models are easier to understand and to apply to different questions.

Computational models serve as repositories of the current knowledge, both established and hypothetical, on how pathways might operate, providing one with quantitative codification of this knowledge and with the ability to simulate the biological processes according to this codification (Levchenko 2003). The attempt to formulate current knowledge and open problems in mathematical terms often uncovers a lack of knowledge and requirements for clarification. On the other hand, computational models can be used to test whether different hypotheses about the true process are reliable.

Many current approaches pay tribute to the fact that biological items are subject to evolution. This concerns on one hand the similarity of biological organisms from different species. This similarity allows for the use of model organisms and for the critical transfer of insights gained from one cell type to other cell types. Applications include, e.g., prediction of protein function from similarity, prediction of network properties from optimality principles, reconstruction of phylogenetic trees, or identification of regulatory DNA sequences through cross-species comparisons. On the other hand, the evolutionary process leads to genetic variations within species. Therefore, personalized medicine and research is an important new challenge for biomedical research.

1.2
Systems Biology is Modeling

Observation of the real world and, especially, of biological processes confronts us with many simple and complex processes that cannot be explained with elementary principles and the outcome of which cannot reliably be foreseen from experience. Mathematical modeling and computer simulations can help us to understand the internal nature and dynamics of these processes and to arrive at well-founded predictions about their future development and the effect of interactions with the environment.

What is a model? The answer will differ among communities of researchers. In the broadest sense, a model is an abstract representation of objects or processes that explains features of these objects or processes. For instance, the strings composed of the letters A, C, G, and T are used as a model for DNA sequences. In some cases a cartoon of a reaction network showing dots for metabolites and arrows for reactions is a model, while in other cases a system of differential equations is employed to describe the dynamics of that network. In experimental biology, the term model is also used to denote species that are especially suitable for experiments. For example the mouse Ts65DN serves as a model for human trisomy 21 (Reeves et al. 1995).

1.2.1
Properties of Models

1.2.1.1 Model Assignment is not Unique
Biological phenomena can be described in mathematical terms. Many examples have been presented during the past few decades (from the description of glycolytic oscillations with ordinary differential equations, to populations growth with difference equations, to stochastic equations for signaling pathways, to Boolean networks for gene expression). It is important to note that a certain process can be described in more than one way.

- A biological object can be investigated with different experimental methods.
- Each biological process can be described with different (mathematical) models.
- A mathematical formalism may be applied to different biological instances.
- The choice of a mathematical model or an algorithm to describe a biological object depends on the problem, the purpose, and the intention of the investigator.
- Modeling has to reflect essential properties of the system. Different models may highlight different aspects of the same instance.

This ambiguity has the advantage that different ways of studying a problem also provide different insights into the system. An important disadvantage is that the diversity of modeling approaches makes it very difficult to merge established models (e.g., for individual metabolic pathways) into larger super-models (e.g., for the complete cellular metabolism).

1.2.1.2 System State
An important notion in dynamical systems theory is the *state*. The state of a system is a snapshot of the system at a given time that contains enough information to predict the behavior of the system for all future times. The state of the system is described by the set of variables that must be kept track of in a model.

Different modeling approaches have different representations of the state: in a differential equation model for a metabolic network, the state is a list of concentrations of each chemical species. In the respective stochastic model, it is a probability distribution and/or a list of the current number of molecules of a species. In a Boolean model of gene regulation, the state is a string of bits indicating for each gene whether it is expressed ("1") or not expressed ("0"). Thus, each model defines what it means by the state of the system. Given the current state, the model predicts which state or states can occur next, thereby describing the change of state.

1.2.1.3 Steady States

The concept of stationary states is important for the modeling of dynamical systems. *Stationary states* (other terms are *steady states* or *fixed points*) are determined by the fact that the values of all state variables remain constant in time. The asymptotic behavior of dynamic systems, i.e., the behavior after a sufficiently long time, is often stationary. Other types of asymptotic behavior are oscillatory or chaotic regimes.

The consideration of steady states is actually an abstraction that is based on a separation of time scales. In nature, everything flows. Fast and slow processes – ranging from formation and release of chemical bonds within nanoseconds to growth of individuals within years – are coupled in the biological world. While fast processes often reach a quasi-steady state after a short transition period, the change of the value of slow variables is often negligible in the time window of consideration. Thus each steady state can be regarded as a quasi-steady state of a system that is embedded in a larger non-stationary environment. Although the concept of stationary states is a mathematical idealization, it is important in kinetic modeling since it points to typical behavioral modes of the investigated system and the respective mathematical problems are frequently easier to solve.

1.2.1.4 Variables, Parameters, and Constants

The quantities involved in a model can be classified as variables, parameters, and constants. A *constant* is a quantity with a fixed value, such as the natural number e or Avogadro's number $N_A = 6.02 \cdot 10^{23}$ (number of molecules per mole). *Parameters* are quantities that are assigned a value, such as the K_m value of an enzyme in a reaction. This value depends on the method used and on the experimental conditions and may change. *Variables* are quantities with a changeable value for which the model establishes relations. The *state variables* are a set of variables that describe the system behavior completely. They are independent of each other and each of them is necessary to define the system state. Their number is equivalent to the dimension of the system. For example, diameter d and volume V of a sphere obey the relation $V = \pi d^3 / 6$. π and 6 are constants and V and d are variables, but only one of them is a state variable, since the mentioned relation uniquely determines the other one.

Whether a quantity is a variable or a parameter depends on the model. The enzyme concentration is frequently considered a parameter in biochemical reaction kinetics. That is no longer valid if, in a larger model, the enzyme concentration may change due to gene expression or protein degradation.

1.2.1.5 Model Behavior

There are two fundamental causes that determine the behavior of a system or its changes: (1) influences from the environment (input) and (2) processes within the system. The system structure, i.e., the relation among variables, parameters, and constants, determines how endogenous and exogenous forces are processed. It must be noted that different system structures may produce similar system behavior (output). The structure determines the behavior, not the other way around. Therefore, the system output is often not sufficient to predict the internal organization. Generally, system limits are set such that the system output has no impact on the input.

1.2.1.6 Process Classification

For modeling, processes are classified with respect to a set of criteria. *Reversibility* determines whether a process can proceed in a forward and backward direction. Irreversible means that only one direction is possible. *Periodicity* indicates that a series of states may be assumed in the time interval $\{t, t + \Delta t)$ and again in the time interval $\{t + i \cdot \Delta t, t + (i + 1) \cdot \Delta t\}$ for $i = 1, 2, ...$ With respect to the randomness of the predictions, deterministic modeling is distinct from stochastic modeling. A description is *deterministic* if the motion through all following states can be predicted from the knowledge of the current state. *Stochastic* description gives instead a probability distribution for the succeeding states. The nature of values that time, state, or space may assume distinguishes a *discrete* model (where values are taken from a discrete set) from a *continuous* model (where values belong to a continuum).

1.2.1.7 Purpose and Adequateness of Models

Models represent only specific aspects of the reality. The intention of modeling is to answer particular questions. Modeling is, therefore, a subjective and selective procedure. It may, for example, aim at predicting the system output. In this case it might be sufficient to obtain precise input-output relation, while the system internals can be regarded as black box. However, if the function of an object is to be elucidated, then its structure and the relations between its parts must be described realistically. One may intend to formulate a model that is generally applicable to many similar objects (e.g., Michaelis-Menten kinetics holds for many enzymes, the promoter-operator concept is applicable to many genes, and gene regulatory motifs are common) or that is specific to one special object (e.g., the 3D structure of a protein, the sequence of a gene, or a model of deteriorating mitochondria during aging). The mathematical part can be kept as simple as possible to allow for easy implementation and comprehensible results. Or it can be modeled very realistically and be much more complicated. None of the characteristics mentioned above makes a model wrong or right, but they determine whether a model is appropriate to the problem to be solved.

1.2.1.8 Advantages of Computational Modeling

Models gain their reference to reality from comparison with experiments, and their benefits are, therefore, somewhat dependent on experimental performance. Nevertheless, modeling has a lot of advantages.

Modeling drives conceptual clarification. It requires that verbal hypotheses be made specific and conceptually rigorous. Modeling also highlights gaps in knowledge or understanding. During the process of model formulation, unspecified components or interactions have to be determined.

Modeling provides independence of the modeled object. Time and space may be stretched or compressed *ad libitum*. Solution algorithms and computer programs can be used independently of the concrete system. Modeling is cheap compared to experiments. Models exert by themselves no harm on animals or plants and help to reduce it in experiments. They do not pollute the environment. Models interact neither with the environment nor with the modeled system.

Modeling can assist experimentation. With an adequate model one may test different scenarios that are not accessible by experiment. One may follow time courses of compounds that cannot be measured in an experiment. One may impose perturbations that are not feasible in the real system. One may cause precise perturbations without directly changing other system components, which is usually impossible in real systems. Model simulations can be repeated often and for many different conditions. Model results can often be presented in precise mathematical terms that allow for generalization. Graphical representation and visualization make it easier to understand the system. Finally, modeling allows for making well-founded and testable predictions.

1.2.1.9 Model Development

For the process of model development, we suggest the following modeling workflow:

1. Formulation of the problem: Before establishing an initial model, it must be clear which questions shall be answered with the approach. A distinct verbal statement about background, problem, and hypotheses is a helpful guide in further analysis.
2. Verification of available information: As a first step, the existing quantitative and structural knowledge has to be checked and collected. This concerns information about the included components and their interactions as well as experimental results with respect to phenotypic changes such as growth and shape after system perturbations such as knockout experiments, RNAi, and variation of environmental conditions.
3. Selection of model structure: Based on the available information and on the problem to solve, the general type of the model is determined: (1) the level of description as macroscopic or microscopic, (2) the choice of a deterministic or stochastic approach, (3) the use of discrete or continuous variables, and (4) the choice of steady-state, temporal, or spatio-temporal description. Furthermore, it must be decided what the determinants for system behavior (external influences, internal structure) are. The system variables must be assigned.
4. Establishing a simple model: The first model can be expressed in words, schematically, or in mathematical formulation. It serves as general test and allows refined hypotheses.
5. Sensitivity analysis: Mathematical models typically contain a number of parameters, and the simulation result can be highly sensitive to parameter changes. It is recommendable to verify the dependence of the model results on the parameter choice.

6. Experimental tests of the model predictions: This is a hard task. Experimental design in biology is usually hypothesis-driven. In fact, hypotheses that state general relations can rarely be verified, but only falsified. These predictions usually concern relationships between different cellular states or biochemical reactions. On the other hand, hypothesis about the existence of items are hard to falsify. The choice of parameters to be measured, how many measurements are to be performed, and at what time intervals is not uniquely defined but depends on the researcher's opinion. These selections are largely based on experience and, in new areas in particular, on intuition.

7. Stating the agreements and divergences between experimental and modeling results: Although the behavior of the model and the experimental system should eventually agree, disagreement drives further research. It is necessary to find out whether the disagreement results from false assumptions, tampering simplifications, wrong model structure, inadequate experimental design, or other inadequately represented factors.

8. Iterative refinement of model: The initial model will rarely explain all features of the studied object and usually leads to more open questions than answers. After comparing the model outcome with the experimental results, model structure and parameters may be adapted.

As stated above, the choice of a model approach is not unique. Likewise, the possible outcome of models differs. Satisfactory results could be the solution to the initially stated problem, the establishment of a strategy for problem solution, or reasonable suggestions for experimental design.

1.2.2
Typical Aspects of Biological Systems and Corresponding Models

A number of notions have been introduced or applied in the context of systems biology or computational modeling of biological systems. Their use is often not unique, but we will present here some interpretations that are helpful in understanding respective theories and manuscripts.

1.2.2.1 Network Versus Elements

A system consists of individual elements that interact and thus form a network. The elements have certain properties. In the network, the elements have certain relations to each other (and, if appropriate, to the environment). The system has properties that rely on the individual properties and relations between the elements. It may show additional systemic properties and dynamic characteristics that often cannot be deduced from the individual properties of the elements.

1.2.2.2 Modularity

Modules are subsystems of complex molecular networks that can be treated as functional units, which perform identifiable tasks (Lauffenburger 2000). Typical examples for assignment of modules are (1) the DNA-mRNA-enzyme-metabolism cascade and (2) signal transduction cascades consisting of covalent modification cycles. The reaction networks at each level are separated as modules by the criterion that mass transfer occurs internally but not between the modules, and they are linked by means of catalytic or regulatory effects from a chemical species of one module to a reaction in another module (Hofmeyr and Westerhoff 2001). Consideration of modules has the advantage that modeling can be performed in a hierarchical, nested, or sequential fashion. The properties of each module can be studied first in isolation and subsequently in a comprehensive, integrative attempt. The concept is appealing since it allows thinking in terms of classes of systems with common characteristics that can be handled with a common set of methods. The disadvantage is that a modular approach has to ignore or at least reduce the high level of connectivity in cellular networks – in particular the variety of positive and negative feedback and feed-forward regulatory loops – which actually contradicts the basic idea of systems biology.

1.2.2.3 Robustness and Sensitivity are Two Sides of the Same Coin

Robustness is an essential feature of biological systems. It characterizes the insensitivity of system properties to variations in parameters, structure, and environment or to other uncertainties. Robust systems maintain their state and functions despite external and internal perturbations. An earlier notion for this observation is homeostasis. Robustness in biological systems is often achieved by a high degree of complexity involving feedback, modularity, redundancy, and structural stability (Kitano 2002). On the one hand, biological systems must protect their genetic information and their mode of living against perturbations; on the other hand, they must adapt to changes, sense and process internal and external signals, and react precisely depending on the type or strength of a perturbation. Sensitivity or fragility characterizes the ability of living organisms for adequately reacting on a certain stimulus. Note that in some areas sensitivity is more rigorously defined as the ratio of the change of a variable by the change of a quantity that caused the change in the variable.

1.3
Systems Biology is Data Integration

The information that we can gain about a biological system appears in practice as an experimental observation, and systems biology research is restricted to the granularity and the precision of the experimental techniques in use. Systems biology has evolved rapidly in the last few years, driven by the new high-throughput technologies. The most important impulse was given by the large sequencing projects such as the human genome project, which resulted in the full sequence of the human and other genomes (Lander et al. 2001; Venter et al. 2001). This knowledge builds the theoretical basis to compute gene regulatory motifs, to determine the exon-intron structure of genes, and to derive the coding sequence of potentially all genes of many organisms. From the exact sequences probes for whole-genome DNA arrays have been constructed that allow us to monitor the transcriptome level of most genes active in a given cell or tissue type. Proteomics technologies have been used to identify translation status on a large scale (2D-gels, mass spectrometry). Protein-protein interaction data involving thousands of components were measured to determine information on the proteome level (von Mering et al. 2002). Data generated by these techniques are the basis for system-wide investigations. However, to validate such data in the system-wide hierarchical context ranging from DNA to RNA to protein to interaction networks and further on to cells, organs, individuals, etc., one needs to correlate and integrate such information. Thus, an important part of systems biology is data integration.

Data integration itself cannot explain the dynamical behavior of the biological system and is not a replacement for a mathematical model. However, it is extremely useful for increasing the information content of the individual experimental observation, enhancing the quality of the data, and identifying relevant components in the model for the biological system. Both the generation and the analysis of genome, transcriptome, and proteome data are becoming increasingly widespread and need to be merged for the generation of biological models.

At the lowest level of complexity, data integration defines common schemas for data storage, data representation, and data transfer. For particular experimental techniques, this has already been established, e.g., in the field of transcriptomics with MIAME (minimum information about a microarray experiment) (Brazma et al. 2001), in proteomics with PEDRo (Proteomics Experiment Data Repository) (Taylor et al. 2003), and the HUPO (The Human Proteome Organization) consortium (Hermjakob et al. 2004). On a more complex level, schemas have been defined for biological models and pathways such as SBML (Hucka et al. 2003) and CellML (Lloyd et al. 2004). Most of these repositories use an XML-like language style.

On a second level of complexity, data integration deals with query-based information retrieval, the connection of different data types (typically stored in different databases), and the visualization and presentation of the data. Here, for example, commercial applications such as SRS (Etzold et al. 1996) are in use. SRS provides a user interface that enables access to hundreds of biological databases. The EnsMart system developed at EBI is an advanced tool for data retrieval from database networks using a powerful query system (Kasprzyk et al. 2004). Both systems allow a simple integration of additional resources and programs so that they are continuously growing.

Data integration at the next level of complexity consists of data correlation. This is a growing research field as researchers combine information from multiple diverse datasets to learn about and explain natural processes (Ideker et al. 2001; Gitton et al. 2002). For example, methods have been developed to integrate insights from transcriptome or proteome experiments with genome sequence annotations. The integration of data enables their explanation and analysis, e.g., the comparison of gene expression patterns for orthologous genes or their evaluation in light of conserved transcription factor binding sites in upstream regions of the corresponding gene sequences (Tavazoie et al. 1999). At this level of complexity, researchers typically face the fact that data from diverse experimental platforms are correlated on a much lower level than assumed. This is partially due to the fact that experimental data generation typically involves a large pipeline of experimental stages with numerous factors of influence that might affect the output. Normalization strategies are therefore indispensable for interpretation of the data. This step requires highly sophisticated analysis tools, data mining models, and algorithms. Data mining defines the process of discovering meaningful new correlations, patterns, and trends by sifting through large amounts of data stored in repositories and by using pattern recognition technologies as well as statistical and mathematical techniques. Taking together, there is no doubt that data handling, storage, integration, and analysis methods and rules must be enforced in order to interpret the experimental outcomes and to transfer the experimental information into functional knowledge. Furthermore, in the case of complex disease conditions, it is clear that an integrated approach is required in order to link clinical, genetic, behavioral, and environmental data with diverse types of molecular phenotype information and to identify correlative associations. Such correlations, if found, are the key to identifying biomarkers and processes that are either causative or indicative of the disease. Importantly, the identification of biomarkers (e.g., proteins, metabolites) associated with the disease will open up the possibility to generate and test hypotheses on the biological processes and genes involved in this condition. The evaluation of disease-relevant data is a multi-step procedure involving a complex pipeline of analysis and data-handling tools such as data normalization, quality control, multivariate statistics, correlation analysis, visualization techniques, and intelligent database systems (Kanehisa and Bork 2003). Recently, several pioneering approaches have indicated the power of integrating datasets from different levels, e.g., the correlation of gene membership of expression clusters and promoter sequence motifs (Tavazoie et al. 1999); the combination of transcriptome and quantitative proteomics data in order to construct models of cellular pathways (Ideker et al. 2001); and the identification of novel metabolite-transcript correlations (Urbanczyk-Wochniak et al. 2003).

The highest level of data integration is the mapping of the integrated experimental data from multiple sources into networks in order to model interactions of the biological objects of the system. These networks represent qualitative models for the biological system. For example, Ideker et al. (2001) studied the galactose utilization pathway in yeast. The authors employed several strains of yeast, each with a different galactose gene knocked out, and a wild type and monitored changes in the levels of yeast genes using DNA arrays with the system in the presence and absence of galactose. Together with known data such as protein-protein interactions and protein-DNA interactions, they were able to construct an entire physical interaction network of that pathway. Davidson and colleagues (2002) studied endomesoderm specification in sea urchin and constructed a large gene regulatory network model comprising 60 genes. Most of the network architecture is based on perturbation experiments and expression data. Several conclusions can be drawn from these and other studies (Lee et al. 2002; Shen-Orr et al. 2002). There appears to be a variety of small modules similar to those found in engineering (feed-forward loops, single-input motifs). Such motifs can be found through different organisms (sea urchin, yeast, *E. coli*). Thus, current research tries to classify motifs into a kind of lexicon for higher-order functioning. By topological analysis, genes can be identified in these networks that may change fundamental properties of the system (hubs, articulation points, etc.)

and give rise to suggestions for further perturbation experiments. Thus, these qualitative models provide fundamental new strategies for systems biology research.

It should be pointed out that the current state of data integration is well elaborated at the lower levels of complexity, in particular with the database networks, whereas the higher stages need far more development. This is due to the fact that system-wide approaches are rare at the current state. These would require a guided and planned set of interacting experimental techniques on a defined experimental model, which is hard to realize. Instead, many data available for computational research are generated under varying experimental conditions with different experimental platforms and without any serious attempt at standardization. For example, it is a well-known fact that DNA array data from different platforms correlate at a very low level (Kuo et al. 2002; Tan et al. 2003), and the same phenomenon is observable with protein-protein interactions (Ito et al. 2000; Uetz et al. 2000). The lack of standardization remains the most important limiting factor of data integration and has to be tackled by future system-wide approaches.

1.4
Systems Biology is a Living Science

Systems biology comprises experimentation and computational modeling. To this end, it integrates approaches from diverse areas of science such as biology, chemistry, physics, mathematics, applied science, engineering, cybernetics, and computer science. By demanding new strategies, it also stimulates their further development and contributes to new solutions.

The integrative and interdisciplinary nature of systems biology necessitates the exchange of information among scientists from different fields. This means, for example, that mathematical formulas have to be made understandable for biologists and that people acquainted with the exact world of computers have to understand the diversity of biological objects and the uncertainty in the outcome of experiments. In the long term, these problems may be solved by education. In the short term, they require presentation of results from different perspectives and at different levels of accuracy.

Information exchange necessitates a *common language* about biological aspects. One seminal example is the gene ontology (GO, see Chapter 13, Section 13.1), which provides a controlled vocabulary that can be applied to all organisms, even as knowledge about gene and protein roles in cells is accumulating and changing. Another example is the Systems Biology Markup Language (SBML, see Chapter 14, Section 14.2.2) as an exchange language for models of biochemical reaction networks.

In addition to statements in mathematical terms or detailed verbal explanations, information and knowledge exchange demand *visualization* of concepts, perceptions, and insights, since it enhances understanding. Important fields for visualization are (1) the spatial organization of cell components and of cellular processes, (2) the representation of complex dynamics, and (3) interactions and regulatory patterns in networks. A traditional, well-known example is the Boehringer chart (Michal 1999), which can be found in the majority of biological labs.

Modeling of biological processes drives the development of concepts. The necessity for specific and mathematically exact formulation has stimulated the development of common model exchange languages (Chapter 14, Section 14.2), metabolic control theory (Chapter 5, Section 5.3), and clustering algorithms (Chapter 9, Section 9.3).

Standardization of experimental conditions and model approaches seems to restrict freedom of research and is hard to achieve. But standardization is essential for comparability of results, for the integration of the efforts of several labs, and for fast exchange of information between theoretical and experimental groups. Promising examples include MIAME and SBML.

The new paradigm of integrated and concerted efforts also demands open access to information. This is given on one hand by the exchange of data via Internet databases and by the exchange of modeling facilities as in SBW (Systems Biology Workbench). On the other hand, published results must be quickly available for the community.

Systems biology might also be the key to publication in biology in the future. Instead of, or in addition to, extensive descriptions of a biological system as text, we might "publish" our view of the biological object we are describing in the form of a working "computer object", which can be "published" over the Internet. This can then be tested by other scientists, in combination with other "computer objects", to see whether the object correctly predicts all aspects of the system, which can be observed experimentally. In many cases, complete agreement of predictions and all experimentally observable parameters of a system might be as close to the "truth" about a complex process in biology as we will be able to get.

References

Brazma, A., Hingamp, P., Quackenbush, J., Sherlock, G., Spellman, P., Stoeckert, C., Aach, J., Ansorge, W., Ball, C.A., Causton, H.C., Gaasterland, T., Glenisson, P., Holstege, F.C., Kim, I.F., Markowitz, V., Matese, J.C., Parkinson, H., Robinson, A., Sarkans, U., Schulze-Kremer, S., Stewart, J., Taylor, R., Vilo, J. and Vingron, M. Minimum information about a microarray experiment (MIAME)-toward standards for microarray data (2001) Nat. Genet. *29*, 365–71.

Davidson, E.H., Rast, J.P., Oliveri, P., Ransick, A., Calestani, C., Yuh, C.H., Minokawa, T., Amore, G., Hinman, V., Arenas-Mena, C., Otim, O., Brown, C.T., Livi, C.B., Lee, P.Y., Revilla, R., Rust, A.G., Pan, Z., Schilstra, M.J., Clarke, P.J., Arnone, M.I., Rowen, L., Cameron, R.A., McClay, D.R., Hood, L. and Bolouri, H. A genomic regulatory network for development (2002) Science *295*, 1669–78.

Etzold, T., Ulyanov, A. and Argos, P. SRS: information retrieval system for molecular biology data banks (1996) Methods Enzymol. *266*, 114–28.

Gitton, Y., Dahmane, N., Baik, S., Ruiz i Altaba, A., Neidhardt, L., Scholze, M., Herrmann, B.G., Kahlem, P., Benkahla, A., Schrinner, S., Yildirimman, R., Herwig, R., Lehrach, H. and Yaspo, M.L. A gene expression map of human chromosome 21 orthologues in the mouse (2002) Nature *420*, 586–90.

Hermjakob, H., Montecchi-Palazzi, L., Bader, G., Wojcik, J., Salwinski, L., Ceol, A., Moore, S., Orchard, S., Sarkans, U., von Mering, C., Roechert, B., Poux, S., Jung, E., Mersch, H., Kersey, P., Lappe, M., Li, Y., Zeng, R., Rana, D., Nikolski, M., Husi, H.,

BRUN, C., SHANKER, K., GRANT, S.G., SANDER, C., BORK, P., ZHU, W., PANDEY, A., BRAZMA, A., JACQ, B., VIDAL, M., SHERMAN, D., LEGRAIN, P., CESARENI, G., XENARIOS, I., EISENBERG, D., STEIPE, B., HOGUE, C. and APWEILER, R. The HUPO PSIs molecular interaction format–a community standard for the representation of protein interaction data (2004) Nat. Biotechnol. *22*, 177–83.

HOFMEYR, J.H. and WESTERHOFF, H.V. Building the cellular puzzle: control in multi-level reaction networks (2001) J. Theor. Biol. *208*, 261–85.

HUCKA, M., FINNEY, A., SAURO, H.M., BOLOURI, H., DOYLE, J.C., KITANO, H., ARKIN, A.P., BORNSTEIN, B.J., BRAY, D., CORNISH-BOWDEN, A., CUELLAR, A.A., DRONOV, S., GILLES, E.D., GINKEL, M., GOR, V., GORYANIN, II, HEDLEY, W.J., HODGMAN, T.C., HOFMEYR, J.H., HUNTER, P.J., JUTY, N.S., KASBERGER, J.L., KREMLING, A., KUMMER, U., LE NOVERE, N., LOEW, L.M., LUCIO, D., MENDES, P., MINCH, E., MJOLSNESS, E.D., NAKAYAMA, Y., NELSON, M.R., NIELSEN, P.F., SAKURADA, T., SCHAFF, J.C., SHAPIRO, B.E., SHIMIZU, T.S., SPENCE, H.D., STELLING, J., TAKAHASHI, K., TOMITA, M., WAGNER, J. and WANG, J. The systems biology markup language (SBML): a medium for representation and exchange of biochemical network models (2003) Bioinformatics *19*, 524–31.

IDEKER, T., THORSSON, V., RANISH, J.A., CHRISTMAS, R., BUHLER, J., ENG, J.K., BUMGARNER, R., GOODLETT, D.R., AEBERSOLD, R. and HOOD, L. Integrated genomic and proteomic analyses of a systematically perturbed metabolic network (2001) Science *292*, 929–34.

ITO, T., TASHIRO, K., MUTA, S., OZAWA, R., CHIBA, T., NISHIZAWA, M., YAMAMOTO, K., KUHARA, S. and SAKAKI, Y. Toward a protein-protein interaction map of the budding yeast: A comprehensive system to examine two-hybrid interactions in all possible combinations between the yeast proteins (2000) Proc. Natl. Acad. Sci. USA *97*, 1143–7.

KANEHISA, M. and BORK, P. Bioinformatics in the post-sequence era (2003) Nat Genet *33 Suppl*, 305–10.

KASPRZYK, A., KEEFE, D., SMEDLEY, D., LONDON, D., SPOONER, W., MELSOPP, C., HAMMOND, M., ROCCA-SERRA, P., COX, T. and BIRNEY, E. EnsMart: a generic system for fast and flexible access to biological data (2004) Genome Res. *14*, 160–9.

KITANO, H. Computational systems biology (2002) Nature *420*, 206–10.

KUO, W.P., JENSSEN, T.K., BUTTE, A.J., OHNO-MACHADO, L. and KOHANE, I.S. Analysis of matched mRNA measurements from two different microarray technologies (2002) Bioinformatics *18*, 405–12.

LANDER, E.S., LINTON, L.M., BIRREN, B., NUSBAUM, C., ZODY, M.C., BALDWIN, J., DEVON, K., DEWAR, K., DOYLE, M., FITZHUGH, W., FUNKE, R., GAGE, D., HARRIS, K., HEAFORD, A., HOWLAND, J., KANN, L., LEHOCZKY, J., LEVINE, R., MCEWAN, P., MCKERNAN, K., MELDRIM, J., MESIROV, J.P., MIRANDA, C., MORRIS, W., NAYLOR, J., RAYMOND, C., ROSETTI, M., SANTOS, R., SHERIDAN, A., SOUGNEZ, C., STANGE-THOMANN, N., STOJANOVIC, N., SUBRAMANIAN, A., WYMAN, D., ROGERS, J., SULSTON, J., AINSCOUGH, R., BECK, S., BENTLEY, D., BURTON, J., CLEE, C., CARTER, N., COULSON, A., DEADMAN, R., DELOUKAS, P., DUNHAM, A., DUNHAM, I., DURBIN, R., FRENCH, L., GRAFHAM, D., GREGORY, S., HUBBARD, T., HUMPHRAY, S., HUNT, A., JONES, M., LLOYD, C., MCMURRAY, A., MATTHEWS, L., MERCER, S., MILNE, S., MULLIKIN, J.C., MUNGALL, A., PLUMB, R., ROSS, M., SHOWNKEEN, R., SIMS, S., WATERSTON, R.H., WILSON, R.K., HILLIER, L.W., MCPHERSON, J.D., MARRA, M.A., MARDIS, E.R., FULTON, L.A., CHINWALLA, A.T., PEPIN, K.H., GISH, W.R., CHISSOE, S.L., WENDL, M.C., DELEHAUNTY, K.D., MINER, T.L., DELEHAUNTY, A., KRAMER, J.B., COOK, L.L., FULTON, R.S., JOHNSON, D.L., MINX, P.J., CLIFTON, S.W., HAWKINS, T., BRANSCOMB, E., PREDKI, P., RICHARDSON, P., WENNING, S., SLEZAK, T., DOGGETT, N., CHENG, J.F., OLSEN, A., LUCAS, S., ELKIN, C., UBERBACHER, E., FRAZIER, M., et al. Initial sequencing and analysis of the human genome (2001) Nature *409*, 860–921.

LAUFFENBURGER, D.A. Cell signaling pathways as control modules: complexity for simplicity? (2000) Proc. Natl. Acad. Sci. USA *97*, 5031–3.

LEE, T.I., RINALDI, N.J., ROBERT, F., ODOM, D.T., BAR-JOSEPH, Z., GERBER, G.K., HANNETT, N.M., HARBISON, C.T., THOMPSON, C.M., SIMON, I., ZEITLINGER, J., JENNINGS, E.G., MURRAY, H.L., GORDON, D.B., REN, B., WYRICK, J.J., TAGNE, J.B., VOLKERT, T.L., FRAENKEL, E., GIFFORD, D.K. and YOUNG, R.A. Transcriptional regulatory networks in *Saccharomyces cerevisiae* (2002) Science *298*, 799–804.

LEVCHENKO, A. Dynamical and integrative cell signaling: challenges for the new biology (2003) Biotechnol. Bioeng. *84*, 773–82.

LLOYD, C.M., HALSTEAD, M.D. and NIELSEN, P.F. CellML: its future, present and past (2004) Prog. Biophys. Mol. Biol. *85*, 433–50.

MICHAL, G. Biochemical pathways (1999) Spektrum Akademischer Verlag, Heidelberg.

REEVES, R.H., IRVING, N.G., MORAN, T.H., WOHN, A., KITT, C., SISODIA, S.S., SCHMIDT, C., BRONSON, R.T. and DAVISSON, M.T. A mouse model for Down syndrome exhibits learning and behaviour deficits (1995) Nat. Genet. *11*, 177–84.

SHEN-ORR, S.S., MILO, R., MANGAN, S. and ALON, U. Network motifs in the transcriptional regulation network of *Escherichia coli* (2002) Nat. Genet. *31*, 64–8.

TAN, P.K., DOWNEY, T.J., SPITZNAGEL, E.L., JR., XU, P., FU, D., DIMITROV, D.S., LEMPICKI, R.A., RAAKA, B.M. and CAM, M.C. Evaluation of gene expression measurements from commercial microarray platforms (2003) Nucleic Acids Res. *31*, 5676–84.

TAVAZOIE, S., HUGHES, J.D., CAMPBELL, M.J., CHO, R.J. and CHURCH, G.M. Systematic determination of genetic network architecture (1999) Nat. Genet. *22*, 281–5.

TAYLOR, C.F., PATON, N.W., GARWOOD, K.L., KIRBY, P.D., STEAD, D.A., YIN, Z., DEUTSCH, E.W., SELWAY, L., WALKER, J., RIBA-GARCIA, I., MOHAMMED, S., DEERY, M.J., HOWARD, J.A., DUNKLEY, T., AEBERSOLD, R., KELL, D.B., LILLEY, K.S., ROEPSTORFF, P., YATES, J.R., 3RD, BRASS, A., BROWN, A.J., CASH, P., GASKELL, S.J., HUBBARD, S.J. and OLIVER, S.G. A systematic approach to modeling, capturing, and disseminating proteomics experimental data (2003) Nat. Biotechnol. *21*, 247–54.

UETZ, P., GIOT, L., CAGNEY, G., MANSFIELD, T.A., JUDSON, R.S., KNIGHT, J.R., LOCKSHON, D., NARAYAN, V., SRINIVASAN, M., POCHART, P., QURESHI-EMILI, A., LI, Y., GODWIN, B., CONOVER, D., KALBFLEISCH, T., VIJAYADAMODAR, G., YANG, M., JOHNSTON, M., FIELDS, S. and ROTHBERG, J.M. A comprehensive analysis of protein-protein interactions in *Saccharomyces cerevisiae* (2000) Nature *403*, 623–7.

URBANCZYK-WOCHNIAK, E., LUEDEMANN, A., KOPKA, J., SELBIG, J., ROESSNER-TUNALI, U., WILLMITZER, L. and FERNIE, A.R. Parallel analysis of transcript and metabolic profiles: a new approach in systems biology (2003) EMBO Rep. *4*, 989–93.

VENTER, J.C., ADAMS, M.D., MYERS, E.W., LI, P.W., MURAL, R.J., SUTTON, G.G., SMITH, H.O., YANDELL, M., EVANS, C.A., HOLT, R.A., GOCAYNE, J.D., AMANATIDES, P., BALLEW, R.M., HUSON, D.H., WORTMAN, J.R., ZHANG, Q., KODIRA, C.D., ZHENG, X.H., CHEN, L., SKUPSKI, M., SUBRAMANIAN, G., THOMAS, P.D., ZHANG, J., GABOR MIKLOS, G.L., NELSON, C., BRODER, S., CLARK, A.G., NADEAU, J., McKUSICK, V.A., ZINDER, N., LEVINE, A.J., ROBERTS, R.J., SIMON, M., SLAYMAN, C., HUNKAPILLER, M., BOLANOS, R., DELCHER, A., DEW, I., FASULO, D., FLANIGAN, M., FLOREA, L., HALPERN, A., HANNENHALLI, S., KRAVITZ, S., LEVY, S., MOBARRY, C., REINERT, K., REMINGTON, K., ABU-THREIDEH, J., BEASLEY, E., BIDDICK, K., BONAZZI, V., BRANDON, R., CARGILL, M., CHANDRAMOULISWARAN, I., CHARLAB, R., CHATURVEDI, K., DENG, Z., DI FRANCESCO, V., DUNN, P., EILBECK, K., EVANGELISTA, C., GABRIELIAN, A.E., GAN, W., GE, W., GONG, F., GU, Z., GUAN, P., HEIMAN, T.J., HIGGINS, M.E., JI, R.R., KE, Z., KETCHUM, K.A., LAI, Z., LEI, Y., LI, Z., LI, J., LIANG, Y., LIN, X., LU, F., MERKULOV, G.V., MILSHINA, N., MOORE, H.M., NAIK, A.K., NARAYAN, V.A., NEELAM, B., NUSSKERN, D., RUSCH, D.B., SALZBERG, S., SHAO, W., SHUE, B., SUN, J., WANG, Z., WANG, A., WANG, X., WANG, J., WEI, M., WIDES, R., XIAO, C., YAN, C., et al. The sequence of the human genome (2001) Science *291*, 1304–51.

VON MERING, C., KRAUSE, R., SNEL, B., CORNELL, M., OLIVER, S.G., FIELDS, S. and BORK, P. Comparative assessment of large-scale data sets of protein-protein interactions (2002) Nature *417*, 399–403.

WESTON, A.D. and HOOD, L. Systems biology, proteomics, and the future of health care: Toward predictive, preventative, and personalized medicine (2004) J. Prot. Res. *3*, 179–196.

2
Biology in a Nutshell

Introduction

This chapter gives a brief overview of biology and its related subjects, such as bio-chemistry, with a focus on molecular biology, since the latter is most relevant to cur-rent systems biology. It will review several basics, and introduce fundamental knowl-edge of biology. The basics are required for the setup of all models for biological sys-tems, and the meaningful interpretation of simulation results and analyses. This chapter might be skipped by readers who are familiar with this subject. For a broader and more detailed introduction to biology, consulting books such as Alberts et al. (2002) or Campbell and Reece (2001) is recommended.

Biology is the science that deals with living organisms and their interrelationships between each other and their environment in light of the evolutionary origin. Some of the main characteristics of organisms are:

- Physiology: All living organisms assimilate nutrients, produce substances them-selves, and excrete the remains.
- Growth and reproduction: All living organisms grow and reproduce their own spe-cies.
- Cellular composition: Cells are the general building blocks of organisms.

Biology is divided into several disciplines, including physiology, morphology, cytol-ogy, ecology, developmental biology, behavioral and evolutionary biology, molecular biology, biochemistry, and classical and molecular genetics. Biology tries to explain characteristics such as the shape and structure of organisms and their change dur-ing time, as well as phenomena of their regulatory, individual, or environmental re-lationships. This chapter gives a brief overview about this scientific field with a focus on biological molecules, fundamental cellular structures, and molecular biology and genetics.

Systems Biology in Practice. Concepts, Implementation and Application.
E. Klipp, R. Herwig, A. Kowald, C. Wierling, H. Lehrach
Copyright © 2005 WILEY-VCH Verlag GmbH & Co. KGaA, Weinheim
ISBN: 3-527-31078-9

2.1
The Origin of Life

The earliest development on earth began $4^1/_2$ billion years ago. Massive volcanism released water (H_2O), methane (CH_4), ammonia (NH_3), sulfur hydrogen (H_2S), and molecular hydrogen (H_2), which formed a reducing atmosphere and the early ocean. By loss of hydrogen into space and gas reactions, an atmosphere consisting of nitrogen (N_2), carbon monoxide (CO), carbon dioxide (CO_2), and water (H_2O) was formed. The impact of huge amounts of energy (e. g., sunlight with a high portion of ultraviolet radiation and electric discharges) onto the reducing atmosphere along with the catalytic effect of solid-state surfaces resulted in an enrichment of simple organic molecules such as amino acids, purines, pyrimidines, and monosaccharides in the early ocean. This is called the prebiotic broth hypothesis and is based on the experiments of Miller and Urey (1959). Another possibility is that the first forms of life formed in the deep sea and utilized the energy of hydrothermal vents, well protected from damaging UV radiation and the unstable environment of the surface (Wächtershäuser 1988). Once simple organic molecules were formed in significant amounts, they presumably assembled spontaneously into macromolecules such as proteins and nucleic acids. Through the formation of molecular aggregates from these colloidally dissolved macromolecules, the development of simple compartmented reaction pathways for the utilization of energy sources was possible. Besides this, enzymes appeared that permitted specific reactions to take place in ordered sequences at moderate temperatures, and informational systems necessary for directed synthesis and reproduction were developed. The appearance of the first primitive cells – the last common ancestors of all past and recent organisms – was the end of abiotic (chemical) evolution and the beginning of biotic (biological) evolution. Later, these first primitive cells evolved into the first prokaryotic cells (prokaryotes). About 3.5 billion years ago, the reducing atmosphere was very slowly enriched by oxygen (O_2) due to the rise of photosynthesis that resulted in an oxidative atmosphere (1.4 billion years ago: 0.2% O_2; 0.4 billion years ago: 2% O_2; today: about 21% O_2).

Prokaryotes (eubacteria and archaebacteria) are mostly characterized by their size and simplistic structure compared to the more evolved eukaryotes. Table 2.1 summarizes several differences between these groups. The evolutionary origin of the eukaryotic cells is explained by the formation of a nucleus and several compartments, and by the inclusion of prokaryotic cells which is described by the endosymbiont hypothesis. This hypothesis states that cellular organelles, such as mitochondria and chloroplasts, are descendants of specialized cells (e. g., specialized for energy utilization) that have been engulfed by the early eukaryotes.

Prokaryotes and these early eukaryotes are single-celled organisms. Later during evolution, single-celled eukaryotes evolved further into multicellular organisms. Their cells are mostly genetically identical but differentiate into several specialized cell types during development. (Genetically identical cells are usually called cell clones. The term clone is used in molecular biology mostly to denote colonies of identical cells in culture, such as bacterial or yeast cells on a petri dish.) Most of these organisms reproduce sexually.

Tab. 2.1   Some important differences between prokaryotic and eukaryotic cells.

	Prokaryotes	**Eukaryotes**
Size	Mostly about 1–10 µm in length.	Mostly about 10–100 µm in length.
Nucleus	Nucleus is missing. The chromosomal region is called nucleolus.	Nucleus is separated from the cytoplasm by the nuclear envelope.
Intracellular organization	Normally, no membrane-separated compartments and no supportive intra-cellular skeletal framework are present in the cells' interior.	Distinct compartments are present, e.g., nucleus, cytosol with a cyto-skeleton, mitochondria, ER, Golgi complex, lysosomes, plastids (chloroplasts, leucoplasts).
Gene structure	No introns; some polycistronic genes.	Introns and exons.
Cell division	Simple cell division.	Mitosis or meiosis.
Ribosome	Consists of a large 50S subunit and a small 30S subunit.	Consists of a large 60S subunit and a small 40S subunit.
Reproduction	Parasexual recombination.	Sexual recombination.
Organization	Mostly single cellular.	Mostly multicellular, and with cell differentiation.

The developmental process that takes place by sexual reproduction starts with a fertilized egg (zygote) that divides several times (the cell division underlying this pro-cess is discussed in more detail in Section 2.5 and in Section 7.2). For instance, in the frog *Xenopus laevis* – which is a vertebrate and belongs to the amphibians – the development starts with the zygote and passes through several developmental phases, i.e., morula (64 cells), blastula (10,000 cells), gastrula (30,000 cells), and neurula (80,000 cells), before forming the tadpole (with a million cells 110 hours after fertilization) that develops into the adult frog later on. This process is geneti-cally determined and several phases are similar among species that are closely re-lated to each other due to their identical evolutionary origin. Figure 2.1 shows a sim-plified tree of life that illustrates major evolutionary relations.

While most places with moderate aerobic conditions were populated by eukar-yotes, the prokaryotic archaebacteria in particular have specialized to survive under extreme conditions (e.g., the thermophile bacteria, which propagate at temperatures of 85–105 °C in the black smokers of the deep sea, or the halobacteria, which live un-der high salt concentrations).

Along with organisms that have their own metabolism, parasitic viruses and vir-oids that utilize cells for reproduction have developed. Viruses consist of a very small genome surrounded by a protein envelope (capsid); viroids are single-stranded circu-lar RNAs. Due to the absence of a metabolism and a cellular structure, these para-sites are usually not regarded as living organisms.

The phenotypical diversity of organisms observed is also displayed in the structure of their hereditary information: the size of this genomic information can vary, as can its organization into different elements, i.e., plasmids and chromosomes. Table 2.2 summarizes some data acquired from commonly investigated organisms.

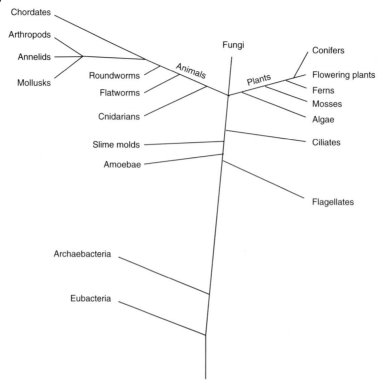

Fig. 2.1 The tree of life shows phylogenetic relations between some major groups of organism.

Tab. 2.2 Genome sizes of different organisms from the prokaryotic and eukaryotic kingdom. Information about further organisms can be found, e. g., at *http://www.cbs.dtu.dk/services/GenomeAtlas.*

Organism	Number of chromosomes (haploid genome)	Genome size (base pairs; genes)
Mycoplasma genitalium (prokaryote)	1 circular chromosome	$580 \cdot 10^3$ bp; 480 genes
Escherichia coli (prokaryote)	1 circular chromosome	$4.6 \cdot 10^6$ bp; 4,290 genes
Saccharomyces cerevisiae (budding yeast; eukaryote)	16 chromosomes	$12.5 \cdot 10^6$ bp; 6,186 genes
Arabidopsis thaliana (flowering plant; eukaryote)	5 chromosomes	$100 \cdot 10^6$ bp; ~25,000 genes
Drosophila melanogaster (fruit fly, eukaryote)	4 chromosomes	$180 \cdot 10^6$ bp; ~14,000 genes
Mus musculus (mouse, eukaryote)	20 chromosomes	$2.5 \cdot 10^9$ bp; ~30,000 genes
Homo sapiens (human, eukaryote)	23 chromosomes	$2.9 \cdot 10^9$; ~30,000 genes

2.2
Molecular Biology of the Cell

Cellular structures and processes result from a complex interaction network of biological molecules. The properties of these molecules determine possible interactions. Although many of these molecules are highly complex, most fall into one of the following four classes or contain substructures that belong to one of these classes: carbohydrates, lipids, proteins, and nucleic acids. Along with these four classes, water is highly important for all living systems. Molecules are held together by and interact through chemical bonds and forces of different types: ionic, covalent and hydrogen bonds, nonpolar associations, and van der Waals forces. The following sections will provide a foundation for the understanding of molecular structures, functions, and interactions by giving a brief introduction to chemical bonds and forces, to the most important classes of biological molecules, and to complex macromolecular structures formed by these molecules.

2.2.1
Chemical Bonds and Forces Important in Biological Molecules

The atom model introduced by Rutherford and significantly extended by Bohr describes the atom as a positively charged nucleus surrounded by one or more shells (or, more exactly, energy levels) that are filled with electrons. Most significant for the chemical properties of an atom is the number of electrons in its outermost shell. Atoms tend to fill up their outermost shell to obtain a stable state. The innermost or first shell is filled up by two electrons. The second and further shells are filled up by $2n^2$ electrons, where n depicts the number of the shell. However, due to reasons of energetic stability, the outermost shell will not contain more than eight electrons. For example, helium, with two electrons in its single shell, or atoms such as neon or argon, with eight electrons in their outermost shells, are essentially chemically inert. Atoms with a number of electrons near to these numbers tend to lose or gain electrons to attain these stable states. For example, sodium (one electron in its outer shell) and chlorine (seven electrons in its outer shell) can both achieve such a stable state by transferring one electron from sodium to chlorine, thus forming the ions Na^+ and Cl^-. The force holding together the oppositely charged ions in solid state is called the ionic or electrostatic bond (Fig. 2.2a). If the number of electrons in the outer shell differs by more than one, atoms tend to share electrons by forming a so-called covalent bond (Fig. 2.2b). Atoms held together by covalent bonds are called molecules. If the shared electron pair is equally distributed between the two atoms, this bond is called nonpolar (e.g., the hydrogen molecule). If one atom has a higher attraction to the shared electron pair, it becomes partially negatively charged. Then the other atom in this polar association becomes partially positively charged, as is the case with the water molecule (H_2O), where the oxygen attracts the shared electron pairs stronger than the hydrogen atoms do. Thus –OH and –NH groups usually form polar regions in which the hydrogen is partially positively charged. A measurement for the affinity of an atom to attract electrons in a covalent bond is given by its electronegativity, which was introduced by

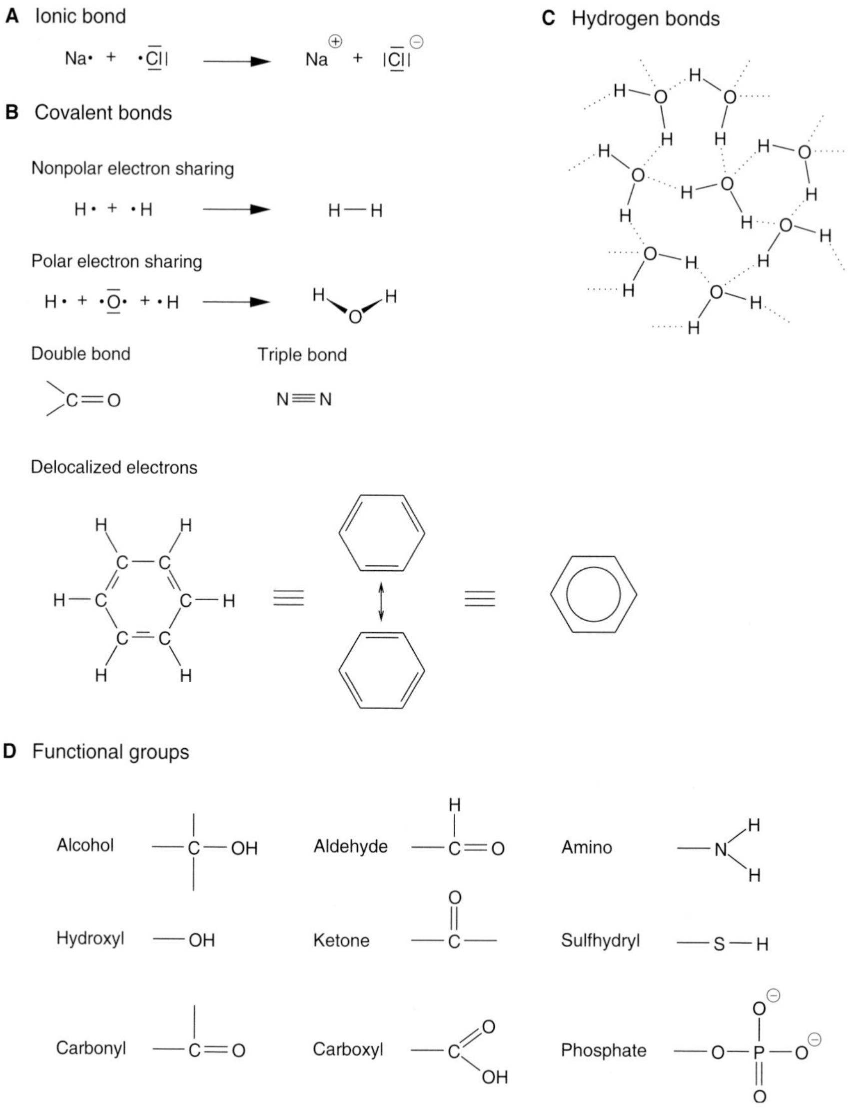

A Ionic bond

$$Na\cdot + \cdot\bar{\underline{Cl}}| \longrightarrow Na^{\oplus} + |\bar{\underline{Cl}}|^{\ominus}$$

C Hydrogen bonds

B Covalent bonds

Nonpolar electron sharing

$$H\cdot + \cdot H \longrightarrow H-H$$

Polar electron sharing

$$H\cdot + \cdot\bar{O}\cdot + \cdot H \longrightarrow H\underset{O}{\diagdown}H$$

Double bond   Triple bond

$$>\!C=O \qquad\qquad N\equiv N$$

Delocalized electrons

D Functional groups

Alcohol	—C—OH	Aldehyde	—C=O (with H)	Amino	—N〈H H
Hydroxyl	—OH	Ketone	—C— (=O)	Sulfhydryl	—S—H
Carbonyl	—C=O	Carboxyl	—C〈O OH	Phosphate	—O—P(—O⁻)(=O)—O⁻

Fig. 2.2 Chemical bonds and functional organic groups. Single electrons in the outer shell are visualized by a dot; electron pairs are replaced by a dash. Shared electron pairs are represented by a dash between two atoms. (a) Single charged Na^+ and Cl^- ions are formed by the transition of the single outermost electron of sodium to chlorine. (b) In a covalent bond, electrons are shared between two atoms. If the shared electron pair is attracted more strongly by one of the participating atoms than by the other, this bond is called a polar bond. Depending on the molecule structure, double and triple bonds can occur as well. Sometimes, binding electron pairs might also be de-localized among several atoms, as is the case in benzol. (c) Unequal electron sharing causes the formation of hydrogen bonds (shown by dotted lines) as found in water. (d) The skeleton of organic molecules essentially consists of carbon atoms bound to each other or to hydrogen. Some of these carbons are bound to or are part of functional groups with special chemical characteristics. Hence, these influence the reactivities and physicochemical properties of the molecule.

Linus Pauling. In addition to single covalent bonds, double and triple bonds also exist. These kinds of bonds are more exactly described by the quantum-mechanical atom model, in which the electron shells of an atom can be described by one of several differently shaped orbitals that represent the areas where the electrons are located with highest probability (electron clouds). A covalent bond is then described by molecule orbitals, which are derived from atom orbitals. Furthermore, if single and double bonds are altered in a single molecule or a double bond is in the direct vicinity of an atom with a free electron pair, then one electron pair of the double bond and the free electron pair can delocalize across the participating atoms, e.g., the three electron pairs in benzol (Fig. 2.2b) or the double bond between C and O and the free electron pair of N in a peptide bond (Fig. 2.6a). Such electrons are called de-localized π-electrons. For a more detailed description, please consult books about general and anorganic chemistry or introductory books about biochemistry.

Hydrogen atoms with a positive partial charge that are bound to oxygen or nitrogen (as in H_2O or NH_3) are able to interact with free electron pairs of atoms with a negative partial charge. These attractions are called hydrogen bonds and are relatively weak compared to solid-state ionic bonds or covalent bonds. To break a hydrogen bond, only about $4\,kJ\,mol^{-1}$ is required. Therefore, hydrogen bonds separate readily at elevated temperatures, which is often the reason that proteins such as enzymes lose their function during heating. Likewise, the hydrogen bonds that hold together the double strands of nucleic acids (see Section 2.2.3) can be separated at high temperatures. This fact is utilized for several molecular biological methods, e.g., polymerase chain reaction (PCR) and radioactive labeling of DNA (deoxyribonucleic acid) fragments. Hydrogen bonds also explain why water is liquid at room temperature and boils at $100\,°C$. Small alcohols, such as methanol or ethanol, are fully soluble in water due to their hydroxyl group, which interacts with the hydrogen bonds of water, whereas larger alcohols, such as hexanol or heptanol, are weakly soluble or insoluble in water due to their longer unpolar carbohydrate tail. As we have seen, polarized functional groups can interact with water, which is why they often are called hydrophilic (or lipophobic), while nonpolar molecules or molecule parts are called hydrophobic (or lipophilic).

Also critical to structures and interactions of biological molecules are the van der Waals forces. The electron clouds surrounding atoms that are held together by covalent bonds are responsible for these forces. Momentary inequalities in the distribution of electrons in any covalent bond, due to chance, can make one end of the covalent bond more negative or positive than the other for a short moment, which results in rapid fluctuations in the charge of the electron cloud. These fluctuations can set up opposite fluctuations in nearby covalent bonds, thus establishing a weak attractive force. This attractive force is stronger the closer the electron clouds are, but if the outermost electron orbitals begin to overlap, the negatively charged electrons strongly repel each other. Thus, van der Waals forces can be either attractive or repulsive. Their binding affinity is, at $0.4\,kJ\,mol^{-1}$ in water, even lower than that of hydrogen bonds. The optimal distance for maximum van der Waals forces of an atom is called its van der Waals contact radius. The van der Waals repulsions have an important influence on the possible conformations of a molecule.

2.2.2
Functional Groups in Biological Molecules

As outlined before, a major characteristic of life are the physiological processes in which nutrients from the outside are converted by the organism to maintain a thermodynamically open system with features such as development or behavior. These physiological processes are realized on the metabolic level by myriads of reactions in which specific molecules are converted into others. These intra- or intermolecular rearrangements often take place at specific covalent bonds that can more readily be disturbed than others. Such covalent bonds are often formed by certain intramolecular substructures called functional groups. Thus, functional groups often serve as reaction centers that convert some molecules into others or link some molecular subunits to form larger molecular assemblies, e.g., polypeptides or nucleic acids. The functional groups most relevant in biological molecules are hydroxyl, carbonyl, carboxyl, amino, phosphate, and sulfhydryl groups (Fig. 2.2 d).

Hydroxyl groups (–OH) are strongly polar and often enter into reactions that link subunits into larger molecular assemblies in which a water molecule is released. These reactions are called condensations. The reverse reaction, in which a water molecule enters a reaction by which a larger molecule is split into two subunits, is called hydrolysis. The formation of a dipeptide from two amino acids is an example of a condensation, and its reverse reaction is the hydrolysis of the dipeptide (Fig. 2.6 a). If the hydroxyl group is bound to a carbon atom, which in turn is bound to other hydrogen and/or carbon atoms, it is called an alcohol. Alcohols can easily be oxidized to form aldehydes or ketones, which are characterized by their carbonyl group (Fig. 2.2 d). Aldehydes and ketones are particularly important for carbohydrates (such as sugars) or lipids (such as fats). In aldehydes the carbonyl group occurs at the end of a carbon chain, whereas in ketones it occurs in its interior. A carboxyl group is strongly polar and is formed by an alcohol group and an aldehyde group. The hydrogen of the hydroxyl part can easily dissociate as H^+ due to the influence of the nearby carbonyl oxygen. In this way, it acts as an organic acid. The carboxyl group (–COOH) is the characteristic group of organic acids such as fatty acids and amino acids. Amino acids are further characterized by an amino group. Amino groups (–NH_2, Fig. 2.2 d) have a high chemical reactivity and can act as a base in organic molecules. They are, for instance, essential for the linkage of amino acids to form proteins and for the establishment of hydrogen bonds in DNA double strands. Moreover, amino acids carrying NH_2 in their residual group often play a crucial role as part of the catalytic domain of enzymes. Another group that has several important roles is the phosphate group (Fig. 2.2 d). As part of large organic molecules, this group acts as a bridging ligand connecting two building blocks to each other, as is the case in nucleic acids (DNA, RNA; see Section 2.2.3) or phospholipids. Furthermore, the di- and triphosphate forms in conjunction with a nucleoside serve as a universal energy unit in cells, e.g., adenosine triphosphate (ATP, Fig. 2.7 a). Phosphate groups are also involved in the regulation of the activity of enzymes, e.g., MAP kinases, which participate in signal transduction (see Section 6.3). Sulfhydryl groups (Fig. 2.2 d) are readily oxidized. If two sulfhydryl residues participate in an

oxidization, a so-called disulfide bond is created (Fig. 2.6 d). These linkages often occur between sulfhydryl residues of amino acids that form a protein. Thus they are responsible for the stable folding of proteins, which is required for their correct functioning.

2.2.3
Major Classes of Biological Molecules

The structural and functional properties of an organism are based on a vast number
of diverse biological molecules and their interplay. The physicochemical properties
of a molecule are determined through their functional groups. In the following sections, four major classes of biological molecules that are ubiquitously present and
are responsible for fundamental structural and functional characteristics of living organisms will be introduced: carbohydrates, lipids, proteins, and nucleic acids.

2.2.3.1 Carbohydrates
Carbohydrates function as energy storage molecules and furthermore can be found
as extracellular structure mediators, e.g., in plants. The chemical formula of carbohydrates is mostly $C_n(H_2O)_n$. The individual building blocks of all carbohydrates are
the monosaccharides, which consist of a chain of three to seven carbon atoms. Depending on the number of carbon atoms, they are categorized as trioses, tetroses,
pentoses, hexoses, or heptoses (cf. Fig. 2.3 a). All monosaccharides can occur in linear form, and with more than four carbons, they exist in equilibrium with a ring
form. In the linear form, all carbons of the chain, except for one, carry a hydroxyl
group (polyalcohol), which makes the carbohydrates hydrophilic. The remaining carbon carries a carbonyl group, and depending on its position–whether it is an aldehyde or ketone–it is called an aldose or a ketose. The circular configuration is attained by an intramolecular reaction between the carbonyl group and one of the hydroxyl groups. Such a compound is called a hemiacetal. An example of the ring formation for the six-carbon monosaccharide glucose is given in Fig. 2.3 b, in which it
forms a so-called glucopyranose ring. Depending on the orientation of the hydroxyl
group at the 1-carbon, i.e., whether it points downwards (α-glucose) or upwards
(β-glucose), two alternate conformations exist. Glucose is one of the most important
energy sources for organisms. It is metabolized during glycolysis (see Section 2.3.3)
into ATP and reduction equivalents (e.g., NADH, NADPH, or $FADH_2$).
   The hydroxyl group at the 1-carbon position of the cyclic hemiacetal can react via a
condensation with the hydroxyl group of another monosaccharide. This linkage
forms a disaccharide from two monosaccharides (Fig. 2.3 c). If this happens subsequently for several carbohydrates, polysaccharides that occur as linear chains or
branching structures are formed.

2.2.3.2 Lipids
Lipids are a very diverse and heterogeneous group. Since they are made up mostly of
nonpolar groups, lipids can be characterized by their higher solubility in nonpolar
solvents, such as acetone. Due to their hydrophobic character, lipids tend to form

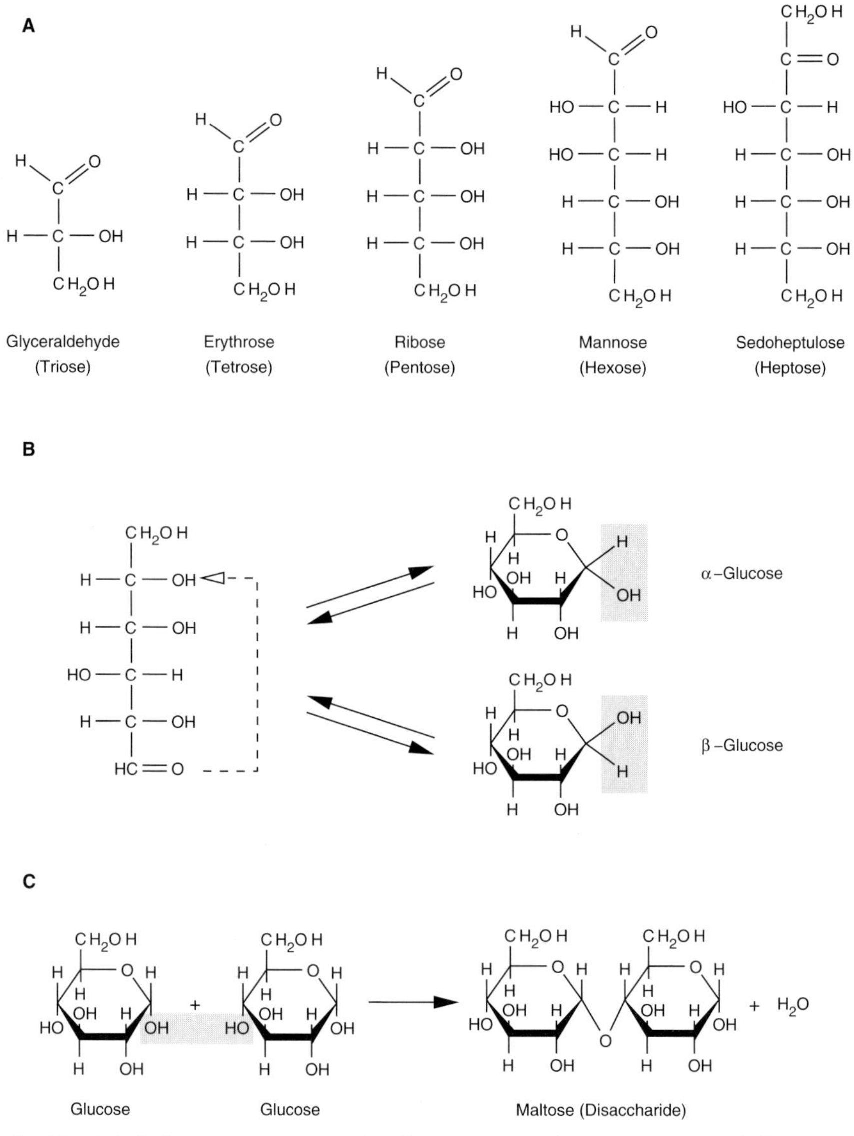

A

Glyceraldehyde
(Triose)

Erythrose
(Tetrose)

Ribose
(Pentose)

Mannose
(Hexose)

Sedoheptulose
(Heptose)

B

α–Glucose

β–Glucose

C

Glucose

Glucose

Maltose (Disaccharide)

Fig. 2.3 Carbohydrates. (a) Some examples of carbohydrates with a backbone of three to seven carbon atoms. (b) Glucose, like other monosaccharides with more than four carbons in their backbone, can form a circular structure, known as hemiacetal, by an intramolecular condensation reaction that can occur in two different conformations. (c) By further condensation reactions, such sugar monomers can form disaccharides or even larger linear or branched molecules called oligomers or polymers, depending on the number of monomers involved.

nonpolar associations or membranes. Eventually, these membranes form cellular hydrophilic compartments. Furthermore, such hydrophobic regions offer a local area for reactions that require a surrounding deprived of water. Three different types of lipids are present in various cells and tissues: neutral lipids, phospholipids, and steroids. Lipids can also be linked covalently to proteins or carbohydrates to form lipoproteins or glycolipids, respectively.

Neutral lipids are generally completely nonpolar and are commonly found as storage fats and oils in cells. They are composed of the alcohol glycerol (an alcohol with three hydroxyl groups), which is covalently bound to fatty acids. A fatty acid is a linear chain of 4 to 24 or more carbon atoms with attached hydrogens (molecules like this are well known as hydrocarbons) and a carboxyl group at one end (Fig. 2.4a). Most frequent are chains with 16 or 18 carbons. Fatty acids can be either saturated or unsaturated (polyunsaturated). Unsaturated fatty acids contain one or more double bonds in their carbon chain and have a more fluid character than do saturated ones. Linkage of the fatty acids to glycerol results from a condensation reaction of the carboxyl group with one of the alcohol groups of glycerol; this is called an ester binding. If all three sites of the glycerol bind a fatty acid, it is called a triglyceride, which is the most frequent neutral lipid in living systems. Triglycerides – in the form of fats or oils – serve mostly as energy reserves.

Phospholipids are the primary lipids of biological membranes (cf. Section 2.3.1). Their structure is very similar to that of the neutral lipids. However, the third carbon of glycerol binds a polar residue via a phosphate group instead of a fatty acid. Polar subunits commonly linked to the phosphate group are ethanolamine, choline, glycerol, serine, threonine, or inositol (Fig. 2.4c). Due to their polar and unpolar parts, phospholipids have dual-solubility properties termed amphipathic or amphiphilic. This property enables phospholipids to form a so-called bilayer in an aqueous environment, which is the fundamental design principle of biological membranes (Fig. 2.9a). Polar and nonpolar parts of the amphipathic molecules are ordered side by side in identical orientation and form a one-molecule thick layer (monolayer) with a polar and a nonpolar side; the aqueous environment forces the lipophilic sides of two such layers to each other, thus creating the mentioned bilayer.

Steroids are based on a framework of four condensed carbon rings that are modified in various ways (Fig. 2.4d). Sterols – the most abundant group of steroids – have a hydroxyl group linked to one end of the ring structure, representing the slightly polar part of the amphiphilic molecule; a nonpolar carbon chain is attached to the opposite end. The steroid cholesterol plays an important part in the plasma membrane of animal cells. Among other things, cholesterol loosens the packing of membrane phospholipids and maintains membrane fluidity at low temperatures. Other steroids act as hormones (substances that regulate biological processes in tissues far away from their own place of production) in animals and are, e.g., involved in regulatory processes concerning sexual determination or cell growth.

In glycolipids, the lipophilic part is constituted of fatty acids bound to the 1-carbon and 2-carbon of glycerol, as is the case with phospholipids. The 3-carbon is covalently attached to one or more carbohydrate groups that confer an amphiphilic character to the molecule. Glycolipids occur, e.g., in the surface-exposed parts of the plasma

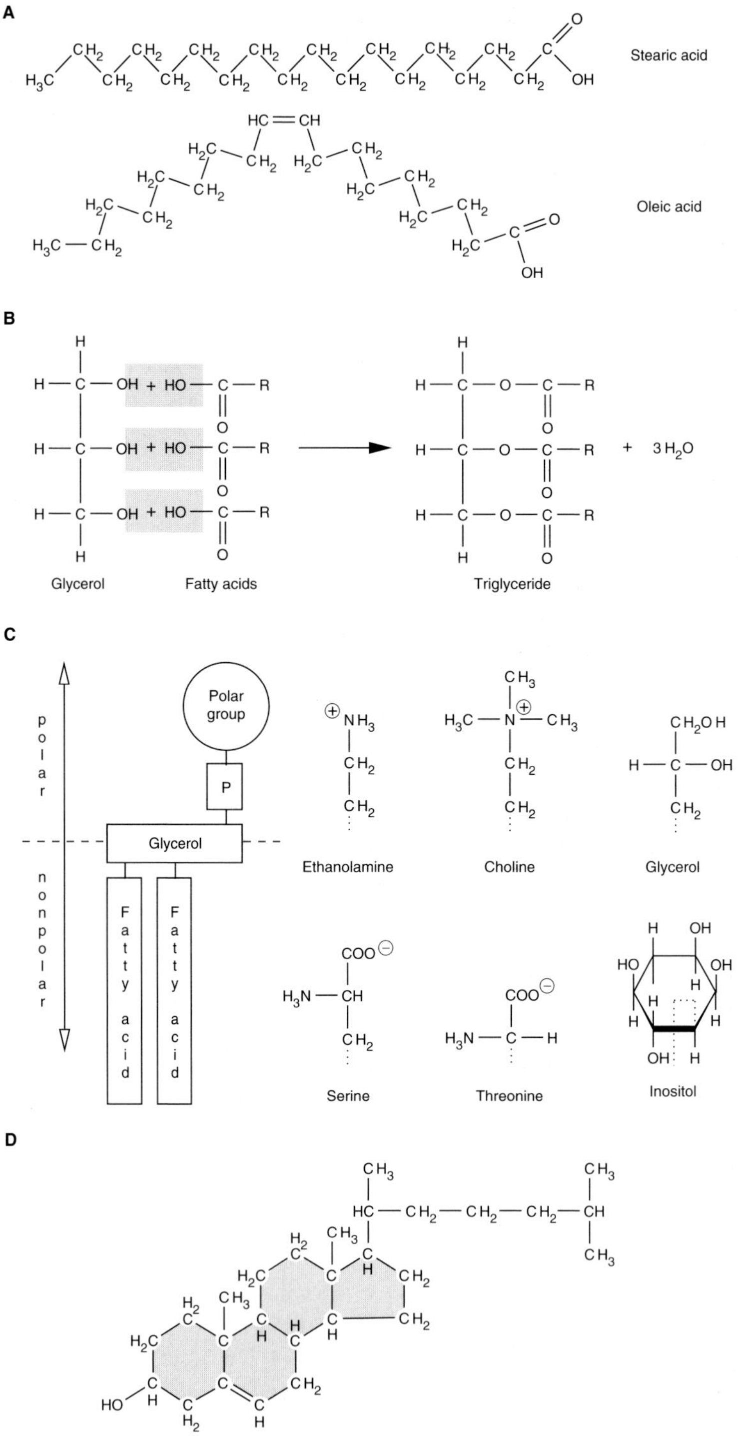
A
Stearic acid
Oleic acid
B
Glycerol
Fatty acids
Triglyceride
+ 3 H2O
C
polar
nonpolar
Polar group
P
Glycerol
Fatty acid
Fatty acid
Ethanolamine
Choline
Glycerol
Serine
Threonine
Inositol
D

membrane bilayer of animal cells that are subject to physical or chemical stress. Furthermore, among several other things, they are responsible for the AB0 blood system of humans.

2.2.3.3 Proteins

Proteins fulfill numerous highly important functions in the cell, of which only a few can be mentioned here. They build up the cytoskeletal framework, which forms the cellular structure and is responsible for cell movements (motility). Proteins are also part of the extracellular supportive framework (extracellular matrix), e. g., as collagen in animals. As catalytic enzymes for highly specific biochemical reactions, they rule and control the metabolism of a single cell or whole organism. Furthermore, proteins regulated by transient modifications are relevant for signal transduction, e. g., proteins controlling cell division such as cyclin-dependent protein kinases (CDK). A further highly important function of proteins is their ability to control the transcription and translation of genes as well as the degradation of proteins (see Section 2.4).

Proteins consist of one or more polypeptides. Each polypeptide is composed of covalently linked amino acids; these covalent bonds are called peptide bonds. Such a bond is formed by a condensation reaction between the amino group of one amino acid and the carboxyl group of another (Fig. 2.6 a). The primary structure of a polypeptide is coded by the genetic information that defines in which order amino acids – chosen from a set of 20 different ones – appear. Figure 2.5 shows the chemical structures of these amino acids. Common to all amino acids is a central carbon (α-carbon), which carries an amino group (except for proline, where this is a ring-forming imino group), a carboxyl group, and a hydrogen. Furthermore, it carries a residual group with different physicochemical properties, due to which the amino acids can be divided into different groups, such as amino acids that carry (1) nonpolar residues that can grant lipophobic characteristics, (2) uncharged polar residues, (3) residues that contain a carboxyl group that is negatively charged at physiological pH and thus act as acids, and (4) residues that are usually positively charged at common pH ranges of living cells and thus show basic characteristics. Due to the combination of possibilities of these amino acids, proteins are very diverse. Usually, proteins are assembled from about 50 to 1000 amino acids, but they might be much smaller or larger. Except for glycine, the α-carbon of amino acids binds four different residues and therefore amino acids can occur in two different isoforms that behave like an image and its mirror image. These two forms are called the L-isoform and the D-isoform, of which only the L-isoform is used in naturally occurring proteins. Furthermore, amino acids of proteins are often altered posttranslational. For in-

---

◀ **Fig. 2.4** (a) Fatty acids represent one part of fats and phospholipids. They are either saturated or unsaturated. (b) Triglycerides are formed by condensation reactions of glycerol and three fatty acids. (c) In phospholipids the third carbon of glycerol is bound to a polar group via a phos-phate group (P), which is usually ethanolamine, choline, glycerol, serine, threonine, or inositol. (d) Steroids constitute another major lipid class. They are formed by four condensed carbon rings. Cholesterol, shown here, is important, e. g., for membrane fluidity of eukaryotic cells.

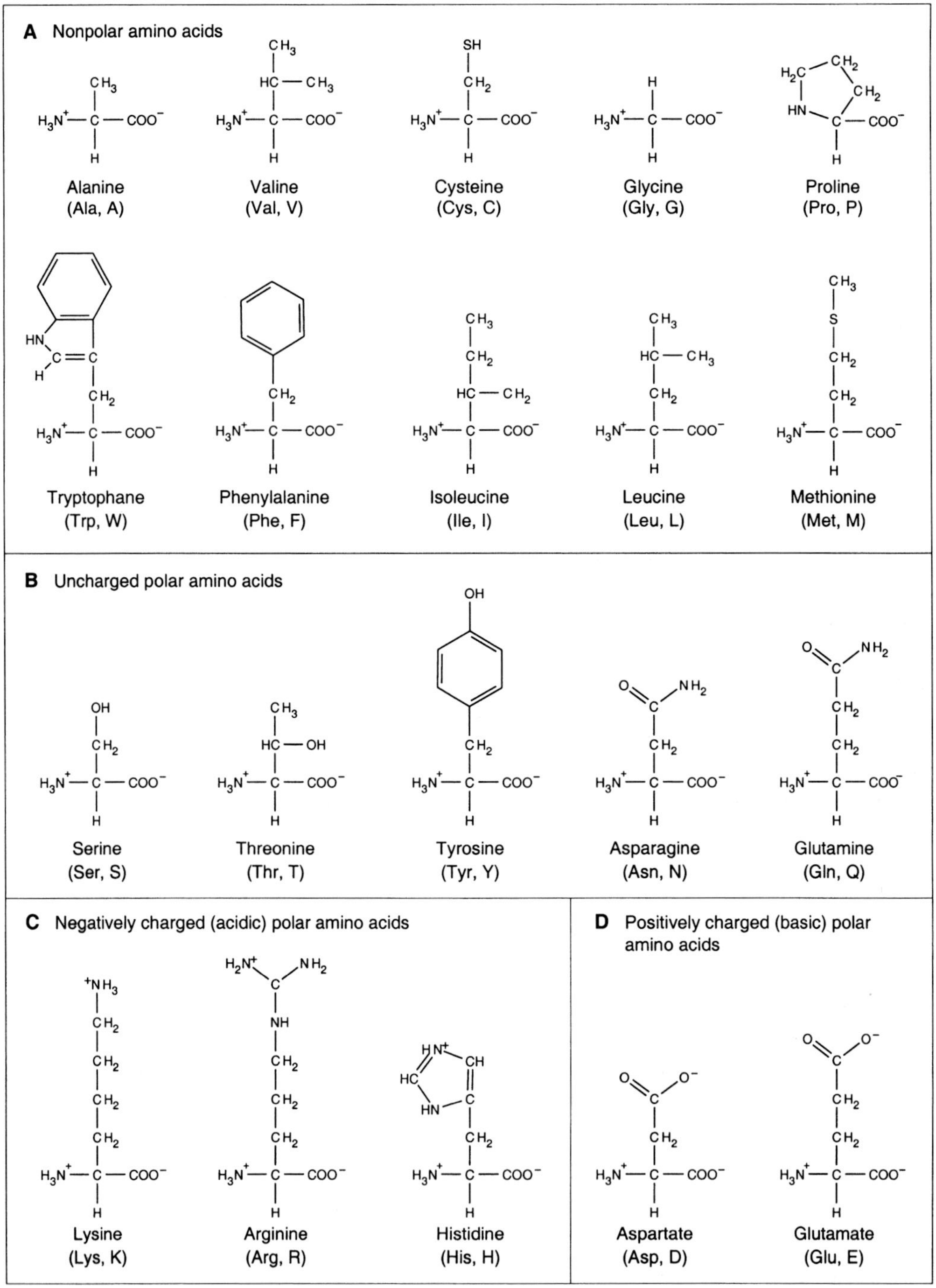

A Nonpolar amino acids

Alanine
(Ala, A)

Valine
(Val, V)

Cysteine
(Cys, C)

Glycine
(Gly, G)

Proline
(Pro, P)

Tryptophane
(Trp, W)

Phenylalanine
(Phe, F)

Isoleucine
(Ile, I)

Leucine
(Leu, L)

Methionine
(Met, M)

B Uncharged polar amino acids

Serine
(Ser, S)

Threonine
(Thr, T)

Tyrosine
(Tyr, Y)

Asparagine
(Asn, N)

Glutamine
(Gln, Q)

C Negatively charged (acidic) polar amino acids

Lysine
(Lys, K)

Arginine
(Arg, R)

Histidine
(His, H)

D Positively charged (basic) polar amino acids

Aspartate
(Asp, D)

Glutamate
(Glu, E)

stance, proline residues in collagen are modified to hydroxyproline by addition of a hydroxyl group.

The primary structure of a protein is given by the sequence of the amino acids linked via peptide bonds. This sequence starts at the N-terminus of the polypeptide and ends at its C-terminus (cf. Fig. 2.6 a). In the late 1930s Linus Pauling and Robert Corey elucidated the exact structure of the peptide bond. They found that the hydrogen of the substituted amino group almost always is in opposite position to the oxygen of the carbonyl group, so that both together, with the carbon of the carbonyl group and the nitrogen of the amino group, build a rigid plane. This is due to the fact that the bond between carbon and nitrogen has a partial double-bond character. In contrast to this, both the bonds of the α-carbon with the nitrogen of the substituted amino group and the carbon of the carbonyl group are flexible since they are pure single bonds. The free rotation around these two bonds is limited only by steric interactions of the amino acid residues. Based on this knowledge, Pauling and Corey proposed two very regular structures: the α-helix and the β-strand. Both are very common in proteins. They are formed by the polypeptide backbone and are supported and stabilized by a specific local amino acid sequence composition. Such regular arrangements are called secondary structures. An α-helix (Fig. 2.6 b) has a cylindrical helical structure in which the carbonyl oxygen atom of each residue (n) accepts a hydrogen bond from the amide nitrogen four residues further in sequence ($n + 4$). Amino acids often found in α-helices are Glu, Ala, Leu, Met, Gln, Lys, Arg, and His. In a β-sheet, parallel peptide strands – β-strands that may be widely separated in the linear protein sequence – are linked side by side via hydrogen bonds between hydrogen and oxygen atoms of their backbone (Fig. 2.6 c). The sequence direction (always read from the amino/N-terminus to the carboxy/C-terminus of the polypeptide) of pairing β-strands can be either parallel or antiparallel. The residual groups of the amino acids point up and down from the β-sheet. Characteristic amino acids of β-sheets are Val, Ile, Tyr, Cys, Trp, Phe, and Thr. The regular secondary structure elements fold into a compact form that is called the tertiary structure of a protein. Its surface topology enables specific interactions with other molecules. Figure 2.6 e shows a model of the three-dimensional structure of the superoxide dismutase (SOD), which detoxifies aggressive superoxide radicals ($O_2^{\bullet-}$). Sometimes the tertiary structure is stabilized by posttranslational modifications such as disulfide bridges (Fig. 2.6 d) or by metal ions such as calcium (Ca^{2+}) or zinc (Zn^{2+}). Some proteins are fibrous, i.e., they form filamentous structures (e.g., the keratin of hair). But most proteins fold into globular, compact shapes. Larger proteins often fold into several independent structural regions: the domains. Domains frequently consist of 50 to 350 residues and are often capable of folding stably enough to exist on their own. Often proteins are composed of assemblies of more than one polypeptide

---

◄ **Fig. 2.5** Amino acids are formed by carbon that is bound to an amino group, a carboxy group, a hydrogen, and a residual group. Depending on the physicochemical characteristics of the residual group, they can be categorized as (a) nonpolar, (b) uncharged polar, (c) acidic, or (d) basic amino acids.

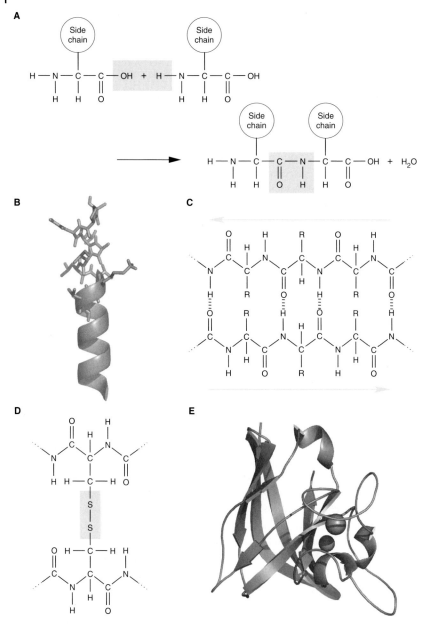

Fig. 2.6 (a) Formation of a peptide linkage by a reaction between the carboxyl group of one amino acid with the amino group of a second. (b) The molecular structure of an α-helix, as shown in the upper part of the image, is often illustrated by a simple helical structure as shown below. (c) An antiparallel β-sheet. (d) A disulfide bridge is formed by oxidation of the SH groups of cysteine residues belonging to either the same or different polypeptides. (e) Three-dimensional illustration of the copper zinc superoxide dismutase (CuZnSOD) of *E. coli* (PDB: 1EOS). α-helices are depicted as helical structures and β-strands are illustrated by arrows. The two metal ions are shown as spheres.

chain. Such a composition is termed the quaternary structure. The subunits can be either identical or different in sequence and the protein is thus referred to as a homo- or heteromer, e. g., a protein composed of four identical subunits such as the *lac* repressor is called a homotetramer.

2.2.3.4 Nucleic Acids

Deoxyribonucleic acid (DNA) is present in all living organisms and is the molecule storing hereditary information, i. e., the genes. Another molecule, ribonucleic acid (RNA), takes part in a vast number of processes. Among these, the transfer of the hereditary information leading from DNA to protein synthesis (via transcription and translation; see Section 2.4) is the most important. Both DNA and RNA are nucleic acids. Nucleic acids are polymers built up of covalently bound mononucleotides. A nucleotide consists of three parts: (1) a nitrogen-containing base, (2) a pentose, and (3) one or more phosphate groups (Fig. 2.7a). Bases are usually pyrimidines such as cytosine (C), thymine (T), or uracil (U) or purines such as adenine (A) or guanine (G) (Fig. 2.7b). In RNA the base is covalently bound to the first carbon (1'-carbon) of the circular pentose ribose. In DNA it is bound to the 1'-carbon of deoxyribose, a pentose that lacks the hydroxyl group of the 2'-carbon. A unit consisting of these parts – a base and a pentose – is named nucleo*side*. If it furthermore carries a mono-, di-, or triphosphate, it is called a nucleo*tide*. Nucleotides are named according to their nucleoside, e. g., adenosine monophosphate (AMP), adenosine diphosphate (ADP), or adenosine triphosphate (ATP); prepending *deoxy* to the name (or *d* in the abbreviation) indicates the deoxy form (e. g., deoxyguanosine triphosphate or dGTP). Nucleotides are not only relevant for nucleic acid construction but also are responsible for energy transfer in several metabolic reactions (e. g., ATP and ADP) or play certain roles in signal transduction pathways, such as 3'-5'-cyclic AMP (cAMP), which is synthesized by the adenylate cyclase and is involved, for instance, in the activation of certain protein kinases.

In DNA and RNA, the 3'-carbon of a nucleotide is linked to the 5'-carbon of the next nucleotide in sequence via a single phosphate group. These alternating sugar and phosphate groups form the backbone of the nucleic acids. Both DNA and RNA can carry the bases adenine, guanine, and cytosine. In DNA thymine can also be present. The sequence of the different bases has a direction – because of the 5'-3'-linkage of its backbone – and is used in living organisms for the conservation of information. DNA contains millions of nucleotides, e. g., a single DNA strand of human chromosome 1 is about 246 million nucleotides long. Each base of the sequence is able to pair with a so-called complementary base by hydrogen bonds. Due to the number and steric arrangement of hydrogen bonds, only two different pairing types are possible (Fig. 2.7b): adenine can bind thymine (A-T, with two hydrogen bonds) and guanine can bind cytosine (G-C, with three hydrogen bonds). In RNA, thymine is replaced by uracil. In 1953, Watson and Crick proposed a double strand for DNA, with an antiparallel orientation of the backbones. Each of the bases of one strand binds to its complementary base on the other strand, and together they form a helical structure (Fig. 2.7d). This so-called double helix is the usual conformation of DNA in cells. RNA usually occurs as a single strand. Occasionally it is paired to a

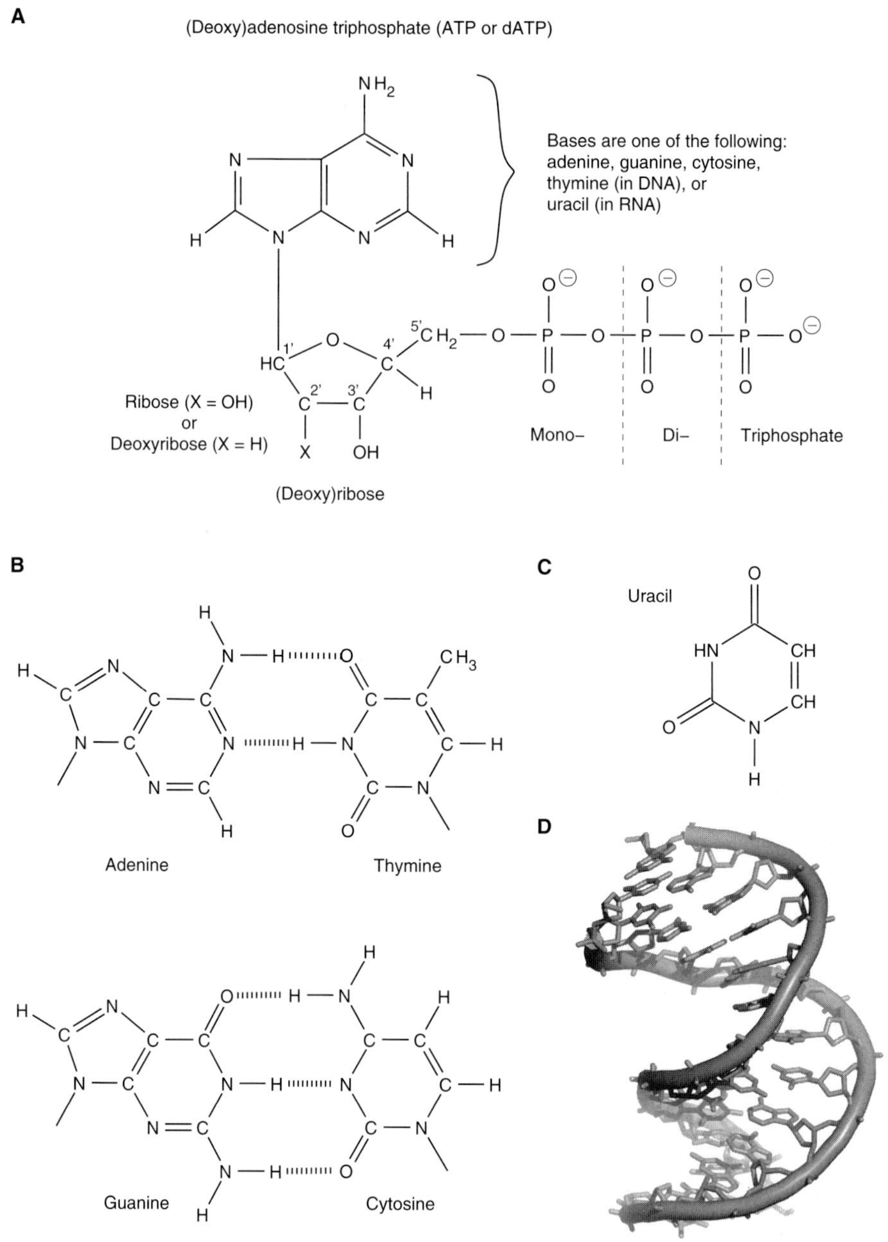

A

(Deoxy)adenosine triphosphate (ATP or dATP)

Bases are one of the following: adenine, guanine, cytosine, thymine (in DNA), or uracil (in RNA)

Ribose (X = OH)
or
Deoxyribose (X = H)

(Deoxy)ribose

Mono–   Di–   Triphosphate

B

Adenine   Thymine

Guanine   Cytosine

C

Uracil

D

Fig. 2.7 (a) Nucleoside phosphates are composed of a ribose or deoxyribose that is linked at its 1'-position to a purine or pyrimidine base. Purines are adenine and guanine, and pyrimidines are thymine, cytosine, or uracil. (b) In DNA, adenine is bound to its complementary base thymine by two hydrogen bonds, and guanine is bound to cytosine by three hydrogen bonds. (c) In RNA, thymine is replaced by uracil. (d) The DNA double helix (PDB: 140D).

DNA single strand, as during mRNA synthesis (see Section 2.4.1), or complementary bases of the same molecule are bound to each other, e. g., as in tRNA.

2.3
Structural Cell Biology

This section gives a general introduction to the structural elements of eukaryotic cells. Fundamental differences between prokaryotic and eukaryotic cells have already been mentioned and are summarized in Table 2.1.

The first microscopic observations of cells were done in the 17th century by Robert Hooke and Anton van Leeuwenhoek. The general cell theory was developed in the 1830s by Theodor Schwann and Matthias Schleiden. It states that all living organisms are composed of nucleated cells that are the functional units of life and that cells arise only from preexisting cells by a process of division (see Section 2.5). Today we know that this is true not only for nucleated eukaryotic cells but also for prokaryotic cells lacking a nucleus. The interior of a cell is surrounded by a membrane that separates it from its external environment. This membrane is called the cell membrane or plasma membrane and it is semipermeable, i. e., the traffic of substances across this membrane in either orientation is restricted to some specific molecule species or is specifically controlled by proteins of the membrane that handle the transport. Fundamental to eukaryotic cells – in contrast to prokaryotic cells – is their subdivision by intracellular membranes into distinct compartments. Figure 2.8 illustrates the general structure of a eukaryotic cell as it is found in animals. Generally, one distinguishes between the storage compartment of the DNA, the nucleus, and the remainder of the cell interior that is located in the cytoplasm. The cytoplasm contains further structures that fulfill specific cellular functions and that are surrounded by the cytosol. Among these cytoplasmatic organelles are the endoplasmatic reticulum (ER), which forms a widely spread intracellular membrane system; the mitochondria, which are the cellular power plants; the Golgi complex; transport vesicles; peroxisomes; and, additionally in plant cells, chloroplasts, which act as sunlight-har-

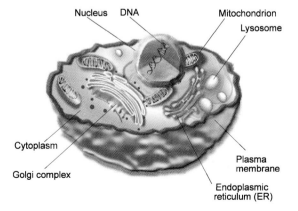

Fig. 2.8 Schematic illustrations of an animal cell with its major organelles.

vesting systems performing photosynthesis, and the vacuole. In the following sections, we will describe the structure and function of biological membranes and the most important cellular compartments that are formed by them.

2.3.1
Structure and Function of Biological Membranes

All cells are surrounded by a plasma membrane. It not only separates the cell plasma from its surrounding environment but also acts as a selective filter for nutrients and byproducts. By active transport of ions, for which the energy source ATP is usually utilized, a chemical and/or electrical potential can be generated across the membrane that is essential, e.g., for the function of nerve cells. Furthermore, receptor proteins of the plasma membrane enable the transmission of external signals that enable the cell to react to its environment. As already mentioned, eukaryotes additionally possess an intracellular membrane system acting as a boundary for different essential compartments.

The assembly of a bilayer, which is the fundamental structure of all biological membranes, is described in the section about lipids (Section 2.2.3; cf. also Fig. 2.9a). Biological membranes are composed of this molecular bilayer of lipids (mainly phospholipids, but also cholesterol and glycolipids) and membrane proteins that are inserted and held in the membrane by noncovalent forces. Besides integral membrane proteins, proteins can also be attached to the surface of the membrane (peripheral proteins). This model of biological membranes is known as the fluid mosaic model and was introduced by Singer and Nicolson (1972) (Fig. 2.9b). They further proposed a possible asymmetric arrangement of adjoining monolayers caused by different lipid composition and orientation of integral proteins, as well as specific occurrence of peripheral proteins in either of the monolayers. In the plasma membrane, for example, glycolipids always point to the exterior. While an exchange of lipid molecules between the two monolayers – a so-called flip-flop – very seldomly occurs by mere chance, lateral movement of lipid molecules takes place frequently. This can also be observed with proteins as long as their movement is not prevented by interaction with other molecules. Lateral movement of lipids depends on the fluidity of the bilayer. The fluidity is strongly enhanced if one of the hydrocarbon chains of the phospholipids is unsaturated and the membrane contains a specific amount of cholesterol.

An important feature of biological membranes is their ability to form a cavity that pinches off as a spherical vesicle, and the reverse process in which the membrane of a vesicle fuses with another membrane and becomes a part of it (Fig. 2.9c). This property is utilized by eukaryotic cells for vesicular transport between different intracellular compartments and for the exchange of substances with the exterior. The latter process

Fig. 2.9 (a) In a lipid bilayer the amphipathic lipids are orientated to both aqueous compartments with their hydrophilic parts. The hydrophobic tails point to the inner membrane space. (b) The fluid mosaic model of a cellular membrane. (c) Formation of a spherical vesicle that is in the process of either pinching off from or fusing with a membrane. Such vesicles are formed during either endo- or exocytosis by peripheral proteins inducing the process. ▶

A

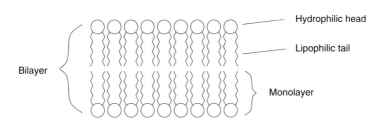

Bilayer

Monolayer

Hydrophilic head

Lipophilic tail

B

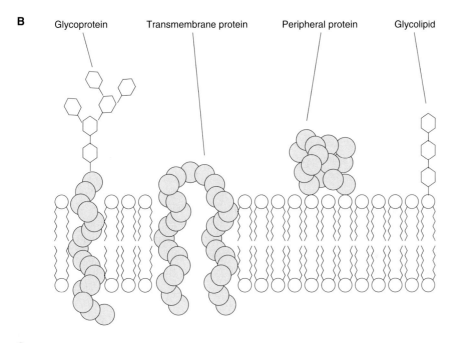

Glycoprotein   Transmembrane protein   Peripheral protein   Glycolipid

C

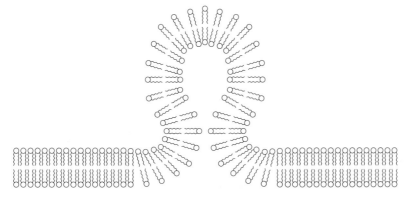

is termed exocytosis when proteins produced by the cell are secreted to the exterior and endocytosis or phagocytosis when extracellular substances are taken up by the cell.

There are two different kinds of exocytoses. The first one is a constitutive secretion: synthesized proteins packed into transport vesicles at the Golgi complex move to the plasma membrane and fuse with it, thereby delivering their payload to the exterior. This happens, e.g., with proteins intended for the extracellular matrix. In the second case termed regulated exocytosis, the proteins coming from the Golgi complex via transport vesicles are enriched in secretory vesicles that deliver their content usually due to an external signal recognized by a receptor and further transmitted via second messengers (e.g., Ca^{2+}). This pathway is common, for example, to neurotransmitters secreted by neurons or digestive enzymes produced by acinus cells of the pancreas.

Vesicular transport is important for large molecules such as proteins. For smaller molecules (e.g., ions or glucose) there are alternative mechanisms. In the case of passive transport, the flux takes place along an osmotic or electrochemical concentration gradient and requires no expenditure of cellular energy. Therefore, either the molecules can diffuse through the membrane or, since especially polar and charged substances cannot pass this hydrophobic barrier, transport is mediated selectively by integral transmembrane proteins. Other transmembrane proteins enable an active transport against a concentration gradient that requires cellular energy (e.g., ATP).

Sensing of exterior conditions and communication with other cells are often mediated by receptors of the cell membrane that tackle the signal transmission. Alternatively, mostly hydrophobic substances like steroid and thyroid hormones can cross the cell membrane directly and interact with receptors in the cell's interior. Signal transduction is discussed in more detail in Chapter 6. A general overview of biochemistry of signal transduction is given, e.g., in Krauss (2003).

Besides the plasma membrane, plant cells are further surrounded by a cell wall with cellulose, a polysaccharide, as the main polymer forming the fundamental scaffold. Prokaryotes also often have a cell wall where different monosaccharides act as building blocks for the polymer.

2.3.2
Nucleus

Prokaryotes store their hereditary information – their genome – in a single circular, double-stranded DNA (located in a subregion of the cell's interior called the nucleoid) and optionally in one or several small, circular DNAs (the plasmids), which code for further genes. The genome of eukaryotes is located in the cell nucleus and forms the chromatin that is embedded into the nuclear matrix and has dense regions (heterochromatin) and less dense regions (euchromatin). The nucleus occupies about 10% of the cellular volume and is surrounded by the nuclear envelope formed by an extension of the ER that creates a double membrane. The nuclear envelope has several protein complexes that form nuclear pores and that are responsible for the traffic between the nucleus and the cytosol. A subregion of the chromatin in which many repeats of genes encoding ribosomal RNAs are located appears as a roughly spherical body called the nucleolus.

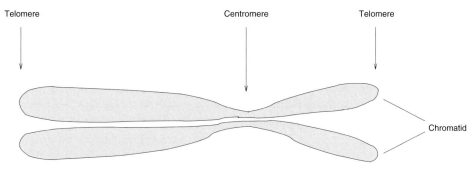

Fig. 2.10 The chromosome consists of two identical chromatids that are connected at the centromere. Both ends of the linear DNA of a chromatid are called telomeres. Each chromatid has a short and a long arm. The DNA is wrapped around histones and coiled further.

The structure of the chromatin usually becomes optically clearer during cell division, when the DNA strands condense into chromosomes, each consisting of two DNA double strands called chromatids. Both chromatids are joined at the centromere (Fig. 2.10). The ends of the chromatids are called telomeres. At the molecular level, the DNA of a chromosome is highly ordered. The double strand is wound around protein complexes, the histones, and each DNA/histone complex is called a nucleosome.

2.3.3
Cytosol

The cytosol fills the space between the organelles of the cytoplasm. It represents about half of the cell volume and contains the cytoskeletal framework. This fibrous network consists of different protein filaments that constitute a general framework and are responsible for the coordination of cytoplasmatic movements. These activities are controlled by three major types of protein filaments: the actin filaments (also called microfilaments), the microtubules, and the intermediate filaments.

The long, stretched actin filaments, with a diameter of about 5–7 nm, are built up of globular actin proteins. One major task of actin filaments is the generation of motility during muscle contraction. For the generation of movement, actin filaments slide along another filament type called myosin. This ATP-consuming process is driven by a coordinated interaction of these proteins. Together with other proteins involved in the regulation of muscle activity, these filaments form very regular structures in muscle cells. Furthermore, in many animal cells, actin filaments associated with other proteins are often located directly under the plasma membrane in the cell cortex and form a network that enables the cell to change its shape and to move.

Another filament type found in eukaryotes are the microtubules. They consist of heterodimers of the proteins α- and β-tubulin, which form unbranched cylinders of about 25 nm in diameter with a central open channel. These filaments are involved, e. g., in rapid motions of flagella and cilia, which are hair-like cell appendages. Flagella are responsible for the movement of, e. g., sperm and many single-celled eukaryotic protists. Cilia occur, for instance, on epithelial cells of the human respiratory system. The motion of cilia or flagella is due to the bending of a complex internal structure called the axoneme. Almost all kinds of cilia and eukaryotic flagella have nearly the same characteristic structure of the axoneme. This is called the 9 + 2 structure, because of its appearance: nine doublets that look like two condensed microtubules form a cylinder together with other associated proteins, the center of which contains two further single microtubules. The flexibility of the axoneme is also an ATP-consuming process that is further assisted by the protein dynein.

The third major filament type of the cytoskeleton is the intermediate filament. In contrast to actin filaments and microtubules, which are built of globular proteins, intermediate filaments consist of fibrous proteins. Several subtypes of these filaments are known, e. g., keratin filaments in the cytosol of epithelial cells, which make these cells resistant to mechanical influence, or lamin filaments, which are involved in the formation of the nuclear lamina.

Furthermore, the cytosol contains ribosomes responsible for protein synthesis (see Section 2.4.3), and it is filled with thousands of metabolic enzymes. A central metabolic pathway that is catalyzed by some of these enzymes is glycolysis. Substrates of this pathway are glucose or some similar six-carbon derivatives of it. These substrates are converted by several reactions into two molecules of the three-carbon compound pyruvate. Each metabolized glucose molecule generates two molecules of ATP, and one NAD^+ (the oxidized form of nicotinamide adenine dinucleotide) is reduced to NADH. But via this pathway – which does not involve molecular oxygen – only a small amount of the energy that can be gained through oxidation of glucose is made available. In aerobic organisms the bulk of ATP is produced from pyruvate in the mitochondria (see Section 2.3.4).

2.3.4
Mitochondria

Mitochondria have a spherical or elongated shape and are about the size of a bacterium. Their interior is surrounded by two membranes: a highly permeable outer membrane and a selective inner membrane. Therefore, mitochondria have two internal compartments, the intermembrane space and the matrix. The outer membrane is permeable for ions and most of the small molecules due to several transmembrane channel proteins called porins. The inner membrane's surface area is strongly increased by numerous folds and tabular projections into the mitochondrial interior, which are called cristae. Mitochondria are partially autonomous: they possess their own DNA and enzymatic complexes required for protein expression (such as ribosomes and mRNA polymerase). Nevertheless, they depend on symbiosis with their cell since most genes of mitochondrial proteins are encoded by the nuclear DNA. These mitochondrial proteins are synthesized in the cytoplasm and are then imported into the organelle.

As mentioned above, the bulk of ATP (34 out of 36 molecules per metabolized glucose molecule) is gained in mitochondria; thus, they can be termed the "power plants" of eukaryotic cells. The underlying oxidative process that involves molecular oxygen and yields CO_2 and ATP is driven mainly by pyruvate from the glycolysis and fatty acids. Both pyruvate and fatty acids can be converted into acetyl-CoA molecules. Acetyl-CoA has an acetyl group (CH_3CO-, a two-carbon group consisting of a methyl group and a carbonyl group) that is covalently liked to coenzyme A (CoA). Cytosolic pyruvate can pass the outer mitochondrial membrane and enter the mitochondrial matrix via a transporter of the inner membrane. Pyruvate is then converted into acetyl-CoA by a huge enzyme complex called pyruvate dehydrogenase. Acetyl-CoA reacts with oxaloacetate and thus enters the citrate cycle, a sequence of several reactions during which two CO_2 molecules and energetic reduction equivalents (mainly NADH, but also $FADH_2$) are produced. Finally, oxaloacetate is regenerated and thus the cycle is closed. The electrons delivered by the reduction equivalents are further transferred step by step onto O_2, which then reacts together with H^+ ions to form water. The huge amount of energy provided by this controlled oxyhydrogen reaction is used subsequently for the transfer of H^+ ions out of the mitochondrial matrix, thus establishing an H^+ gradient across the inner membrane. The energy provided by this very steep gradient is used by another protein complex of the inner mitochondrial membrane – the ATP synthetase – for the production of ATP inside the mitochondrial matrix by a flux of H^+ from the intermembrane space back into the matrix. This coupled process of an oxidation and a phosphorylation is called oxidative phosphorylation. The complete aerobic oxidation of glucose produces as many as 36 molecules of ATP:

$$C_6H_{12}O_6 + 6\,O_2 + 36\,P_i^- + 36\,ADP^{3-} + 36\,H^+ \rightarrow 6\,CO_2 + 36\,ATP^{4-} + 42\,H_2O$$

2.3.5
Endoplasmatic Reticulum and Golgi Complex

The endoplasmatic reticulum (ER) is a widely spread cytosolic membrane system that forms tubular structures and flattened sacs. Its continuous and unbroken membrane encloses a lumen that stays in direct contact with the perinuclear space of the nuclear envelope. The ER occurs in two forms: the rough ER and the smooth ER. The rough ER forms mainly flattened sacs and has many ribosomes that are attached to its cytosolic surface; the smooth ER lacks ribosomes and forms mostly tubular structures. Proteins destined for secretion but also intended for the ER itself, the Golgi complex, the lysosomes, or the outer plasma membrane enter the lumen of the ER directly after being synthesized by ribosomes of the rough ER. The total number of ER membranes of a cell and the ratio of smooth and rough ER vary strongly depending on species and cell type. All enzymes required for biosynthesis of membrane lipids, such as phosphatidylcholine, phosphatidylethanolamine, or phosphatidylinositol, are located in the ER membrane, their active centers facing the cytosol. Membrane lipids synthesized by these enzymes are integrated into the cytosolic part of the ER bilayer. Since this would result in an imbalance of lipids in the two layers of the membrane, phospholipid translocators can increase the flip-flop rate for specific membrane lipids; thus, the lipid imbalance can be compensated and the membrane asymmetry concerning specific membrane lipids can be established. Furthermore, the ER can form transport vesicles responsible for the transfer of membrane substances and proteins to the Golgi complex.

The Golgi complex (also called Golgi apparatus), usually located in the vicinity of the nucleus, consists of piles of several flat membrane cisternae. ER transport vesicles enter these piles at its *cis*-side. Substances leave the Golgi complex at the opposite *trans*-site. Transport between the different cisternae is mediated by Golgi vesicles. Some modifications of proteins by the addition of a specific oligosaccharide happen in the ER, but further glycosylations of various types take place in the lumen of the Golgi complex. Since such modified membrane proteins and lipids point to the organelles' inner space, they will be exposed to the cell's outer space when they are transported to the plasma membrane. The synthesis of complex modifications by several additions of carbohydrates requires a special enzyme for each specific addition. Therefore, these reaction pathways become very complex.

2.3.6
Other Organelles

Eukaryotic cells have further compartments for certain functions. Some of these organelles and their major functions will be mentioned briefly here.

Lysosomes are responsible for the intracellular digestion of macromolecules. These vesicular organelles contain several hydrolyzing enzymes (hydrolases), e.g., proteases, nucleases, glycosidases, lipases, phosphatases, and sulfatases. All of them have their optimal activity at pH 5. This pH value is maintained inside the lysosomes via ATP-dependent H^+ pumps (for comparison, the pH of the cytosol is about 7.2).

Peroxisomes (also called microbodies) contain enzymes that oxidize organic substances (R) and therefore use molecular oxygen as an electron acceptor. This reaction produces hydrogen peroxide (H_2O_2).

$$RH_2 + O_2 \rightarrow R + H_2O_2$$

H_2O_2 is used by peroxidase to further oxidize substances such as phenols, amino acids, formaldehyde, and ethanol, or it is detoxified by catalase ($2\ H_2O_2 \rightarrow 2\ H_2O + O_2$).

In contrast to the ER, the Golgi cisternae, lysosomes, peroxisomes, and vesicles, which are surrounded by a single membrane, chloroplasts as well as mitochondria have a double membrane of which the inner one is not folded into cristae as in mitochondria. Instead, a chloroplast has a third membrane that is folded several times and forms areas that look like piles of coins. This membrane contains light-harvesting complexes and ATP synthases that utilize the energy of the sunlight for the production of cellular energy and reduction equivalents used for the fixation of carbon dioxide (CO_2) into sugars, amino acids, fatty acids, or starch. Chloroplasts, as well as mitochondria, have their own circular DNA and ribosomes.

2.4
Expression of Genes

Classically, a gene is defined as the information encoded by the sequence of a DNA region that is required for the construction of an enzyme or – more generally – of a protein. We will see that this is a simplified definition, since, e.g., mature products of some genes are not proteins but RNAs with specific functions; eukaryotic gene sequences in particular also contain non-coding information. The term gene expression commonly refers to the whole process during which the information of a particular gene is translated into a particular protein. This process involves several steps (cf. Chapter 8). First, during transcription (Fig. 2.11 ①), the DNA region encoding the gene is transcribed into a complementary messenger RNA (mRNA). In eukaryotic cells this mRNA is further modified (②) inside the nucleus and transferred to the cytosol (③). In the cytosol, the mRNA binds to a ribosome that uses the sequence as a template for the synthesis of a specific polypeptide that can fold into the three-dimensional protein structure (④). In prokaryotic cells the mRNA is not further modified and ribosomes can bind to the nascent mRNA during transcription.

In eukaryotic cells the synthesized proteins can either remain in the cytosol (⑤) or, if they have a specific signaling sequence, be synthesized by ribosomes of the rough ER and enter its lumen (⑦). However, there are several mechanisms of directing each protein to its final destination. During this sorting, proteins are often modified, e.g., by cleavage of signaling peptides or by glycosylation.

All the genes of a single organism make up its genome. But only a subset of these genes will be expressed at a particular time or in a specific cell type. Some genes fulfill basic functions of the cell and are always required; these are called constitutive or housekeeping genes. Others are expressed only under certain conditions. The amount of a gene product, e.g., a protein, depends mainly on its stability and the number of its mRNA templates. The number of the latter depends on the transcription rate, which is influenced by regulatory regions of the gene and transcription factors that control the initialization of transcription. Thus, quantitative changes in gene expression can be monitored by mRNA and protein concentrations (see Chapter 4 on experimental techniques used for this purpose). Rate changes in any production or degradation step of a specific gene, which might happen in different cell types or at developmental stages, can lead to differential gene expression.

The whole procedure of gene expression, protein sorting, and posttranslational modifications is summarized in Fig. 2.11 and will be described in more detail in the following section.

2.4.1
Transcription

The synthesis of an RNA polymer from ATP, GTP, CTP, and UTP employing a DNA region as a template is called transcription. RNA synthesis is catalyzed by the RNA polymerase. In eukaryotic cells there are different types of this enzyme that are responsible for the synthesis of different RNA types, including messenger RNA

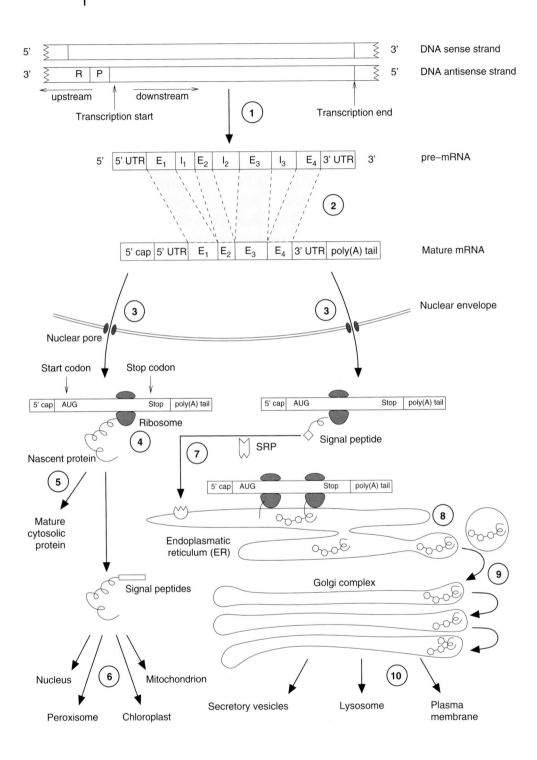

(mRNA), ribosomal RNA (rRNA), or transfer RNA (tRNA). In prokaryotic cells all these different RNA types are synthesized by the same polymerase. This enzyme has an affinity to a specific DNA sequence, the promoter, that also indicates the first base to be copied. During initiation of transcription, the RNA polymerase binds to the promoter with a high affinity that is supported by further initiation factors. Complete formation of the initiation complex causes the DNA to unwind in the promoter region. Now the enzyme is ready to add the first RNA nucleoside triphosphate to the template strand of the opened DNA double strand. In the subsequent elongation phase, the RNA polymerase moves along the unwinding DNA and extends the newly developing mRNA continuously with nucleotides complementary to the template strand. During this phase a moving transient, double-stranded RNA-DNA hybrid is established. As the polymerase moves along, the DNA rewinds again just behind it. As RNA synthesis always proceeds in $5' \rightarrow 3'$ direction, only one of the DNA chains acts as a template, the so-called antisense (–) strand. The other one, the sense (+) strand, has the same sequence as the transcribed RNA, except for the thymine nucleotides that are replaced by uracil nucleotides in RNA. As much as the promoter is responsible for initiation of transcription, the terminator – another specific DNA sequence – is responsible for its termination. For the bacterium *E. coli* two different termination mechanisms are described: the Rho-independent and Rho-dependent terminations. In Rho-independent termination, the transcribed terminator region shows two short GC-rich and self-complementary sequences that can bind to each other and thus form a so-called hairpin structure. This motif is followed by a block of uracil residues that bind the complementary adenine residues of the DNA only weakly. Presumably, this RNA structure causes the RNA polymerase to terminate and release the RNA. In Rho-dependent termination, a protein – the Rho factor – can bind the newly synthesized RNA near the terminator and mediate the RNA release. Termination in eukaryotic cells shows both, similarities to and differences from the mechanisms found in bacteria.

2.4.2
Processing of the mRNA

In eukaryotic cells the primary mRNA transcript (precursor mRNA or pre-mRNA) is further processed before being exported into the cytosol and entering translation (Fig. 2.11 ②). The protein-coding sequence lies internally in the mRNA and is flanked on both sides by nucleotides that are not translated. During processing, a so-called 5' cap is attached to the flanking 5' untranslated region (5' UTR, about 10 to 200 nucleotides) preceding, or lying upstream of, the coding sequence. This 5' cap consists of three nucleotides that are further modified. The 3' untranslated region (3' UTR) of most mRNAs is also modified after transcription by addition of a series of about 30 to 200

◀ **Fig. 2.11** Gene expression in eukaryotic cells comprises several steps from the DNA to the mature protein at its final destination. This involves the ① transcription of the gene, ② splicing and processing of the pre-mRNA, ③ export of the mature mRNA into the cytosol, ④ translation of the genetic code into a protein, and ⑤–⑩ several steps of sorting and modification. More details are given in the text.

adenine nucleotides that are known as the poly(A) tail. Furthermore, the pre-mRNA is often much longer than the mature RNA because the coding sequence is often interrupted by one or several intervening sequences called introns, which do not occur in the mature mRNA exported to the cytosol. These intron sequences are removed during processing by a mechanism called splicing. The remaining sequences are called exons. The final coding sequence thus consists of a series of exons joined together. It starts with AUG, which is the first triplet translated into an amino acid, and it stops with a stop codon (UGA, UAA, or UAG). Via the pores of the nuclear envelope, the mature mRNA is finally exported to the cytoplasm, where the translation process takes place.

2.4.3
Translation

Translation of the genetic information encoded by the mRNA into the amino acid sequence of a polypeptide is done by ribosomes in the cytosol. To encode the 20 different amino acids occurring in polypeptides, at least three bases out of the four possibilities (G, U, T, C) are necessary ($4^3 = 64 > 20$). During evolution, a code developed that uses such triplets of exactly three bases, which are called codons, to code the amino acids and signals for start and end of translation. By using three bases for each codon, more than 20 amino acids can be coded, and hence some amino acids are encoded by more than one triplet. The genetic code is shown in Tab. 2.3. It is

Tab. 2.3 The genetic code. Each codon of the genetic code – read in the 5′ → 3′ direction along the mRNA – encodes a specific amino acid or a starting or termination signal of translation.

Position 1 (5′ end)	Position 2				Position 3 (3′ end)
	U	*C*	*A*	*G*	
U	Phe	Ser	Tyr	Cys	U
	Phe	Ser	Tyr	Cys	C
	Leu	Ser	Stop	Stop	A
	Leu	Ser	Stop	Trp	G
C	Leu	Pro	His	Arg	U
	Leu	Pro	His	Arg	C
	Leu	Pro	Gln	Arg	A
	Leu	Pro	Gln	Arg	G
A	Ile	Thr	Asn	Ser	U
	Ile	Thr	Asn	Ser	C
	Ile	Thr	Lys	Arg	A
	Met	Thr	Lys	Arg	G
G	Val	Ala	Asp	Gly	U
	Val	Ala	Asp	Gly	C
	Val	Ala	Glu	Gly	A
	Val	Ala	Glu	Gly	G

highly conserved across almost all prokaryotic and eukaryotic species except for some mitochondria or chloroplasts. For translation of the genetic information, adapter molecules are required. These are the transfer RNAs (tRNAs). They consist of about 80 nucleotides and are folded into a characteristic form similar to an "L". Each tRNA can recognize a specific codon by a complementary triplet, called an anticodon, and it can also bind the appropriate amino acid. For each specific tRNA, a certain enzyme (aminoacyl-tRNA synthetase) attaches the right amino acid to the tRNA's 3' end. Such a loaded tRNA is called an aminoacyl-tRNA.

During translation (Fig. 2.12), the genetic information of the mRNA is read codon by codon in a 5'→3' direction of the mRNA, starting with an AUG codon. AUG codes for methionine, and therefore newly synthesized proteins always begin with this amino acid at their amino terminus. Protein biosynthesis is catalyzed by ribosomes. Both eukaryotic and prokaryotic ribosomes consist of a large and a small subunit, and both subunits are composed of several proteins and rRNAs. In eukaryotic cells the small ribosomal subunit first associates with an initiation tRNA (Met-tRNA$_i$) and binds the mRNA at its 5' cap. Once attached, the complex scans along the mRNA until reaching the start AUG codon. In most cases this is the first AUG codon in the 5'→3' direction. This position indicates the translation start and determines the reading frame. Finally, during initiation the large ribosomal subunit is added to the complex and the ribosome becomes ready for protein synthesis. Each ribosome has three binding sites: one for the mRNA and two for tRNAs. In the beginning the first tRNA binding site, also called P site, contains

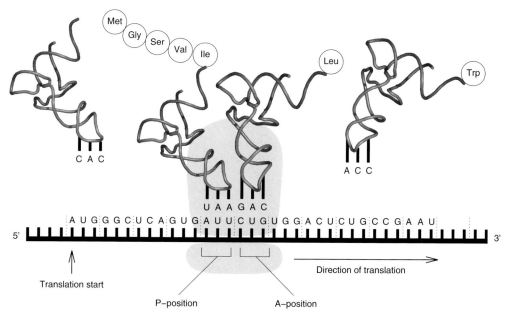

Fig. 2.12 During translation the genetic information of the mRNA is converted into the corresponding polypeptide. More details are given in the text.

the initiation tRNA. The second or A site is free to be occupied by an aminoacyl tRNA that carries an anticodon complementary to the second codon. Once the A site is filled, the amino acid at the P site, which is the methionine, establishes a peptide bond with the amino group of the amino acid at the A site. Now the unloaded tRNA leaves the P site and the ribosome moves one codon further downstream. Thus, the tRNA carrying the dipeptide enters the P site and the A site is open for another aminoacyl tRNA, which is complementary to the third codon in sequence. This cycle is repeated until a stop codon (UAA, UAG, or UGA) is reached. Then the newly synthesized polypeptide detaches from the tRNA and the ribosome releases the mRNA. It is obvious that the addition or alteration of nucleotides of a gene can lead to changes in the reading frame or to the insertion of false amino acids, which might result in malfunctioning proteins. Such changes can happen by mutations, which are random changes of the genomic sequence of an organism that either occur spontaneously or are caused by chemical substances or radiation. A mutation can be either an exchange of a single nucleotide by another or some larger rearrangement. Even the exchange of a single nucleotide by another might severely influence the function of an enzyme, if it occurs e.g. in the sequence coding for its active center.

2.4.4
Protein Sorting and Posttranslational Modifications

Cells possess a sorting and distribution system that routes newly synthesized proteins to their intra- or extracellular location. This is mediated by signal peptides – short sequences of the polypeptide occurring at diverse positions. The sorting begins during translation when the polypeptide is synthesized by either a free ribosome or by one that becomes attached to the ER membrane. The latter occurs if the nascending polypeptide has a signal sequence at its amino terminus that can be recognized by a specific signal-recognition particle (SRP) that routes it to a receptor located in the ER membrane (Fig. 2.11 ⑦). Such polypeptides are transferred into the ER lumen, where the signal peptide is cleaved off.

Peptides synthesized in the cytosol (Fig. 2.11 ④) either remain in the cytosol (⑤), if not possessing a specific signal sequence, or are routed further to a mitochondrion, chloroplast, peroxisome, or the nucleus (⑥). The nuclear localization sequence (NLS) is usually located inside the primary sequence of the protein and is not found terminally; thus, it is not cleaved from the protein as happens with many other signal peptides. Similarly, some transmembrane proteins synthesized by ribosomes of the rough ER have internal signal peptides that are required for correct routing to the membrane.

Polypeptides entering the ER after synthesis are usually further modified by glycosylations, where oligosaccharides are bound to specific positions of the newly synthesized proteins (⑧). Most proteins entering the ER do not remain in the ER but are transferred via transport vesicles to the Golgi complex (⑨), where further modifications of the bound oligosaccharides and additional glycosylations take place. If the proteins are not intended to remain in the Golgi complex, they are further transferred into lysosomes or secretory vesicles or they become transmembrane protein complexes of the plasma membrane (⑩).

2.4.5
Regulation of Gene Expression

The human genome presumably contains about 30,000–35,000 protein-coding genes, with an average coding length of about 1400 bp and an average genomic extent of about 30 kb (1 kb = 1000 bp). This would mean that only about 1.5% of the human genome consists of coding sequences and only one-third of the genome would be transcribed in genes (Lander et al. 2001, Venter et al., 2001). Besides coding sequences also regulatory sequences are known, that play important roles, in particular through control of replication and transcription. The remaining non-coding genomic DNA, that do not yet appear to have any function, is often referred to as "junk DNA".

Since only a small subset of all the genes of an organism must be expressed in a specific cell (e. g., detoxification enzymes produced by liver cells are not expressed in epidermal cells), there must be regulatory mechanisms that repress or specifically induce the expression of genes. This includes mechanisms that control the level of gene expression.

In 1961 François Jacob and Jacques Monod proposed a first model for the regulation of the *lac* operon, a genetic region of the *E. coli* genome that codes for three genes required for the utilization of the sugar lactose by this bacterium (cf. Chapter 8.4). These genes are activated only when glucose is missing but lactose, as an alternative carbon source, is present in the medium. The transcription of the *lac* genes is under the control of a single promoter, which overlaps with a regulatory region lying downstream called operator to which a transcription factor, a repressor, can bind. Jacob and Monod introduced the term operon for such a polycistronic gene. (The term cistron is defined as the functional genetic unit within which two mutations cannot complement. The term is often used synonymously with gene and describes the region of DNA that encodes a single polypeptide [or functional RNA]. Thus, the term polycistronic refers to a DNA region encoding several polypeptides. Polycistronic genes are known only for prokaryotes.)

Besides the negative regulations or repressions mediated by a repressor, positive regulations or activations that are controlled by activators are also known. An activator found in *E. coli* that is also involved in the catabolism of alternative carbon sources is the catabolite activator protein (CAP). Since the promoter sequence of the *lac* operon shows only low agreement with the consensus sequence of normal *E. coli* promoters, the RNA polymerase has only a weak affinity to it. (The consensus sequence of a promoter is a sequence pattern that shows highest sequence similarity to all promoter sequences to which a specific RNA polymerase can bind.) The presence of CAP, which indicates the lack of glucose, enhances the binding affinity of RNA polymerase to the *lac* promoter and thus supports the initiation of transcription. The regulation of the *lac* operon is described in more detail in Section 8.4.1.

The regulation of gene expression in eukaryotic cells is more complicated than in prokaryotic cells. In contrast to the bacterial RNA polymerase that recognizes specific DNA sequences, the eukaryotic enzymes require a protein/DNA complex that is established by general transcription factors. One of these transcription factors (TFIIB) binds the so-called TATA box – a promoter sequence occurring in most protein-coding genes with the consensus sequence TATAAA. Besides these general transcription factor-binding sites, most genes are further regulated by a combination of sequence elements lying in the vicinity of the promoter and enhancer sequence elements located up to 1000 nucleotides or more upstream of the promoter.

Regulation of gene expression is not only carried out by transcriptional control but can also be controlled during processing and export of the mRNA into the cytosol, by the translation rate, by the decay rates of the mRNA and the protein, and by control of the protein activity.

2.5
Cell Cycle

Growth and reproduction are major characteristics of life. Crucial for these is the cell division by which one cell divides into two and all parts of the mother cell are distributed to the daughter cells. This also requires the genome be duplicated in advance, which is performed by the DNA polymerase, an enzyme that utilizes deoxynucleotide triphosphates (dNTPs) for the synthesis of two identical DNA double strands from one parent double strand. In this case each single strand acts as a template for one of the new double strands. Several types of DNA polymerases have been found in prokaryotic and eukaryotic cells, but all of them synthesize DNA only in the $5' \rightarrow 3'$ direction. In addition to DNA polymerase, several other proteins are involved in DNA replication: proteins responsible for the unwinding and opening of the mother strand (template double strand); proteins that bind the open, single-stranded DNA and prevent it from rewinding during synthesis; an enzyme called primase that is responsible for the synthesis of short RNA primers that are required by the DNA polymerase for the initialization of DNA polymerization; and a DNA ligase that is responsible for linkage of DNA fragments that are synthesized discontinuously on one of the two template strands, because of the limitation to $5' \rightarrow 3'$ synthesis.

The cell cycle is divided into two major phases: the interphase and the M-phase (Fig. 2.13). The interphase is often a relatively long period between two subsequent cell divisions. Cell division itself takes place during the M-phase and consists of two steps: (1) the nuclear division in which the duplicated genome is separated into two parts and (2) the cytoplasmatic division or cytokinesis, where the cell divides into two cells. The latter not only distributes the two separated genomes between each of the newly developing cells but also the cytoplasmatic organelles and substances. Finally, the centrosome is replicated and distributed between both cells as well.

Most eukaryotic cells have two copies of each chromosome and hence are called diploid. For example, human cells carry 22 pairs of chromosomes coding for the same genes (one set of chromosomes coming from each parent). These chromosomes are called autosomes. The two chromosomes of such a pair are called homolo-

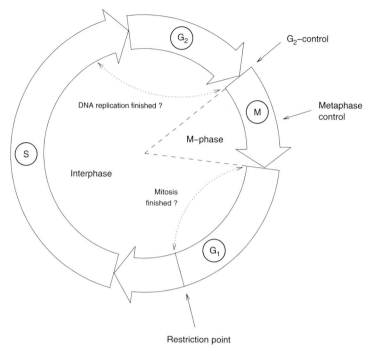

Fig. 2.13 The cell cycle is divided into the interphase, which is the period between two subsequent cell divisions, and the M-phase, during which one cell separates into two. Major control points of the cell cycle are indicated by arrows. More details are given in the text.

gous chromosomes, and their corresponding genes are called homologous genes or homologues. The remaining chromosome pair consists of two X chromosomes in females and of an X and Y chromosome in males. These so-called heterosomes are responsible for sexual determination. Germ cells (or gametes) such as the unfertilized egg of a woman or the sperm of a man have only a single chromosome set (e. g., 23 chromosomes in human), which is called haploid. Some organisms also have four (tetraploid), six (hexaploid), or many more (polyploid) chromosome sets in their cells, a situation often occurring in crops. Several genes show homology not only to their direct counterpart on the homologous chromosome but also to genes located somewhere else in the genome. This might be the case due to a duplication of genetic regions during evolution. Such genes are called paralogs. Homologous genes occurring in different species are called orthologs.

During division of a normal body cell, the whole diploid set of chromosomes is distributed equally between both daughter cells, such that these cells are also diploid. Such a cell division is called mitosis. Even haploid cells can also perform mitotic cell divisions. Germ cells are produced from diploid cells by a cell division process called meiosis that yields haploid cells. Both division mechanisms are described in more detail in the following sections.

2.5.1
Mitosis

DNA replication takes place during interphase in the so-called S-phase (S = synthesis) of the cell cycle (Fig. 2.13). This phase is usually preceded by a gap phase, G_1, and followed by another gap phase, G_2. From the G_1 phase, cells can also leave the cell cycle and enter a rest phase, G_0. The interphase normally represents 90% of the cell cycle. During interphase the chromosomes are dispersed as chromatin in the nucleus. Cell division occurs during the M-phase, which follows the G_2 phase, and consists of mitosis and cytokinesis. Mitosis is divided into different stages. During the first stage – the prophase – chromosomes condense into their compact form and the two centrosomes of a cell begin recruiting microtubules for the formation of the mitotic spindle. In later stages of mitosis, this spindle is used for the equal segregation of the chromatids of each chromosome to opposite cellular poles. During the following prometaphase, the nuclear envelope dissolves and the microtubules of the mitotic spindle attach to protein structures, called kinetochores, at the centromeres of each chromosome. In the following metaphase, all chromosomes line up in the middle of the spindle and form the metaphase plate. Now, during anaphase, the proteins holding together both sister chromatids are degraded and each chromatid of a chromosome segregates into opposite directions. Finally, during telophase, new nuclear envelopes are re-created around the separated genetic materials and form two new nuclei. The chromosomes unfold again into chromatin. The mitotic reaction is often followed by a cytokinesis where the cellular membrane pinches off between the two newly separated nuclei and two new cells are formed.

The cell cycle is strictly controlled by specific proteins. When a certain checkpoint, the restriction point, in the G_1 phase is passed, this leads to a series of specific steps that end up in cell division. At this point the cell checks whether it has achieved a sufficient size and whether the external conditions are suitable for reproduction. The control system ensures that a new phase of the cycle is entered only if the preceding phase has been finished successfully. For instance, to enter a new M-phase it has to be assured that DNA replication during the S-phase has correctly been brought to an end. Similarly, entering of the S-phase requires a preceding mitosis. A detailed description of cell cycle regulation and its molecular mechanisms is given in Section 7.2.

2.5.2
Meiosis and Genetic Recombination

Single-celled organisms and some multicellular organisms reproduce asexually by simple mitotic cell division. Evolution of such organisms is driven mostly by mutations of genes and less by recombination of existing genes or genetic regions. In contrast to this, sexual reproduction is an efficient method for the recombination of beneficial mutations from different organisms. Therefore, diploid organisms can produce haploid germ cells via meiosis. By fertilization of an egg by a sperm, an organism with a rearranged genome can develop. During meiosis the chromosomes inherited from each parent are rearranged, such that a single germ cell might contain some chromosomes originating from one parent and the others from the other parent. Eventually, all germ cells have a full haploid chromosome set.

During meiosis the diploid cell is divided into two haploid cells that in turn divide into four haploid cells. During the first stage of meiosis – prophase I – the chromosomes of a replicated diploid cell condense and each chromosome pairs to its homologous chromosome, each of which consists of two sister chromatids. During this process of chromosome alignment, it sometimes happens that a part of a chromatid arm of one chromosome is exchanged with the according chromatid arm of its homologues chromosome. This process is called crossover and it is another mechanism of genetic rearrangement. Once this elaborate and time-consuming alignment process has finished, metaphase I is entered and two consecutive cell divisions occur (meiosis I and meiosis II). During meiosis I a segregation of the homologous chromosomes takes place. Meiosis II occurs in a manner similar to normal mitotic division, except that the cells are haploid. At the end of a meiotic cycle, four haploid cells have been generated.

References

ALBERTS, B., JOHNSON, A., LEWIS, J., RAFF, M., ROBERTS, K. and WALTER, P. Molecular biology of the cell (2002) Fourth Edition Edition Garland Science Publishing.

CAMPBELL, N.A. and REECE, J.B. Biology (2001) Sixth Edition, Benjamin Cummings.

JACOB, F. and MONOD, J. Genetic regulatory mechanisms in the synthesis of proteins (1961) J. Mol. Biol. 3, 318–356.

KRAUSS, G. Biochemistry of signal transduction and regulation (2003) Third Edition, Wiley-VCH.

LANDER, E.S., LINTON, L.M., BIRREN, B., NUSBAUM, C., ZODY, M.C., BALDWIN, J., DEVON, K., DEWAR, K., DOYLE, M., FITZHUGH, W., FUNKE, R., GAGE, D., HARRIS, K., HEAFORD, A., HOWLAND, J., KANN, L., LEHOCZKY, J., LEVINE, R., MCEWAN, P., MCKERNAN, K., MELDRIM, J., MESIROV, J.P., MIRANDA, C., MORRIS, W., NAYLOR, J., RAYMOND, C., ROSETTI, M., SANTOS, R., SHERIDAN, A., SOUGNEZ, C., STANGE-THOMANN, N., STOJANOVIC, N., SUBRAMANIAN, A., WYMAN, D., ROGERS, J., SULSTON, J., AINSCOUGH, R., BECK, S., BENTLEY, D., BURTON, J., CLEE, C., CARTER, N., COULSON, A., DEADMAN, R., DELOUKAS, P., DUNHAM, A., DUNHAM, I., DURBIN, R., FRENCH, L., GRAFHAM, D., GREGORY, S., HUBBARD, T., HUMPHRAY, S.,

HUNT, A., JONES, M., LLOYD, C., MCMURRAY, A., MATTHEWS, L., MERCER, S., MILNE, S., MULLIKIN, J.C., MUNGALL, A., PLUMB, R., ROSS, M., SHOWNKEEN, R., SIMS, S., WATERSTON, R.H., WILSON, R.K., HILLIER, L.W., MCPHERSON, J.D., MARRA, M.A., MARDIS, E.R., FULTON, L.A., CHINWALLA, A.T., PEPIN, K.H., GISH, W.R., CHISSOE, S.L., WENDL, M.C., DELEHAUNTY, K.D., MINER, T.L., DELEHAUNTY, A., KRAMER, J.B., COOK, L.L., FULTON, R.S., JOHNSON, D.L., MINX, P.J., CLIFTON, S.W., HAWKINS, T., BRANSCOMB, E., PREDKI, P., RICHARDSON, P., WENNING, S., SLEZAK, T., DOGGETT, N., CHENG, J.F., OLSEN, A., LUCAS, S., ELKIN, C., UBERBACHER, E., FRAZIER, M., et al. Initial sequencing and analysis of the human genome (2001) Nature 409, 860–921.

MILLER, S.L. and UREY, H.C. Organic compound synthesis on the primitive earth (1959) Science 130, 245–51.

SINGER, S.J. and NICOLSON, G.L. The fluid mosaic model of the structure of cell membranes (1972) Science 175(23), 720–731.

VENTER, J.C., et al. The sequence of the human genome (2001) Science 291, 1304–1351.

WÄCHTERSHÄUSER, G. Before enzymes and templates: theory of surface metabolism (1988) Microbiol. Rev. 52, 452–484.

3
Mathematics in a Nutshell

Introduction

In this chapter we sum up necessary and basic relations, tools, and algorithms, which are well known to some readers and hard to recall for others. We will abandon long derivations and proofs and instead present proven tools and recipes. References to further reading are given.

3.1
Linear Algebra

In the modeling of biochemical systems, many relations do not hold just for one quantity but also for several. For example, all metabolites of a pathway have concentrations that may be concisely represented in a vector of concentrations. These metabolites are involved in a subset of the reactions occurring in this pathway; the respective stoichiometric coefficients may be presented in a matrix. Using techniques of linear algebra helps us to understand properties of biological systems. In Section 3.1.1 we will briefly recall the classical problem of how to solve a system of linear equations, since the solution algorithm represents a basic strategy. Afterwards we will introduce our notions for vectors, matrices, rank, null space, eigenvalues, and eigenvectors.

3.1.1
Linear Equations

A linear equation of n variables $x_1, x_2, ..., x_n$ is an equation of the form

$$a_1 x_1 + a_2 x_2 + ... + a_n x_n = b, \tag{3-1}$$

where $a_1, a_2, ..., a_n, b$ are real numbers. For example, $2x_1 + 5x_2 = 10$ describes a line passing through the points $(x_1, x_2) = (5,0)$ and $(x_1, x_2) = (0,2)$. A system of m linear equations of n variables $x_1, x_2, ..., x_n$ is a system of linear equations as follows

Systems Biology in Practice. Concepts, Implementation and Application.
E. Klipp, R. Herwig, A. Kowald, C. Wierling, H. Lehrach
Copyright © 2005 WILEY-VCH Verlag GmbH & Co. KGaA, Weinheim
ISBN: 3-527-31078-9

$$a_{11} x_1 + a_{12} x_2 + \ldots + a_{1n} x_n = b_1$$
$$a_{21} x_1 + a_{22} x_2 + \ldots + a_{2n} x_n = b_2$$
$$\vdots$$
$$a_{m1} x_1 + a_{m2} x_2 + \ldots + a_{mn} x_n = b_m .$$

(3-2)

If $b_1 = b_2 = \ldots = b_m = 0$, the system is *homogeneous*. We wish to determine whether the system in Eq. (3-2) has a solution, i.e., if there exist numbers $x_1, x_2, \ldots, x_n$, which satisfy each of the equations simultaneously. We say that the system is *consistent* if it has a solution. Otherwise the system is called *inconsistent*.

In order to find the solution, we employ the matrix formalism (Section 3.1.2). The matrix A_c is the coefficient matrix of the system and has the dimension $m \times n$, while the matrix A_a of dimension $m \times n + 1$ is called the augmented matrix of the system:

$$A_c = \begin{pmatrix} a_{11} & a_{12} & \cdots & a_{1n} \\ a_{21} & a_{22} & \cdots & a_{2n} \\ \vdots & \vdots & \ddots & \vdots \\ a_{m1} & a_{m2} & \cdots & a_{mn} \end{pmatrix} \qquad A_a = \left(\begin{array}{cccc|c} a_1 & a_{12} & \cdots & a_{1n} & b_1 \\ a_{21} & a_{22} & \cdots & a_{2n} & b_2 \\ \vdots & \vdots & \ddots & \vdots & \vdots \\ a_{m1} & a_{m2} & \cdots & a_{mn} & b_m \end{array} \right).$$

(3-3)

The solution of a single linear equation with one unknown is easy. A system of linear equations can be solved using the Gaussian elimination algorithm. The following terms are needed. A matrix is in row-echelon form if (1) all zero rows (if any) are at the bottom of the matrix and (2) if two successive rows are nonzero, the second row starts with more zeros than the first (moving from left to right).

Example 3-1

Matrix B_r is in row-echelon form and matrix B_n in non-row-echelon form:

$$B_r = \begin{pmatrix} 3 & 0 & 0 & 1 \\ 0 & 2 & 2 & 3 \\ 0 & 0 & 0 & 4 \\ 0 & 0 & 0 & 0 \end{pmatrix} \qquad B_n = \begin{pmatrix} 3 & 0 & 0 & 1 \\ 0 & 2 & 2 & 3 \\ 0 & 0 & 0 & 4 \\ 0 & 1 & 2 & 0 \end{pmatrix}$$

(3-4)

A matrix is in reduced row-echelon form if (1) it is in row-echelon form, (2) the leading (leftmost nonzero) entry in each nonzero row is 1, and (3) all other elements of the column in which the leading entry 1 occurs are equal to zero.

Example 3-2

A_1 and A_2 are matrices in reduced row-echelon form, while A_3 is not:

$$A_1 = \begin{pmatrix} 1 & 4 & 0 & 7 \\ 0 & 0 & 1 & 2 \end{pmatrix} \qquad A_2 = \begin{pmatrix} 1 & 0 & 0 & -2 \\ 0 & 1 & 0 & 4 \\ 0 & 0 & 1 & -5 \\ 0 & 0 & 0 & 0 \end{pmatrix} \qquad A_3 = \begin{pmatrix} 1 & 0 \\ 0 & 0 \\ 0 & 1 \end{pmatrix}. \qquad (3\text{-}5)$$

The zero matrix of any size is always in reduced row-echelon form.

The following operations are used on systems of linear equations and do not change the solutions. There are three types of elementary row operations that can be performed on matrices.

1. Interchanging two rows: $R_i \leftrightarrow R_j$.
2. Multiplying a row by a real number: $R_i \rightarrow \alpha \cdot R_i$.
3. Adding a multiple of one row to another row: $R_j \rightarrow R_j + \alpha \cdot R_i$.

A matrix A is row-equivalent to matrix B if B is obtained from A by a sequence of elementary row operations.

Example 3-3

Elementary row operations

$$A = \begin{pmatrix} 2 & 4 \\ 7 & 5 \\ 1 & 2 \end{pmatrix} \rightarrow \begin{pmatrix} 1 & 2 \\ 7 & 5 \\ 2 & 4 \end{pmatrix} \quad \rightarrow \quad \begin{pmatrix} 1 & 2 \\ 0 & -9 \\ 2 & 4 \end{pmatrix} \quad \rightarrow \quad \begin{pmatrix} 1 & 2 \\ 0 & -9 \\ 1 & 2 \end{pmatrix} = B \quad (3\text{-}6)$$

$$R_1 \leftrightarrow R_3 \qquad R_2 \rightarrow R_2 - 7\,R_1 \qquad R_3 \rightarrow 1/2 \cdot R_3$$

Thus, A and B are row-equivalent.

If A and B are row-equivalent matrices of two systems of linear equations, then the two systems have the same solution sets – a solution of one system is a solution of the other. In other words, each row of A is a linear combination of the rows of B.

3.1.1.1 The Gaussian Elimination Algorithm

The Gaussian elimination algorithm is a method for solving linear equation systems by transforming the systems augmented matrix A into its row-equivalent reduced row-echelon form B by elementary row operations. B is simpler than A, and it allows one to read off the consistency or inconsistency of the corresponding equation system and even the complete solution of the equation system.

1. Sort the rows so that the upper rows always have fewer than or the same number of zero entries before the first nonzero entry (counting from the left) as the lower

rows. Perform the following row operations. If the mentioned matrix element is zero, continue with its next nonzero right neighbor.

2. Divide the first row by a_{11} (or by its next nonzero right neighbor a_{1C_1}) and then subtract $a_{i1} \cdot R_1$ (or $a_{iC_1} \cdot R_1$) from all other rows i. Now all elements of the first (C_1-th) column apart from the first are zero.

3. Divide the second row by the new value of a_{22} (or a_{2C_2}); subtract $a_{i2} \cdot R_2$ (or $a_{iC_2} \cdot R_2$) from all other rows i. Now all elements of the second (C_2-th) column apart from the second are zero.

4. Repeat this for all lower rows until the lowest row or all lower rows contain only zeros.

Example 3-4

$$\begin{pmatrix} 2 & 2 & 2 \\ 1 & 0 & -1 \\ 3 & 2 & 1 \end{pmatrix} \rightarrow \begin{pmatrix} 1 & 1 & 1 \\ 1 & 0 & -1 \\ 3 & 2 & 1 \end{pmatrix} \rightarrow \begin{pmatrix} 1 & 1 & 1 \\ 0 & -1 & -2 \\ 0 & -1 & -2 \end{pmatrix} \rightarrow \begin{pmatrix} 1 & 1 & 1 \\ 0 & 1 & 2 \\ 0 & -1 & -2 \end{pmatrix} \rightarrow \begin{pmatrix} 1 & 0 & -1 \\ 0 & 1 & 2 \\ 0 & 0 & 0 \end{pmatrix}$$

$$R_1 \rightarrow R_1/2 \qquad \begin{matrix} R_2 \rightarrow R_2 - R_1 \\ R_3 \rightarrow R_3 - 3\,R_1 \end{matrix} \qquad R_2 \rightarrow R_2/-1 \qquad \begin{matrix} R_1 \rightarrow R_1 - R_2 \\ R_3 \rightarrow R_3 + R_2 \end{matrix} \qquad (3\text{-}7)$$

The reduced row-echelon form of a given matrix is unique.

3.1.1.2 Systematic Solution of Linear Systems

Suppose a system of m linear equations of n unknowns $x_1, x_2, \ldots, x_n$ has the augmented matrix A and A is row-equivalent to the matrix B, which is in reduced row-echelon form. A and B have the dimension $m \times (n + 1)$. Suppose that B has r nonzero rows and that the leading entry 1 in row i occurs in column number C_i for $1 \le i \le r$. Then

$$1 \le C_1 < C_2 < \ldots < C_r \le n + 1 \,. \tag{3-8}$$

The system is inconsistent if $C_r = n + 1$. The last nonzero row of B has the form $(0, 0, \ldots, 0, 1)$. The corresponding equation is

$$0\,x_1 + 0\,x_2 + \ldots + 0\,x_n = 1 \,. \tag{3-9}$$

This equation has no solution. Consequently, the original system has no solution.

The system of equations corresponding to the nonzero rows of B is consistent if $C_r \le n$. It holds that $r \le n$.

If $r = n$ then $C_1 = 1, C_2 = 2, \ldots, C_n = n$, and the corresponding matrix is

$$B = \begin{pmatrix} 1 & 0 & \ldots & 0 & | & d_1 \\ 0 & 1 & \ldots & 0 & | & d_2 \\ \vdots & & & \vdots & | & \vdots \\ 0 & 0 & \ldots & 1 & | & d_n \\ 0 & 0 & \ldots & 0 & | & 0 \\ \vdots & \vdots & \ddots & \vdots & | & \vdots \\ 0 & 0 & \ldots & 0 & | & 0 \end{pmatrix}. \tag{3-10}$$

There is a unique solution $x_1 = d_1$, $x_2 = d_2$, ..., $x_n = d_n$, which can be directly read off from B.

If $r < n$, the system is underdetermined. There will be more than one solution (in fact, infinitely many solutions). To obtain all solutions, take x_{C_1}, ..., x_{C_r} as *dependent* variables and use the r equations corresponding to the nonzero rows of B to express these variables in terms of the remaining *independent* variables $x_{C_{r+1}}$, ..., x_{C_n}, which can assume arbitrary values:

$$x_{C_1} = b_{1n+1} - b_{1C_{r+1}} x_{C_{r+1}} - \ldots - b_{1C_n} x_{C_n}$$

$$\vdots \tag{3-11}$$

$$x_{C_r} = b_{rn+1} - b_{rC_{r+1}} x_{C_{r+1}} - \ldots - b_{rC_n} x_{C_n}.$$

In particular, taking $x_{C_{r+1}} = 0$, ..., $x_{C_{n+1}} = 0$ and $x_{C_n} = 0$ or $x_{C_n} = 1$ produces at least two solutions.

Example 3-5

Solving the system

$$\begin{aligned} x_1 + x_2 + x_3 &= 0 \\ x_1 - x_2 - x_3 &= 1 \end{aligned} \tag{3-12}$$

with the following augmented and reduced row-echelon-form matrices

$$A = \begin{pmatrix} 1 & 1 & 1 & | & 0 \\ 1 & -1 & -1 & | & 1 \end{pmatrix} \qquad B = \begin{pmatrix} 1 & 0 & 0 & | & 1/2 \\ 0 & 1 & 1 & | & -1/2 \end{pmatrix} \tag{3-13}$$

leads with the choice $x_3 = 1$ to the solution $x_2 = -3/2$ and $x_1 = 1/2$.

A system of linear equations (Eq. (3-2)) with $b_1 = 0$, ..., $b_m = 0$ (i.e., a homogeneous system) is always consistent, as $x_1 = 0$, ..., $x_n = 0$ is always a solution, which is called the *trivial* solution. Any other solution is called a *nontrivial* solution. It holds that a homogeneous system of m linear equations of n unknowns always has a nontrivial solution if $m < n$.

3.1.2
Matrices

3.1.2.1 Basic Notions

Let us consider the space of real numbers $\mathfrak{R}$. A scalar is a quantity whose value can be expressed by a real number, i.e., by an element of $\mathfrak{R}$. It has a magnitude, but no direction. A vector is an element of the space $\mathfrak{R}^n$. It contains numbers for each coordinate of this space, e.g., $\boldsymbol{x} = \begin{pmatrix} x_1 \\ x_2 \\ \vdots \\ x_n \end{pmatrix}$.

A matrix is a rectangular array of $m \times n$ elements of $\mathfrak{R}$ in m rows and n columns, such as

$$A = \begin{pmatrix} a_{11} & a_{12} & \cdots & a_{1n} \\ a_{21} & a_{22} & \cdots & a_{2n} \\ \vdots & \vdots & \ddots & \vdots \\ a_{m1} & a_{m2} & \cdots & a_{mn} \end{pmatrix} = [a_{ik}]. \tag{3-14}$$

Here and below, it holds that $i = 1, ..., m$ and $k = 1, ..., n$.

For our purposes, a vector can be considered as a matrix comprising only one column ($m \times 1$).

In a zero matrix $\boldsymbol{0}$ all elements are zero ($a_{ik} = 0$ for all i, k). The matrix is a square matrix if it holds that $m = n$. A square matrix is a diagonal matrix if $a_{ik} = 0$ for all $i \neq k$. A diagonal matrix is called an identity matrix $\boldsymbol{I}_n$, if it holds that $a_{ik} = 1$, for $i = k$ or $\boldsymbol{I}_n = \begin{pmatrix} 1 & 0 & \cdots & 0 \\ 0 & 1 & & 0 \\ \vdots & & \ddots & \vdots \\ 0 & 0 & \cdots & 1 \end{pmatrix}$.

3.1.2.2 Linear Dependency

The vectors $\boldsymbol{x}_1, ..., \boldsymbol{x}_m$ of type $n \times 1$ are said to be linearly dependent if scalars $\alpha_1, ..., \alpha_m$ exist, not all zero, such that $\alpha_1 \boldsymbol{x}_1 + ... + \alpha_m \boldsymbol{x}_m = 0$. In other words, one of the vectors can be expressed as a sum over certain scalar multiples of the remaining vectors, or one vector is a linear combination of the remaining vectors. If $\alpha_1 \boldsymbol{x}_1 + ... + \alpha_m \boldsymbol{x}_m = 0$ has only the trivial solution $\alpha_1 = ... = \alpha_m = 0$, the vectors are linearly independent. A set of m vectors of type $n \times 1$ is linearly dependent if $m > n$. Equivalently, a linearly independent set of m vectors must have $m \leq n$.

3.1.2.3 Basic Matrix Operations

The transpose A^T of a matrix A is obtained by interchanging rows and columns:

$$A^T = [a_{ik}]^T = [a_{ki}]. \tag{3-15}$$

The sum of two matrices A and B of the same size $m \times n$ is

$$A + B = [a_{ik}] + [b_{ik}] = [a_{ik} + b_{ik}] . \tag{3-16}$$

The matrix product of matrix A with sizes $m \times n$ and matrix B with size $n \times p$ is

$$A.B = \left[\sum_{j=1}^{n} a_{ij} \cdot b_{jk} \right] . \tag{3-17}$$

A scalar multiple of a matrix A is

$$\alpha \cdot A = \alpha \cdot [a_{ik}] = [\alpha \cdot a_{ik}] . \tag{3-18}$$

Subtraction of matrices is composed of scalar multiplication with –1 and summation:

$$A - B = A + (-1) \cdot B . \tag{3-19}$$

Division of two matrices is not possible. However, for a square matrix A of size $n \times n$, one may in some cases find the inverse matrix A^{-1}, fulfilling

$$A.A^{-1} = A^{-1}.A = I_n . \tag{3-20}$$

If the respective inverse matrix A^{-1} exists, then A is called nonsingular (regular) and invertible. If the inverse matrix A^{-1} does not exist, then A is called singular. The inverse matrix of an invertible matrix is unique. For invertible matrices it holds that:

$$(A^{-1}) = A \tag{3-21}$$

and

$$(A.B)^{-1} = B^{-1}.A^{-1} . \tag{3-22}$$

Matrix inversion: for the inverse of a 1×1 matrix, it holds that $(a_{11})^{-1} = (a_{11}^{-1})$; the inverse of a 2×2 matrix is calculated as:

$$\begin{pmatrix} a & b \\ c & d \end{pmatrix}^{-1} = \frac{1}{ad - bc} \begin{pmatrix} d & -b \\ -c & a \end{pmatrix} . \tag{3-23}$$

In general the inverse of an $n \times n$ matrix is given as

$$A^{-1} = \frac{1}{Det\,A} \begin{pmatrix} A_{11} & A_{21} & \cdots & A_{n1} \\ A_{12} & A_{22} & \cdots & A_{n2} \\ \vdots & \vdots & & \vdots \\ A_{1n} & A_{2n} & \cdots & A_{nn} \end{pmatrix} , \tag{3-24}$$

where A_{ik} are the adjoints of A. For $Det\,A$, see below.

If a square matrix A is invertible, its rows (or columns) are linearly independent. In this case, the linear equation system $A.x = 0$ with $x = (x_1, ..., x_m)^T$ has only the trivial solution $x = 0$. If A is singular, i.e., rows (or columns) are linearly dependent, then the linear equation system $A.x = 0$ has a nontrivial solution.

The determinant of A ($DetA$) is a real or complex number that can be assigned to every square matrix. For the 1×1 matrix (a_{11}), it holds that $DetA = a_{11}$. For a 2×2 matrix, it is calculated as

$$Det \begin{pmatrix} a_{11} & a_{12} \\ a_{21} & a_{22} \end{pmatrix} = \begin{vmatrix} a_{11} & a_{12} \\ a_{21} & a_{22} \end{vmatrix} = a_{11} a_{22} - a_{12} a_{21}. \tag{3-25}$$

The value of a determinant of higher order can be obtained by an iterative procedure, i.e., by expanding the determinant with respect to one row or column: sum up every element of this row (or column) multiplied by the value of its adjoint. The adjoint A_{ik} of element a_{ik} is obtained by deleting the i-th row and the k-th column of the determinant (forming the (i,k) minor of A), calculating the value of the (i,k) minor and multiplying by $(-1)^{i+k}$. For example, a determinant of third order is

$$\begin{vmatrix} a_{11} & a_{12} & a_{13} \\ a_{21} & a_{22} & a_{23} \\ a_{31} & a_{32} & a_{33} \end{vmatrix} = a_{11}A_{11} + a_{12}A_{12} + a_{13}A_{13}$$

$$= a_{11} \cdot (-1)^2 \cdot \begin{vmatrix} a_{22} & a_{23} \\ a_{32} & a_{33} \end{vmatrix} + a_{12} \cdot (-1)^3 \cdot \begin{vmatrix} a_{21} & a_{23} \\ a_{31} & a_{33} \end{vmatrix} + a_{13} \cdot (-1)^4 \cdot \begin{vmatrix} a_{21} & a_{22} \\ a_{31} & a_{32} \end{vmatrix} \tag{3-26}$$

$$= a_{11} \cdot (a_{22} a_{33} - a_{23} a_{32}) - a_{12} \cdot (a_{21} a_{33} - a_{23} a_{31}) + a_{13} \cdot (a_{21} a_{32} - a_{22} a_{31}).$$

The value of a determinant is zero (1) if it contains a zero row or a zero column or (2) if one row (or column) is a linear combination of the other rows (or columns). In this case, the respective matrix is singular.

3.1.2.4 Dimension and Rank

Subspace of a vector space: Let us further consider the vector space V^n of all n-dimensional column vectors ($n \times 1$). A subset S of V^n is called a subspace of V^n (1) if the zero vector belongs to S, (2) if with two vectors belonging to S their sum also belongs to S, and (3) if with one vector belonging to S its scalar multiples also belong to S. Vectors $x_1, ..., x_m$ belonging to a subspace S form a basis of a vector subspace S if they are linearly independent and if every vector in S is a linear combination of x_1, ..., x_m. A subspace where at least one vector is nonzero has a basis. In general, a subspace will have more than one basis. Every linear combination of basis vectors is itself a basis. The number of vectors making up a basis is called the dimension of S (*dim S*). For the n-dimensional vector space, it holds that *dim S* $\leq n$.

The rank of a matrix is an important integer associated with a matrix A of size $m \times n$. $RankA$ is equal to the number of linearly independent columns or rows in A and equal to the number of nonzero rows in the reduced row-echelon form of the matrix A. It holds that $Rank\,A \leq m, n$.

Example 3-6

The matrix

$$A = \begin{pmatrix} 2 & 1 & 1 \\ 4 & 2 & 2 \end{pmatrix} \quad \text{with} \quad R_2 \rightarrow R_2 - 2R_1 \begin{pmatrix} 2 & 1 & 1 \\ 0 & 0 & 0 \end{pmatrix}$$

has $m = 2$ rows, $n = 3$ columns, and $Rank\,A = 1$.

Null space of a vector space: The solution of a homogeneous linear equation system, $Ax = 0$, leads to the notion null space (or kernel) of matrix A. Nontrivial solutions for the vector x exist if $Rank\,A < m$, i.e., if there are linear dependencies between the columns of A. A kernel matrix K with

$$AK = 0 \tag{3-27}$$

can express these dependencies. The m-$Rank\,A$ columns, k_i, of K are particular, linearly independent solutions of the homogeneous linear equation system and span the null space of matrix A. K is not uniquely determined: all linear combinations of the vectors k_i again constitute a valid solution. In other terms, post-multiplying matrix K by a nonsingular square matrix Q of matching type gives another null space matrix K'.

3.1.2.5 Eigenvalues and Eigenvectors of a Square Matrix

Let A be an $(n \times n)$ square matrix. If λ is a complex number and b is a nonzero complex vector satisfying

$$Ab = \lambda b, \tag{3-28}$$

then b is called an eigenvector of A, while λ is called an eigenvalue of A. Equation (3-28) can be rewritten as $(A - \lambda I_n)b = 0$. This equation has nontrivial solutions only if

$$Det\,(A - \lambda I_n) = 0. \tag{3-29}$$

In this case there are at most n distinct eigenvalues of A. Equation (3-29) is called the characteristic equation of A and $Det\,(A - \lambda I_n)$ is the characteristic polynomial of A. The eigenvalues are the roots of the characteristic polynomial.

For a (2×2) matrix $A = \begin{pmatrix} a_{11} & a_{12} \\ a_{21} & a_{22} \end{pmatrix}$ the characteristic polynomial is $\lambda^2 - \lambda \cdot Trace\,A$ + $Det\,A$ where $Trace\,A = a_{11} + a_{22}$ is the sum of the diagonal elements of A.

Example 3-7

For the matrix $A = \begin{pmatrix} 2 & 1 \\ 1 & 2 \end{pmatrix}$ the characteristic equation reads $\lambda^2 - \lambda \cdot 4 + 3 = (\lambda - 1)$ $\cdot (\lambda - 3) = 0$ and the eigenvalues are $\lambda_1 = 1$, $\lambda_2 = 3$. The eigenvector equation reads $\begin{pmatrix} 2 - \lambda & 1 \\ 1 & 2 - \lambda \end{pmatrix} \begin{pmatrix} b_1 \\ b_2 \end{pmatrix} = \begin{pmatrix} 0 \\ 0 \end{pmatrix}$. Taking $\lambda_1 = 1$ results in the equation system $\begin{cases} b_1 + b_2 = 0 \\ b_1 + b_2 = 0 \end{cases}$. Thus it holds that $b_1 = -b_2$ with arbitrary values $b_1 \neq 0$. The eigenvectors corresponding to λ_1 are the vectors $\begin{pmatrix} b_1 \\ -b_1 \end{pmatrix}$. For $\lambda_2 = 3$ $\begin{pmatrix} b_1 \\ b_1 \end{pmatrix}$ is the corresponding eigenvector.

3.2
Ordinary Differential Equations

An important problem in the modeling of biological systems is to characterize the dependence of certain properties on time and space. One frequently applied strategy is the description of the change of state variables by differential equations. If only temporal changes are considered, ordinary differential equations (ODEs) are used. For changes in time and space, partial differential equations are appropriate. In this section we will deal with solutions, analysis, numerical integration of ordinary differential equations, and basic concepts of dynamical systems theory as state space, trajectory, steady states, and stability.

The time behavior of biological systems in a deterministic approach can be described by a set of differential equations

$$\frac{dx_i}{dt} = \dot{x} = f_i(x_1, \ldots, x_n, p_1, \ldots, p_l, t) \quad i = 1, \ldots, n, \tag{3-30}$$

where x_i represents the variables, e.g., concentrations, p_j represents the parameters, e.g., enzyme concentrations or kinetic constants, and t is the time. We will use the notions $\frac{dx}{dt}$ and $\dot{x}$ interchangeably. In vector notation, Eq. (3-30) reads

$$\frac{d}{dt} x = \dot{x} = f(x, p, t), \tag{3-31}$$

with $x = (x_1, \ldots, x_n)^T$, $f = (f_1, \ldots, f_n)^T$, and $p = (p_1, \ldots, p_l)^T$.

Example 3-8

The linear pendulum is the classical example: the back propagation force, which is proportional to acceleration $\ddot{s} = \dfrac{d^2 s}{dt^2}$, is proportional to the amplitude s or $\ddot{s}(t) = \omega^2 s(t)$.

An important example for metabolic modeling is substance degradation: the concentration change $\dot{c}$ is proportional to the actual concentration c, i.e. $\dot{c}(t) = k \cdot c(t)$.

3.2.1
Notions

Ordinary differential equations (ODEs) depend on one variable (e.g., time t). Otherwise, they are called partial differential equations (PDEs). PDEs are not considered here.

An *implicit* ODE

$$F\left(x, y, y', \ldots, y^{(n)}\right) = 0 \tag{3-32}$$

includes the variable x, the unknown function y, and its derivatives up to the n-th order. An *explicit* ODE of n-th order has the form

$$y^{(n)} = f\left(x, y, y', \ldots, y^{(n-1)}\right). \tag{3-33}$$

The highest derivative (here n) determines the order of the ODE.

Studying the time behavior of our system, we may be interested in finding solutions of the ODE, i.e., finding an n times differentiable function y fulfilling Eq. (3-33). Such a solution may depend on parameters, so-called integration constants, and represents a set of curves. A solution to an ODE of the n-th order depending on n integration parameters is a *general* solution. Specifying the integration constants, for example, by specifying n initial conditions (for $n = 1$: $x(t = 0) = x^0$), leads to a special or *particular* solution. Rather than showing all possibilities of solving ODEs here, we will focus on some cases relevant to the following chapters.

If the right sites of the explicit ODEs are not explicitly dependent on time t ($\dot{x} = f(x, p)$), the system is called autonomous. Otherwise it is non-autonomous. This case will not be considered here.

The system state is a snapshot of the system at a given time that contains enough information to predict the behavior of the system for all future times. The state of the system is described by the set of variables. The set of all possible states is the state space. The number n of independent variables is equal to the dimension of the state space. For $n = 2$ the two-dimensional state space can be called phase plane.

A particular solution to the ODE system $\dot{x} = f(x, p, t)$, determined from the general solution by specifying parameter values p and initial conditions $x(t_0) = x^0$, describes a path through the state space and is called trajectory.

Stationary (or steady) states are points $\bar{x}$ in the phase plane, where the condition $\dot{x} = 0$ ($x_1 = 0$, ..., $x_n = 0$) is met. At steady state, the system of n differential equations is represented by a system of n algebraic equations for n variables. $\dot{x} = 0$ can have multiple solutions referring to multiple steady states. The change in number or character of steady states upon changes in parameter values p is called a bifurcation.

Linear systems of ODEs have linear functions of the variables as right sides, such as

$$\frac{dx_1}{dt} = a_{11} x_1 + a_{12} x_2 + z_1$$

$$\frac{dx_2}{dt} = a_{21} x_1 + a_{22} x_2 + z_2 ,$$

(3-34)

or, in general, $\dot{x} = Ax + z$. The matrix $A = \{a_{ik}\}$ is the system matrix containing the system coefficients $a_{ik} = a_{ik}(p)$, and the vector $z = (z_1, ..., z_n)^T$ contains inhomogeneities. The linear system is homogeneous if $z = 0$ holds. Linear systems can be solved analytically. Although in real-world problems the functions are usually nonlinear, linear systems are important as linear approximations in the investigation of steady states.

Example 3-9

The simple linear system

$$\frac{dx_1}{dt} = a_{12} x_2$$

$$\frac{dx_2}{dt} = -x_1$$

(3-35)

has the general solution

$$x_1 = \frac{1}{2} e^{-i\sqrt{a_{12}}t} \left(1 + e^{2i\sqrt{a_{12}}t}\right) C_1 - \frac{1}{2} i e^{-i\sqrt{a_{12}}t} \left(-1 + e^{2i\sqrt{a_{12}}t}\right) \sqrt{a_{12}} C_2$$

$$x_2 = \frac{i}{2\sqrt{a_{12}}} e^{-i\sqrt{a_{12}}t} \left(1 + e^{2i\sqrt{a_{12}}t}\right) C_1 + \frac{1}{2} e^{-i\sqrt{a_{12}}t} \left(1 + e^{2i\sqrt{a_{12}}t}\right) C_2$$

with the integration constants C_1, C_2. Choosing $a_{12} = 1$ simplifies the system to

$$x_1 = C_1 \cos t + C_2 \sin t, \quad x_2 = C_2 \cos t - C_1 \sin t .$$

Specification of the initial conditions to $x_1(0) = 2$, $x_2(0) = 1$ gives the particular solution

$$x_1 = 2 \cos t + \sin t, \quad x_2 = \cos t - 2 \sin t .$$

The solution can be presented in the phase plane or directly as functions of time (see Fig. 3.1).

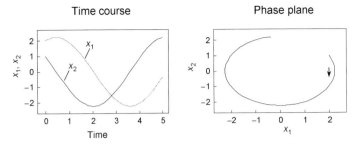

Fig. 3.1 Time course and phase plane for the linear system of ODEs represented in Eq. (3-35). In the time course panel, gray line, x_1 (t); black line, x_2 (t). Parameters: $a_{12} = 1$, x_1 (0) = 1, x_2 (0) = 2.

3.2.2
Linearization of Autonomous Systems

In order to investigate the behavior of a system close to steady state, it may be useful to linearize it. Considering the deviation ξ (t) from steady state with x (t) = $\bar{x} + \xi$ (t), it follows that

$$\dot{x} = f\left(\bar{x} + \xi(t)\right) = \frac{d}{dt}\left(\bar{x} + \xi(t)\right) = \frac{d}{dt}\,\xi(t).$$ (3-36)

Taylor expansion of the temporal change of the deviation, $\frac{d}{dt}\,\xi_i = f_i\left(\bar{x}_1 + \xi_1, \ldots,\right.$ $\left.\bar{x}_n + \xi_n\right)$, gives

$$\frac{d}{dt}\,\xi_i = f_i\left(\bar{x}_1, \ldots, \bar{x}_n\right) + \sum_{j=1}^{n}\frac{\partial f_i}{\partial x_j}\,\xi_j + \frac{1}{2}\sum_{j=1}^{n}\sum_{k=1}^{n}\frac{\partial^2 f_i}{\partial x_j\,\partial x_k}\,\xi_j\,\xi_k + \ldots .$$ (3-37)

Since we consider steady state, it holds that $f_i(\bar{x}_1, \ldots, \bar{x}_n) = 0$. Neglecting terms of higher order, we have

$$\frac{d}{dt}\,\xi_i = \sum_{j=1}^{n}\frac{\partial f_i}{\partial x_j}\,\xi_j = \sum_{j=1}^{n} a_{ij}\,\xi_j.$$ (3-38)

The coefficients a_{ij} are calculated at steady state and are constant. They form the so-called Jacobian matrix:

$$J = \{a_{ij}\} = \begin{pmatrix} \dfrac{\partial f_1}{\partial x_1} & \dfrac{\partial f_1}{\partial x_2} & \cdots & \dfrac{\partial f_1}{\partial x_n} \\[2mm] \dfrac{\partial f_2}{\partial x_1} & \dfrac{\partial f_2}{\partial x_2} & \cdots & \dfrac{\partial f_2}{\partial x_n} \\[2mm] \vdots & \vdots & \ddots & \vdots \\[2mm] \dfrac{\partial f_n}{\partial x_1} & \dfrac{\partial f_n}{\partial x_2} & \cdots & \dfrac{\partial f_n}{\partial x_n} \end{pmatrix}.$$ (3-39)

For linear systems it holds that $J = A$.

3.2.3
Solution of Linear ODE Systems

We may be interested in two different types of problems: describing the temporal evolution of the system and finding its steady state. The problem of finding the steady state $\bar{x}$ of a linear ODE system $\dot{x} = 0$ implies that $A\bar{x} + z = 0$. The solution necessitates inversion of the system matrix A:

$$\bar{x} = -A^{-1} z. \tag{3-40}$$

The time course solution of homogeneous linear ODEs is described below. The systems can be solved using an exponential function as approach. In the simplest case $n = 1$, we have

$$\frac{dx_1}{dt} = a_{11} x_1. \tag{3-41}$$

Introducing the approach $x_1(t) = b_1 e^{\lambda t}$ with constant b_1 into Eq. (3-41) yields:

$$b_1 \lambda e^{\lambda t} = a_{11} b_1 e^{\lambda t}. \tag{3-42}$$

Equation (3-42) is true if $\lambda = a_{11}$. This leads to the general solution

$$x_1(t) = b_1 e^{a_{11} t}. \tag{3-43}$$

To find a particular solution, we must specify the initial conditions $x_1(t = 0) = x_1^0 = b_1 e^{a_{11} t}|_{t=0} = b_1$. Thus, the solution is

$$x_1(t) = x_1^0 e^{a_{11} t}. \tag{3-44}$$

For a linear homogeneous system of n differential equations, $\dot{x} = Ax$, the approach is $x = be^{\lambda t}$. This gives $\dot{x} = b\lambda e^{\lambda t} = Abe^{\lambda t}$. The scalar factor $e^{\lambda t}$ can be cancelled out, leading to $b\lambda = Ab$ or the characteristic equation

$$(A - \lambda I_n) b = 0. \tag{3-45}$$

The solution of this equation is described in Section 3.1.2.

For homogeneous linear systems, the superposition principle holds: if x_1 and x_2 are solutions of this ODE system, then their linear combination is also a solution. This leads to the general solution of the homogeneous linear ODE system:

$$x(t) = \sum_{i=1}^{n} c_i b^{(i)} e^{\lambda_i t}, \tag{3-46}$$

where $b^{(i)}$ are the eigenvectors of the system matrix A corresponding to the eigenvalues λ_i. A particular solution specifying the coefficients c_i can be found considering the initial conditions $x(t=0) = x^0 = \sum_{i=1}^{n} c_i b^{(i)}$. This constitutes an inhomogeneous linear equation system to be solved for c_i.

For the solution of inhomogeneous linear ODEs, the system $\dot{x} = Ax + z$ can be transformed into a homogeneous system by the coordination transformation $\hat{x} = x - \bar{x}$.

Since $\frac{d}{dt}\bar{x} = A\bar{x} + z = 0$, it holds that $\frac{d}{dt}\hat{x} = A\hat{x}$. Therefore, we can use the solution algorithm for homogeneous systems for the transformed system.

3.2.4
Stability of Steady States

If a system is at steady state it should stay there, at least until an external perturbation occurs. Depending on systems behavior after perturbation, their steady states are

- *stable* (the system returns to this state),
- *unstable* (the system leaves this state), or
- *metastable* (the system behavior is indifferent).

A steady state is asymptotically stable if it is stable and nearby initial conditions tend to this state for $t \to \infty$. Local stability describes the behavior after small perturbations, global stability after any perturbation.

To investigate whether a steady state $\bar{x}$ of the ODE system $\dot{x} = f(x)$ is asymptotically stable, we consider the linearized system $\dot{\xi} = A\xi$ (Section 3.2.1.2) with $\xi(t) = x(t) - \bar{x}$. The steady state $\bar{x}$ is asymptotically stable if the Jacobian A has n eigenvalues with strictly negative real parts each. The steady state is unstable if at least one eigenvalue has a positive real part. This will be explained in more detail for one- and two-dimensional systems.

We start with one-dimensional systems, i.e., $n = 1$. Without a loss of generality $\bar{x}_1 = 0$ or $x_1 = \xi_1$. To the system $\dot{x}_1 = f_1(x_1)$ belongs the linearized system $\dot{x}_1 = \frac{\partial f_1}{\partial x_1}\Big|_{\bar{x}_1}$ $x_1 = a_{11}x_1$. The Jacobian matrix $A = \{a_{11}\}$ has only one eigenvalue, $\lambda_1 = a_{11} = \frac{\partial f_1}{\partial x_1}\Big|_{\bar{x}_1}$.

The solution is $x_1(t) = x_1^0 e^{\lambda_1 t}$. It is obvious that $e^{\lambda_1 t}$ increases for $\lambda_1 > 0$ and that the system runs away from the steady state. For $\lambda_1 < 0$, the deviation from steady state decreases and $x_1(t) \to \bar{x}_1$ for $t \to \infty$. For $\lambda_1 = 0$, consideration of the linearized system allows no conclusion about stability of the original system.

Consider the two-dimensional case $n = 2$. To the system

$$\dot{x}_1 = f_1(x_1, x_2)$$
$$\dot{x}_2 = f_2(x_1, x_2)$$

$(3\text{-}47)$

belongs the linearized system

$$\dot{x}_1 = \left.\frac{\partial f_1}{\partial x_1}\right|_{\bar{x}} x_1 + \left.\frac{\partial f_1}{\partial x_2}\right|_{\bar{x}} x_2$$

$$\text{or}\quad \dot{x} = \begin{pmatrix} \left.\frac{\partial f_1}{\partial x_1}\right|_{\bar{x}} & \left.\frac{\partial f_1}{\partial x_2}\right|_{\bar{x}} \\ \left.\frac{\partial f_2}{\partial x_1}\right|_{\bar{x}} & \left.\frac{\partial f_2}{\partial x_2}\right|_{\bar{x}} \end{pmatrix} x = \begin{pmatrix} a_{11} & a_{12} \\ a_{21} & a_{22} \end{pmatrix} x = Ax \quad (3\text{-}48)$$

$$\dot{x}_2 = \left.\frac{\partial f_2}{\partial x_1}\right|_{\bar{x}} x_1 + \left.\frac{\partial f_2}{\partial x_2}\right|_{\bar{x}} x_2$$

To find the eigenvalues of A, we have to solve the characteristic polynomial

$$\lambda^2 - \underbrace{(a_{11} + a_{22})}_{Trace\ A}\lambda + \underbrace{a_{11}\,a_{22} - a_{12}\,a_{21}}_{Det\ A} = 0 \qquad (3\text{-}49)$$

and get

$$\lambda_{1/2} = \frac{Trace\ A}{2} \pm \sqrt{\frac{(Trace\ A)^2}{4} - Det\ A}\,. \qquad (3\text{-}50)$$

The eigenvalues are either real for $(Trace\ A)^2/4 - Det\ A \geq 0$) or complex (otherwise). For complex eigenvalues, the solution contains oscillatory parts.

For stability it is necessary that $Trace\ A < 0$ and $Det\ A > 0$. Depending on the sign of the eigenvalues, steady states of a two-dimensional system may have the following characteristics:

1. $\lambda_1 < 0$, $\lambda_2 < 0$, both real: stable node;
2. $\lambda_1 > 0$, $\lambda_2 > 0$, both real: unstable node;
3. $\lambda_1 > 0$, $\lambda_2 < 0$, both real: saddle point, unstable;
4. $Re(\lambda_1) < 0$, $Re(\lambda_2) < 0$, both complex with negative real parts: stable focus;
5. $Re(\lambda_1) > 0$, $Re(\lambda_2) > 0$, both complex with positive real parts: unstable focus; or
6. $Re(\lambda_1) = 0$, $Re(\lambda_2) = 0$, both complex with zero real parts: center, unstable.

Graphical representation of stability depending on trace and determinant is given in Fig. 3.2.

Up to now we have considered only the linearized system. For the stability of the original system, the following holds. If the steady state of the linearized system is asymptotically stable, then the steady state of the complete system is also asymptotically stable. If the steady state of the linearized system is a saddle, an unstable node, or an unstable focus, then the steady state of the complete system is also unstable. This means that statements about the stability remain true, but the character of the steady state is not necessarily kept. No statement about the center is possible.

The Routh-Hurwitz theorem (Bronstein and Semendjajew 1987) states: For systems with $n > 2$ differential equations, it holds that the characteristic polynomial

$$a_n\,\lambda^n + a_{n-1}\,\lambda^{n-1} + \ldots + a_1\,\lambda + a_0 = 0 \qquad (3\text{-}51)$$

is a polynomial of degree n, which frequently cannot be solved analytically (at least for $n < 4$). We can use the Hurwitz criterion to test whether the real parts of all eigenvalues are negative. We have to form the Hurwitz matrix H, containing the coefficients of the characteristic polynomial:

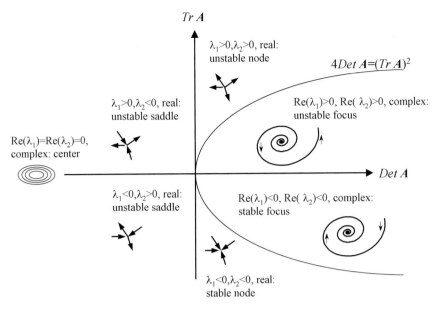

Fig. 3.2 Stability of steady states in two-dimensional systems. The character of steady-state solutions is represented depending on the value of the determinant (x-axis) and the trace (y-axis) of the Jacobian matrix. Phase plane behavior of trajectories in the different cases is schematically represented.

$$H = \begin{pmatrix} a_{n-1} & a_{n-3} & a_{n-5} & \cdots & 0 \\ a_n & a_{n-2} & a_{n-4} & \cdots & 0 \\ 0 & a_{n-1} & a_{n-3} & \cdots & 0 \\ 0 & a_n & a_{n-2} & \cdots & 0 \\ \vdots & \vdots & \vdots & \ddots & \vdots \\ 0 & 0 & 0 & \cdots & a_0 \end{pmatrix} = \{h_{ik}\}, \tag{3-52}$$

where h_{ik} follows the rule

$$h_{ik} = \begin{cases} a_{n+i-2k}, & \text{if } 0 \le 2k - i \le n \\ 0, & \text{else} \end{cases} . \tag{3-53}$$

It can be shown that all solutions of the characteristic polynomial have negative real parts if all coefficients a_i of the polynomial as well as all principal leading minors of H have positive values.

3.2.4.1 Global Stability of Steady States

A state is globally stable if the trajectories for all initial conditions approach it for $t \to \infty$. The stability of a steady state of an ODE system can be tested with a method of Lyapunov.

1. Transfer the steady state into the point of origin by coordination transformation $\hat{x} = x - \bar{x}$.

2. Find a Lyapunov function $V_L(x_1, ..., x_n)$ with the following properties: $V_L(x_1, ..., x_n)$ has steady derivatives with respect to all variables x_i and $V_L(x_1, ..., x_n)$ is positive definite, i.e., $V_L(x_1, ..., x_n) = 0$ for $x_i = 0$ and $V_L(x_1, ..., x_n) > 0$ for $x_i \neq 0$.

3. The time derivative of V_L is given by

$$\frac{dV_L}{dt} = \sum_{i=1}^{n} \frac{\partial V_L}{\partial x_i} \frac{dx_i}{dt} = \sum_{i=1}^{n} \frac{\partial V_L}{\partial x_i} f_i(x_1, \ldots, x_n). \tag{3-54}$$

It holds that a steady state $\bar{x} = 0$ is stable if the time derivative of V_L in a certain region around this state has no positive values. The steady state is asymptotically stable if the time derivative of V_L in this region is negative definite, i.e., $dV_L/dt = 0$ for $x_i = 0$ and $dV_L/dt < 0$ for $x_i \neq 0$.

Example 3-10

The system $\dot{x}_1 = -x_1$, $\dot{x}_2 = -x_2$ has the solution $x_1(t) = x_1^0 e^{-t}$, $x_2(t) = x_2^0 e^{-t}$, and the state $x_1 = x_2 = 0$ is asymptotically stable. The global stability can also be shown using the positive definite function $V_L = x_1^2 + x_2^2$ as a Lyapunov function. It holds that $dV_L/dt = (\partial V_L/\partial x_1)\dot{x}_1 + (\partial V_L/\partial x_2)\dot{x}_2 = 2x_1(-x_1) + 2x_2(-x_2)$, which is negative definite.

3.2.4.2 Limit Cycles

Oscillatory behavior is a typical phenomenon in biology. The cause of the oscillation may be different, either externally imposed or internally implemented. Internally caused stable oscillations as a function of time can be found if we have a limit cycle in the phase space.

A limit cycle is an isolated closed trajectory. All trajectories in its vicinity are periodic solutions winding towards (stable limit cycle) or away from (unstable) the limit cycle for $t \to \infty$.

Example 3-11

The nonlinear system $\dot{x}_1 = x_1^2 x_2 - x_1$, $\dot{x}_2 = p - x_1^2 x_2$ has a steady state at $\bar{x}_1 = p$, $\bar{x}_2 = 1/p$.

Choosing, e.g., $p = 0.98$, this steady state is unstable since $Trace\, A = 1 - p^2 > 0$. Time course and phase plane behavior are shown in Fig. 3.3.

For two-dimensional systems there are two criteria for determining whether a limit cycle exists. Consider the following system of differential equations:

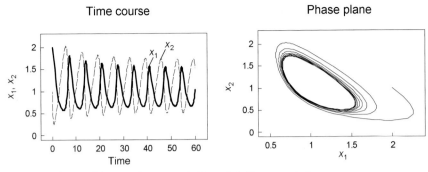

Fig. 3.3 Solution of the equation system in Example 3-11 represented as time course and phase plane. Initial conditions: $x_1(0) = 2$, $x_2(0) = 1$.

$$\dot{x}_1 = f_1(x_1, x_2)$$

$$\dot{x}_2 = f_2(x_1, x_2).$$

(3-55)

The negative criterion of Bendixson states: if the expression $Trace = \dfrac{\partial f_1}{\partial x_1} + \dfrac{\partial f_2}{\partial x_2}$ does not change its sign in a certain region of the phase plane, then there is no closed trajectory in this area. Hence, a necessary condition for the existence of a limit cycle is a change in the sign of *Trace*.

Example 3-12

In Example 3-11 it holds that $Trace = (2 x_1 x_2 - 1) + (-x_1^2)$. Therefore, $Trace = 0$ is fulfilled at $x_2 = \dfrac{x_1^2 + 1}{2 x_1}$ and *Trace* may assume positive or negative values for varying x_1, x_2 and the necessary condition for the existence of a limit cycle is met.

The criteria of Poincaré-Bendixson states: if a trajectory in the phase plane remains within a finite region without approaching a singular point (a steady state), then this trajectory either is a limit cycle or it approaches a limit cycle. This criterion gives a sufficient condition for the existence of a limit cycle. Nevertheless, the limit cycle trajectory can be computed analytically only in very rare cases.

3.3
Difference Equations

Modeling with difference equations employs a discrete timescale, in contrast to the continuous timescale in ODEs. For some processes, the value of the variable x at a discrete time point t depends directly on the value of this variable at a former time point. For example, the actual number of individuals in a population of birds in one year can be related to the number of individuals last year.

A general (first-order) difference equation takes the form

$$x_i = f(t, x_{i-1}) \quad \text{for all } t. \tag{3-56}$$

We can solve such an equation by successive calculation: given x_0, we have

$$
\begin{aligned}
x_1 &= f(1, x_0) \\
x_2 &= f(2, x_1) = f(2, f(1, x_0)) .
\end{aligned} \tag{3-57}
$$
$$\vdots$$

In particular, given any value x_0, there exists a unique solution path x_1, x_2, ... For simple forms of the function f, we can also find general solutions.

Example 3-13

Consider the exponential growth of a bacterial population with a doubling of the population size x_i in each time interval. The recursive equation $x_i = 2 x_{i-1}$ is equivalent to the explicit equation $x_i = x_0 \cdot 2^i$ and also to the difference equation $x_i - x_{i-1} = \Delta x = x_{i-1}$.

The difference equation expresses the relation between values of a variable at discrete time points. We are interested in the dynamics of the variable. For the general case $x_i = r x_{i-1}$, it can be easily shown that $x_i = r^i x_0$. This corresponds to the law of exponential growth (Malthus' law). The dynamic behavior depends on the parameter r:

$1 < r$:	exponential growth
$r = 1$:	x remains constant, steady state
$0 < r < 1$:	exponential decay
$-1 < r < 0$:	alternating decay
$r = -1$:	periodic solution
$r < -1$:	alternating increase

Example time courses are shown in Fig. 3.4.

A difference equation of the form

$$x_{i+k} = f(x_{i+k}, \ldots, x_{i+1}, x_i) \tag{3-58}$$

is a k-th order difference equation. Like ODEs, difference equations may have stationary solutions that might be stable or unstable, which are defined as follows. The value $\bar{x}$ is a stationary solution or fix point of the difference equation (Eq. (3-58)) if $\bar{x} = f(\bar{x})$. A fix point is stable (or unstable), if there is a neighborhood $N = \{x : |x - \bar{x}| < \varepsilon\}$ such that every series that begins in N converges against $\bar{x}$ (leaves N). The following sentence is practically applicable: the fix point is stable under the condition that f is continuously differentiable if $\left| \dfrac{df(x)}{dx} \right|_{\bar{x}} < 1$.

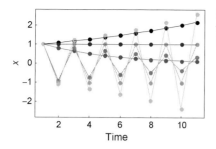

Fig. 3.4 Temporal behavior of a difference equation describing exponential growth for various values of parameter r (r drops with the gray level).

Example 3-14

The simplest form of the logistic equation, which plays a role in population dynamics, is $x_{n+1} = r x_n (1 - x_n)$, with $f(x) = rx(1-x)$ where r is a positive valued parameter. This difference equation has two fix points, $\bar{x}_1 = 0$ and $\bar{x}_2 = 1 - \dfrac{1}{r}$.

Stability analysis yields that fix point $\bar{x}_1$ is stable if $\left| \dfrac{df(x)}{dx} \right|_{\bar{x}_1} = r < 1$ and fix point $\bar{x}_2$ is stable if $\left| \dfrac{df(x)}{dx} \right|_{\bar{x}_2} = |2 - r| < 1$; hence, $1 < r < 3$.

For $r > 3$ there are stable oscillations of period 2, i.e., successive generations alternate between two values. Finding the steady states $\bar{\bar{x}}_1$ and $\bar{\bar{x}}_2$ is enabled by the new function $g(x) = f(f(x))$. The equation $g(x) = x$ has the two solutions

$$\bar{\bar{x}}_{1,2} = \frac{r + 1 \pm \sqrt{(3 - r)(r + 1)}}{2r}.$$

They are stable if $\left| \dfrac{dg(x)}{dx} \right|_{\bar{\bar{x}}_i} < 1$ holds for $i = 1, 2$ or

$$\left| \left(\frac{df(x)}{dx} \right)_{\bar{\bar{x}}_1} \cdot \left(\frac{df(x)}{dx} \right)_{\bar{\bar{x}}_2} \right| < 1,$$

i.e., for $3 < r < 3.3$. For $r > 3.3$, oscillations of higher period occur, which can be treated in a manner analogous to oscillations of period 2. For $r > r_{crit}$ chaos arises, i.e., albeit a deterministic description, the system trajectories in fact cannot be reliably predicted and may differ remarkably for close initial conditions. The points $r = 1$, $r = 3$, and $r = 3.3$ are bifurcation points since the number and stability of steady states change. A graphical representation is given in Fig. 3.5.

3.4
Statistics

In this section we give an introduction to basic concepts of probability theory and statistics. In practice, experimental measurements undergo some uncertainty (concentrations, RNA levels, etc.), and statistical concepts give us a framework to quantify this uncertainty. Concepts of probability theory (Section 3.4.1) provide the necessary mathematical models for computing the significance of the experimental out-

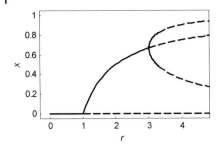

Fig. 3.5 Bifurcation diagram of the logistic equation. For increasing parameter r, the number of steady-states increments are shown. At the points $r = 1$, $r = 3$, and $r = 3.3$, stability changes from stable (solid lines) to unstable (dashed lines) occur. Only the constant solution and the solution of periods 1 and 2 are shown.

come. The focus of elementary statistics (Section 3.4.2) is to describe the underlying probabilistic parameters by functions on the experimental sample, the sample statistics, and to provide tools for visualization of the data. Statistical test theory (Section 3.4.3) provides a framework for judging the significance of statements (hypotheses) with respect to the data. Linear models (Section 3.4.4) are one of the most prominent tools for analyzing complex experimental procedures.

3.4.1
Basic Concepts of Probability Theory

The quantification and characterization of uncertainty are formally described by the concept of a probability space for a random experiment. A random experiment is an experiment that consists of a set of possible outcomes with a quantification of the possibility of such an outcome. For example, when a coin is tossed, one cannot deterministically predict the outcome of "heads" or "tails" but rather assigns a probability that either of the outcomes will occur. Intuitively, one will assign a probability of 0.5 if the coin is fair (i.e., both outcomes are equally likely). Random experiments are described by a set of probabilistic axioms.

A probability space is a triplet (Ω, A, P) where Ω is a nonempty set, A is a σ-algebra of subsets of Ω, and P is a probability measure on A. A σ-algebra is a family of subsets of Ω that (1) contains Ω itself, (2) contains for every element $B \in A$ the complementary element $B^c \in A$, and (3) contains for every series of elements $B_1, B_2, \dots$, $\in A$ their union, i.e., $\bigcup_{i=1}^{\infty} B_i \in A$. The pair (Ω, A) is called a measurable space. An element of A is called an event. If Ω is discrete, i.e., it has at most countable many elements, then a natural choice of A would be the power set of Ω, $P(\Omega)$, i.e., the set of all subsets of Ω.

A probability measure $P: A \to [0,1]$ is a real-valued function that has the properties

$$P(B) \geq 0 \text{ for all } B \in A \text{ and } P(\Omega) = 1$$

and

$$P(\bigcup_{i=1}^{\infty} B_i) = \sum_{i=1}^{\infty} P(B_i) \text{ for all series of disjoint sets } B_1, B_2, \dots, \in A \text{ (σ-additivity)}. \quad (3\text{-}59)$$

Example 3-15: Urn models

Many practical problems can be described with urn models. Consider an urn containing N balls of which K are red and $N - K$ are black. The random experiment consists of n draws from that urn. If the ball is replaced in the urn after each draw we call the experiment drawing with replacement; otherwise, it is called drawing without replacement. Here, Ω is the set of all n-dimensional binary sequences $\Omega = \{(x_1, ..., x_n); x_i \in \{0,1\}\}$, where a "1" means that a red ball was drawn and a "0" means that a black ball was drawn. Since Ω is discrete, a suitable σ-algebra is the power set of Ω. Of practical interest is the calculation of the probability of having exactly k red balls among the n balls drawn. This is given by

$$P(k) = \binom{n}{k} p^k (1 - p)^{n-k}, \text{ with } p = \frac{K}{N}, \text{ if we draw with replacement and}$$

$$P(k) = \frac{\binom{K}{k}\binom{N - K}{n - k}}{\binom{N}{n}} \text{ if we draw without replacement. Here for all numbers,}$$

$a \geq b \geq 0$ it is defined (binomial coefficients)

$$\binom{a}{b} = \frac{a!}{(a - b)! b!}. \tag{3-60}$$

We can define the concept of conditional dependency. Let (Ω, A, P) be a probability space and let $B_1, B_2 \in A$ be two events. In general, there will be some dependency between the two events that influences the probability that both events will occur simultaneously. For example, consider B_1 as the event that a randomly picked person has lung cancer and let B_2 be the event that the person is a smoker. If both events were independent of each other, then the joint event $B_1 \cap B_2$ would be the product of the probabilities, i.e., $P(B_1 \cap B_2) = P(B_1) P(B_2)$. This would mean that the probability that a randomly picked person has lung cancer is independent of the fact that he is a smoker. Otherwise, the probability of B_1 would be higher dependent on B_2 (Fig. 3.6).

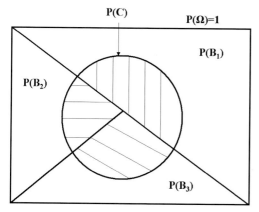

Fig. 3.6 Illustration of conditional probabilities. Three events, B_1, B_2, B_3, build a partition of the probability space Ω with *a priori* probabilities $P(B_1) = 0.5$, $P(B_2) = P(B_3) = 0.25$. Any event C defines a conditional probability measure with respect to C. Here, the *a posteriori* probabilities given C are $P(B_1) = 0.5$, $P(B_2) = 0.17$, $P(B_3) = 0.33$, respectively.

We can generalize this to define another probability measure with respect to any given event C with positive probability. For any event $B \in A$, define $P(B|C) = \dfrac{P(B \cap C)}{P(C)}$, which is the conditional probability of B given C. The measure $P(.|C)$ is a probability measure on the measurable space (Ω, A).

If we have a decomposition of Ω into disjoint subsets $\{B_1, B_2, ...\}$ with $P(B_1) > 0$, then the probability of any event C can be retrieved by the sum of probabilities with respect to the decomposition, i.e.,

$$P(C) = \sum_i P(C|B_i) P(B_i).$$ (3-61)

Conversely, if $P(C) > 0$, the probability for each B_i conditioned on C can be calculated by Bayes' rule, i.e.

$$P(B_i|C) = \frac{P(C|B_i) P(B_i)}{\sum_j P(C|B_j) P(B_j)}.$$ (3-62)

In the Bayesian setup, the probabilities $P(B_i)$ are called *a priori* probabilities. These describe the probability of the events with no additional information. If we consider now an event C with positive probability, one can ask about the *a posteriori* probabilities $P(B_i|C)$ of the events in light of event C. In practice, Eq. (3-62) is very important since many problems do not allow a direct calculation of the probability of an event but rather the probability of the event conditioned on another event or series of other events.

Example 3-16: Power of diagnostics

Consider a specific disease affecting 0.5% of the population. A diagnostic test with a false positive rate of 5% and a true positive rate of 90% is conducted with a randomly picked person. The test result is positive. What is the probability that this person has the disease? Let B_1 be the event that a person has the disease (B_1^c is the complementary event). Let B_2 be the event that the test is positive. Thus, we are asking for the conditional probability that the person has the disease given that the test is positive, i.e., $P(B_1 | B_2)$. From Eq. (3-62) we get

$$P(B_1|B_2) = \frac{P(B_2|B_1) P(B_1)}{P(B_2|B_1) P(B_1) + P\left(B_2|B_1^c\right) P\left(B_1^c\right)} = \frac{0.9 \cdot 0.005}{0.9 \cdot 0.005 + 0.05 \cdot 0.995} = 0.083.$$

That means that only 8% of persons with a positive test result will actually have the disease!

The above effect is due to the fact that the disease is rare and thus that a randomly picked person will have a low chance *a priori* of having the disease. The diagnostic test, however, will produce a high number of false positives in this sample. The diagnostic power of the test can be improved by decreasing the error rate. For example, decreasing the false positive rate to 1% would give a predictive success rate of 31.142% (0.5% would give 47.493%).

3.4.1.1 Random Variables, Densities, and Distribution Functions

Let (Ω, A) and (Ω', A') be two measurable spaces. A function $f : \Omega \to \Omega'$ is called measurable if $f^{-1}(B') \in A$ for all $B' \in A'$. A measurable function defined on a probability space is called a random variable. Random variables are used to describe outcomes of random experiments. A particular result of a random experiment will occur with a given probability.

Of practical interest are real- or vector-valued random variables, i.e., $\Omega' = \mathfrak{R}$ or $\Omega' = \mathfrak{R}^n$. In this case a σ-algebra can be defined straightforwardly. Let $\mathfrak{I}$ be the family of all n-dimensional intervals $Q = (a_1, b_1] \times ... \times (a_n, b_n]$. Then there exists a minimal σ-algebra that contains $\mathfrak{I}$, the Borel σ-algebra. This σ-algebra contains all sets that one can typically imagine, such as all open, closed, or semi-open intervals and arbitrary mixtures of these. Indeed, it is not straightforward to define sets in $\mathfrak{R}^n$ that are not contained in the Borel σ-algebra! A random variable is commonly denoted as $x : \Omega \to \mathfrak{R}$ in order to point to the outcomes (or realizations) of x. The probability measure P defined on Ω induces a probability measure, P_x, on the Borel σ-algebra on $\mathfrak{R}$ through the equality $P_x(B') = P(x \in B') = P(x^{-1}(B'))$.

If x is a random vector, then the distribution of x is uniquely defined by assigning a probability to each n-dimensional vector z by $F(z) = P(x \le z) = P(x_1 \le z_1, ..., x_n \le z_n)$. F is called the cumulative distribution function of x. If F admits the n-th-order mixed partial derivative, then the density function of x is defined as $f(z) = f(z_1, ..., z_n) = \dfrac{\partial^n}{\partial z_1 ... \partial z_n} F(z_1, ..., z_n)$ and the relation holds that

$$F(z) = F(z_1, ..., z_n) = \int_{-\infty}^{z_1} ... \int_{-\infty}^{z_n} f(t_1, ..., t_n) \, dt_1 ... dt_n. \tag{3-63}$$

If x is a discrete random vector, i.e., if x can adopt only countable many outcomes, then the density function can be denoted as $f(z) = P(x = z) = P(x_1 = z_1, ..., x_n = z_n)$. In the discrete case, f is often called the probability mass function of x.

Example 3-17

In the one-dimensional case, the distribution function of a random variable is defined by $F(t) = P(x \le t) = P_x((-\infty, t])$. If x is a continuous random variable, the density function f is defined as $P_x((-\infty, t]) = \int_{-\infty}^{t} f(z) \, dz$; if x is a discrete random variable, then we have $P_x((-\infty, t]) = \sum_{x \le t} f(x)$.

Important characteristics of a probability distribution are the mean outcome that one would expect if all possible outcomes together with their respective probabilities were considered (expectation) and the mean deviation of the outcomes from the mean outcome (variance). The expectation of a random variable is defined as

$$E(x) = \int_{-\infty}^{\infty} t f(t)\, dt = \mu \tag{3-64}$$

and the variance as

$$Var(x) = \int_{-\infty}^{\infty} (t - \mu)^2 f(t)\, dt. \tag{3-65}$$

The variance is equal to $Var(x) = E(x^2) - E(x)^2$. The covariance of two random variables x and y is defined as

$$Cov(x, y) = E((x - E(x))(y - E(y))). \tag{3-66}$$

Note that $Var(x) = Cov(x, x)$. If $x_1, \ldots, x_n$ are random variables with means $E(x_i) = \mu_i$, variances $Var(x_i) = \sigma_{ii}$ and covariances $Cov(x_i, x_j) = \sigma_{ij} = \sigma_{ji}$, then the random vector $x = (x_1, \ldots, x_n)^T$ has expectation $E(x) = \mu$, where $\mu = (\mu_1, \ldots, \mu_n)^T$, and covariance matrix

$$\mathbf{Cov}(\mathbf{x}) = E((\mathbf{x} - \boldsymbol{\mu})(\mathbf{x} - \boldsymbol{\mu})^T) = \begin{pmatrix} \sigma_{11} & \ldots & \sigma_{1n} \\ \ldots & \ldots & \ldots \\ \sigma_{n1} & \ldots & \sigma_{nn} \end{pmatrix}. \tag{3-67}$$

A random vector is called nonsingular (singular) when its covariance matrix is nonsingular (singular). If x is an n-dimensional random vector, A is a $p{\times}n$ matrix, and b is a p-dimensional vector, we get the following transformation rules

$$E(\mathbf{Ax} + \mathbf{b}) = \mathbf{A}E(\mathbf{x}) + \mathbf{b} \quad \text{and} \quad \mathbf{Cov}(\mathbf{Ax} + \mathbf{b}) = \mathbf{A}\,\mathbf{Cov}(\mathbf{x})\,\mathbf{A}^T. \tag{3-68}$$

Equation (3-68) gives the expectation of a random vector under an affine transformation. Under general transformations, the expectation cannot be calculated straightforwardly from the expectation of x. However, in some cases one can give a lower bound for the expectation of the transformation that is useful in practice. Let x be a random variable and let g be a real-valued convex function, i.e., a function for which $g(\sum_{i=1}^{n} \lambda_k x_k) \le \sum_{i=1}^{n} \lambda_k g(x_k)$ where $0 \le \lambda_k \le 1$, $\sum_{i=1}^{n} \lambda_k = 1$ (if the inequality is reversed, we call g a concave function). Then the inequality holds that (Jensen's inequality)

$$g(E(x)) \le E(g(x)). \tag{3-69}$$

Example 3-18

The variance of a random variable is always nonnegative because $g(x) = x^2$ is a convex function; thus, it follows from Eq. (3-69) that $(Ex)^2 \le E(x^2)$.

Example 3-19

The normal distribution is the most important distribution in probability theory. Numerous methods in test theory and multivariate statistics rely on calculus with the normal distribution (compare also Sections 3.4.3 and 3.4.4). x has a one-dimensional normal (or Gaussian) distribution with parameters μ, σ^2 if the density of x is equal to

$$f(t) = \frac{1}{\sqrt{2\pi\sigma^2}} e^{-\frac{(t-\mu)^2}{2\sigma^2}}.$$

(3-70)

This is also denoted as $x \sim N(\mu, \sigma^2)$. The special case $\mu = 0$, $\sigma^2 = 1$ is called the standard normal distribution. The expectation and the variance of the standard normal distribution can be calculated as $E(x) = 0$ and $Var(x) = 1$. If z is standard normally distributed, then the random variable $x = \sigma z + \mu$ is distributed with parameters $x \sim N(\mu, \sigma^2)$. From Eq. (3-68) it follows that $E(x) = \mu$ and $Var(x) = \sigma^2$. The normal distribution can be easily generalized. Let x be an n-dimensional random vector that follows a normal distribution; then the density of x is

$$f(z) = \frac{1}{(2\pi)^{n/2}} (det(\Sigma))^{1/2} exp\left(-\frac{1}{2}(z-\mu)^T \Sigma^{-1}(z-\mu)\right),$$

(3-71)

where μ is the mean vector and Σ is the covariance matrix composed of the components $x_1, ..., x_n$ of x.

Example 3-20

The exponential distribution is important in modeling decay rates and in the characterization of stochastic processes. A random variable is exponentially distributed with parameter $\lambda > 0$ if the density of x is equal to

$$f(t) = \lambda e^{-\lambda t},$$

(3-72)

where $t \geq 0$. The expectation and variance of x are equal to $E(x) = \frac{1}{\lambda}$ and $Var(x) = \frac{1}{\lambda^2}$, respectively.

Example 3-21

An example of a discrete distribution is the binomial distribution. The binomial distribution is used to describe urn models with replacement (cf. Example 3–15) where we ask specifically for the number of successes in n independent repetitions of a random experiment with binary outcomes (a Bernoulli experiment). If x_i is the random variable that describes the outcome of the i-th experiment, then the random variable $x = \sum_{i=1}^{n} x_i$ has a binomial distribution with probability mass function of

$$f(x = k) = \binom{n}{k} p^k (1-p)^{n-k}, \tag{3-73}$$

where p is the probability for succes.
The expectation and variance are $E(x) = np$ and $Var(x) = np(1-p)$, respectively.

3.4.1.2 Transforming Probability Densities

Let x be a random variable with probability density f; then for each measurable function h, $y = h(x)$ is also a random variable. The transformation rule states that if h is a function with strictly positive (negative) derivation with inverse function h^{-1}, then y has the density $g(y) = \dfrac{f(h^{-1}(y))}{|h'(h^{-1}(y))|}$. More generally, let x be an n-dimensional random vector and h a vector-valued function $h : \Re^n \to \Re^n$ that is differentiable, i.e., h admits the partial derivatives. Let h^{-1} be the inverse function with $\det(J_{h^{-1}}(y)) \neq 0$ for all $y \in \Re^n$, where $J_{h^{-1}}$ is the Jacobian matrix of h^{-1}. Then, the density of the random vector $y = h(x)$ is given by

$$g(y) = f(h^{-1}(y)) |\det(J_{h^{-1}}(y))|. \tag{3-74}$$

Example 3-22: Affine transformations of a probability density

Let x be a random vector with density function f, let h be a vector-valued affine function $h : \Re^n \to \Re^n$, i.e., $h(x) = \Sigma x + \mu$ for an $n \times n$ matrix Σ and an n-dimensional vector μ; then, the density function of the random vector $y = h(x)$ is equal to $g(y) = f(A^{-1}(y - \mu))|\det(A^{-1})|$. In particular, in the one-dimensional case we have the transformation $h(x) = ax + b$ and the corresponding probability density

$$g(y) = f\left(\frac{y-b}{a}\right) \frac{1}{|a|}.$$

Example 3-23: The density function of a log-normal distribution

A random variable y is log-normally distributed if the random variable $\ln(y) = x$ is Gaussian distributed with parameters $x \sim N(\mu, \sigma^2)$. The density of y can be calculated according to the transformation rule; we then have $y = h(x) = e^x$ and $h^{-1}(y) = \ln(y)$, and we get the density function of y as $g(y) = \dfrac{1}{\sqrt{2\pi\sigma^2}} e^{-\frac{(\ln(y)-\mu)^2}{2\sigma^2}} \dfrac{1}{y}$.

3.4.1.3 Product Experiments and Independence

Consider n different probability spaces (Ω_i, A_i, P_i). In many applications the actual interesting probability space would be the product space $(\otimes \Omega_i, \otimes A_i, \prod P_i)$. Here, the product set and the product σ-algebra denote the Cartesian products. The product measure is defined as the product of the individual probability measures. Implicitly, we have used this definition before; for example, an experiment described by the binomial distribution is the product experiment of individual Bernoulli experiments.

Let $x = (x_1, ..., x_n)^T$ and $y = (y_1, ..., y_m)^T$ be two n- and m-dimensional random vectors, respectively; in this case, the joint probability density of the vector $(x^T, y^T)^T$ is defined as $f_{xy}(x_1, ..., x_n, y_1, ..., y_m)$ and the marginal density f_x of x is defined as

$$f_x(x) = f_x(x_1, ..., x_n) = \int_{-\infty}^{+\infty} ... \int_{-\infty}^{+\infty} f_{xy}(x_1, ..., x_n, y_1, ..., y_m) dy_1 ... dy_m. \tag{3-75}$$

Two random vectors x and y are independent of each other when the joint probability function is the product of the marginal probability functions, i.e.,

$$f_{xy}(x, y) = f_x(x) f_y(y). \tag{3-76}$$

Let x_1, x_2 be two independent real-valued random variables with probability densities f_1, f_2. Many practical problems require the distribution of the sum of the random variables, $y = g(x_1, x_2) = x_1 + x_2$. For each realization c of y, we have $g^{-1}(c) = \{(a, b); a + b = c\}$ and we get

$$P(y \le c) = \iint_{\{(a,b); a+b \le c\}} f_1(a) f_2(b) \, da \, db = \int_{-\infty}^{c} \left(\int_{-\infty}^{+\infty} f_1(u-b) f_2(b) \, db \right) du = \int_{-\infty}^{c} (f_1 * f_2)(u) \, du.$$

The function $f_1 * f_2$ is called the convolution of f_1 and f_2.

Example 3-24: Convolution rule of the normal distribution

Let x_1, ..., x_n be independent random variables that are Gaussian distributed with $x_i \sim N(\mu_i, \sigma_i^2)$. Then, $y = x_1 + ... + x_n$ is Gaussian distributed $y \sim N(\mu_1 + ... + \mu_n, \sigma_1^2 + ... + \sigma_n^2)$.

3.4.1.4 Limit Theorems

In this section we list some fundamental theorems of probability theory that describe the convergence properties of series of random variables. The first states that the empirical distribution function (compare Section 3.4.2) is converging against the true underlying (but unknown) distribution function. The second tells us that the sample mean (Section 3.4.2) is an estimator for the distribution moment. The third states that all distributions converge asymptotically against a Gaussian distribution if they are transformed conveniently.

All convergence properties are defined "almost everywhere". This technical term of measure theory is introduced to indicate that a result for a probability space is valid everywhere except on subsets of probability zero.

Theorem of Glivenko-Cantelli

Let x_1, ..., x_n be random variables that are independently and identically distributed with distribution function F. Then, the empirical distribution function $F_n(t)$ converges (almost everywhere) to the true distribution function, i.e.,

$$\sup_{t\in\Re}\left|F_n(t) - F(t)\right| \to_{n\to+\infty} 0 \text{ (almost everywhere).}\tag{3-77}$$

Strong Law of the Large Numbers

Let $x_1, x_2, \ldots$ be a series of uncorrelated real-valued random variables with $Var(x_i) \le M < +\infty$ for all i; then, the series of random variables

$$z_n = \frac{1}{n}\sum_{i=1}^{n}(x_i - E(x_i))\tag{3-78}$$

converges to zero (almost everywhere).

Central Limit Theorem

Let Φ be the distribution function of the standard Gaussian distribution. Let $x_1, x_2, \ldots$ be a series of independently identically distributed random variables with finite and nonzero variance, i.e., $0 < Var(x_i) < +\infty$. Define the series of random variables

$$z_n = \frac{\sum_{i=1}^{n} x_i - nE(x_1)}{\sqrt{Var(x_1)}\sqrt{n}}; \text{ then, } z_n \text{ converges to } \Phi \text{ (almost everywhere), i.e.,}$$

$$\sup_{t\in\Re}\left|z_n(t) - \Phi(t)\right| \to_{n\to+\infty} 0.\tag{3-79}$$

3.4.2
Descriptive Statistics

The basic object of descriptive statistics is the sample. A sample is a subset of data measured from an underlying population, e.g., repeated measurements of DNA array levels from the same gene. A numerical function of a sample is called a statistic. Commonly, a statistic is used to compress the information inherent in the sample and to describe certain properties of the sample. Interesting features that characterize the sample are (1) statistics for sample location, (2) statistics for sample variance, and (3) statistics for sample distribution. In the following sections, the main concepts are introduced.

3.4.2.1 Statistics for Sample Location
Measures of location describe the center of gravity of the sample. The most commonly used measures of location are the mean and the median. Let $x_1, \ldots, x_n$ be a sample of n values; the mean of the sample is defined as

$$\bar{x} = \frac{1}{n}\sum_{i=1}^{n} x_i\tag{3-80}$$

and the median is defined as the value that is greater than or equal to 50% of the sample. For the proper definition of the median, it is necessary to introduce the definition of a percentile. Consider the ordered sample $x^{(1)} \le \ldots \le x^{(n)}$ derived from $x_1, \ldots, x_n$ by sorting the sample in increasing order. Then, the p-th percentile is the value that is larger than $p\%$ of the measurements. It is clear that the 0-percentile and the 100-percentile are the minimum and the maximum of the sample. The median is the 50th percentile. If the sample size is odd, then the median is defined as $x^{\left(\frac{n+1}{2}\right)}$; if the sample size is even, the median is not unique. It can be any value between $x^{\left(\frac{n}{2}\right)}$ and $x^{\left(\frac{n}{2}+1\right)}$, e. g., the average of both values $\left(x^{\left(\frac{n}{2}\right)} + x^{\left(\frac{n}{2}+1\right)}\right)/2$. An important characteristic of the median is its robustness against outlier values. In contrast, the mean value is biased to a large extent by outlier values. In order to robustify the mean value, we define the α-trimmed mean. Here, the $\alpha\%$ lowest and highest values are simply deleted from the dataset and the mean is calculated of the remaining sample values. Common values of α are between 10% and 20%. Note that the median is the 50%-trimmed mean of the sample.

Example 3-25

Consider the measurements of gene expression for a particular gene in a certain tissue in 12 individuals. These individuals represent a common group (control type), and we want to derive the mean expression level.

Sample	x_1	x_2	x_3	x_4	x_5	x_6	x_7	x_8	x_9	x_{10}	x_{11}	x_{12}
Value	2434	2289	5599	2518	1123	1768	2304	2509	14820	2489	1349	1494

We get $\bar{x} = 3391.33$ for the mean and $x_{med} = 0.5\,(2304 + 2434) = 2369$ for the median. If we look more deeply into the sample, we would rather prefer the median as sample location since most values scatter around the median. The overestimation of the sample location by the mean results from the high values of the outlier value x_9 (and probably x_3). The 10%-trimmed mean of the sample is $\bar{x} = 2475.3$, which is comparable with the median.

Another measure of location that is preferably used if the sample values represent proportions rather than absolute values is the geometric mean. The geometric mean is defined as

$$\bar{x}_g = \sqrt[n]{\prod_{i=1}^{n} x_i}\,. \tag{3-81}$$

Note that it always holds that $\bar{x} \geq \bar{x}_g$.

3.4.2.2 Statistics for Sample Variability

Once we have determined the center of the sample, another important bit of information is how the sample values scatter around that center. A very simple way of measuring sample variability is the range, the difference between the maximum and the minimum values, $x_{max} - x_{min}$. The most common statistic for sample variability is the standard deviation,

$$s_n = \sqrt{\frac{1}{n-1}\sum_{i=1}^{n}(x_i - \bar{x})^2}. \tag{3-82}$$

s_n^2 is called the variance of the sample. The standard deviation measures the individual difference of each sample value and the sample mean. Similar to the mean, it is influenced by outlier values. Standard deviations cannot directly be compared since they are dependent on the scale of the values. For example, if two series of distance values were measured in m and mm, the latter one would have a higher standard deviation. In order to compare sample variability from different samples, one instead compares the relative standard deviations. This measure is called coefficient of variation:

$$cv_n = \frac{s_n}{\bar{x}}. \tag{3-83}$$

The interpretation of the coefficient of variation is variability relative to location. A more robust measure of variability is the interquartile range, IQR, i.e., the difference of the upper and lower quartile of the sample: $IQR_n = x^{(\lceil 0.75n \rceil)} - x^{(\lceil 0.25n \rceil)}$. Here $\lceil \alpha n \rceil$ denotes the smallest integer that is greater than or equal to αn. Analogue to the median, another measure is the median absolute deviation from the median (MAD):

$$MAD = median\left(|x_1 - x_{med}|, ..., |x_n - x_{med}|\right). \tag{3-84}$$

Both measures of location, $\bar{x}$ and $\bar{x}_{med}$ are related to their corresponding measure of variability and can be derived as solutions of a minimization procedure. We have

$$\bar{x} \in \arg\min\left\{a; \sum_{i=1}^{n}(x_i - a)^2\right\} \quad \text{and} \quad x_{med} \in \arg\min\left\{a; \sum_{i=1}^{n}|x_i - a|\right\}.$$

The sample characteristics are commonly condensed and visualized by a box plot (Fig. 3.7).

3.4.2.3 Density Estimation
In order to have a description of the distribution of the sample values across the sample range, one commonly defines the histogram. Let $I_1, ..., I_M$ be disjoint intervals, $I_m = (a_{m-1}, a_m]$, and let $n_m = |\{x_i; x_i \in I_m\}|$ be the number of sample values that fall in the respective interval. Then, the weighted histogram statistic

$$f_n(t) = \begin{cases} \dfrac{n_m}{n}\dfrac{1}{a_m - a_{m-1}}, & t \in I_m \\ 0, & \text{else} \end{cases} \tag{3-85}$$

can be used to estimate the density of the distribution.

A fundamental statistic of the sample is the empirical distribution function. This is defined as

Box-plots of Gaussian distributions

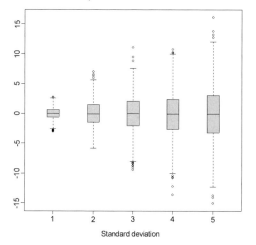

Standard deviation

Box-plots of replicated array measurements

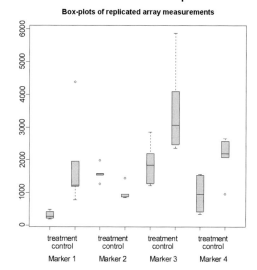

Fig. 3.7 Visualization of sample characteristics by box plots. Left graph: Five different samples from Gaussian distributions with mean $\mu = 0$ and standard deviations $\sigma = 1, 2, 3, 4,$ and 5, respectively, were randomly generated. The box displays the IQR, and the line is the median of the samples. The whiskers denote an area defined by a multiple of the IQR. Sample values outside this area are marked as outliers (circles). Graphics were generated with the R-statistical software package. Right graph: Four marker genes determined in a study on Down syndrome. Samples are based on six (treatment) and five (control) individuals, respectively. Three markers are downregulated (markers 1, 3 and 4), and one marker gene is upregulated.

$$F_n(t) = \frac{1}{n} \sum_{i=1}^{n} 1_{(-\infty,t]}(x_i) \tag{3-86}$$

where $1_{(-\infty,t]}(x_i) = \begin{cases} 1, \text{ if } x_i \leq t \\ 0, \text{ else} \end{cases}$ denotes the indicator function. This function is a real-valued step function with values in the interval [0,1] that has a step at each point x_i. In Section 3.4.1.4 we showed that the two statistics above converge to the probability density and the distribution function, respecttively, with respect to an underlying probability law. Figure 3.8 shows as an example the density, cumulative distribution function, and empirical distribution function of a Gaussian distribution.

3.4.2.4 Correlation of Samples

So far we have discussed statistics for samples measured on one variable. Let us now consider a sample measured on two variables, i.e., $z_1, ..., z_n$, where $z_i = (x_i, y_i)$ is a two-dimensional observation. A fundamental question is whether the two individual samples $x_1, ..., x_n$ and $y_1, ..., y_n$ correlate with each other, i.e., have a similar trend. A measure of correlation is Pearson's correlation (PC) coefficient. This is defined as

$$PC = \frac{\sum_{i=1}^{n}(x_i - \bar{x})(y_i - \bar{y})}{\sqrt{\sum_{i=1}^{n}(x_i - \bar{x})^2 \sum_{i=1}^{n}(y_i - \bar{y})^2}} \; . \tag{3-87}$$

The Pearson correlation measures the linear relationship of both samples. It is close to one if both samples have strong linear correlation, it is negative if the samples are anti-correlated, and it scatters around zero if there is no linear trend observable. Outliers can influence the Pearson correlation to a large extent. Therefore, ro-

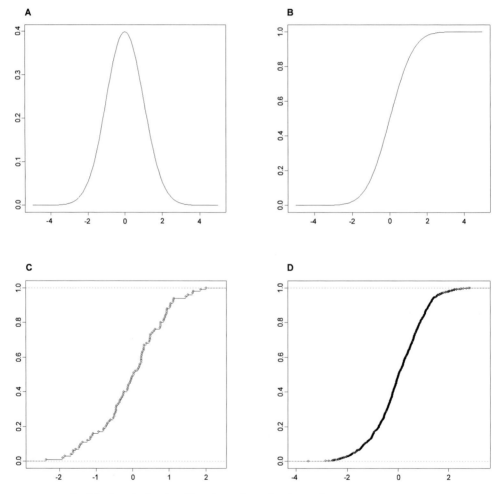

Fig. 3.8 Density function (A) and cumulative distribution function (B) of a standard normal distribution with parameters $\mu = 0$ and $\sigma = 1$. Empirical distribution function of a random sample of 100 (C) and 1000 (D) values drawn from a standard normal distribution.

bust statistics for sample correlation have been defined. We call $r_i^x = |\{x_j; x_j \leq x_i\}|$ the rank of x_i within the sample $x_1, ..., x_n$. It denotes the number of sample values smaller or equal to the i-th value. Note that the minimum, the maximum, and the median of the sample have ranks, $1, n,$ and $\frac{n}{2}$, respectively, and that the ranks and the ordered sample have the correspondence that $x_i = x^{(r_i^x)}$. A more robust measure of correlation than Pearson's correlation coefficient is Spearman's rank correlation (SC):

$$SC = \frac{\sum_{i=1}^{n}(r_i^x - \bar{r}^x)(r_i^y - \bar{r}^y)}{\sqrt{\sum_{i=1}^{n}(r_i^x - \bar{r}^x)^2 \sum_{i=1}^{n}(r_i^y - \bar{r}^y)^2}} \ . \tag{3-88}$$

Here, $\bar{r}^x$ denotes the mean rank. SC is derived from PC by replacing the actual sample values by their ranks within the respective sample. Another advantage of this measure is the fact that SC can measure relationships other than linear ones. For example, if the second sample is derived from the first by any monotonic function (square root, logarithm), then the correlation is still high (Fig. 3.9). Measures of correlation are extensively used in many algorithms of multivariate statistical analysis, such as pairwise similarity measures for gene expression profiles (cf. Chapter 9).

3.4.3
Testing Statistical Hypotheses

Many practical applications imply statements such as "It is very likely that two samples are unequal" or "This fold change of gene expression is significant". Consider the following problems.

1. We observe the expression of a gene in replicated measurements of cells with a chemical treatment and control cells. Can we quantify whether a certain fold change in gene expression is significant?
2. We observe the expression of a gene in different individuals suffering from a certain disease and a control group. Is the variability in the two samples equal?
3. We measure gene expression of many genes. Does the signal distribution of these genes resemble a specific distribution?

Statistical test theory provides a unique framework to tackle these questions and to give numerical estimates for the significance of these differences.

3.4.3.1 Statistical Framework
Replicated measurements of the same object in a treatment and a control condition typically yield two series of values, $x_1, ..., x_n$ and $y_1, ..., y_m$. The biological problem of judging differences from replicated measurements can be formulated as statistical hypotheses: the null hypothesis, H_0, and the alternative, H_1.

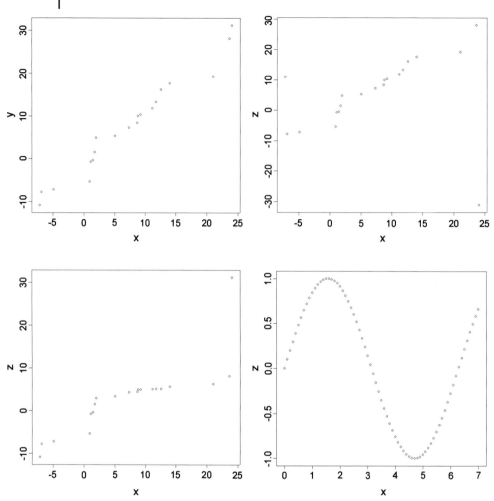

Fig. 3.9 Correlation plots and performance of correlation measures. Top left: linear correlation of two random variables (PC = 0.98, SP = 1.00); top right: presence of two outliers (PC = 0.27, SP = 0.60); bottom left: nonlinear, monotonic correlation (PC = 0.83, SP = 1.00); bottom right: nonlinear, non-monotonic correlation (PC = –0.54, SP = –0.54).

An important class of tests is the two-sample location test. Here, the null hypothesis states that the difference between the two samples is zero, i.e., there is no difference, and the alternative states that there is a difference.

$$H_0 : \mu_x = \mu_y \quad \text{versus} \quad H_1 : \mu_x \neq \mu_y,$$

where μ_x, μ_y are the mean values of the respective samples.

A very simple argument would be to calculate the averages of the two series and compare the ratios. However, this would not allow judging whether the ratio has any significance. If we make some additional assumptions, we can describe the problem using an appropriate probability distribution. We regard the two series as realizations of random variables $x_1, ..., x_n$ and $y_1, ..., y_m$. Statistical tests typically have two constraints: it is assumed that (1) repetitions are independent and (2) the random variables are identically distributed within each sample. Test decisions are based upon a reasonable test statistic, a real-valued function T, on both samples. For specific functions and using the distributional assumptions, it has been shown that they follow a quantifiable probability law given the null hypothesis H_0. Suppose that we observe a value of the test statistic $T(x_1, ..., x_n, y_1, ..., y_m) = \hat{t}$. If T could be described with a probability law, we can then judge the significance of the observation by $prob(T$ more extreme than $\hat{t}|H_0)$. This probability is called a P-value. Thus, if one assigns a P-value of 0.05 to a certain observation, this means that under the distributional assumptions, the probability of observing an outcome more extreme than the observed one is 0.05 given the null hypothesis. Observations with a small P-value typically give incidence that the null hypothesis should be rejected. This makes it possible to quantify statistically, using a probability distribution, whether the result is significant. In practice, significance levels of 0.01, 0.05, and 0.1 are used as upper bounds for significant results.

In such a test setup, two types of error occur: error of the first kind and error of the second kind.

	H_0 is true	H_1 is true
Test does not reject H_0	No error (TN)	Error of the second kind (FN)
Test rejects H_0	Error of the first kind (FP)	No error (TP)

The error of the first kind is the false-positive (FP) rate of the test. Usually, this error can be controlled by the analysis by assuming a significance level of α and judging only those results where the probability is lower than α as significant. The error of the second kind is the false-negative (FN) rate of the test. The power of a test (TP) (given a significance level α) is defined as the probability of rejecting H_0 across the parameter space that is under consideration. It should be low in the subset of the parameter space that belongs to H_0 and high in the subset H_1. The quantities $\frac{TP}{TP + FN}$ and $\frac{TN}{FP + TN}$ are called *sensitivity* and *specificity*, respectively. An optimal test procedure would give a result of 1 to both quantities.

3.4.3.2 Two-sample Location Tests

Assume that both series are independently Gaussian distributed, $N(\mu_x, \sigma^2)$ and $N(\mu_y, \sigma^2)$ respectively, with equal variances. Thus we interpret each series value x_i as an outcome of independent random variables that are Gaussian distributed with the respective parameters (y_i likewise). We want to test the hypothesis of whether the sample means are equal, i.e.,

$$H_0 : \mu_x = \mu_y \quad \text{versus} \quad H_1 : \mu_x \neq \mu_y,$$

Under the above assumptions, the test statistic

$$T(x_1, ..., x_n, y_1, ..., y_m) = \frac{\bar{x}_. - \bar{y}_.}{\sqrt{\dfrac{(n-1)s_x^2 + (m-1)s_y^2}{n+m-2}}\sqrt{\dfrac{1}{n} + \dfrac{1}{m}}} \tag{3-89}$$

(compare Sections 3.4.2.1 and 3.4.2.2) and is distributed according to a t-distribution with $m + n - 2$ degrees of freedom. Here, s_x^2, s_y^2 denote the variances of the samples. The test based on this assumption is called Student's t-test.

For a calculated value of the t-statistic, $\hat{t}$, we can now judge the probability of having an even more extreme value by calculating the probability $P(|T| > |\hat{t}|) = 2P(T > |\hat{t}|) = \int_{\hat{t}}^{\infty} f_{T,p}(z)\,dz$, where

$$f_{T,p}(z) = \frac{\Gamma\left(\dfrac{p+1}{2}\right)}{\Gamma\left(\dfrac{p}{2}\right)\Gamma\left(\dfrac{1}{2}\right)\sqrt{p}}\left(1 + \frac{z^2}{p}\right)^{-(p+1)/2} \tag{3-90}$$

is the probability distribution of the respective t-distribution with p degrees of freedom. Here, $\Gamma(z) = \int_0^{\infty} t^{z-1}e^{-t}dt$ is the gamma function.

For most practical applications, the assumptions of the Student's t-test are too strong, and data are not Gaussian distributed with equal variances. Furthermore, since the statistic is based on the mean sample values, the test is not robust against outliers. In cases where the underlying distribution is unknown and in order to define a more robust alternative, we introduce Wilcoxon's rank sum test. Here, instead of evaluating the signal values, only the ranks of the signals are taken into consideration. Consider the combined series $x_1, ..., x_n, y_1, ..., y_m$. Under the null hypothesis this series represents $m + n$ independent identically distributed random variables. The test statistic of the Wilcoxon test is

$$T = \sum_{i=1}^{n} R_i^{x,y}, \tag{3-91}$$

where $R_i^{x,y}$ is the rank of x_i in the combined series. The minimum and maximum values of T are $\dfrac{n(n+1)}{2}$ and $\dfrac{(m+n)(m+n+1)}{2} - \dfrac{n(n+1)}{2}$, respectively. The expected value under the null hypothesis is $E_{H_0}(T) = \dfrac{n(m+n+1)}{2}$ and the variance is $Var_{H_0}(T) = \dfrac{mn(m+n+1)}{12}$. Thus, under the null hypothesis, values for T will scatter around the expectation, and unusually low or high values will indicate that the null hypothesis should be rejected. For small sample sizes, P-values of the Wilcoxon test can be calculated exactly; for larger sample sizes, we have the following approximation:

$$
P\left(\frac{T - \dfrac{n\,(n+m+1)}{2}}{\sqrt{\dfrac{mn\,(m+n+1)}{12}}} \leq z\right) \to \Phi\,(z) \quad \text{for} \quad n, m \to \infty. \tag{3-92}
$$

The P-values of the Wilcoxon test statistic can be approximated by the standard normal distribution. This approximation has been shown to be accurate for $n + m > 25$.

In practice, some of the series values might be equal, e. g., because of the resolution of the measurements. Then, the Wilcoxon test statistic can be calculated using ties. Ties can be calculated by the average rank of all values that are equal. Ties have an effect on the variance of the statistic since this might be underestimated and should be corrected in the normal approximation. The correction is calculated by replacing the original variance by

$$
Var_{H_0,corr}\,(T) = Var_{H_0}(T) - \frac{mn}{12\,(m+n)(m+n-1)}\sum_{i=1}^{r}(b_i^3 - b_i). \tag{3-93}
$$

Here, r is the number of different values in the combined series of values and b_i is the frequency.

Example 3-26

Expression of a specific gene was measured in cortex brain tissue from control mice and Ts65Dn mice – a mouse model for Down syndrome (Kahlem et al. 2004). Repeated array hybridization experiments yield the following series of measurements for control mice
2434 2289 5599 2518 1123 1768 2304 2509 14820 2489 1349 1494
and for trisomic mice
3107 3365 4704 3667 2414 4268 3600 3084 3997 3673 2281 3166.
Due to two outlier values in the control series (*5599* and *14820*) the trisomic versus control ratio is close to one, *1.02*, and the P-value of Student's t-test is not significant, $p = 9.63\,e - 01$. For the Wilcoxon statistic, we get $T = \sum_{i=1}^{n} R_i^{x,y} = 14 + 16 +$ 22 + 18 + 8 + 21 + 17 + 13 + 20 + 19 + 5 + 15 = 188, $E_{H_0}(T) = 150$, $Var_{H_0}(T) = 300$, and for the Z-score we have $z = \dfrac{38}{\sqrt{300}} \sim 2.19$, which indicates that the result is significant. The exact P-value of the Wilcoxon test is $p = 2.84\,e - 02$.

3.4.4
Linear Models

The general linear model has the form $y = X\beta + \varepsilon$, with the assumptions $E(\varepsilon) = 0$ and $Cov(\varepsilon) = \sigma^2 I$. Here y is an n-dimensional vector of observations, β is a p-dimensional vector of unknown parameters, X is an nxp dimensional matrix of known constants (the design matrix), and ε is a vector of random errors. Since the errors are random, y is a random vector as well. Thus, the observations are separated into a deterministic part and a random part. The rationale behind linear models is that the deterministic part of the experimental observations is a linear function of the design matrix and the unknown parameter vector. Note that linearity is required in the parameters, not in the design matrix. For example, problems such as $x_{ij} = x_i^j$ for $i = 1, ..., n$ and $j = 0, ..., p - 1$ are also linear models. Here, for each coordinate i we have the equation $y_i = \beta_0 + \sum_{j=1}^{p-1} \beta_j x_i^j + \varepsilon_i$ and the model is called the polynomial regression model.

The goal of linear models is testing of complex statistical hypotheses and parameter estimation (cf. Chapter 9). In the following sections we introduce two classes of linear models: analysis of variance (ANOVA) and regression.

3.4.4.1   ANOVA

In Section 3.4.3.2 we introduced a particular test problem, the two-sample location test. The purpose of this test is to judge whether or not two samples are drawn from the same population by comparison of the centers of these samples. The null hypothesis was $H_0 : \mu_1 = \mu_2$ and the alternative hypothesis was $H_1 : \mu_1 \neq \mu_2$, where μ_i is the mean of the i-th sample. A generalization of the null hypothesis is targeted in this section. Assume n different samples where each sample measures the same interesting factor. Within each sample, i, the factor is measured n_i times. This results in a table of the following form

$$
\begin{array}{cccc}
x_{11} & x_{21} & \cdots & x_{n1} \\
\cdots & \cdot\cdot & \cdots & \cdots \\
x_{1n_1} & x_{2n_2} & \cdots & x_{nn_n}
\end{array}
$$

Here, the columns correspond to the different individual samples, and the rows correspond to the individual repetitions within each sample (the number of rows within each sample can vary!). The interesting question now is whether there is any difference in the sample means or, alternatively, whether the samples represent the same population. We thus test the null hypothesis $H_0 : \mu_1 = \mu_2 = ... = \mu_n$ against the alternative $H_1 : \mu_i \neq \mu_j$ for at least one pair, $i \neq j$. This question is targeted by the so-called one-way ANOVA. As in the case of Student's t-test, additional assumptions on the data samples are necessary:

1. The n samples are drawn independently from each other representing populations with mean values $\mu_1, \mu_2, ..., \mu_n$.
2. All population variances have the same variance σ^2 (homoscedasticity).
3. All populations are Gaussian distributed, $N(\mu_i, \sigma^2)$.

Although, the one-way ANOVA is based on the analysis of variance, it is essentially a test for location. This is exemplified in Fig. 3.10. The idea of ANOVA is the comparison of between- and within-group variability. If the variance between the groups is not different from the variance within the groups, we cannot reject the null hypotheses (Fig. 3.10, left). If the variances differ, we would reject the null hypothesis and conclude that the means are different (Fig. 3.10, right).

The calculation of the one-way ANOVA is based on the partition of the sample variance $\sum_{i=1}^{n}\sum_{j=1}^{n_i}(x_{ij} - \bar{x}_{..})^2$ into two parts that account for the between- and within-group variability, i. e.,

$$SS_{total} = \sum_{i=1}^{n}\sum_{j=1}^{n_i}(x_{ij} - \bar{x}_{..})^2 = \sum_{i=1}^{n}\sum_{j=1}^{n_i}(\bar{x}_{i.} - \bar{x}_{..})^2 + \sum_{i=1}^{n}\sum_{j=1}^{n_i}(x_{ij} - \bar{x}_{i.})^2 = SS_{between} + SS_{within}.$$

$$(3\text{-}94)$$

It can be shown that under H_0 the test statistic $T = \dfrac{SS_{between}}{SS_{within}}\dfrac{M-n}{n-1}$, where $M = \sum_{i=1}^{n} n_i$, is distributed according to an F distribution with degrees of freedom $v_1 = n - 1$ and $v_2 = M - n$, respectively. The multiplicative constant accounts for the degrees of freedom of the two terms. Thus, we can quantify experimental outcomes

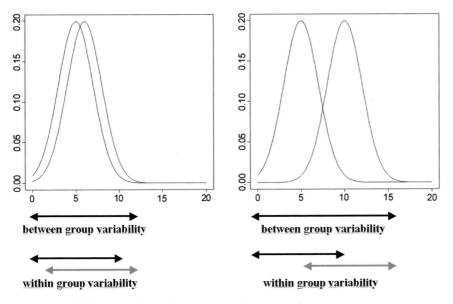

between group variability

within group variability

between group variability

within group variability

Fig. 3.10 ANOVA test for differential expression. Left: two normal distributions with means $\mu_1 = 5$, $\mu_2 = 6$ and equal variances. The variability between the groups is comparable with the variability within the groups. Right: two normal distributions with means $\mu_1 = 5$, $\mu_2 = 10$ and equal variances. The variability between the groups is higher than the variability within the groups.

according to this distribution. If μ_i are not equal, $SS_{between}$ will be high compared to SS_{within}, and, conversely, if all μ_i are equal, then the two factors will be similar and T will be small.

3.4.4.2 Multiple Linear Regression

Let $\mathbf{y}$ be an n-dimensional observation vector and let $\mathbf{x}_1, ..., \mathbf{x}_{p-1}$ be independent n-dimensional variables. We assume that the number of observations is greater than the number of variables, i.e., $n > p$. The standard model here is

$$\mathbf{y} = \mathbf{X}\boldsymbol{\beta} + \boldsymbol{\varepsilon} \tag{3-95}$$

or, in matrix notation,

$$\begin{pmatrix} y_1 \\ \vdots \\ y_n \end{pmatrix} = \begin{pmatrix} 1 & x_{11} & \cdots & x_{p-1,1} \\ \vdots & \vdots & \vdots & \vdots \\ 1 & x_{1n} & \cdots & x_{p-1,n} \end{pmatrix} \begin{pmatrix} \beta_0 \\ \vdots \\ \beta_{p-1} \end{pmatrix} + \begin{pmatrix} \varepsilon_1 \\ \vdots \\ \varepsilon_n \end{pmatrix}$$

where $E(\varepsilon) = 0$ and $Var(\varepsilon) = \sigma^2 I_n$. In our model we are interested in an optimal estimator for the unknown parameter vector $\boldsymbol{\beta}$. The least-squares method defines this optimization as a vector $\hat{\boldsymbol{\beta}}$ that minimizes the Euclidean norm of the residuals, i.e.,

$$\hat{\boldsymbol{\beta}} \in arg\ min\ \left\{ \boldsymbol{\beta};\ \|\mathbf{y} - \mathbf{X}\boldsymbol{\beta}\|^2 \right\}$$

Using partial derivatives, we can transform this problem into a linear equation (cf. Section 3.1.1) system by

$$\mathbf{X}^T\mathbf{X}\boldsymbol{\beta} = \mathbf{X}^T\mathbf{y} \tag{3-96}$$

and get the solution

$$\hat{\boldsymbol{\beta}} = (\mathbf{X}^T\mathbf{X})^{-1}\mathbf{X}^T\mathbf{y}. \tag{3-97}$$

The solution is called the least-squares estimator for $\boldsymbol{\beta}$. The least-squares estimator is unbiased, i.e., $E(\hat{\boldsymbol{\beta}}) = \boldsymbol{\beta}$ and the covariance matrix $\Sigma_{\hat{\beta}}$ of $\hat{\boldsymbol{\beta}}$ is equal to $\Sigma_{\hat{\beta}} = \sigma^2 (\mathbf{X}^T\mathbf{X})^{-1}$. Through the estimator for $\boldsymbol{\beta}$, we have an immediate estimator for the error vector ε using the residuals

$$\hat{\varepsilon} = \mathbf{y} - \mathbf{X}\hat{\boldsymbol{\beta}} = \mathbf{y} - \mathbf{X}(\mathbf{X}^T\mathbf{X})^{-1}\mathbf{X}^T\mathbf{y} = \mathbf{y} - \mathbf{P}\mathbf{y}. \tag{3-98}$$

Geometrically, $\mathbf{P}$ is the projection of $\mathbf{y}$ in the p-dimensional subspace of $\mathfrak{R}^n$ that is spanned by the column vectors of $\mathbf{X}$.

An unbiased estimator for the unknown standard deviation σ^2 is given by

$$\hat{s}^2 = \frac{\left\| y - X\hat{\beta} \right\|^2}{n - p}. \qquad (3\text{-}99)$$

Thus, $E(\hat{s}^2) = \sigma^2$.

Example 3-27: Simple linear regression

An important application is the simple linear regression of two samples $x_1, ..., x_n$ and $y_1, ..., y_n$. Here Eq. (3-95) reduces to $\begin{pmatrix} y_1 \\ \vdots \\ y_n \end{pmatrix} = \begin{pmatrix} 1 & x_1 \\ \vdots & \vdots \\ 1 & x_n \end{pmatrix} \begin{pmatrix} \beta_0 \\ \beta_1 \end{pmatrix} + \begin{pmatrix} \varepsilon_1 \\ \vdots \\ \varepsilon_n \end{pmatrix}$ and the parameters of interest are β_0, β_1, the intercept and the slope of the regression line. Minimizing the Euclidean norm of the residuals computes the line that minimizes the vertical distances of all points to the regression line. Solving according to Eq. (3-97) gives

$$X^T X = \begin{pmatrix} n & \sum_{i=1}^{n} x_i \\ \sum_{i=1}^{n} x_i & \sum_{i=1}^{n} x_i^2 \end{pmatrix} \quad \text{and} \quad X^T y = \begin{pmatrix} \sum_{i=1}^{n} y_i \\ \sum_{i=1}^{n} x_i y_i \end{pmatrix}, \quad \text{and thus we have}$$

$$\hat{\beta} = \frac{1}{n \sum_{i=1}^{n} x_i^2 - \left(\sum_{i=1}^{n} x_i \right)^2} \begin{pmatrix} \sum_{i=1}^{n} x_i^2 & -\sum_{i=1}^{n} x_i \\ -\sum_{i=1}^{n} x_i & n \end{pmatrix} \begin{pmatrix} \sum_{i=1}^{n} y_i \\ \sum_{i=1}^{n} x_i y_i \end{pmatrix} =$$

$$= \frac{1}{n \sum_{i=1}^{n} x_i^2 - \left(\sum_{i=1}^{n} x_i \right)^2} \begin{pmatrix} \sum_{i=1}^{n} x_i^2 \sum_{i=1}^{n} y_i - \sum_{i=1}^{n} x_i \sum_{i=1}^{n} x_i y \\ n \sum_{i=1}^{n} x_i y_i - \sum_{i=1}^{n} x_i \sum_{i=1}^{n} y_i \end{pmatrix}$$

The slope of the regression line is the correlation of the samples divided by the variance of the variables. It is called the empirical regression coefficient.

3.5
Graph and Network Theory

Many kinds of data arising in systems biology applications can be represented as graphs (metabolic pathways, signaling pathways, or gene regulatory networks). Other examples are taxonomies, e.g., of enzymes or organisms; protein interaction networks; DNA, RNA, or protein sequences; chemical structure graphs; or gene co-expression. In this section we give a brief overview of the formalization of graph problems (Section 3.5.1) and introduce specifically the framework of gene regulatory networks (Section 3.5.2) that are essential for the analysis of transcriptome data.

3.5.1
Introduction

A graph, $G(V, E)$, is composed of a set of vertices (or nodes), V, and a binary relation, E, on V. A visual representation of a graph consists of a set of vertices, whereby each pair is connected by an edge whenever the binary relation holds. If there is an edge from vertex i to j, we denote it with $(i, j) \in E$. If the edges have a specific direction, then $G(V, E)$ is called a directed graph; otherwise, it is called an undirected graph. A directed graph allows so-called self-loops, i.e., edges from a vertex to itself.

Computationally, a graph containing n vertices can be represented in two ways: as an adjacency list or as an adjacency matrix (Cormen et al. 2001). An adjacency list stores for each vertex i the list of vertices connected to vertex i. An adjacency matrix is an $n \times n$ binary matrix defined as $A = [a_{ij}]$, where

$$a_{ij} = \begin{cases} 1 & \text{there is an edge from vertex i to vertex j} \\ 0 & \text{else} \end{cases}$$. In the case of an undirected

graph, A is symmetric. Commonly, the adjacency-list presentation is preferred if the graph structure is sparse and there are not many edges compared to the number of vertex pairs, i.e., $|E| << |V|^2$, because then the amount of memory is far less than when using a matrix representation. A weighted graph consists of a graph, $G(V, E)$, together with a real-valued weight function $w : E \to \Re$. Weighted graphs are used, e.g., to represent gene regulatory networks (cf. Chapter 9).

The degree of a vertex i, $d(i)$, in an undirected graph is the number of edges connected to i, $d(i) = |\{(i, j) \in E; j = 1, ..., n\}|$. The degree of a vertex i in a directed graph is defined as the sum of its in-degree and out-degree. The in-degree of vertex i is defined as the number of edges entering vertex i, and the out-degree is the number of edges leaving it. The degree of a vertex i can be computed from the adjacency matrix as the sum of the i-th row (out-degree) and the i-th column sums (in-degree).

Topological properties of interaction graphs are commonly used in applications to characterize biological function (Jeong et al. 2001; Stelling et al. 2002; Przulj et al. 2004). For example, lethal mutations in protein-protein interactions are defined by highly connected parts of a protein interaction graph whose removal disrupts the graph structure.

A path of length l from a vertex v_0 to a vertex v_i in a graph $G(V, E)$ is a sequence of vertices $v_0, ..., v_l$ such that $(v_{i-1}, v_i) \in E$ for $i = 1, ..., l$. A path is a cycle if $l \geq 1$ and $v_0 = v_l$. A directed graph that contains no cycle is called a directed acyclic graph. The weight of a path in a weighted directed graph is the sum of the weights of all edges constituting the path. The shortest path from vertex v_0 to vertex v_l is the path with the minimal weight. If all weights are equal, then the shortest path is the path from vertex v_0 to vertex v_l with the minimal number of edges.

An important practical problem consists of the identification of substructures of a given graph. An undirected graph is connected when a path exists for each pair of vertices. If a subset of a graph is connected, it is called a connected component.

3.5.2
Regulatory Networks

Regulatory networks are graph-based models for a simplified view on gene regulation (cf. Chapter 8). Transcription factors are stimulated by upstream signaling cascades and bind on *cis*-regulatory positions of their target genes. Bound transcription
factors promote or inhibit RNA polymerase assembly and thus determine whether
and to what extent the target gene is expressed. The modeling of gene regulation via
genetic networks has been widely used in practice (for a review, see de Jong 2002).
We give here a brief introduction to some basic principles.

3.5.2.1 Linear Networks
The general model of gene regulation assumes that the change of gene expression of
gene x_i at time t can be described by the following equation

$$\frac{dx_i(t)}{dt} = r_i f\left(\sum_{j=1}^{n} w_{ij}\, x_j(t) + \sum_{k=1}^{m} v_{ik}\, u_k(t) + b_i\right) - \lambda_i\, x_i(t),\qquad (3\text{-}100)$$

where
f is the activation function,
$x_i(t)$ is the gene expression of gene i at time t,
r_i is the reaction rate of gene i,
w_{ij} is the weight that determines the influence of gene j on gene i,
$u_k(t)$ are the external inputs (e. g., a chemical compound) at time t,
v_{ik} is the weight that determines the influence of external compound k on gene i,
b_i is a lower base level of gene i, and
λ_i is the degradation constant for gene i.

The activation function, f, is a monotone function, assuming that the concentration of the gene is monotonically dependent on the concentrations of its regulators.
Often, these functions have sigmoid form, such as $f(z) = (1 + e^{-z})^{-1}$. If this function
is the identity, i. e., $f(z) = z$, then the network is linear. Additionally, common simplifications include constancy in the reaction rates, no external influence, and no degradation, so that Eq. (3-100) reduces to

$$\frac{dx_i(t)}{dt} = \sum_{j=1}^{n} w_{ij}\, x_j(t) + b_i.\qquad (3\text{-}101)$$

These models have been investigated, for example, by D'Haeseleer et al. (1999).
The interesting parameters are the weights w_{ij}, which are estimated by statistical
methods (cf. Section 3.4.4).

3.5.2.2 Boolean Networks
Boolean networks are qualitative descriptions of gene regulatory interactions. Gene
expression has two states: on (1) and off (0) (Kauffman 1993; Akutsu et al. 1999,

2000, Cormen et al. 2001). Let x be an n-dimensional binary vector representing the state of a system of n genes. Thus, the state space of the system consists of 2^n possible states. Each component, x_i, determines the expression of the i-th gene. With each gene i we associate a Boolean rule, b_i. Given the input variables for gene i at time t, this function determines whether the regulated element is active or inactive at time $t + 1$, i.e.,

$$x_i(t+1) = b_i(x(t)), 1 \le i \le n.$$ (3-102)

Equation (102) describes the dynamics of the Boolean network. The practical feasibility of Boolean networks is heavily dependent on the number of input variables, k, for each gene. The number of possible input states of k inputs is 2^k. For each such combination, a specific Boolean function must determine whether the next state would be on or off. Thus, there are 2^{2k} possible Boolean functions (or rules). This number rapidly increases with the connectivity. For $k = 2$ we have four possible input states and 16 possible rules; for $k = 3$, we have eight possible input states and 256 possible rules, etc.

In a Boolean network each state has a deterministic output state. A series of states is called a trajectory. If no difference occurs between the transitions of two states, i.e., output state equals input state, then the system is in a point attractor. Point attractors are analogous to steady states (cf. Section 3.2.3). If the system is in a cycle of states, then we have a dynamic attractor. The Boolean rules for one and two inputs as well as examples for the dynamic behavior of Boolean networks are given in Chapter 10, Section 10.3.3.

There have been algorithms to reconstruct or reverse engineer (cf. Chapter 9) Boolean networks from time series of gene expression data, i.e., from a limited number of states. Among the first was *REVEAL* developed by Liang et al. (1999). Additionally, properties of random Boolean networks were intensively investigated by Kauffman (1993), e.g., global dynamics, steady states, connectivity, and the specific types of Boolean functions.

3.5.2.3 Bayesian Networks

Bayesian networks are probabilistic descriptions of the regulatory network (Heckerman 1998; Friedman et al. 2000; Jensen 2001). A Bayesian network consists of (1) a directed acyclic graph, $G(V, E)$ (cf. Section 3.5.1), and (2) a set of probability distributions. The n vertices (n genes) correspond to random variables x_i, $1 \le i \le n$. For example, in regulatory networks the random variables describe the gene expression level of the respective gene. For each x_i, a conditional probability $p(x_i | L(x_i))$ is defined, where $L(x_i)$ denotes the parents of gene i, i.e., the set of genes that have a direct regulatory influence on gene i. Figure 3.11 gives an example of a Bayesian network consisting of five vertices.

The set of random variables is completely determined by the joint probability distribution. Under the Markov assumption, i.e., the assumption that each x_i is conditionally independent of its non-descendants given its parents, this joint probability distribution can be determined by the factorization via

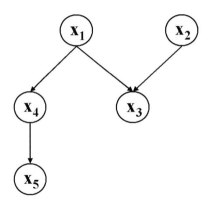

Fig. 3.11 Bayesian network. The network structure determines, e. g., the conditional independencies $i(x_1, x_2)$, $i(x_3, x_4 | x_1)$, $i(x_5, x_3 | x_4)$. The joint probability distribution has the form

$$p(x) = \prod_{i=1}^{n} p(x_i | L(x_i)).$$

(3-103)

Here, conditional independence of two random variables x_i and x_j given a random variable x_k means that $p(x_i, x_j | x_k) = p(x_i | x_k) p(x_j | x_k)$ or, equivalently, $p(x_i | x_j, x_k) = p(x_i | x_k)$. The conditional distributions given in Eq. (3-103) are typically assumed to be linearly normally distributed, i.e., $p(x_i | L(x_i)) \sim N\left(\sum_k a_k x_k, \sigma^2\right)$, where x_k is in the parent set of x_i. Thus, each x_i is assumed to be normally distributed around a mean value that is linearly dependent on the values of its parents.

The typical application of Bayesian networks is learning from observations. Given a training set T of independent realizations of the n random variables $x^1, ..., x^n$, the problem is to find a Bayesian network that best matches T. A common solution is to assign a score to each calculated network using the *a posteriori* probability of the calculated network, N, given the training data (cf. Section 3.4.1) by $\log P(N | T) = \log \frac{P(T|N) P(N)}{P(T)} = \log P(T|N) + \log P(N) + const$, where the constant is independent of the calculated network and $P(T|N) = \int P(T|N, \Theta) P(\Theta|N) d\Theta$ is the marginal likelihood that averages the probability of the data over all possible parameter assignments to the network. The choice of the *a priori* probabilities $P(N)$ and $P(\Theta|N)$ determines the exact score. The optimization of the *a posteriori* probability is beyond the scope of this introduction. For further reading, see e.g., Friedman et al. 2000; Jensen 2001; and Chickering 2002.

3.6
Stochastic Processes

The use of differential equations for describing biochemical processes makes certain assumptions that are not always justified. One assumption is that variables can attain continuous values. This is obviously a simplification, since the underlying biological objects, molecules, have a discrete nature. As long as molecule numbers are sufficiently large this is no problem, but if the involved molecule numbers are only on the order of dozens or hundreds, the discreteness should be taken into account. Another important assumption of differential equations is that they treat the described process as deterministic. Random fluctuations are normally not part of differential equations. Again, this presumption does not hold for very small systems.

A solution to both limitations is to use a stochastic simulation approach that explicitly calculates the change of the number of molecules of the participating species during the time course of a chemical reaction. If we consider the following set of chemical reactions

$$A \xrightarrow{k_1} B + C$$

$$C + D \xrightarrow{k_2} E$$

and denote the number of molecules of the different species X_i with $\#X_i$, then the state of the system is given by $S = (\#A, \#B, \#C, \#D, \#E)$. If the first reaction takes place, the system changes into a new state given by $S^* = (\#A-1, \#B+1, \#C+1, \#D, \#E)$. The probability that a certain reaction μ occurs within the next time interval dt is given by the following equation, where a_μ is given by the product of a mesoscopic rate constant and the current particle number, and $o(dt)$ describes other terms that can be neglected for small dt (Gillespie 1992).

$$P(S^*, t + dt \,|\, S, t) = a_\mu dt + o(dt). \tag{3-104}$$

One approach to proceed within this stochastic framework is to develop a so-called master equation. For each possible state $(\#A, \#B, \#C, \#D, \#E)$ a probability variable is created. Using Eq. (3-104) and the definition of the a_μ's, a system of coupled differential equations can be developed that describes the reaction system. The variables of this system represent transition probabilities, and the equation system itself is called a master equation. However, because each state requires a separate variable, the system becomes quickly intractable as the number of chemical species and the number of each kind of molecule grows.

It was therefore a major breakthrough when Gillespie developed exact stochastic simulation algorithms (Gillespie 1977). These algorithms are exact in the sense that they are equivalent to the results of the master equation, but instead of solving the probabilities for all trajectories simultaneously, the simulation method calculates single trajectories. Calculating many individual trajectories and studying the statistics of these trajectories can provide the same insights as obtained with the master equation. Gillespie developed two exact stochastic simulation algorithms, the direct method and the first reaction method. For this introductory text, we will discuss in detail only the direct method.

3.6.1
Gillespie's Direct Method

At a given moment in time, the system is in a certain state S and the algorithm computes which reaction happens next and how long it takes until it occurs. Once this is known, there is enough information to update the state and current time. Both questions are answered by picking random numbers from appropriate probability distributions. It can be shown (Gillespie 1977) that in a system with n reactions, the probability that the next reaction is μ and that it occurs at time τ is given by

$$P(\mu, \tau)\, dt = a_\mu\, e^{-\tau \sum_{i=1}^{n} a_i}\, d\tau . \qquad (3\text{-}105)$$

Integrating this equation over all possible reaction times gives us the probability distribution for the reactions (Eq. (3-106)), and integration over all n possible reactions yields the probability distribution for the waiting times (Eq. (3-107)).

$$P(reaction = \mu) = \frac{a_\mu}{\sum\limits_{i=1}^{n} a_i} \qquad (3\text{-}106)$$

$$P(\tau)\, d\tau = \sum_{i=1}^{n} a_i \cdot e^{-\tau \sum_{i=1}^{n} a_i}\, d\tau . \qquad (3\text{-}107)$$

The pseudocode for the direct method can now be written as follows:

1. Initialize (define mesoscopic rate constants, set initial numbers of molecules, set time to zero).
2. Calculate a_μ's (given by the product of mesoscopic rate constants and molecule number).
3. Choose next reaction μ according to Eq. (3-106), i.e., proportional to normalized reaction rate.
4. Obtain waiting time τ by picking a random number from an exponential distribution with parameter $\sum_i a_i$ according to Eq. (3-107).
5. Update the number of molecules (state) according to the stoichiometry of reaction μ. Advance time by τ.
6. Go to step 2.

3.6.2
Other Algorithms

The direct method described above requires the generation of two random numbers per iteration, and the computation time is proportional to the number of possible reactions. Gillespie's other algorithm, the first reaction method, works slightly differently in that it generates a putative waiting time for each possible reaction (again chosen from an exponential distribution). The reaction to occur is the one with the smallest waiting time. The algorithm requires n random numbers per iteration (n = number of reactions) and the computation time is again proportional to the number of reactions. Gibson and Bruck (2000) succeeded in considerably improving the efficiency of the first reaction method. Their elegant algorithm, called the next reaction method, uses only a single random number per iteration, and the computation time is proportional to the logarithm of the number of reactions. This makes the stochastic approach amenable for much larger systems.

However, notwithstanding these improvements, stochastic simulations are computationally very demanding, especially if the reaction system of interest contains a mixture of participating species with large and small molecule numbers. In this case the simulation will spend most of its time performing reactions of the species with large molecule numbers (large a_μ's), although for these species a stochastic treatment is not really necessary. Even worse, the high reaction rates of those species lead to very short time intervals, τ, between individual reactions, so that the simulated reaction time advances very slowly. Gillespie has formulated another approximate method that achieves significant speed improvements with only moderate losses in accuracy (Gillespie 2001). This τ-leap method can in principle also be used in cases of mixed reaction systems, but it loses efficiency because the length of the appropriate time step is determined by the species with the smallest number of molecules and is on the order of waiting times for exact algorithms. However, a recent software development using the τ-leap method for the fast reactions of a mixed system and the next reaction method for the slow reactions provides a solution to these problems (Puchalka and Kierzek 2004). The use of this software package, STOCKS, is described in Chapter 14, Section 14.1.8.

3.6.3
Stochastic and Macroscopic Rate Constants

The mesoscopic rate constants used for stochastic simulations and the macroscopic rate constants used for deterministic modeling are related but not identical. Macroscopic rate constants depend on concentrations, while the stochastic constants depend on the number of molecules. A dimension analysis shows how the classical rate constants for reactions of the first and second orders have to be transformed to be suitable for stochastic simulations.

3.6.3.1 First-order Reaction
Imagine a first-order decay of a substance X. The reaction rate, v, is given by $v = -k \cdot X$, with k being the rate constant. The dimensions for the deterministic description are $\dfrac{mol}{L \cdot s} = \dfrac{1}{s} \cdot \dfrac{mol}{L}$ and for the stochastic framework $\dfrac{molecules}{s} = \dfrac{1}{s} \cdot molecules$. The dimension of the rate constant is in both cases $1/s$, and thus no conversion is necessary.

3.6.3.2 Second-order Reaction

This time we imagine a substance that is produced by the reaction of one molecule of X and one molecule of Y. The reaction rate is given by $v = k \cdot X \cdot Y$. The dimensions for the deterministic equation are $\dfrac{mol}{L \cdot s} = \dfrac{L}{s \cdot mol} \cdot \dfrac{mol^2}{L^2}$ and for the stochastic case $\dfrac{molecules}{s} = \dfrac{1}{s \cdot molecules} \cdot molecules^2$. To convert the macroscopic rate constant from $\dfrac{L}{s \cdot mol}$ into $\dfrac{1}{s \cdot molecules}$, the numerical value has to be divided by the reaction volume and the Avogadro constant (to convert moles into molecules). Thus, a classical second-order rate constant of $1\ \mathrm{M}^{-1}\ \mathrm{s}^{-1}$, which has been measured, e.g., in a reaction volume of 10^{-15} L, converts to a mesoscopic rate constant of $1.66 \times 10^{-9}\ \mathrm{molecule}^{-1}\ \mathrm{s}^{-1}$.

References

AKUTSU, T., MIYANO, S. and KUHARA, S. Identification of genetic networks from a small number of gene expression patterns under the Boolean network model (1999) In: R. B. Altman et al., eds. Proceedings of the Pacific Symposium on Biocomputing ,99. Singapore, pp 17–28.

AKUTSU, T., MIYANO, S. and KUHARA, S. Inferring qualitative relations in genetic networks and metabolic pathways (2000) Bioinformatics 16, 727–734.

BRONSTEIN, I.N. and SEMENDJAJEW, K.A. Taschenbuch der Mathematik (1987) 23rd edition Edition Nauka, Moscow.

CHICKERING, D.M. Learning equivalence classes of Bayesian network structures (2002) J. Machine Learning Res. 2, 445–498.

CORMEN, T.H., LEISERSON, C.E., RIVEST, R.L. and STEIN, C. Introduction to algorithms (2001) 2nd Edition Edition MIT Press, Cambridge, Mass.

DE JONG, H. Modeling and simulation of genetic regulatory systems: a literature review (2002) J. Comput. Biol. 9, 67–103.

D'HAESELEER, P., WEN, X., FUHRMAN, S., and SOMOGYI, R. (1999) Linear modeling of mRNA expression levels during CNS development and injury. In: Pacific Symposium on Biocomputing 1999, eds. Altman, R.B. et al., pp. 41–52.

FRIEDMAN, N., LINIAL, M., NACHMAN, I. and PE'ER, D. Using Bayesian networks to analyze expression data (2000) J. Comput. Biol.7, 601–620.

GIBSON, M.A. and BRUCK, J. Efficient exact stochastic simulation of chemical systems with many species and many channels (2000) J. Phys. Chem. 104, 1876–1889.

GILLESPIE, D.T. Exact stochastic simulation of coupled chemical reactions (1977) J. Phys. Chem. 81, 2340–2361.

GILLESPIE, D.T. A rigorous derivation of the chemical master equation (1992) Physica A 188, 404–425.

GILLESPIE, D.T. Approximate accelerated stochastic simulation of chemically reacting systems (2001) J. Chem. Phys. 115, 1716–1733.

HECKERMAN, D. A tutorial on learning with Bayesian networks (1998) In: M. I. Jordan, ed. Learning in graphical models, Kluwer, Dordrecht, the Netherlands

JENSEN, F.V. Bayesian networks and decision graphs (2001) Springer, New York.

JEONG, H., MASON, S.P., BARABASI, A.L. and OLTVAI, Z.N. Lethality and centrality in protein networks (2001) Nature 411, 41–42.

KAHLEM, P., SULTAN, M., HERWIG, R., STEINFATH, M., BALZEREIT, D., EPPENS, B., SARAN, N.G., PLETCHER, M.T., SOUTH, S.T., STETTEN, G., LEHRACH, H., REEVES, R.H. and YASPO, M.L. Transcript level alterations reflect gene dosage effects across multiple tissues in a mouse model of down syndrome (2004) Genome Res. 14, 1258–67.

KAUFFMAN, S.A. The origins of order: Self-organization and selection in evolution (1993) Oxford University Press, New York.

LIANG, S., FUHRMAN, S. and SOMOGYI, R. REVEAL, a general reverse engineering algorithm for inference of genetic network architecture' (1999) in R. B. Altman et al., ed. Proceedings of the Pacific Symposium on Biocomputing '98. Singapore, pp 18–28.

PRZULJ, N., WIGLE, D.A. and JURISICA, I. Functional topology in a network of protein interactions (2004) Bioinformatics *20*, 340–348.

PUCHALKA, J. and KIERZEK, A.M. 'Bridging the gap between stochastic and deterministic regimes in the kinetic simulations of the biochemical reaction networks' (2004) Biophysical Journal *86*, 1357–1372.

STELLING, J., KLAMT, S., BETTENBROCK, K., SCHUSTER, S. and GILLES, E.D. Metabolic network structure determines key aspects of functionality and regulation (2002) Nature *420* 190–193.

4
Experimental Techniques in a Nutshell

Introduction

In this chapter we will give a brief description of the experimental techniques used in modern molecular biology. In the same way that Chapter 2 is only an introduction to biology, this chapter is only an introduction to the large arsenal of experimental techniques that are used and is not meant to be a comprehensive overview. However, we felt that for readers without an experimental background it might be interesting and helpful to get a basic idea of the techniques that are used to actually acquire the immense biological knowledge that is nowadays available. A basic knowledge of the techniques is also indispensable for understanding experimental scientific publications or for simply discussing experiments with colleagues.

In the first part of this chapter, elementary techniques will be explained that have already existed for many years but nevertheless still form the basic workhorses of every day lab work. In the second part, techniques that have been developed more recently are discussed. Some of these techniques are of special interest because they are able to generate large quantities of data (high-throughput techniques) that can be used for quantitative modeling in systems biology.

4.1
Elementary Techniques

4.1.1
Restriction Enzymes and Gel Electrophoresis

We have seen in Chapter 2 that the genes that code for the proteins of a cell are all located on very long pieces of DNA, the chromosomes. To isolate individual genes, it is therefore necessary to break up the DNA and isolate the fragment of interest. However, until the early 1970s this was a very difficult task. DNA consists of only four different building blocks – the nucleotides adenine, thymine, guanine, and cytosine – making it a very homogeneous and monotonous molecule. In principle the DNA can be broken into smaller pieces by mechanical shear stress. This can be achieved

Systems Biology in Practice. Concepts, Implementation and Application.
E. Klipp, R. Herwig, A. Kowald, C. Wierling, H. Lehrach
Copyright © 2005 WILEY-VCH Verlag GmbH & Co. KGaA, Weinheim
ISBN: 3-527-31078-9

by ultrasound treatment or intensive vortexing. However, this results in random fragments, which are not useful for further processing.

This situation began to change when the first restriction endonucleases were isolated from bacteria at the end of the 1960s. These enzymes recognize specific short sequences of DNA and cut the molecule only at these positions. At first sight it seems surprising that organisms contain enzymes that cut DNA into small pieces. But it turns out that restriction enzymes are part of a bacterial defense system against bacteriophages (prokaryote-specific viruses). This system consists of two components. The first part, the restriction enzymes, cuts double-stranded DNA at their recognition sequences. These sequences are typically between four and eight base pairs long. The second component, the methylases, modifies DNA molecules at specific sequences by adding methyl groups to the nucleotides of the target sequence. In order to work, a pair consisting of a methylase and a restriction enzyme has to recognize the same sequence stretch. The DNA of the bacterium is methylated by the methylase, and this protects it against the nuclease activity of the restriction enzyme. However, the DNA of a phage that enters the cell is not methylated and hence is degraded by the restriction enzyme.

Over the years several hundred different restriction enzymes have been isolated from different bacterial strains with many different recognition sequences. Restriction enzymes can cut the double helix in three different ways, as depicted by Fig. 4.1. Some produce blunt ends, but others cut the DNA in a staggered way, resulting in short stretches (here 4 bp) of single-stranded DNA. Depending on the way the enzyme cuts the DNA, the single-stranded overhang can have either a 5′ end (if cut by Bam HI) or a 3′ end (if cut by Kpn I). Because these overhanging single strands can base pair with other complementary single strands, they are also called sticky ends.

The following table provides an overview of some of the available restriction enzymes, the organism from which they have been isolated, and their recognition sequence. Restriction enzymes are normally named after the organism and strain in which they were discovered. Eco RI, for instance, originates from *Escherichia coli* strain RY13. The final Roman numeral indicates the order in which the enzymes were isolated from single bacteria (i. e., Eco RI vs. Eco RV). If different enzymes recognize the same sequence but produce different cuts, they are called isoschizomers.

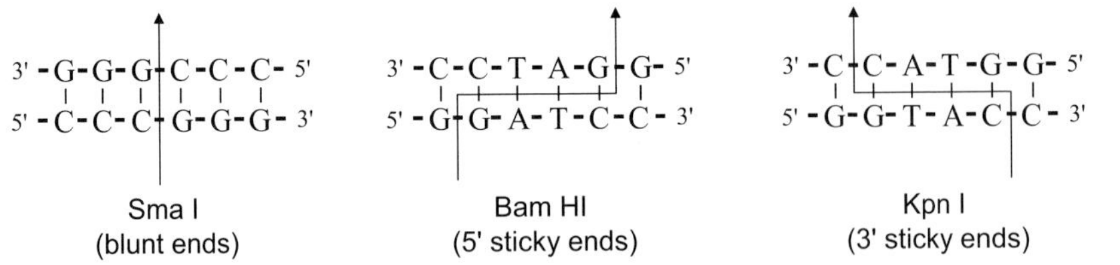

```
3'-G-G-G┼C-C-C- 5'      3'-C-C-T-A-G┼G- 5'      3'-C┼C-A-T-G-G- 5'
    | | | | | |               | | | | |  |           | | | | |  |
5'-C-C-C┼G-G-G- 3'      5'-G┼G-A-T-C-C- 3'      5'-G-G-T-A-C┼C- 3'

     Sma I                    Bam HI                   Kpn I
  (blunt ends)            (5' sticky ends)         (3' sticky ends)
```

Fig. 4.1 Restriction enzymes recognize short stretches of DNA that often have a palindromic structure. The enzyme then cuts the DNA in one of three ways, producing either blunt ends or sticky ends. This behavior is shown here for the enzymes Sma I, Bam HI, and Kpn I. The arrow indicates where the enzymes cut the double helix.

For instance, the enzymes Sma I and Xma I in the table are isoschizomers. Finally, the "N" in the recognition sequence for Sau96 I indicates that it does not matter which nucleotide is at this position; the enzyme will accept all of them.

Name	Organism	Recognition sequence
Alu I	*Arthrobacter luteus*	5′ A G ↑ C T 3′
Bam HI	*Bacillus amyloliquefaciens*	5′ G ↑ G A T C C 3′
Bgl II	*Bacillus globigii*	5′ A ↑ G A T C T 3′
Eco RI	*Escherichia coli*	5′ G ↑ A A T T C 3′
Eco RV	*Escherichia coli*	5′ G A T ↑ A T C 3′
Hind III	*Haemophilus influenzae*	5′ A ↑ A G C T T 3′
Kpn I	*Klebsiella pneumonia*	5′ G G T A C ↑ C 3′
Pme I	*Pseudomonas mendocina*	5′ G T T T ↑ A A A C 3′
Sau96 I	*Staphylococcus aureus*	5′ G ↑ G N C C 3′
Sma I	*Serratia marcescens*	5′ C C C ↑ G G G 3′
Xma I	*Xanthomonas malvacearum*	5′ C ↑ C C G G G 3′

Why are restriction enzymes so useful? They generate reproducibly specific fragments from large DNA molecules. This is a very important advantage over the random fragments that can be generated by shear forces. If the restriction fragments that result from an enzymatic digestion are separated according to size, they form a specific pattern that represents a fingerprint of the digested DNA. Changes in this fingerprint indicate that the number or position of the recognition sites of the used restriction enzyme has changed. Restriction enzyme patterns can therefore be used to characterize mutational changes or to compare orthologous genes from different organisms.

The size separation of digested DNA is also a prerequisite to isolate and clone specific fragments. If the sequence of the DNA is known, the number and size of the restriction fragments for a given restriction enzyme can be predicted. By choosing the right enzyme from the large number of available restriction enzymes, it is often possible to produce a fragment that contains the gene, or region of DNA, of interest. This fragment can then be separated from the others and cloned into a vector (see Section 4.1.2) for further investigation.

Electrophoresis is one of the most convenient and most often used methods of molecular genetics to separate molecules that differ in size or charge. Many different forms of electrophoresis exist, but they all work by applying an electrical field to the charged molecules. Depending on the type of charge, the molecules will move towards one of the two electrodes. Since each nucleotide of DNA (or RNA) carries a negative charge, nucleic acids move from the anode to the cathode. The separation is carried out in a gel matrix to prevent convection currents and to present a barrier to the moving molecules, which causes a sieving effect. The size, charge, and shape of the molecules decide how fast they move through the gel. Generally it holds that the smaller the molecule, the faster it moves. The pore size of the gel controls the size range of the DNA fragments that can be separated successfully. For a typical restriction fragment, i.e., between 0.5 kb and 20 kb, agarose gels are used. Agarose is a linear polysaccharide that is extracted from seaweed. Agarose gels are not suited for DNA fragments smaller than 500 bp. In this case, polyacrylamide gels that have smaller pores are used. For such small molecules size differences of a single base pair can be detected. Another problem are very large DNA molecules that are completely retarded by the gel matrix. Those fragments are not separated by the usual type of electrophoresis. In this case, a special type of electrophoresis, the so-called pulse field electrophoresis, can be used, which allows the separation of DNA molecules of up to 10^7 bp. This technique varies the direction of the electric field periodically, so that the molecules follow a zigzag path through the gel. Very long DNA fragments move head-on through the gel, which results in a velocity that is independent of size. Because of the oscillating field, the molecules have to re-orientate themselves. This is easier for the smaller fragments, and the larger ones therefore lag behind. A typical application of this technique is the separation of whole chromosomes of microorganisms (mammalian chromosomes are too large even for this technique).

Whatever type of electrophoresis or gel is used, the DNA is invisible unless it is specially labeled or stained. A commonly used dye for staining is ethidium bromide, which intercalates between DNA bases. In the intercalated state, ethidium exposed to UV light fluoresces a bright orange. Figure 4.2 sketches the different processing steps from the DNA to the size-separated restriction fragments on an agarose gel. On the gel (Fig. 4.2, right) different lanes can be seen, where different DNA probes are separated in parallel. The concentrated solution of DNA fragments is filled in the pockets at the top of the gel, and the fragments migrate during electrophoresis to the bottom. The smallest fragments move fastest and appear at the bottom of the gel. The lanes on the left and right sides contain fragments of known length that serve as size markers.

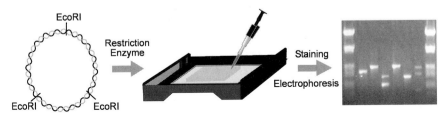

Fig. 4.2 Agarose gel electrophoresis of DNA restriction fragments. A plasmid containing several recognition sites for a restriction enzyme (here, Eco RI) is digested with the enzyme and the resulting fragments are placed on an agarose gel (middle). An applied electrical field moves the charged molecules through the gel (here, from top to bottom) and separates them according to size. After staining, the individual fragments appear under UV light as bright bands (right). (Courtesy of Dr. P. Weingarten, Protagen AG.)

4.1.2
Cloning Vectors and DNA Libraries

In the last section we discussed how restriction enzymes generate DNA fragments by cutting the DNA at short, specific recognition sites. However, this is not the end of the cloning procedure. In this section we will see how the generated fragments can be used to generate billions of identical copies. But first we should clarify what is meant by cloning, because, unfortunately, the terms clone and cloning have multiple meanings. To create a clone of an organism means to generate a copy of an organism such that both individuals are genetically identical. The first and most famous example of such a clone generated from another adult organism is the sheep Dolly (Wilmut et al. 1997). Another example is of course monozygotic twins, which are natural clones. Surprisingly, rough calculations show that currently approximately 60 million human clones exist (Colletto et al. 2003)! However, most often the term cloning is used in a different context, meaning to create an identical copy of a DNA molecule or to isolate a specific DNA fragment from the total DNA content of a cell. In the remainder of this chapter and the whole book, it is this second meaning that we are referring to.

For the actual cloning (amplification) step, a restriction fragment has to be inserted into a self-replicating genetic element. This can be, for instance, a virus or a plasmid. Plasmids are small circular rings of DNA that occur naturally in many bacteria. They often carry a few genes for resistance to antibiotics or to enable the degradation of unusual carbon sources and are normally only a few thousand base pairs long (Fig. 4.3). Genetic elements that are used in the laboratory to amplify DNA fragments of interest are called cloning vectors and the amplified DNA is said to be cloned. In the following we will concentrate on the use of plasmids as vectors. The actual insertion process requires that the DNA to be cloned and the vector be cut with the same restriction enzyme and that the vector has only one recognition site for this enzyme. This creates a linearized plasmid that has the same type of sticky ends as the DNA to be cloned. If the linearized vector and the digested DNA are now mixed at the right concentration and temperature, the complementary sticky ends base pair and form a new recombinant DNA molecule. Initially, the resulting molecule is held together only by hydrogen bonds. This is made permanent by adding the enzyme DNA ligase that forms covalent bonds between the phosphodiester backbones of the DNA molecules. This procedure enables the combination of DNA from arbitrary sources. It is in principle no problem to clone mammalian or plant DNA into bacterial vectors, because the genetic code is universal (with a few exceptions in mitochondrial DNA).

Finally, the vector is introduced into bacterial cells, which are then grown in culture. Every time the bacteria double (approximately every 30 min), the recombinant plasmids also double. Each milliliter of the growth medium can eventually contain up to 10^7 bacteria, an immense amplification! The actual process of introducing the vector into the bacteria is called transformation. For this end the cells are specially treated so that they are temporarily permeable for the DNA molecules.

But loss occurs at all steps of this genetic engineering. Not all vector molecules will have received an insert, because it is possible that the sticky ends of some vectors

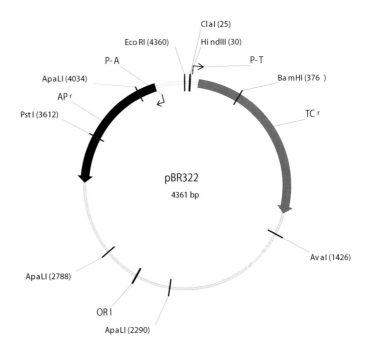

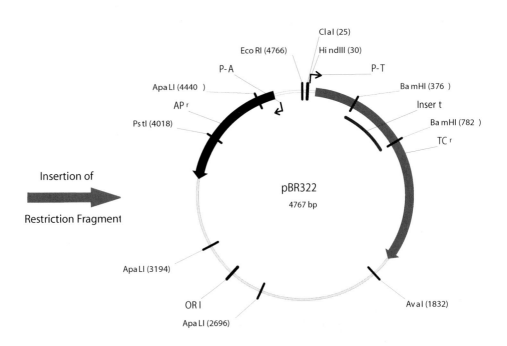

self-ligate without insert. Furthermore, not all bacteria used in the transformation step will have received a vector molecule. It can therefore be that there is only a small proportion of cells that contain a vector with insert in the growing cell population. There are different strategies to cope with this problem, but normally one tries to make use of genes in the original vector that can be used as selection markers. Figure 4.3 shows pBR322, a typical cloning vector. Apart from a DNA sequence that enables the cell machinery to replicate the plasmid (ori), it also contains two genes for resistance against the antibiotics ampicillin and tetracycline. If the DNA fragment is cloned into a restriction site that lies within one of the resistance genes, e.g., the Bam HI site, simple selection steps can be used to end up with cells that contain the desired construct. For this purpose the bacteria are grown in a medium that contains ampicillin so that only cells that carry the plasmid can survive. The next step is more complicated since we are interested in all those bacteria that contain a vector with a nonfunctional tetracycline gene (caused by an insert). The cells are plated in high dilution on the surface of an agar plate, where each individual cell forms a colony. After the colonies become visible, some bacteria of each colony are copied onto a second agar plate by a stamping technique (which preserves the spatial arrangement of colonies). This second plate contains tetracycline; therefore, only those cells with an intact resistance gene can grow. By comparing the colony pattern of the two plates, it is now possible to identify those colonies that exist on the first plate but not on the second. These are the colonies that we are interested in.

For many years plasmid vectors have been used very successfully. However, there is an upper size limit for the DNA one can clone into such a vector. Above 10 kb, the cloning efficiency declines so much that other vectors are required. The following table lists some of the types of vectors currently used. Lambda is a linear bacteriophage of approximately 48 kb, and up to 20 kb of the original phage DNA can be replaced by foreign DNA. Cosmids are artificial constructs that combine some features of the phage lambda and of the classical plasmids. The advantage is that fragments up to 45 kb can be cloned. For really large fragments of up to one million base pairs, yeast artificial chromosomes (YACs) have been developed (Burke et al. 1987), which are now gradually being replaced by bacterial artificial chromosomes (BACs) (Shizuya et al. 1992). BACs are based on the naturally occurring F-plasmid, which itself is around 100 kb in length. While the copy number per cell of most smaller plasmids is rather large, the F-plasmid and the derived BACs are maintained at only one to two copies per cell. This reduces the risk of unwanted recombination events between different copies and contributes to the stability of such large inserts.

◀ **Fig. 4.3** pBR322 is a circular plasmid of 4.3 kb that is often used as cloning vector. The diagram on the top shows several important genetic elements of the plasmid. *ORI* marks a region of DNA that controls the replication of the plasmid; it is the origin of replication. The boxes represent genes that confer resistance to the plasmid for the antibiotics ampicillin (APr) and tetracycline (TCr). P-A and P-R are the promoters of the resistance genes, and the lines and text mark recognition sites for the corresponding restriction enzyme. The lower part shows pBR322 after a restriction fragment has been inserted into the Bam HI restriction site.

Vector	Maximum insert size	Required number of clones in library of *Arabidopsis thaliana (115.4 Mb)*
Plasmid	10 kb	53,141
Phage lambda	20 kb	26,570
Cosmid	45 kb	11,800
BAC	Approx. 1 Mb	530
YAC	Approx. 1 Mb	530

Because the average fragment size of restriction enzymes is much smaller than 1 Mb, the enzyme reaction is allowed to proceed for only a very short time. This time is not long enough to cut all recognition sites, and therefore the resulting fragments are much longer. This technique is called a partial digest.

So far we have discussed the situation when we want to clone a specific fragment after a restriction digest. The DNA is separated on an agarose gel, and the desired fragment is excised from the gel and cloned into an appropriate vector. However, often the situation is different insofar as we do not know in advance the fragment that contains our gene of interest. In this case we can construct a so-called DNA library by simply cloning all fragments that result from a digest into vectors. Such a library is maintained in a population of bacteria that now contain vectors with many different inserts. Bacteria with different inserts are either kept together or separated, so that the library consists of thousands of clones (each kept in a separate plastic tube), each carrying a specific fragment. This is, for instance, important for the construction of DNA chips (cf. Section 4.2.2). This strategy is also known as shotgun cloning. To be sure that the library does contain the fragment of interest, it has to cover the complete genome of the organism we are interested in. Because by chance some fragments can occur more frequently than others in the library, more clones than expected are needed. The number of clones required to have a probability of P that a particular fragment is represented by a clone in the library depends on the insert size, I, and the genome size, GS, and is given by the following equation (Clarke and Carbon 1976). The number of required clones in the above table has been calculated for a probability of 99%.

$$N = \frac{\ln(1 - P)}{\ln\left(1 - \dfrac{I}{GS}\right)} \tag{4-1}$$

There are two basic types of DNA libraries that are extensively used in molecular genetics. The first type is the genomic DNA library, which is exactly what we have described so far. This type of library is directly created from the genetic material of an organism. Restriction enzymes cut DNA regardless of the start and end points of genes, and hence there is no guarantee that the gene of interest completely fits on a single clone. Furthermore, in Chapter 2 we have seen that the genome of most higher organisms contains large amounts of junk DNA. These sequences also end up in the genomic DNA library and increase the number of required clones.

A different type of library, the cDNA library, circumvents these problems. This technique does not use DNA as source material, but starts from the mRNA pool of the cells or tissue of interest. The trick is that the mRNA molecules are a copy of exactly those parts of the genome that are the most interesting. They represent the coding regions of the genes and contain neither introns nor inter-gene junk DNA. Using the enzyme reverse transcriptase that exists in some viruses, mRNA can be converted into cDNA. The resulting DNA is called complementary DNA (cDNA) because it is complementary to the mRNA. cDNA libraries differ from genomic libraries in several important points: (1) they contain only coding regions; (2) they are tissue-specific since they represent a snapshot of the current gene expression pattern; and (3) because they are an image of the expression pattern, the frequency of specific clones in the library is an indicator of the expression level of the corresponding gene. cDNA libraries have many different applications. By sequencing cDNA libraries, it is possible to experimentally determine the intron-exon boundaries of eukaryotic genes. Constructing cDNA libraries from different tissues helps us to understand which genes are expressed in which parts of the body. A derivative of the cDNA library is the expression library. This type of library is constructed in such a way that it contains a strong promoter in front of the cloned cDNAs. This makes it possible not only to amplify the DNA of interest but also to synthesize the protein that is encoded by this DNA insert. This technique is important especially for proteins that are normally expressed only in very small amounts

4.1.3
1D and 2D Protein Gels

The basic principle of electrophoresis works for all charged molecules. This means not only nucleic acids but also other kinds of cellular macromolecules, such as proteins, can be separated by electrophoresis. But the distribution of charges in a typical protein is quite different from the distribution in nucleic acids. DNA molecules carry a negative charge that is proportional to the length of the DNA, since the overall charge is controlled by the phosphodiester backbone. The net charge of proteins, however, varies from protein to protein since it depends on the amount and type of charged amino acids that are incorporated into the polypeptide chain. If proteins are separated in this native form, their velocity is controlled by a difficult-to-predict function of charge, size, and shape.

It was a major improvement when Shapiro et al. (1967) introduced the strong detergent sodium dodecyl sulfate (SDS) to protein electrophoresis in the 1960s. SDS has a hydrophilic sulfate group and a hydrophobic part that binds to the hydrophobic backbone of polypeptides. This has important consequences: (1) the negative charge of the protein/detergent complex is now proportional to the protein size because the number of SDS molecules that bind to a protein is proportional to the number of its amino acids, (2) all proteins denature and adopt a linear conformation, and (3) even very hydrophobic, normally insoluble proteins can be separated by gel electrophoresis. Under these conditions the separation of proteins is reduced to a function of their size, as in the case of nucleic acids. Small proteins travel quickly, while large proteins are more strongly retained by the gel matrix. Images of protein gels are normally presented such that the large polypeptides are at the top and smaller ones at the bottom.

For proteins, a different gel matrix is used than for nucleic acids. Acrylamide monomers are polymerized to give a polyacrylamide gel. During the polymerization step, the degree of cross-linking and thus the pore size of the network can be controlled to be optimal for the size range of interest. Proteins often contain sulfide bridges that connect either different parts of the same polypeptide or different peptide chains of a multi-subunit protein complex. Therefore, in addition to SDS, a reducing substance such as mercaptoethanol is often added, which reduces the sulfide bridges to sulfhydryl groups. This linearizes single peptides and separates multi-subunit complexes into the individual proteins. Over the years, SDS polyacrylamide gel electrophoresis (SDS-PAGE) has become an easy-to-use standard technique for separating proteins by size. As in the case of DNA, the gel has to be stained to make the protein bands visible. The most frequently used dye is Coomassie blue, which can detect quantities of proteins down to 100 ng. A more sensitive technique is so-called silver staining, which can detect 5–10 ng of protein. However, Coomassie blue staining is much simpler to perform and is therefore often the technique of choice. Figure 4.4 top sketches the basic steps required for SDS-PAGE. In this example, the outermost lanes contain protein size markers (large proteins at the top, small ones at the bottom), and the middle lanes contain different samples of interest.

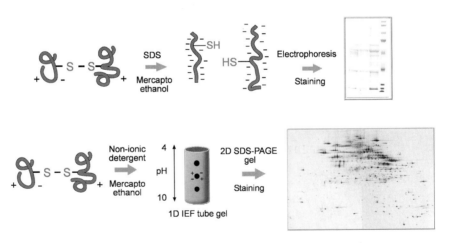

Fig. 4.4 (Top) SDS-PAGE: Native proteins are treated with the negatively charged detergent SDS and the reducing agent mercaptoethanol to break up disulfide bridges and unfold the protein. After this treatment even extremely hydrophobic proteins can be separated on a polyacrylamide gel according to their size. (Courtesy of Dr. P. Weingarten, Protagen AG.) (Bottom) 2D gel electrophoresis: For the first dimension, proteins are separated in a tube gel according to their isoelectric point. To preserve the native charge of the proteins, a nonionic detergent is used to unfold the polypeptides. For the second dimension, the tube gel is placed on top of a standard SDS-PAGE slab gel and the proteins are now separated by size. Up to 2000 proteins can be separated with this technique. (Courtesy of Dr. L. Mao and Prof. J. Klose, Charité Berlin.)

On the gel shown in Fig. 4.4 top, only a few protein bands can be seen. This will be the case after several protein purification steps. However, a cell or subcellular fraction contains hundreds or thousands of different proteins. If such a mixture is used for SDS-PAGE, individual bands overlap and proteins cannot be separated clearly. The solution to this problem is the two-dimensional polyacrylamide gel electrophoresis (O'Farrell 1975). The idea is to separate the proteins in a second dimension according to a property other than size.

Isoelectric focusing (IEF) is such a separation technique. The net charge of a protein depends on the number of charged amino acids, but also on the pH of the medium. At a very low pH, the carboxy groups of aspartate and glutamate are uncharged ($-COOH$), while the amino groups of lysine and arginine are fully ionized ($-NH_3^+$), conferring a positive net charge to the protein. At a very basic pH, by contrast, the carboxy groups are charged ($-COO^-$) and the amino groups are neutral ($-NH_2$), resulting in a negative net charge. Accordingly, for each protein a pH exists that results in an equal amount of negative and positive charges. This is the isoelectric point of the protein, at which it has no net charge. For isoelectric focusing, the proteins are treated with a nonionic detergent so that the proteins unfold but retain their native charge distribution (Fig. 4.4 bottom). Then they are placed onto a rod-like tube gel, which has been prepared such that it has a pH gradient from one end to the other. After a voltage is applied, the proteins travel until they reach the pH that corresponds to their isoelectric point.

For the second dimension, the tube gel is soaked in SDS and then placed on top of a normal SDS slab gel. A voltage is applied perpendicular to the direction of the first dimension and the proteins are now separated according to size. The result is a two dimensional (2D) distribution of proteins in the gel, as shown in Fig. 4.4 bottom. This technique makes it possible to separate all proteins of a typical prokaryote in a single experiment!

4.1.4
Hybridization and Blotting Techniques

Hybridization techniques are based on the specific recognition of a probe and target molecule. The aim is to use such techniques to detect and visualize only those molecules in a complex mixture that are of interest to the researcher. The base pairing of complementary single-stranded nucleic acids is the source of specificity for Southern blotting, Northern blotting, and *in situ* hybridization, which are described in the following sections. A short fragment of DNA, the probe, is labeled in such a way that it can later easily be visualized. Originally, radioactive labeling was used, but in recent years this has often been replaced by fluorescent labels. The probe is incubated with the target sample, and after the recognition of probe and target molecules is completed, the location of the probe shows the location and existence of the sought-after target molecule. In principle 16 nucleotides are sufficient to ensure that the sequence is unique in a typical mammalian genome ($4^{16} \approx 4.29 \cdot 10^9$), but in practice much longer probes are used. The Western blot is not a hybridization technique, since it is not based on the formation of double-stranded DNA, RNA, or DNA/RNA hybrids by complementary base pairing. Instead, it is based on the specific interaction between antibody and antigen.

4.1.4.1 Southern Blotting

The technique of Southern blotting was invented in 1975 and is used to analyze complex DNA mixtures (Southern 1975). Normally, the target DNA is digested by restriction enzymes and separated by gel electrophoresis. If the DNA is of genomic origin, the number of resulting fragments will be so large that no individual bands are visible. If we are interested in a certain gene and know its sequence, small DNA fragments can be synthesized, which are complementary to the gene. However, before the actual hybridization step, the digested DNA has to be transferred from the gel onto the surface of a nitrocellulose or nylon membrane so that the DNA molecules are accessible for the hybridization. This is achieved with the help of a blotting apparatus, as shown in Fig. 4.5. Originally the transfer was achieved by placing the nitrocellulose filter between the gel and a stack of blotting paper. Capillary forces lead to a flow of water and DNA fragments from the gel onto the blotting paper. In this way, the DNA gets trapped by a nitrocellulose or nylon filter. Nowadays, blotting machines that transfer the DNA by applying a voltage across the gel and membrane are used. Once the DNA is blotted, the membrane is placed into a plastic bag and incubated for several hours with a solution containing the labeled DNA probe. In the case of a radioactive label, the membrane is placed against an X-ray film. The radioactive DNA fragments expose the film and form black bands that indicate the location of the target DNA.

With this technique, not only can the presence of the gene of interest be tested, but also modifications of the gene structure (in the case of a mutation) can be studied. By performing several Southern blots with DNA probes that correspond to different regions of the gene, modifications such as deletions and insertions can be detected. Point mutations, however, cannot be identified with Southern blotting.

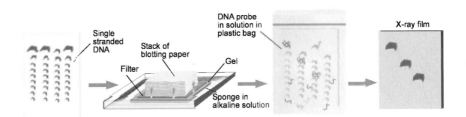

Fig. 4.5 Elementary steps required for Southern blotting. Following gel electrophoresis, the DNA fragments are treated with an alkaline solution to make them single-stranded. The nitrocellulose or nylon membrane is sandwiched between the gel and a stack of blotting paper and the DNA is transferred onto the membrane through capillary forces. Finally, the membrane is incubated with the labeled DNA probe (here, radioactive labeling) and the bands are then visualized by X-ray film exposure. (Courtesy of Dr. P. Weingarten, Protagen AG.)

4.1.4.2 **Northern Blotting**

Northern blotting is very similar to Southern blotting. The only difference is that mRNA, not DNA, is used for blotting. Although the experimental technique is very similar, Northern blotting can be used to answer different questions than Southern blotting. Even though mRNA is only an intermediate product on the way from the gene to the protein, it is normally a reasonable assumption that the amount of mRNA is correlated to the amount of the corresponding protein in the cell. Northern hybridization is therefore used not only to verify the existence of a specific mRNA but also to estimate the amount of the corresponding protein via the amount of mRNA. Since the expression profile of genes varies among tissues, Northern blotting gives different results for different organs, in contrast to Southern blotting, which is based on genomic DNA.

Surprisingly, the technique did not get its name from the researcher who invented it; rather, it was named as a humorous allusion to the double meaning of the name of E. M. Southern, who gave his name to the Southern blot.

4.1.4.3 **Western Blotting**

So far we have seen techniques for blotting different types of nucleic acids. A similar type of technique exists for proteins, the Western blot. As with the Northern blot, its name indicates only that it is a special type of blotting technique. Depending on the problem at hand, 1D or 2D protein gels can be used for blotting. It is more difficult to obtain specific probes for proteins than for nucleic acids. Apart from special cases, antibodies that are directed against the desired protein are used. If no commercial antibodies are available for the protein of interest, they have to be produced, e. g., by immunizing rabbits.

Once the protein is transferred to the nitrocellulose membrane, it is incubated with the primary antibody. The primary antibody recognizes the protein and forms an antibody-protein complex with the protein of interest. In a further step, the membrane is incubated with the so-called secondary antibody, which is an antibody against the primary antibody. If the primary antibody was obtained by immunizing a rabbit, the secondary antibody could be a goat-anti-rabbit antibody. This is an antibody from a goat that recognizes all rabbit antibodies. The secondary antibody is chemically linked to an enzyme, such as horseradish peroxidase, that catalyzes a chemiluminescence reaction, and exposure of an X-ray film finally produces bands, indicating the location of the protein-antibody complex. The intensity of the band is proportional to the amount of protein. Unlike Northern blotting, Western blotting gives a direct estimate of the protein content. The secondary antibody serves as signal amplification step. This is the reason that the enzyme is not linked directly to the primary antibody.

4.1.4.4 *In situ* **Hybridization**

The described blotting and hybridization techniques are applied to mixtures of nucleic acids or proteins that have been extracted from cells or tissues. During this process, all information about the spatial location is lost. *In situ* hybridization solves this problem by applying DNA probes directly to cells or tissue slices.

One common application is the location of specific genes on chromosomes. For this purpose metaphase chromosomes, which have been exposed to a high pH to separate the double strands, are incubated with labeled DNA probes. This makes it possible to directly see where and how many copies of the gene are located on the chromosome. If the label is a fluorescent dye, the technique is called FISH (fluorescent *in situ* hybridization). Not only chromosomes but also slices of whole tissues and organisms can be hybridized to DNA probes. This can be used to study the spatial and temporal expression pattern of genes by using probes specific to certain mRNAs. This method is often used to study gene expression patterns during embryogenesis. Finally, immunostaining uses antibodies to localize proteins within cells. Knowledge about the subcellular localization often helps one to better understand the functioning or lack of functioning of the studied proteins.

4.1.5
Further Protein Separation Techniques

4.1.5.1   Centrifugation

One of the oldest techniques for the separation of cell components is centrifugation. This technique fractionates molecules (and larger objects) according to a combination of size and shape. However, in general it is true that the larger the object, the faster it moves to the bottom. A typical low-speed centrifugation (around 1000-fold gravitational acceleration, g) collects cell fragments and nuclei in the pellet, at medium speeds (50,000 g) cell organelles and ribosomes are collected, and at ultrahigh speeds (up to 500,000 g) even typical enzymes end up in the pellet. Of course, such a separation is not quantitative, but repeating the centrifugation after re-dissolving the pellet improves the purity. The sedimentation rate for macromolecules is measured in Svedberg units, S, after Theodor Svedberg, who invented ultracentrifugation in 1925. S depends on the mass (m) and density of the particle (ρ_{par}), as well as on the density (ρ_{sol}) and friction (f) of the medium. These properties control the velocity (v) of the particle (ω^2 = angular velocity, r = distance from center of rotation).

$$S = \frac{v}{\omega^2 r} = \frac{m(1 - \rho_{sol}/\rho_{par})}{f} \tag{4-2}$$

The ribosomal subunits, for instance, got their name from their sedimentation coefficient (40S subunit and 60S subunit). Because the friction is controlled not only by the size of the particle but also by its shape, S values are not additive. The complete ribosome (40S plus 60S) sediments at 80S and not at 100 S.

From Eq. (2) it also follows that the sedimentation rate is zero if the densities of the particle and the surrounding medium are identical. This is the basis for the equilibrium centrifugation method, in which the medium forms a stable density gradient (caused by the gravitational forces) such that the density of the studied particles lies within the density range of the gradient. If the centrifugation is run long enough, the particles move to the position where the densities of the medium and the particle are identical and form stable bands there. Thus, equilibrium centrifugation separates the molecules by density, independent of their size. The necessary density gradients are typically formed with saccharose or cesium chloride (CsCl).

4.1.5.2 Column Chromatography

Other classical separation techniques include the different forms of column chromatography (Fig. 4.6). A column (often made of glass, a few centimeters wide and a few dozen centimeters tall) is filled with a solid carrier material and the protein mixture is placed on top of it. Then a buffer is slowly washed through the column and takes the protein mixture along with it. However, different proteins are held back to a different degree by the column material and arrive at different times at the bottom of the column. The eluate can be fractionated and tested for the presence of the desired protein. The ratio of desired protein to total protein is a measure of the purity, which can additionally be checked on normal SDS gels. Different column materials are available and the success of a separation often depends critically on the choice of material.

The material for ion exchange chromatography (Fig. 4.6a) contains negatively (carboxymethyl or phosphor cellulose) or positively (diethylaminoethyl cellulose) charged beads that can be used to separate hydrophilic proteins according to charge. The binding between the proteins and the beads is also controlled by the salt concentration and pH of the elution buffer. Some proteins possess hydrophobic surfaces that can be used to separate proteins by hydrophobic interaction chromatography (Fig. 4.6b). For this purpose short aliphatic side chains are attached to the surface of the column material. Gel filtration chromatography (Fig. 4.6c) is also often used to separate proteins according to size. The beads contain a range of pores and channels that

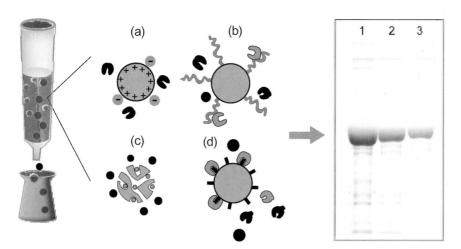

Fig. 4.6 In column chromatography a protein mixture is placed on top of the column material and then eluted with buffer. Different types of material are available to separate the proteins according to (a) charge, (b) hydrophobicity, (c) size, or (d) affinity to a specific target molecule. Often, different chromatographic steps have to be used successively to purify the desired protein to homogeneity (lanes 1–3 of the gel). (Courtesy of Dr. P. Weingarten, Protagen AG.)

allow small molecules to enter, which increases their retention times. This allows not only their separation by size but also estimation of the absolute size of a protein or protein complex. A more recent development is affinity chromatography (Fig. 4.6 d), which makes use of highly specific interactions between a protein and the column material. This can be achieved, for instance, by chemically linking antibodies to the column material. For affinity chromatography the column is loaded with the protein mixture in the first step. The proteins of interest bind, while the other proteins pass through the column. In the second step, the elution process is started by using a high-salt or high-pH buffer that frees the bound protein from the column.

A major improvement regarding speed and separating power was achieved through the development of high performance liquid chromatography (HPLC). The columns are much smaller and the carrier material is packed more densely and homogenously. To achieve reasonable buffer flow rates, very high pressures (up to several hundred atmospheres) are needed. Therefore, special pumps are used and the column housing is made of steel.

The enrichment factor of a single chromatographic step is normally between 10- and 20-fold. However, since many proteins represent only a tiny fraction of the total protein content of a cell, different chromatographic columns often have to be used consecutively. A notable exception is affinity chromatography, which can achieve enrichments up to 10^4 in a single step. In combination with modern recombinant DNA techniques, affinity chromatography has many applications. Recombinant proteins can be designed to contain special short sequences of amino acids that do not compromise the functionality of the protein but can serve as molecular tags. A short stretch of histidine residues is called a His-tag and is specifically recognized by a nickel surface or special His antibodies.

4.2
Advanced Techniques

4.2.1
PCR

The polymerase chain reaction (PCR) was invented in the mid-1980s and allows the billion-fold amplification of specific DNA fragments (typically up to 10 kbp) directly from genomic DNA (Saiki et al. 1985). A pair consisting of short oligonucleotides (15–25 bp), the primers, is synthesized chemically such that they are complementary to an area upstream and downstream of the DNA of interest. DNA is made single-stranded by heating, and during the cooling phase primers are added to the mixture, which then hybridize to the single-stranded DNA (Fig. 4.7). In the next step a DNA polymerase extends the primers, doubling the copy number of the desired DNA fragment. This concludes one PCR cycle. Each additional cycle (denaturation, annealing, and amplification) doubles the existing amount of DNA that is located between the primer pair. Thus, 30 cycles correspond to a $2^{30} = {\sim}10^9$-fold amplification step (30–40 cycles are typically used). A special heat-stable DNA polymerase is used that remains

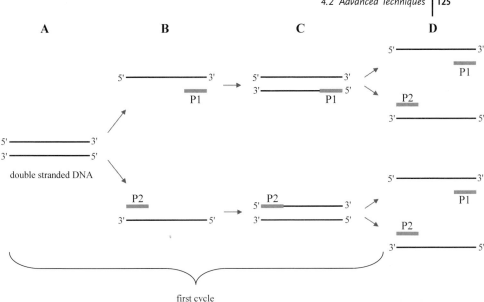

A   B   C   D

double stranded DNA

P1

P2

first cycle

Fig. 4.7 The polymerase chain reaction. (a) After double-stranded DNA is heated to obtain single strands, (b) short DNA primers (P1 and P2) are hybridized to a region that is upstream or downstream, respectively, of the DNA of inter- est. (c) A DNA polymerase is then used to extend the primers. (d) Then the cycle is repeated by melting the DNA and annealing new primers. For clarity the primers that were used in the first cycle are not drawn in bold in the second cycle.

active during the heating step and thus obviates the need to add fresh enzyme after each cycle. Today, the different steps of the PCR reaction don't have to be performed manually. Small, automated PCR machines, also called thermal cyclers, can perform dozens of PCR reactions in parallel, and the typical 30 cycles are finished in roughly half an hour.

In the last few years, sequence information for many complete genomes has become available, which allows one to use PCR to clone genes directly from genomic DNA without the use of DNA libraries. PCR has revolutionized modern molecular genetics and has many applications. For instance, by combining reverse transcriptase (which makes a DNA copy from RNA) with PCR, it is also possible to clone mRNA with this technique. The extreme sensitivity of PCR also makes it the method of choice for forensic studies. Highly variable tandem repeats are amplified and used to determine whether genetic material that comes from hair follicle cells, saliva, or blood stains belongs to a certain suspect. This is possible because different individuals have tandem repeats of different length, which results in amplified DNA fragments of different length. By looking at a large number of different tandem repeats, the chances of a false positive result can be made arbitrarily small. This principle is also the basis of paternity tests.

Another type of application is the use of multiple, or degenerate, primers. This can be useful when a consensus sequence is known and the aim is to amplify genes that contain this conserved sequence. Degenerate primers are also used if a stretch of the amino acid sequence of a new protein is known (e.g., through protein sequencing) and the corresponding gene has to be found. Because of the degeneracy of the genetic code, several nucleotide sequences can code for a given amino acid sequence. The use of degenerate PCR can solve this problem.

An important, more recent, development is the technique of real-time PCR, which is especially suited to quantify the amount of template that was initially present. Classical PCR is normally unable to give quantitative results because of saturation problems during the later cycles. Real-time PCR circumvents these problems by using fluorescent dyes that either intercalate in double-stranded DNA or are bound to sequence-specific oligonucleotides (TaqMan probe). The increase of fluorescence with time is used, in real time, as an indicator of product generation during each PCR cycle.

4.2.2
DNA and Protein Chips

4.2.2.1 DNA Chips
DNA chips, also called DNA microarrays, are a recently developed method for the high-throughput analysis of gene expression (DeRisi et al. 1997). Instead of looking at the expression of a single gene, microarrays allow one to monitor the expression of several thousand genes in a single experiment, resulting in a global picture of the cellular activity. This idea is also the basis of the systems biological modeling approach, and chip data can therefore be a very important source of data.

A microarray experiment starts with the construction of the chip (Fig. 4.8) from a DNA library (see Section 4.1.2). The inserts of individual clones are amplified by PCR (a single primer pair that is specific for the vector used to construct the library can be used) and spotted in a regular pattern on a glass slide or nylon membrane. These steps are normally automated and performed by robots. Then, total mRNA is extracted from two samples that we would like to compare (e.g., yeast cells before and after osmotic shock). Using reverse transcriptase, the mRNA is transcribed into

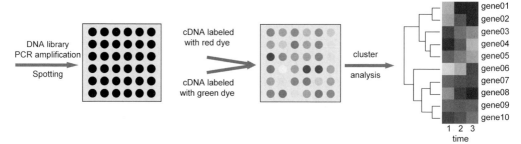

Fig. 4.8 DNA chips are used to study the expression level of thousands of genes in parallel. Individual genes from a DNA library are amplified by PCR and spotted onto glass slides. cDNA is prepared from the cells or tissues that are to be compared and is labeled with red and green fluorescent dyes. The color reveals, after hybridization, the relative mRNA amounts in the two sources. Finally, the expression data are clustered.

cDNA and labeled with a fluorescent dye. It is important that the dyes emit light at different wavelengths; red and green dyes are commonly used. The cDNAs are now incubated with the chip where they hybridize to the spot that contains the complementary DNA fragment. After washing, the ratio of the fluorescence intensities for red and green are measured and displayed as false color pictures (Fig. 4.8, middle). Red or green spots indicate a large excess of mRNA from one or the other sample, while yellow spots show that the amount of this specific mRNA was roughly equal in both samples. Very low amounts of both mRNA samples result in dark spots. These ratios can, of course, also be quantified numerically and used for further calculations, such as the generation of a clustergram. For this analysis, a complete linkage cluster of the genes that were spotted on the chip is generated and the mRNA ratio (represented as color) is displayed in this order (Fig. 4.8, right). This helps to test whether groups of related genes (maybe all involved in fatty acid synthesis) also show a similar expression pattern.

Oligonucleotide chips, a variant of DNA chips, are based on an alternative experimental design. Instead of spotting cDNAs, short oligonucleotides (25–50mer) are used. Approximately a dozen different and specific oligonucleotides are used per gene. In this case only one probe of mRNA is hybridized per chip, and the ratio of fluorescence intensity of different chips is used to estimate the relative abundance of each mRNA. Chips from the companies Affymetrix or Agilent are most commonly used for this approach.

During the past several years, this technique has been used to study such diverse problems as the effects of caloric restriction and aging in mice (Lee et al. 1999), influence of environmental changes on yeast (Causton et al. 2001), and the consequences of serum withdrawal on human fibroblasts (Eisen et al. 1998).

4.2.2.2 Protein Chips

Despite the large success of DNA chips, it is clear that the function of the genes is realized through the proteins and not by the mRNAs. Therefore, efforts are under way to construct chips that consist of spotted proteins instead of DNA. In this case the starting point is an expression library for obtaining large quantities of the recombinant proteins. The proteins are spotted and fixed on a glass slide and can then be incubated with interaction partners. These could be (1) other proteins to study protein complexes, (2) antibodies to quantify the spotted proteins or to identify the recognized antigens, (3) DNA to find DNA-binding proteins, or (4) drugs to identify compounds of pharmaceutical interest (Cahill and Nordhoff 2003).

However, the generation of protein chips poses more problems than DNA chips because proteins are not as uniform as DNA. One challenge is to express sufficient amounts of recombinant proteins in a high-throughput approach. Another problem is that the optimal conditions (temperature, ionic strength, etc.) for interaction with the reaction partner are not identical for different proteins. But the field is making rapid progress, and protein chips will be used more often in the near future.

The main advantage of DNA and protein chips is the huge amount of data that can be gathered in a single experiment. However, there are also points that need careful consideration. The quality of an expression profile analysis based on array data is highly dependent on the number of repeated sample measurements and on the array preparation, hybridization, and signal quantification procedure (Wierling et al. 2002). The many samples on the chip also pose a problem regarding multiple testing. If care is not taken, a large number of false positives is to be expected.

4.2.3
Yeast Two-hybrid System

The yeast two-hybrid (Y2H) system is a technique for the high-throughput detection of protein-protein interactions. It rests on the fact that some transcription factors (TF), such as the yeast *Gal4* gene, have a modular design. The DNA-binding domain is separated from the activating domain. To test whether two proteins (we will call them bait and prey) interact, their genes are fused to the DNA-binding or DNA-activating domain, respectively, of the TF (Fig. 4.9). The bait binds to the DNA via its TF fragment. If bait and prey do interact, the two domains of the transcription factor come close enough together to stimulate the expression of a reporter gene. If bait and prey do not interact, the reporter gene is silent. This technique can be used to find all interacting partners of the bait protein. For this purpose yeast cells are transformed with an expression library containing prey proteins fused to the activating part of the TF. Although the detection occurs in yeast, the bait and prey proteins can come from any organism. This single-bait–multiple-prey system can even be extended to a multiple-bait–multiple-prey approach, which makes it possible to obtain the complete protein interactome of yeast (Uetz et al. 2000). However, as with most high-throughput techniques, the two-hybrid system is prone to false positives, as indicated by the fact that a second study using the same technique derived a quite dissimilar yeast interactome (Ito et al. 2001). To corroborate the interactions obtained with Y2H, affinity chromatography or co-immunoprecipitation can be used.

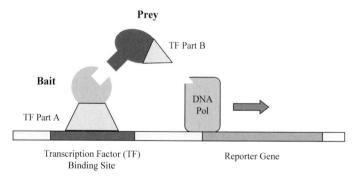

Fig. 4.9 The yeast two-hybrid system identifies protein-protein interactions. The genes of the bait and prey proteins are fused to parts of a yeast transcription factor. If bait and prey interact, the different parts of the transcription factor come close enough together to activate the expression of a reporter gene.

4.2.4
Mass Spectrometry

The identification of individual proteins of a cell is an essential part for studying biological processes. The first step towards identification often involves a separation of the protein broth. 2D gels (see Section 4.1.3) or the different forms of column chromatography (see Section 4.1.5.2) are frequently the method of choice. The separated proteins can then be identified by cleaving them enzymatically or chemically into specific peptides and determining the exact size of these fragments. The resulting size distribution, the fingerprint of the protein, is compared to the theoretical fingerprints that are calculated for all proteins in the sequence databanks. This is possible because it is known at which amino acid sequence proteases like trypsin cut a protein.

Mass spectrometry (MS) has been used for the past 50 years to measure the masses of small molecules with high accuracy. However, its application to large biomolecules has been limited by the fragility and low volatility of these materials. But these problems have been solved with the development of the matrix-assisted laser desorption/ionization time-of-flight (MALDI-TOF) technique. The polypeptide is mixed with a solvent and an excess of the matrix material and is placed inside the mass spectrometer, where the solvent evaporates. The probe is then targeted with a laser beam that transfers most of its energy to the matrix material, which heats up and is vaporized. During this process the intact polymer is charged and carried into the vapor phase. An electrical field accelerates the molecules, which then traverse down an evacuated tube, (smaller ions arrive in a shorter time at the detector than massive ions), and the time of flight is recorded. The masses of the different ions can then be calculated, taking into account that the TOF is proportional to the square root of the mass divided by the charge of the ion (TOF $\sim \sqrt{m/z}$).

The accuracy of MALDI-TOF is extremely high. The error is less than 1 part in 10^5. That means the error in determining the mass of a 100-kDa protein is less than 1 Dalton! Because of this very high accuracy, MS can also be used for sequencing of peptide fragments. In this case two mass spectrometers have to be used in succession. The first one separates the peptides (according to their time of flight) and feeds them individually into the second MS, where they are further fragmented at their peptide bonds. The output of the second spectrometer is therefore mass peaks that are separated by the mass of a single amino acid, which can be used to construct the sequence of the peptide. With the use of degenerate primers (see Section 4.2.1), the gene for the protein can then be cloned. This is useful if the fingerprint of the protein is not found in the database and the protein cannot be identified this way.

Finally, MS-based peptide sequencing also yields information about posttranslational modifications. If an amino acid is chemically modified (i.e., phosphorylated or glycosylated), this results in a characteristic change of the mass and thus it can be identified.

4.2.5
Transgenic Animals

Genetic material can be introduced into single-celled organisms (bacteria, yeast) by transformation (see Section 4.1.2), and it is then automatically passed down to the offspring during each cell division. To achieve the same outcome in a multicellular organism is much more complicated.

The first method applied successfully to mammals was DNA microinjection (Gordon and Ruddle 1981). This technique is based upon the observation that in mammalian cells linear DNA fragments are rapidly assembled into tandem repeats which are then integrated into the genomic DNA. This integration occurs at a single random location within the genome. A linearized gene construct is therefore injected into the pronucleus of a fertilized ovum. After introduction into foster mothers, embryos containing the foreign DNA in some cells of the organism develop; this is known as a chimera. If the construct is also present in germ line cells, some animals of the daughter generation (F_1 generation) will carry the transgene in all of its body cells and a transgenic animal has been created. The advantage of DNA microinjection is that it is applicable to a wide range of species. The disadvantage is that the integration is a random process and thus the genomic neighborhood of the insert is unpredictable. This often means that the expression of the recombinant DNA is suppressed by silencers or by an unfavorable chromatin structure. If a mutant form of an endogenous gene has been introduced, it has to be considered that, generally, the wild type will also be present, which restricts this approach to the investigation of dominant mutants.

This problem can be overcome by using the method of embryonic stem cell–mediated transfer (Gossler et al. 1986). In rare cases (approximately 0.1%), the integration of a gene variant into the genome does not occur randomly, but actually replaces the original gene via homologous recombination. This paves the way to modify or inactivate any gene. In the latter case, this results in knockout animals. For this technique the gene construct is introduced into embryonic stem cells (ES cells), which are omnipotent and can give rise to any cell type. With the help of PCR or Southern blotting, the few ES cells that undergo homologous recombination can be identified. Some of these cells are then injected into an early embryo at the blastocyst stage, which leads to chimeric animals that are composed of wild-type cells and cells derived from the manipulated ES cells. As in the case of DNA microinjection, an F_1 generation of animals has to be bred to obtain genetically homogeneous animals. ES cell–mediated transfer works particularly well in mice and is the method of choice to generate knockout mice, which are invaluable in deciphering the function of unknown genes.

The random integration that accompanies DNA microinjection often has negative effects on the expression of the transgene. To circumvent this obstacle, the method of retrovirus-mediated gene transfer has been developed. In this case the recombinant DNA is inserted into a vector that originates from a retrovirus before it is injected. Retroviruses have developed methods to express their own genes regardless of the location in the host genome, and this ability can be hijacked to increase the expression of the transgene of interest.

4.2.6
RNA Interference

We have seen that the generation of transgenic animals and the use of homologous recombination to produce knockout animals is one way to elucidate the function of a gene. However, this approach is time-consuming, technically demanding, and expensive. A new convenient method for transiently downregulating arbitrary genes makes use of the phenomenon of RNA interference (RNAi). In 1998 it was discovered that the injection of double-stranded RNA (dsRNA) into the nematode *Caenorhabditis elegans* led to a sequence-specific downregulation of gene expression (Fire et al. 1998). It turned out that this effect is part of a natural defense system of eukaryotes against viruses and selfish genetic elements that propagate via long, double-stranded RNA intermediates.

The dsRNA is recognized by a cellular endoribonuclease of the RNase III family, called DICER. This cuts the dsRNA into short pieces of 21–23 bp in length with a 2-bp, single-stranded overhang at the 3′ end. These short fragments are called short interfering RNAs (siRNAs). After phosphorylation they are assembled (as single strands) into a riboprotein complex called RISC (RNA-induced silencing complex). If RISC encounters an mRNA complementary to its siRNA, the mRNA is enzymatically cut at a position that corresponds to the middle of the siRNA (Fig. 4.10). In mammals, long dsRNA also induces the interferon response, which causes unspecific degradation of mRNA and a general shutdown of translation. This would severely hamper the use of RNA interference as research tool, but, luckily, artificial siRNAs can also be used to activate the RNA interference machinery (Dykxhoorn et al. 2003).

Artificial siRNAs are synthesized chemically and can in principle be targeted against any mRNA. However, currently there are no clear design rules that would yield the most effective siRNAs, and positional effects can lead to suppression levels that vary between 10% and 70% (Holen et al. 2002). Because the transfection of siRNA is only transient (it lasts only a few days in mammals), there might also be problems in silencing genes that encode for long-lived proteins, but in general RNAi is a very versatile technique.

If siRNAs are expressed from plasmids or viral vectors, their effects are more persistent and they can be used as therapeutic agents by downregulating specific disease genes. Applications to HIV and other targets have been discussed (Dykxhoorn et al. 2003; Stevenson 2003). They can also be used to study regulatory interactions among proteins by targeting individual components and then measuring the effects on global gene expression. By following this approach, is was possible to study the structure of a signaling pathway involved in the immune response of *Drosophila melanogaster* (Boutros et al. 2002). Finally, RNA interference would also be very useful for the model building of metabolic or gene networks. After a network has been formulated by a set of equations, it can be tested by silencing genes individually or in combination and then measuring the resulting new expression levels. This type of network perturbation can be used to iteratively improve agreement of the model predictions with the experimental data.

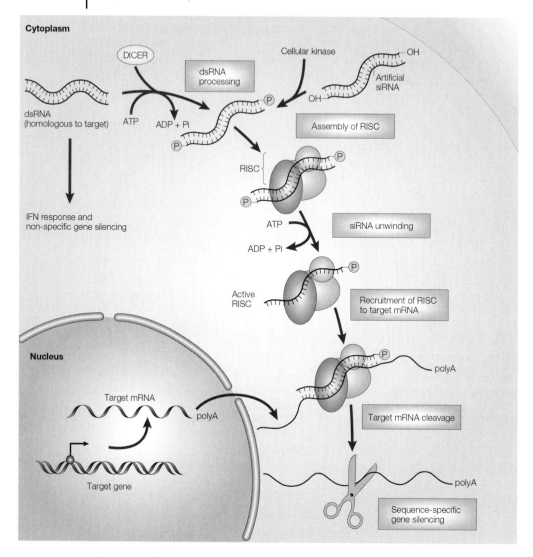

Fig. 4.10 Mechanism of RNA interference (RNAi). Double-stranded RNA (dsRNA) is cleaved by the endoribonuclease DICER into small fragments of 21–23 nucleotides, which are subsequently phosphorylated at the 5′ end. To become functional, these small interfering RNAs (siRNAs) form an RNA-induced silencing com-

plex (RISC) with cellular proteins. If the RISC complex encounters an mRNA that is complementary to the siRNA, this mRNA is cleaved in the middle of the complementary sequence, leading to gene silencing (from Stevenson 2003). Exogenously added siRNAs are also functional in triggering RNAi.

References

Boutros, M., Agaisse, H. and Perrimon, N. Sequential activation of signaling pathways during innate immune responses in Drosophila (2002) Dev. Cell *3*, 711–22

Burke, D.T., Carle, G.F. and Olson, M.V. Cloning of large segments of exogenous DNA into yeast by means of artificial chromosome vectors (1987) Science *236*, 806–812

Cahill, D.J. and Nordhoff, E. Protein arrays and their role in proteomics (2003) Adv. Biochem. Eng. Biotechnol. *83*, 177–87.

Causton, H.C., Ren, B., Koh, S.S., Harbison, C.T., Kanin, E., Jennings, E.G., Lee, T.I., True, H.L., Lander, E.S. and Young, R.A. Remodeling of yeast genome expression in response to environmental changes (2001) Mol. Biol. Cell. *12*, 323–37

Clarke, L. and Carbon, J. A colony bank containing synthetic Col El hybrid plasmids representative of the entire *E. coli* genome (1976) Cell *9*, 91–99

Colletto, G.M., Segre, C.A., Rielli, S.T. and Rosario, H. Multiple birth rates according to different socioeconomic levels: an analysis of four hospitals from the city of Sao Paulo, Brazil (2003) Twin Res. *6*, 177–82

DeRisi, J.L., Iyer, V.R. and Brown, P.O. Exploring the metabolic and genetic control of gene expression on a genomic scale (1997) Science *278*, 680–6

Dykxhoorn, D.M., Novina, C.D. and Sharp, P.A. Killing the messenger: short RNAs that silence gene expression (2003) Nat. Rev. Mol. Cell. Biol. *4*, 457–67

Eisen, M.B., Spellman, P.T., Brown, P.O. and Botstein, D. Cluster analysis and display of genome-wide expression patterns (1998) Proc. Natl. Acad. Sci. USA *95*, 14863–8

Fire, A., Xu, S., Montgomery, M.K., Kostas, S.A., Driver, S.E. and Mello, C.C. Potent and specific genetic interference by double-stranded RNA in *Caenorhabditis elegans* (1998) Nature *391*, 806–11

Gordon, J.W. and Ruddle, F.H. Integration and stable germ line transmission of genes injected into mouse pronuclei (1981) Science *214*, 1244–6

Gossler, A., Doetschman, T., Korn, R., Serfling, E. and Kemler, R. Transgenesis by means of blastocyst-derived embryonic stem cell lines (1986) Proc. Natl. Acad. Sci. USA *83*, 9065–9

Holen, T., Amarzguioui, M., Wiiger, M.T., Babaie, E. and Prydz, H. Positional effects of short interfering RNAs targeting the human coagulation trigger Tissue Factor (2002) Nucleic Acids Res. *30*, 1757–66

Ito, T., Chiba, T., Ozawa, R., Yoshida, M., Hattori, M. and Sakaki, Y. A comprehensive two-hybrid analysis to explore the yeast protein interactome (2001) Proc. Natl. Acad. Sci. USA *98*, 4569–74

Lee, C.-K., Klopp, R.G., Weindruch, R. and Prolla, T.A. Gene expression profile of aging and its retardation by caloric restriction (1999) Science *285*, 1390–1393

O'Farrell, P.H. High resolution two-dimensional electrophoresis of proteins (1975) J. Biol. Chem. *250*, 4007–4021

Saiki, R.K., Scharf, S., Faloona, F., Mullis, K.B., Horn, G.T., Erlich, H.A. and Arnheim, N. Enzymatic amplification of beta-globin genomic sequences and restriction site analysis for diagnosis of sickle cell anemia (1985) Science *230*, 1350–1354

Shapiro, A.L., Vinuela, E. and Maizel, J.V.J. Molecular weight estimation of polypeptide chains by electrophoresis in SDS-polyacrylamide gels (1967) Biochem. Biophys. Res. Comm. *28*, 815–820

Shizuya, H., Birren, B., Kim, U.J., Mancino, V., Slepak, T., Tachiiri, Y. and Simon, M. Cloning and stable maintenance of 300-kilobase-pair fragments of human DNA in *Escherichia coli* using an F-factor-based vector (1992) Proc. Natl. Acad. Sci. USA *89*, 8794–8797

Southern, E.M. Detection of specific sequences among DNA fragments separated by gel electrophoresis (1975) J. Mol. Biol. *98*, 503–517

Stevenson, M. Dissecting HIV-1 through RNA interference (2003) Nat Rev Immunol *3*, 851–8

Uetz, P., Giot, L., Cagney, G., Mansfield, T.A., Judson, R.S., Knight, J.R., Lockshon, D., Narayan, V., Srinivasan, M., Pochart, P., Qureshi-Emili, A., Li, Y., Godwin, B., Conover, D., Kalbfleisch, T., Vijayadamodar, G., Yang, M., Johnston, M., Fields, S. and Rothberg, J.M. A comprehensive analysis of protein-protein interactions in *Saccharomyces cerevisiae* (2000) Nature *403*, 623–7

Wierling, C.K., Steinfath, M., Elge, T., Schulze-Kremer, S., Aanstad, P., Clark, M.,

LEHRACH, H. and HERWIG, R. Simulation of DNA array hybridization experiments and evaluation of critical parameters during subsequent image and data analysis (2002) BMC Bioinformatics *3*, 29

WILMUT, I., SCHNIEKE, A.E., McWHIR, J., KIND, A.J. and CAMPBELL, K.H.S. Viable offspring derived from fetal and adult mammalian cells (1997) Nature *385*, 810–813

Part II
Standard Models and Approaches in Systems Biology

Systems Biology in Practice. Concepts, Implementation and Application.
E. Klipp, R. Herwig, A. Kowald, C. Wierling, H. Lehrach
Copyright © 2005 WILEY-VCH Verlag GmbH & Co. KGaA, Weinheim
ISBN: 3-527-31078-9

5
Metabolism

Introduction

Living cells require energy and material for building membranes, storing molecules, replenishing enzymes, replication and repair of DNA, movement, and many other processes. Through metabolism cells acquire energy and use it to build new cells. Metabolism is the means by which cells survive and reproduce. Metabolism is the general term for two kinds of reactions: (1) catabolic reactions (breakdown of complex compounds to get energy and building blocks) and (2) anabolic reactions (construction of complex compounds used in cellular functioning). Metabolism is a highly organized process. It involves thousands of reactions that are catalyzed by enzymes.

Metabolic networks consist of reactions transforming molecules of one type into molecules of another type. In modeling terms, the concentrations of the molecules and their rates of change are of special interest. The basic concepts of reaction networks, which are outlined here, may also be applied for other types of cellular reaction networks, e. g., signal transduction pathways. In this chapter metabolism will be studied on three levels of abstraction:

1. Enzyme kinetics investigates the dynamic properties of the individual reactions in isolation.
2. The network character of metabolism is studied with stoichiometric analysis considering the balance of compound production and degradation.
3. Metabolic control analysis quantifies the effect of perturbations in the network employing the individual dynamics of concentration changes and their integration in the network.

Note that most modeling approaches for individual biochemical reactions or networks of such reactions that are presented in this chapter also apply for other types of networks, such as signaling cascades or binding of transcription factors to DNA. Since the modeling of metabolic networks is the most elaborate, it is subsumed here.

In order to illustrate the theoretical concepts, we will apply a running example throughout this chapter. This example comprises a subset of reactions of glycolysis

Systems Biology in Practice. Concepts, Implementation and Application.
E. Klipp, R. Herwig, A. Kowald, C. Wierling, H. Lehrach
Copyright © 2005 WILEY-VCH Verlag GmbH & Co. KGaA, Weinheim
ISBN: 3-527-31078-9

in yeast as represented by Hynne and colleagues (2001). You can also find the complete model and many other models in modeling databases (Snoep and Olivier 2002).

Example 1

We will consider the first four reactions from the upper part of glycolysis as well as reactions balancing the energy currency ATP and ADP as represented in Fig. 5.1.

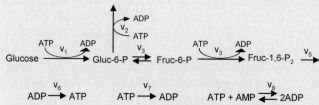

Fig. 5.1 Schematic representation of the upper part of glycolysis, i.e., the degradation of glucose in order to yield energy and building blocks for cellular processes. Abbreviations: Gluc6P: glucose-6-phosphate; Fruc6P: fructose-6-phosphate; Fruc1,6P$_2$: fructose-1,6-bisphosphate; ATP: adenosine-triphosphate; ADP: adenosine-diphosphate: AMP: adenosine-monophosphate. Reactions: v_1: hexokinase; v_2: consumption of glucose-6-phosphate in other pathways; v_3: phosphoglucoisomerase; v_4: phosphofructokinase; v_5: aldolase; v_6: ATP production in lower glycolysis; v7: ATP consumption in other pathways; v_8: adenylate kinase.

The ODE system for this reaction system is given by

$$\frac{d}{dt} Gluc6P = v_1 - v_2 - v_3$$

$$\frac{d}{dt} Fruc6P = v_3 - v_4$$

$$\frac{d}{dt} Fruc1,6P_2 = v_4 - v_5$$

$$\frac{d}{dt} ATP = -v_1 - v_2 - v_4 + v_6 - v_7 - v_8$$

$$\frac{d}{dt} ADP = v_1 + v_2 + v_4 - v_6 + v_7 + 2 v_8$$

$$\frac{d}{dt} AMP = -v_8 . \tag{5-1}$$

Abbreviations are explained in the legend of Fig. 5.1. The individual rate expressions read

$$v_1 = \frac{V_{max,1}\, ATP(t) \cdot Glucose}{1 + \dfrac{ATP(t)}{K_{ATP,1}} + \dfrac{Glucose}{K_{Glucose,1}} + \dfrac{ATP(t)}{K_{ATP,1}} \cdot \dfrac{Glucose}{K_{Glucose,1}}} \quad \text{or} \quad v_1 = \frac{V_{max,1}\, ATP(t)}{K_{ATP,1} + ATP(t)} \tag{5-2}$$

$$v_2 = k_2\, ATP(t) \cdot Gluc6P(t) \tag{5-3}$$

$$v_3 = \frac{\dfrac{V_{max,3}^{f}}{K_{Gluc6P,3}}\, Gluc6P(t) - \dfrac{V_{max,3}^{r}}{K_{Fruc6P,3}}\, Fruc6P(t)}{1 + \dfrac{Gluc6P(t)}{K_{Gluc6P,3}} + \dfrac{Fruc6P(t)}{K_{Fruc6P,3}}} \tag{5-4}$$

$$v_4 = \frac{V_{max,4}\,(Fruc6P(t))^2}{K_{Fruc6P,4}\left(1 + \kappa \left(\dfrac{ATP(t)}{AMP(t)}\right)^2\right) + (Fruc6P(t))^2} \tag{5-5}$$

$$v_5 = k_5\, Fruc1,6P_2(t) \tag{5-6}$$

$$v_6 = k_6\, ADP(t) \tag{5-7}$$

$$v_7 = k_7\, ATP(t) \tag{5-8}$$

$$v_8 = k_{8f}\, ATP(t) \cdot AMP(t) - k_{8r}\,(ADP(t))^2, \tag{5-9}$$

with the following parameters:

$Glucose = 12.8174\,\text{mM}$, $V_{max,1} = 1398.00\,\text{mM} \cdot \text{min}^{-1}$, $K_{ATP,1} = 0.10\,\text{mM}$,
$K_{Glucose,1} = 0.37\,\text{mM}$, $V_{max,1} = 50.2747\,\text{mM} \cdot \text{min}^{-1}$

$k_2 = 2.26\,\text{mM}^{-1} \cdot \text{min}^{-1}$

$V_{max,3}^{f} = 140.282\,\text{mM} \cdot \text{min}^{-1}$, $V_{max,3}^{r} = 140.282\,\text{mM} \cdot \text{min}^{-1}$, $K_{Gluc6P,3} = 0.80\,\text{mM}$,
$K_{Fruc6P,3} = 0.15\,\text{mM}$

$V_{max,4} = 44.7287\,\text{mM} \cdot \text{min}^{-1}$, $K_{Fruc6P,4} = 0.021\,\text{mM}^2$, $\kappa = 0.15$

$k_5 = 6.04662\,\text{min}^{-1}$

$k_6 = 68.48\,\text{min}^{-1}$

$k_7 = 3.21\,\text{min}^{-1}$

$k_{8f} = 432.9\,\text{mM}^{-1} \cdot \text{min}^{-1}$, $k_{8r} = 133.33\,\text{mM}^{-1} \cdot \text{min}^{-1}$

The temporal evolution of the concentrations starting from arbitrarily given values is shown in Fig. 5.2.

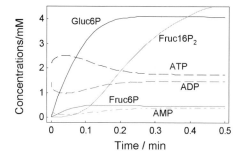

Fig. 5.2 Time courses of concentrations for the running model presented (Example 5-1). Parameters are stated there. Initial values: $Gluc6P(0) = 1$ mM, $Fruc6P(0) = 0$ mM, $Fruc1,6P_2(0) = 0$ mM, $ATP(0) = 2.1$ mM, $ADP(0) = 1.4$ mM, $AMP(0) = 0.1$ mM.

In this chapter it will be illustrated how metabolic models such as this model of upper glycolysis can be described and analyzed. We will present possible choices for rate equations and give reasoning for these choices. The information contained in the network structure, i.e., in the stoichiometry, shall be extracted: Are there main routes through the network? Which fluxes are possible in steady state? Will substances be produced or consumed, or are there conservation relations for metabolite concentrations? Metabolic control analysis will enable us to assess the influence of parameter changes in one part of the network on changes of variables (here, steady-state fluxes or concentrations) at any place of the network.

5.1
Enzyme Kinetics and Thermodynamics

This chapter deals with the deterministic kinetic modeling of individual biochemical reactions. The basic quantities are the concentration S of a substance S (i.e., the number n of molecules of this substance per volume V) and the rate v of a reaction (i.e., the change of concentration S per time t). This type of modeling is macroscopic or phenomenological compared to the microscopic approach, where single molecules and their interactions are considered.

Chemical and biochemical kinetics rely on the assumption that the reaction rate v at a certain point in time and space can be expressed as a unique function of the concentrations of all substances at this point in time and space. Classical enzyme kinetics assumes for simplicity's sake a spatial homogeneity (the "well-stirred" test tube) and no direct dependency of the rate on time:

$$v(t) = v(S(t)). \tag{5-10}$$

In more advanced modeling approaches moving towards whole-cell modeling, spatial inhomogeneities are taken into account, paying tribute to the fact that many components are membrane-bound or that cellular structures hinder the free movement of molecules. However, in most cases one can assume that diffusion is rapid enough to allow for an even distribution of all substances in space.

Enzymes catalyze biochemical reactions. Enzymes are proteins, often in complex with cofactors (Chapter 2, Section 2.1). They have a catalytic center, are usually highly specific, and remain unchanged by the reaction. One enzyme molecule catalyzes about a thousand reactions per second (the so-called turnover number ranges from $10^2\,s^{-1}$ to $10^7\,s^{-1}$). This leads to a rate acceleration of about 10^6- to 10^{12}-fold compared to the uncatalyzed, spontaneous reaction.

5.1.1
The Law of Mass Action

Biochemical kinetics is based on the mass action law, introduced by Guldberg and Waage in the 19th century (Waage and Guldberg 1864; Guldberg and Waage 1867, 1879). It states that the reaction rate is proportional to the probability of a collision of the reactants. This probability is in turn proportional to the concentration of reactants to the power of the molecularity, i. e., the number in which they enter the specific reaction. For a simple reaction like

$$S_1 + S_2 \rightleftharpoons 2P,\tag{5-11}$$

the reaction rate reads

$$v = v_+ - v_- = k_+ S_1 \cdot S_2 - k_- P^2.\tag{5-12}$$

v is the net rate, v_+ the rate of the forward reaction, v_- the rate of the backward reaction, and k_+ and k_- are the respective proportionality factors, the so-called kinetic or rate constants. The molecularity is 1 for each substrate of the forward reaction and 2 for the backward reaction. If we measure the concentration in moles per liter (mol $\cdot$ L^{-1} or M) and the time in seconds (s), then the rates have the unit M $\cdot$ s^{-1}. Accordingly, the rate constants for bimolecular reactions have the unit M $\cdot$ s^{-1}. Rate constants of monomolecular reactions have the dimension s^{-1}. The general mass action rate law for a reaction with substrate concentrations S_i and product concentrations P_j reads

$$v = v_+ - v_- = k_+ \prod_i S_i^{m_i} - k_- \prod_j P_j^{m_j},\tag{5-13}$$

where m_i and m_j denote the respective molecularities of S_i and P_j in this reaction (Heinrich and Schuster 1996).

The equilibrium constant K_{eq} (we will also use the simpler symbol q) characterizes the ratio of substrate and product concentrations in equilibrium (S_{eq} and P_{eq}), i.e., the state with equal forward and backward rates. The rate constants are related to K_{eq} in the following way:

$$K_{eq} = \frac{k_+}{k_-} = \frac{\prod P_{eq}}{\prod S_{eq}}.\tag{5-14}$$

The relation between the thermodynamic description and the kinetic description of biochemical reactions will be outlined in Section 5.1.2.

The dynamics of the concentrations for Eq. (5-11) is described by the ODEs

$$\frac{d}{dt} S_1 = \frac{d}{dt} S_2 = -v$$

$$\frac{d}{dt} P = 2v. \tag{5-15}$$

The time course of S_1, S_2 and P is obtained by integration of these ODEs.

Example 5-2

The kinetics of a simple decay such as

$$S \longrightarrow \tag{5-16}$$

is described by $v = kS$ and $\dfrac{d}{dt} S = -kS$. Integration of this ODE from time $t = 0$ with the initial concentration S_0 to an arbitrary time t with concentration $S(t)$, $\displaystyle\int_{S_0}^{S} \frac{dS}{S} = -\int_{t=0}^{t} k\,dt$, yields the temporal expression $S(t) = S_0 e^{-kt}$.

5.1.2
Reaction Kinetics and Thermodynamics

An important purpose of metabolism is to extract energy from nutrients, which is necessary for the synthesis of molecules, for growth, and for proliferation. We distinguish between energy-supplying reactions, energy-demanding reactions, and energetically neutral reactions. The principles of reversible thermodynamics and their application to chemical reactions allow understanding of energy circulation in the cell. This is eased by the assumption that biological reactions usually occur in hydrous solution at constant pressure and constant temperature with negligible volume changes.

Whether a reaction occurs spontaneously or not, in which direction a reaction proceeds, and the position of the equilibrium are important characteristics of a biochemical process. The first law of thermodynamics, i.e., the law of energy conservation, tells us only that the total energy of a system remains constant during any process. The second law of thermodynamics declares that a process occurs spontaneously only if it increases the total entropy of the system. Unfortunately, entropy is usually not directly measurable. A more suitable measure is the Gibbs free energy G, which is the energy capable of carrying out work under isotherm-isobar conditions, i.e., at constant temperature and constant pressure. The change of the free energy is given as

$$\Delta G = \Delta H - T \Delta S, \tag{5-17}$$

where ΔH is the change in enthalpy, ΔS is the change in entropy, and T is the absolute temperature in Kelvin. ΔG is a measure for the driving force, the spontaneity of a chemical reaction. If $\Delta G < 0$ then the reaction proceeds spontaneously under release of energy (exergonic process). If $\Delta G > 0$ then the reaction is energetically not favorable and will not occur spontaneously (endergonic process). $\Delta G = 0$ means that the system has reached its equilibrium. Endergonic reactions may proceed if they obtain energy from a strictly exergonic reaction by energetic coupling. Free energy is usually given for standard conditions (ΔG^0), i.e., for a concentration of the reaction partners of 1 M, temperature $T = 298$ K, and, for gaseous reactions, a pressure of $p = 98.1$ kPa = 1 atm. The unit is kJ mol^{-1}. For the free energy difference, a set of relations holds as follows. The free energy difference is related to redox potential $E_{red/ox}$:

$$\Delta G = -nF \cdot E_{red/ox} , \qquad (5\text{-}18)$$

where n is the number of transferred charges and F is the Faraday constant (96,500 coulomb). The free energy difference for a reaction can be calculated from the difference of the sums of free energies of its products P and its substrates S:

$$\Delta G = \sum G_P - \sum G_S . \qquad (5\text{-}19)$$

The enzyme cannot change the free energies of the substrates and products of a reaction, nor their differences, but it changes the so-called reaction path, thereby lowering the activation energy for the reaction. The transition state theory explains this (Haynie 2001). It has been observed that many substances or mixtures are thermodynamically unstable, since $\Delta G \ll 0$ (see Tab. 5.1). Nevertheless, they can be stored under normal conditions for a long time. The reason is that during the course of a reaction, the metabolites must pass one or more transition states of maximal free energy, in which bonds are solved or newly formed. The transition state is unstable; the respective molecule configuration is called an activated complex. It has a lifetime of around one molecule vibration, $10^{-14} \ldots 10^{-13}$ s, and it can hardly be experimentally verified. The difference $\Delta G^{\neq}$ of free energy between the reactants and

Tab. 5.1 Values of $\Delta G^{0\prime}$ for some important reactions

Reaction	$\Delta G^{0\prime}/(\text{kJ mol}^{-1})$
$2H_2 + O_2 \rightarrow 2\,H_2O$	-474
$2H_2O_2 \rightarrow 2\,H_2O + O_2$	-99
$PP_i + H_2O \rightarrow 2\,P_i$	-33.49
$ATP + H_2O \rightarrow ADP + P_i$	-30.56
Glucose-6-phosphate + H_2O → Glucose + P_i	-13.82
Glucose + P_i → Glucose-6-phosphate + H_2O	$+13.82$
Glucose-1-phosphate → Glucose-6-phosphate	-7.12
Glucose-6-phosphate → Fructose-6-phosphate	$+1.67$
Glucose + $6\,O_2 \rightarrow 6\,CO_2 + 6\,H_2O$	-2890

Source: Lehninger 1975

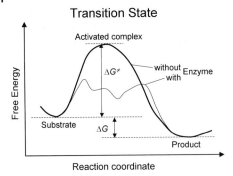

Transition State

Fig. 5.3 Presentation of the change of free energy along the course of reaction. The substrate and the product are situated in local minima of the free energy; the active complex is assigned to the local maximum. The enzyme may change the reaction path and thereby lower the barrier of free energy.

the activated complex determines the dynamics of a reaction: the higher this difference, the lower the probability that the molecules may pass this barrier and the lower the rate of the reaction. The value of $\Delta G^{\neq}$ depends on the type of altered bonds, on steric, electronic, or hydrophobic demands, and on temperature.

Figure 5.3 presents a simplified view of the reaction course. The substrate and the product are situated in local minima of the free energy; the active complex is assigned to the local maximum. The free energy difference ΔG is proportional to the logarithm of the equilibrium constant of the respective reaction:

$$\Delta G = -RT \ln K_{eq}, \tag{5-20}$$

(R – gas constant, $8.314 \, J \, mol^{-1} K^{-1}$). The value of $\Delta G^{\neq}$ corresponds to the kinetic constant k_+ of the forward reaction (Eqs. (12)–(14)) by $\Delta G^{\neq} = -RT \ln k_+$, while $\Delta G^{\neq} + \Delta G$ is related to the rate constant k_- of the backward reaction.

The interaction of the reactants with an enzyme may alter the reaction path and thereby lead to lower values of $\Delta G^{\neq}$. Furthermore, the free energy may assume more local minima and maxima along the path of reaction. They are related to unstable intermediary complexes. Values for the difference of free energy for some biologically important reactions are given in Tab. 5.1.

The detailed consideration of enzyme mechanisms by applying the mass action law for single events has led to a number of standard kinetic descriptions, which will be explained in the following sections.

5.1.3
Michaelis-Menten Kinetics

Brown (1902) proposed the first enzymatic mechanism for the reaction of invertase, which holds for all one-substrate reactions without backward reaction and without effectors in general:

$$E+S \underset{k_{-1}}{\overset{k_1}{\rightleftharpoons}} ES \overset{k_2}{\longrightarrow} E+P. \tag{5-21}$$

It comprises a reversible formation of an enzyme-substrate complex ES from the free enzyme E and the substrate S and an irreversible release of the product P from the enzyme E. The respective system of ODEs for the dynamics of this reaction reads as follows:

$$\frac{dS}{dt} = -k_1\, E \cdot S + k_{-1} ES \tag{5-22}$$

$$\frac{dES}{dt} = k_1\, E \cdot S - (k_{-1} + k_2)\, ES \tag{5-23}$$

$$\frac{dE}{dt} = -k_1\, E \cdot S + (k_{-1} + k_2)\, ES \tag{5-24}$$

$$\frac{dP}{dt} = k_2\, ES\,. \tag{5-25}$$

The rate of the reaction is equal to the negative rate of decay of the substrate as well as to the rate of product formation:

$$v = -\frac{dS}{dt} = \frac{dP}{dt}\,. \tag{5-26}$$

This ODE system (Eqs. (5-22)–(5-26)) cannot be solved analytically. Assumptions have been used to simplify this system in a satisfactory way. Michaelis and Menten (1913) assumed that the conversion of E and S to ES and vice versa is much faster than the decomposition of ES into E and P (so-called *quasi-equilibrium* between the free enzyme and the enzyme-substrate complex), or in terms of the constants

$$k_1, k_{-1} \gg k_2\,. \tag{5-27}$$

Briggs and Haldane (1925) assumed that during the course of reaction a state is reached where the concentration of the ES complex remains constant. This assumption is justified only if the initial concentration of the substrate is much larger than the concentration of the enzyme, $S(t = 0) \gg E$; otherwise, this steady state will never be reached. They suggested the more general assumption of a *quasi-steady state* of the ES complex:

$$\frac{dES}{dt} = 0\,. \tag{5-28}$$

An expression for the reaction rate will be derived using the ODE system in Eqs. (5-22)–(5-25) and the assumption of a quasi-steady state for ES. Adding Eqs. (5-23) and (5-24) results in

$$\frac{dES}{dt} + \frac{dE}{dt} = 0 \quad \text{or} \quad E_{total} = E + ES\,. \tag{5-29}$$

In this reaction, enzyme is neither produced nor consumed; it may be free or involved in the complex, but its total concentration remains constant.

Introducing Eq. (5-29) into Eq. (5-23) under the steady-state assumption (Eq. (5-28)) yields

$$ES = \frac{k_1 \, E_{total} \, S}{k_1 S + k_{-1} + k_2} = \frac{E_{total} \, S}{S + \dfrac{k_{-1} + k_2}{k_1}} \; . \tag{5-30}$$

For the reaction rate, this yields

$$v = \frac{k_2 \, E_{total} \, S}{S + \dfrac{k_{-1} + k_2}{k_1}} \; . \tag{5-31}$$

In enzyme kinetics it is convention to present Eq. (5-31) in a simpler form, which is important in both theory and practice:

$$v = \frac{V_{max} \, S}{S + K_m} \; . \tag{5-32}$$

Equation (5-32) is the expression for Michaelis-Menten kinetics. The parameters have the following meaning: the *maximal velocity*,

$$V_{max} = k_2 \, E_{total} \; , \tag{5-33}$$

is the maximal rate that can be attained when the enzyme is completely saturated with substrate. The *Michaelis constant*,

$$K_m = \frac{k_{-1} + k_2}{k_1} \; , \tag{5-34}$$

is equal to the substrate concentration that yields the half-maximal reaction rate. For the quasi-equilibrium assumption (Eq. (5-27)), it holds that $K_m \cong k_{-1}/k_1$. The meaning of the parameters can be seen from the plot of rate versus substrate concentration (Fig. 5.4). The plot has a hyperbolic shape.

Reaction v_1, Eq. (5-2), is described with Michaelis-Menten kinetics.

5.1.3.1 How to Derive a Rate Equation

Below we will present some enzyme kinetic standard examples. Individual mechanisms for your specific enzyme of interest may be more complicated or merely differ from these standards. Therefore, we summarize here the general way of deriving a rate equation.

1. Draw an illustration of all steps to consider (e.g., Eq. (5-21)). It contains all substrates and products (S and P) and n free or bound enzyme species (E and ES).

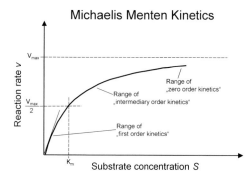

Fig. 5.4 Dependence of reaction rate v on substrate concentration S in Michaelis-Menten kinetics. V_{max} denotes the maximal reaction rate that can be reached for a large substrate concentration. K_m is the substrate concentration that results in a half-maximal reaction rate. For low substrate concentrations, v increases almost linearly with S, while for high substrate concentrations v is almost independent of S.

2. The right sites of the ODEs for the concentrations changes sum up the rates of all steps leading to or away from a certain substance (e.g., Eqs. (5-22)–(5-25)). The rates follow mass action kinetics (Eq. (5-12)).
3. The sum of all enzyme-containing species is equal to the total enzyme concentration E_{total} (the right side of all differential equations for enzyme species sum up to zero). This constitutes one equation.
4. The assumption of a quasi-steady state for $n-1$ enzyme species (i.e., setting the right sides of the respective ODEs equal to zero) together with step 3 results in n algebraic equations for the concentrations of the n enzyme species.
5. The reaction rate is equal to the rate of product formation (e.g., Eq. (5-26)). Introduce the respective concentrations of enzyme species resulting from step 4.

5.1.3.2 Parameter Estimation and Linearization of the Michaelis-Menten Equation

To assess the values of the parameters V_{max} and K_m for an isolated enzyme, one measures the initial rates for different initial concentrations of the substrate. Since the rate is a nonlinear function of the substrate concentration, one has to determine the parameters by nonlinear regression. Another way is to transform Eq. (5-32) to a linear relation between variables and then apply linear regression.

The advantage of the transformed equations is that one may read the parameter values more or less directly from the graph obtained by linear regression of the measurement data. In the Lineweaver-Burk plot (Lineweaver and Burk 1934) (Tab. 5.2), the values for V_{max} and K_m can be obtained from the intersections of the graph with the ordinate and the abscissa, respectively. The Lineweaver-Burk plot is also helpful for discrimination of different types of inhibitions (see below). The drawback of the transformed equations is that they may be sensitive to errors for low or high substrate concentrations or rates. Eadie and Hofstee (Eadie 1942) and Hanes and Woolf (Hanes 1932) have introduced other types of linearization to overcome this limitation.

Tab. 5.2 Different approaches for the linearization of Michaelis-Menten enzyme kinetics.

	Lineweaver-Burk	Eadie-Hofstee	Hanes-Woolf
Transformed equation	$\dfrac{1}{v} = \dfrac{K_m}{V_{max}} \dfrac{1}{S} + \dfrac{1}{V_{max}}$	$v = V_{max} - K_m \dfrac{v}{S}$	$\dfrac{S}{v} = \dfrac{S}{V_{max}} + \dfrac{K_m}{V_{max}}$
New variables	$\dfrac{1}{v}, \dfrac{1}{S}$	$v, \dfrac{v}{S}$	$\dfrac{S}{v}, S$
Graphical representation			

5.1.3.3 The Michaelis-Menten Equation for Reversible Reactions

In practice, many reactions are reversible. The enzyme may catalyze the reaction in both directions. Consider the following mechanism:

$$E + S \underset{k_{-1}}{\overset{k_1}{\rightleftharpoons}} ES \underset{k_{-2}}{\overset{k_2}{\rightleftharpoons}} E + P . \tag{5-35}$$

The product formation is given by

$$\frac{dP}{dt} = k_2 ES - k_{-2} P = v , \tag{5-36}$$

and the respective rate equation reads

$$v = E_{total} \frac{Sq - P}{\dfrac{Sk_1}{k_{-1}k_{-2}} + \dfrac{1}{k_{-2}} + \dfrac{k_2}{k_{-1}k_{-2}} + \dfrac{P}{k_{-1}}} = \frac{\dfrac{V_{max}^{for}}{K_{mS}} S - \dfrac{V_{max}^{back}}{K_{mP}} P}{1 + \dfrac{S}{K_{mS}} + \dfrac{P}{K_{mP}}} . \tag{5-37}$$

While the parameters k_{+1} and k_{+2} are the kinetic constants of the individual reaction steps, the phenomenological parameters V_{max}^{for} and V_{max}^{back} denote the maximal velocity in forward or backward direction, respectively, under zero product or substrate concentration, and the phenomenological parameters K_{mS} and K_{mP} denote the substrate or product concentration causing half maximal forward or backward rate. They are related in the following way:

$$K_{eq} = \frac{V_{max}^{for} K_{mP}}{V_{max}^{back} K_{mS}} \tag{5-38}$$

(Haldane 1930). Reaction v_3, Eq. (5-4), is of the reversible Michaelis-Menten type.

5.1.4

Regulation of Enzyme Activity by Protein Interaction

Enzymes can immensely increase the rate of a reaction, but this is not their only function. Enzymes are involved in metabolic regulation in various ways. Their production and degradation are often adapted to the current requirements of the cell. Furthermore, they may be targets of effectors, both inhibitors and activators.

The effectors are proteins or other molecules that influence the performance of the enzymatic reaction. The interaction of effector and enzyme changes the reaction rate. Such regulatory interactions that are crucial for the fine-tuning of metabolism will be considered here (Schellenberger 1989).

Basic types of inhibition are distinguished by the enzyme's state, in which the enzyme may bind the effector (i.e., the free enzyme E, the enzyme-substrate complex ES, or both), and by the ability of different complexes to release the product. The general pattern of inhibition is schematically represented in Fig. 5.5. The different types result if some of the reactions cannot occur.

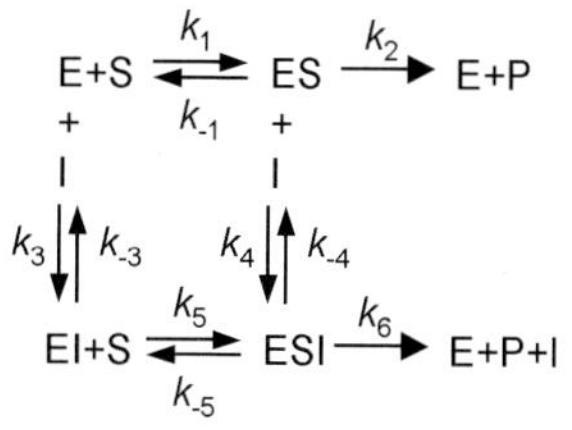

Fig. 5.5 General scheme of inhibition in Michaelis-Menten kinetics. Reactions 1 and 2 belong to the standard scheme of Michaelis-Menten kinetics. Competitive inhibition is given if in addition reaction 3 (and not reactions 4, 5, or 6) occurs. Uncompetitive inhibition involves reactions 1, 2, and 4, and noncompetitive inhibition comprises reactions 1, 2, 3, 4, and 5. Appearance of reaction 6 indicates partial inhibition.

The rate equations are derived according to the following scheme:

1. Consider binding equilibriums between compounds and their complexes:

$$K_m \cong \frac{k_{-1}}{k_1} = \frac{E \cdot S}{ES}, \quad K_{I,3} = \frac{k_{-3}}{k_3} = \frac{E \cdot I}{EI}, \quad K_{I,4} = \frac{k_{-4}}{k_4} = \frac{ES \cdot I}{ESI}, \quad K_{I,5} = \frac{k_{-5}}{k_5} = \frac{EI \cdot S}{ESI}$$

$$(5\text{-}39)$$

Note that if all reactions can occur, the Wegscheider condition (Wegscheider 1902) holds in the form

$$\frac{k_1 \, k_4}{k_{-1} \, k_{-4}} = \frac{k_3 \, k_5}{k_{-3} \, k_{-5}},$$

$$(5\text{-}40)$$

which means that the difference in the free energies between E and ESI is independent of the choice of the reaction path (via ES or EI).

2. Take into account the moiety conservation for the total enzyme (include only those complexes that occur in the course of reaction):

$$E_{total} = E + ES + EI + ESI.$$

$$(5\text{-}41)$$

3. The reaction rate is equal to the rate of product formation:

$$v = \frac{dP}{dt} = k_2 ES + k_6 ESI. \qquad (5\text{-}42)$$

Equations (5-39)–(5-41) comprise four independent equations for the four unknown concentrations of E, ES, EI, and ESI. Their solution can be inserted into Eq. (5-42). The effect of the inhibitor depends on the concentrations of substrate and inhibitor and on the relative affinities to the enzyme. Table 5.3 lists the different types of inhibition for irreversible and reversible Michaelis-Menten kinetics together with the respective rate equations.

In the case of competitive inhibition, the inhibitor competes with the substrate for the binding site (or inhibits substrate binding by binding elsewhere to the enzyme) without being transformed itself. An example of this type is the inhibition of succinate dehydrogenase by malonate. The enzyme converts succinate to fumarate, forming a double bond. Malonate has two carboxyl groups, like the proper substrates, and may bind to the enzyme, but the formation of a double bond cannot take place. Since substrates and the inhibitor compete for the binding sites, a high concentration of one of them may displace the other one. For very high substrate concentrations, the same maximal velocity as without inhibitor is reached, but the effective K_m value is increased.

In the case of uncompetitive inhibition, the inhibitor I binds only to the ES complex. The reason may be that the substrate binding causes a conformational change, which opens a new binding site. Since S and I do not compete for binding sites, an increase in the concentration of S cannot displace the inhibitor. In the presence of inhibitor, the original maximal rate cannot be reached (lower V_{max}). For example, an inhibitor concentration of $I = K_{I,4}$ halves the K_m value as well as V_{max}. Uncompetitive inhibition occurs rarely for one-substrate reactions, but more frequently in the case of two substrates. One example is inhibition of arylsulfatase by hydrazine.

Noncompetitive inhibition is present if substrate binding to the enzyme does not alter the binding of the inhibitor. There must be different binding sites for substrate and inhibitor. In the classical case, the inhibitor has the same affinity to the enzyme with or without bound substrate. If the affinity changes, this is called mixed inhibition. A standard example is inhibition of chymotrypsin by H^+ ions.

If the product can also be formed from the enzyme-substrate-inhibitor complex, the inhibition is only partial. For high rates of product release (high values of k_6), this can even present an activating instead of an inhibiting effect.

Competitive, uncompetitive, and noncompetitive inhibition also apply for the reversible Michaelis-Menten mechanism. The respective rate equations are also listed in Tab. 5.3.

Tab. 5-3 Types of inhibition for irreversible and reversible Michaelis-Menten kinetics.

Name	Implementation	Equation – irreversible	Equation – reversible case	Characteristics
Competitive inhibiton	I binds only to free E; P-release only from ES-complex $k_{\pm4} = k_{\pm5} = k_6 = 0$	$v = \dfrac{V_{max}\, S}{K_m \cdot i_3 + S}$	$v = \dfrac{V_{max}^f\, \dfrac{S}{K_{mS}} - V_{max}^r\, \dfrac{P}{K_{mP}}}{\dfrac{S}{K_{mS}} + \dfrac{P}{K_{mP}} + i_3}$	K_m changes, V_{max} remains; S and I compete for the binding place; high S may out compete I
Uncompetitive inhibition	I binds only to the ES-complex; P-release only from ES-complex $k_{\pm3} = k_{\pm5} = k_6 = 0$	$v = \dfrac{V_{max}\, S}{K_m + S \cdot i_4}$	$v = \dfrac{V_{max}^f\, \dfrac{S}{K_{mS}} - V_{max}^r\, \dfrac{P}{K_{mP}}}{1 + \left(\dfrac{S}{K_{mS}} + \dfrac{P}{K_{mP}}\right) \cdot i_4}$	K_m and V_{max} change, but their ratio remains; S may not out compete I
Noncompetitive inhibition	I binds to E and ES; P-release only from ES $K_{I,3} = K_{I,4},\ k_6 = 0$	$v = \dfrac{V_{max}\, S}{(K_m + S) \cdot i_3}$	$v = \dfrac{V_{max}^f\, \dfrac{S}{K_{mS}} - V_{max}^r\, \dfrac{P}{K_{mP}}}{\left(1 + \dfrac{S}{K_{mS}} + \dfrac{P}{K_{mP}}\right) \cdot i_4}$	K_m remains, V_{max} changes; S may not out compete I
Mixed inhibition	I binds to E and ES; P-release only from ES $K_{I,3} \neq K_{I,4},\ k_6 = 0$	$v = \dfrac{V_{max}\, S}{K_m \cdot i_4 + S \cdot i_3}$		K_m and V_{max} change; $K_{I,3} > K_{I,4}$: competitive-noncompetitive inhibition; $K_{I,3} < K_{I,4}$: noncompetitive-uncompetitive inhibition
Partial inhibition	I may bind to E and ES; P-release from ES and ESI $K_{I,3} \neq K_{I,4},\ k_6 \neq 0$	$v = \dfrac{V_{max}\, S \left(1 + \dfrac{k_6 \cdot I}{k_2 K_{I,3}}\right)}{K_m \cdot i_4 + S \cdot i_3}$		K_m and V_{max} change; if $k_6 > k_2$, activation instead of inhibition.

Abbreviations: $K_{I,3} = \dfrac{k_{-3}}{k_3}$, $K_{I,4} = \dfrac{k_{-4}}{k_4}$, $i_3 = 1 + \dfrac{I}{K_{I,3}}$, $i_4 = 1 + \dfrac{I}{K_{I,4}}$

5.1.5
Inhibition by Irreversible Binding of Inhibitor to Enzyme

An irreversible inhibitor binds irreversibly to the active site of the enzyme:

$$E + I \longrightarrow EI .$$ (5-43)

This prevents binding of the appropriate substrate and may destroy the catalytic center and lead to a denaturation of the enzymes. In any case, an initial inhibitor concentration of I_0 decreases the effective concentration of the enzyme from the initial concentration E_0 to the value $E_0 - I_0$. A molar excess of inhibitor leads to complete loss of catalytic activity. At a molar excess of enzyme, this yields a reduction of maximal velocity to $V'_{max} = k_2(E_0 - I_0)$.

Example 5-3

Covalent binding of iodacetate to SH groups of proteins:

$$E - SH + I \cdot CH_2 \cdot CO_2^- \longrightarrow E - S - CH_2 \cdot CO_2^- + HI$$

5.1.6
Substrate Inhibition

A common characteristic of enzymatic reactions is the increase of the reaction rate with increasing substrate concentration S up to the maximal velocity V_{max}. But in some cases, a decrease of the rate above a certain value of S is recorded. A possible reason for this is the binding of a further substrate molecule to the enzyme-substrate complex, yielding the complex ESS, which cannot form a product. This kind of inhibition is reversible if the second substrate can be released. The rate equation can be derived using the scheme of uncompetitive inhibition by replacing the inhibitor by another substrate. It reads,

$$v = k_2\, ES = \frac{V_{max}\, S}{K_m + S\left(1 + \dfrac{S}{K_I}\right)} .$$ (5-44)

This expression has a maximum at

$$S_{opt} = \sqrt{K_m K_I} \quad \text{with} \quad v_{opt} = \frac{V_{max}}{1 + 2\sqrt{K_m/K_I}} .$$ (5-45)

The dependence of v on S is shown in Fig. 5.6. A typical example for substrate inhibition is the binding of two succinate molecules to malonate dehydrogenase, which possesses two binding pockets for the carboxyl group. This is schematically represented in Fig. 5.6.

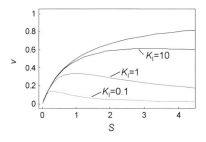 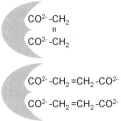

Fig. 5.6 Plot of reaction rate v against substrate concentration S for the case of substrate inhibition. The upper curve shows Michaelis-Menten kinetics without inhibition, and the lower curves show kinetics for the indicated values of binding constant K_I. Parameter values: $V_{max} = 1$, $K_m = 1$. The left part visualizes a possible mechanism for substrate inhibition. The enzyme (gray object) has two binding pockets to bind different parts of a substrate molecule (upper scheme). In the case of high substrate concentration, two different molecules may enter the binding pockets, thereby preventing the specific reaction (lower scheme).

5.1.7
Inhibition by Binding of Inhibitor to Substrate

The reaction rate is also decreased if an inhibitor forms a tight complex with the substrate:

$$S + I \longrightarrow SI. \tag{5-46}$$

The effective substrate concentration is decreased to $S_{eff} = S_0 - SI$. According to the mass action law, for the actual concentrations it holds that

$$\frac{(I_0 - SI)(S_0 - SI)}{SI} = K_I. \tag{5-47}$$

This allows calculating of the effective enzyme concentration:

$$S_{eff} = S_0 - \frac{I_0 + S_0 + K_I}{2} + \sqrt{\left(\frac{I_0 + S_0 + K_I}{2}\right)^2 - S_0 \cdot I_0}. \tag{5-48}$$

At high substrate concentrations, the reaction rate in the presence of an inhibitor reaches the maximal velocity of the non-inhibited reaction. The Lineweaver-Burk plot is nonlinear.

5.1.8
Binding of Ligands to Proteins

Every molecule that binds to a protein is a ligand, irrespective of whether it is the subject of a reaction or not. Below we consider binding to monomer and oligomer proteins. In oligomers, there may be interactions between the binding sites on the subunits.

Consider binding of one ligand (S) to a protein (E) with only one binding site:

$$E+S \rightleftharpoons ES. \tag{5-49}$$

The binding constant K_B is given by

$$K_B = \frac{ES}{E \cdot S}. \tag{5-50}$$

The reciprocal of K_B is the dissociation constant K_D. The fractional saturation Y of the protein is determined by the number of subunits that have bound ligands, divided by the total number of subunits. The fractional saturation for one subunit is

$$Y = \frac{ES}{E_{total}} = \frac{ES}{ES + E} = \frac{K_B \cdot S}{K_B \cdot S + 1}. \tag{5-51}$$

The plot of Y versus S at a constant total enzyme concentration is a hyperbola, like the plot of v versus S in the Michaelis-Menten kinetics. In a process where the binding of S to E is the first step, followed by product release, and where the initial concentration of S is much higher than the initial concentration of E, the rate is proportional to the concentration of ES and it holds that

$$\frac{v}{V_{max}} = \frac{ES}{E_{total}} = Y. \tag{5-52}$$

If the protein has several binding sites, then interactions may occur between these sites, i.e., the affinity to further ligands may change after binding of one or more ligands. This phenomenon is called cooperativity. Positive or negative cooperativity denotes an increase or decrease, respectively, in the affinity of the protein to a further ligand. Homotropic or heterotropic cooperativity denotes that the binding to a certain ligand influences the affinity of the protein to a further ligand of the same or another type, respectively.

5.1.9
Positive Homotropic Cooperativity and the Hill Equation

Consider a dimeric protein with two identical binding sites. The binding to the first ligand facilitates the binding to the second ligand:

$$E_2 + S \xrightarrow{slow} E_2 S$$
$$E_2 S + S \xrightarrow{fast} E_2 S_2, \tag{5-53}$$

where E is a monomer and E_2 a dimer. The fractional saturation is given by

$$Y = \frac{E_2 S + 2 E_2 S_2}{2 E_{2,total}} = \frac{E_2 S + E_2 S_2}{2 E_2 + 2 E_2 S + 2 E_2 S_2}. \tag{5-54}$$

If the affinity to the second ligand is strongly increased by binding to the first ligand, then E_2S will react with S as soon as it is formed, and the concentration of E_2S can be neglected. In the case of complete cooperativity, i.e., every protein is either empty or fully bound, Eq. (5-53) reduces to

$$E_2 + 2S \longrightarrow E_2S_2. \qquad (5\text{-}55)$$

The binding constant reads

$$K_B = \frac{E_2 S_2}{E_2 \cdot S^2}, \qquad (5\text{-}56)$$

and the fractional saturation is

$$Y = \frac{2\,E_2 S_2}{2\,E_{2,total}} = \frac{E_2 S_2}{E_2 + E_2 S_2} = \frac{K_B S^2}{1 + K_B S^2}. \qquad (5\text{-}57)$$

Generally, for a protein with n subunits it holds that

$$v = V_{max} Y = \frac{V_{max} K_B S^n}{1 + K_B S^n}. \qquad (5\text{-}58)$$

This is the general form of the *Hill equation*. It implies complete homotropic cooperativity. Plotting the fractional saturation Y versus substrate concentration S yields a sigmoid curve with the inflection point at $1/K_B$. The quantity n (often "h" is used instead) is termed the Hill coefficient.

The derivation of this expression was based on experimental findings concerning the binding of oxygen to hemoglobin (Hb) (Hill 1910, 1913). In 1904 Bohr and co-workers found that the plot of the fractional saturation of Hb with oxygen against the oxygen partial pressure had a sigmoid shape. Hill (1909) explained this with interactions between the binding sites located at the hem subunits. At this time it was already known that every subunit hem binds one molecule of oxygen. Hill assumed complete cooperativity and predicted an experimental Hill coefficient of 2.8. Today it is known that hemoglobin has four binding sites but that the cooperativity is not complete. The sigmoidal binding characteristic has the advantage that Hb binds strongly to oxygen in the lung with a high oxygen partial pressure, while it can release O_2 easily in the body with low oxygen partial pressure.

5.1.10
The Monod-Wyman-Changeux Rate Expression for Enzymes with Sigmoid Kinetics

In 1965 Monod and colleagues presented a model explaining sigmoidal enzyme kinetics taking into account the interaction of subunits of an enzyme (Monod et al. 1965). A more comprehensive model has been presented by Koshland et al. (1966). The model of Monod et al. uses the following assumptions: (1) the enzyme consists of n identical subunits, (2) each subunit can assume an active (R) or an inactive (T) conformation, (3) all subunits change their conformations at the same time (concerted change), and (4) the equilibrium between the R and the T conformations is given by an allosteric constant:

$$L = \frac{T_0}{R_0} \, . \tag{5-59}$$

The index i for T_i and R_i denotes the number of bound substrate molecules. The binding constants for the active and inactive conformations are given by K_R and K_T, respectively. If substrate molecules can bind only to the active form, i.e., if $K_T = 0$, then the rate can be given as

$$V = \frac{V_{max} K_R S}{(1 + K_R S)} \frac{1}{\left(1 + \dfrac{L}{(1 + K_R S)^n}\right)} \, , \tag{5-60}$$

where the factor $\dfrac{V_{max} K_R S}{(1 + K_R S)}$ corresponds to the Michaelis-Menten rate expression, while the factor $\left(1 + \dfrac{L}{(1 + K_R S)^n}\right)^{-1}$ is a regulatory factor.

For $L = 0$ the plot v versus S is a hyperbola as in Michaelis-Menten kinetics. For $L > 0$ one gets a sigmoid curve shifted to the right. A typical value for the allosteric constant is $L \cong 10^4$.

In the case that the substrate can also bind to the inactive state ($K_T \neq 0$), one gets

$$V = \frac{V_{max} S}{(1 + K_R S)} \frac{K_R + K_T L \left(\dfrac{1 + K_T S}{1 + K_R S}\right)^{n-1}}{\left(1 + L \left(\dfrac{1 + K_T S}{1 + K_R S}\right)^n\right)} \, . \tag{5-61}$$

Up to now we have considered only homotropic and positive effects in the model of Monod, Wyman, and Changeux. But this model is also well suited to explain the dependence of the reaction rate on activators and inhibitors. Activators A bind only to the active conformation, and inhibitors I bind only to the inactive conformation. This shifts the equilibrium to the respective conformation. Effectively, the binding to effectors changes L:

$$L' = L \frac{(1 + K_I I)^n}{(1 + K_A A)^n} \, . \tag{5-62}$$

K_I and K_A denote binding constants. The interaction with effectors is a heterotropic effect. An activator weakens the sigmoidity, while an inhibitor strengthens it as shown in Figure 5.7.

As an example, the kinetics of the enzyme phosphofructokinase, which catalyzes the transformation of fructose-6-phosphate and ATP to fructose-1,6-bisphosphate,

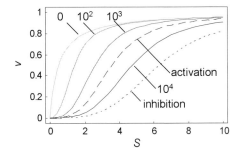

Fig. 5.7 Model of Monod, Wyman, and Changeux: Dependence of the reaction rate on substrate concentration for different values of the allosteric constant L, according to Eq. (5-60). Parameters: $V_{max} = 1$, $n = 4$, $K_R = 2$, $K_T = 0$. The value of L is indicated at the curves. Obviously, increasing the value of L causes stronger sigmoidity. The influence of activators or inhibitors (compare Eq. (5-62)) is illustrated with the dotted line for $K_I I = 2$ and with the dashed line for $K_A A = 2$ ($L = 10^4$ in both cases).

can be described by the model of Monod, Wyman, and Changeux. AMP, NH_4, and K+ are activators, while ATP is an inhibitor (see Example 5-1).

5.2
Metabolic Networks

In this section we will discuss basic structural and dynamic properties of metabolic networks. We will introduce a stoichiometric description of networks and learn how moieties and fluxes are balanced within networks.

The basic elements of a metabolic network model are (1) the substances with their concentrations and (2) the reactions or transport processes changing the concentrations of the substances. In biological environments, reactions are usually catalyzed by enzymes, and transport steps are carried out by transport proteins or by pores. Thus they can be assigned to identifiable biochemical compounds.

Stoichiometric coefficients denote the proportion of substrate and product molecules involved in a reaction. For example, for the reaction depicted in Eq. (5-11), the stoichiometric coefficients of S_1, S_2, and P are –1, –1, and 2. The assignment of stoichiometric coefficients is not unique. We could also argue that for the production of one mole P, half a mole of each S_1 and S_2 have to be used and therefore choose –1/2, –1/2, and 1. Or, if we change the direction of the reaction, then we may choose 1, 1, and –2.

The change of concentrations in time can be described using ODEs. For the reaction depicted in Eq. (5-11) and the first choice of stoichiometric coefficients, we have

$$\frac{dS_1}{dt} = -v, \quad \frac{dS_2}{dt} = -v, \quad \text{and} \quad \frac{dP}{dt} = 2v. \tag{5-63}$$

This means that the degradation of S_1 with rate v is accompanied by the degradation of S_2 with the same rate and by the production of P with the double rate.

5.2.1
Systems Equations

For a metabolic network consisting of m substances and r reactions, the systems dynamics is described by systems equations (or balance equations, since the balance of substrate production and degradation is considered):

$$\frac{dS_i}{dt} = \sum_{j=1}^{r} n_{ij} v_j \quad \text{for} \quad i = 1, .., m \tag{5-64}$$

(Glansdorff and Prigogine 1971; Reder 1988). The quantities n_{ij} are the stoichiometric coefficients of metabolite i in reaction j. Here, we assume that the reactions are the only reason for concentration changes and that no mass flow occurs due to convection or to diffusion. The balance equations (Eq. (5-64)) can also be applied if the system consists of several compartments. In this case, every compound in different compartments has to be considered as an individual compound, and transport steps are formally considered as reactions transferring the compound belonging to one compartment into the same compound belonging to the other compartment.

The stoichiometric coefficients n_{ij} assigned to the substances S_i and the reactions v_j can be combined into the so-called *stoichiometric matrix*

$$N = \{n_{ij}\} \quad \text{for} \quad i = 1, .., m \quad \text{and} \quad j = 1, .., r, \tag{5-65}$$

where each column belongs to a reaction and each row to a substance.

Example 5-4

For the simple network

$$\xrightarrow{v_1} S_1 \xleftrightarrow{v_2} 2S_2 \xleftrightarrow{v_3} , \\ \Big\downarrow v_4 \\ S_3 \tag{5-66}$$

the stoichiometric matrix reads

$$N = \begin{pmatrix} 1 & -1 & 0 & -1 \\ 0 & 2 & -1 & 0 \\ 0 & 0 & 0 & 1 \end{pmatrix}. \tag{5-67}$$

Note that in Eq. (5-66) all reactions may be reversible. In order to determine the signs of N, the direction of the arrows is artificially assigned as positive "from left to right" and "from the top down." If, for example, the net flow proceeds from S_3 to S_1, the value of rate v_4 is negative.

Altogether, the mathematical description of the metabolic system consists of a vector $S = (S_1, S_2, ..., S_n)^T$ of concentration values, a vector $v = (v_1, v_2, ..., v_r)^T$ of reaction rates, a parameter vector $p = (p_1, p_2, ..., p_m)^T$, and the stoichiometric matrix N. If the system is in steady state, we can also consider the vector $J = (J_1, J_2, ..., J_r)^T$ containing the steady state fluxes. With these notions, the balance equation reads

$$\frac{dS}{dt} = Nv.$$ (5-68)

Example 5-5

For our running example (Example 5-1) of the upper glycolysis model, the concentration vector is

$$S = \begin{pmatrix} Gluc6P \\ Fruc6P \\ Fruc1,6P_2 \\ ATP \\ ADP \\ AMP \end{pmatrix},$$ (5-69)

the vector of reaction rates is $v = (v_1, v_2, ..., v_8)^T$, the parameter vector is given by

$$p = \Big(Glucose, V_{max,1}, K_{ATP,1}, K_{Glucose,1}, k_2, V_{max,3}^f, V_{max,3}^r, K_{Gluc6P,3}, K_{Fruc6P,3}, \\ V_{max,4}, K_{F6P,4}, \kappa_4, k_5, k_6, k_7, k_{8f}, k_{8r} \Big)^T,$$ (5-70)

and the stoichiometric matrix reads

$$N = \begin{pmatrix} 1 & -1 & -1 & 0 & 0 & 0 & 0 & 0 \\ 0 & 0 & 1 & -1 & 0 & 0 & 0 & 0 \\ 0 & 0 & 0 & 1 & -1 & 0 & 0 & 0 \\ -1 & -1 & 0 & -1 & 0 & 1 & -1 & -1 \\ 1 & 1 & 0 & 1 & 0 & -1 & 1 & 2 \\ 0 & 0 & 0 & 0 & 0 & 0 & 0 & -1 \end{pmatrix}.$$ (5-71)

5.2.2
Information Contained in the Stoichiometric Matrix N

The stoichiometric matrix contains important information about the structure of the metabolic network. Using the stoichiometric matrix, we can calculate which combinations of individual fluxes are possible in steady state (i.e., calculate the admissible steady-state flux space). We may easily discover dead ends and unbranched reaction pathways. In addition, we may find out the conservation relations for the included reactants.

In steady state it holds that

$$\frac{dS}{dt} = Nv = 0 \tag{5-72}$$

(Reder 1988). The right equality sign denotes a linear equation system for determination of the rates v. This equation has nontrivial solutions only for *Rank $N < r$* (Chapter 3, Section 3.1). The kernel matrix K fulfilling

$$NK = 0 \tag{5-73}$$

can express the respective linear dependencies (Heinrich and Schuster 1996). The choice of the kernel is not unique. It can be determined using the Gauss algorithm described in Chapter 3 (Section 3.1). It contains as columns $r - $ *Rank N* basis vectors. Every possible set of steady-state fluxes can be expressed as a linear combination of the columns k_i of K

$$J = \sum_{i=1}^{r-RankN} \alpha_i \cdot k_i . \tag{5-74}$$

The coefficients must have respective units ($M \cdot s^{-1}$ or $mol \cdot L^{-1} \cdot s^{-1}$).

Example 5-6

For the system

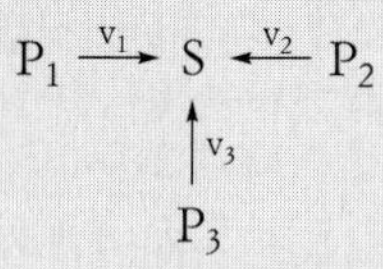

$$P_1 \xrightarrow{v_1} S \xleftarrow{v_2} P_2$$
$$\uparrow v_3 \tag{5-75}$$
$$P_3$$

the stoichiometric matrix is $N = (1 \ 1 \ 1)$. We have $r = 3$ reactions and *Rank $N = 1$*. Each representation of the kernel matrix contains $3 - 1 = 2$ basis vectors, e.g.,

$$K = \begin{pmatrix} k_1 & k_2 \end{pmatrix} \quad \text{with} \quad k_1 = \begin{pmatrix} 1 \\ -1 \\ 0 \end{pmatrix}, \ k_2 = \begin{pmatrix} 1 \\ 0 \\ 1 \end{pmatrix}, \tag{5-76}$$

and for the steady state flux it holds that

$$J = \alpha_1 \cdot k_1 + \alpha_2 \cdot k_2 . \tag{5-77}$$

Example 5-7

The stoichiometric matrix for the running example is given in Eq. (5-71). It comprises $r = 8$ reactions and has $Rank = 5$. Thus the kernel matrix has three linearly independent columns. A possible solution of Eq. (5-73) is

$$K = \begin{pmatrix} k_1 & k_2 & k_3 \end{pmatrix} \quad \text{with} \quad k_1 = \begin{pmatrix} -1 \\ -1 \\ 0 \\ 0 \\ 0 \\ 0 \\ 2 \\ 0 \end{pmatrix}, \quad k_2 = \begin{pmatrix} 1 \\ 1 \\ 0 \\ 0 \\ 0 \\ 2 \\ 0 \\ 0 \end{pmatrix}, \quad k_3 = \begin{pmatrix} 0 \\ -1 \\ 1 \\ 1 \\ 1 \\ 0 \\ 0 \\ 0 \end{pmatrix}. \qquad (5\text{-}78)$$

If the entries in a certain row are zero in all basis vectors, we have found an equilibrium reaction. In any steady state, the net rate of the respective reaction must be zero.

Example 5-8

For the reaction system in Eq. (5-66), the stoichiometric matrix reads

$$N = \begin{pmatrix} 1 & -1 & 0 & -1 \\ 0 & 2 & -2 & 0 \\ 0 & 0 & 0 & 1 \end{pmatrix}$$ with $r = 4$ and $Rank\ N = 3$. Its kernel consists only of one

column $K = (1\ 1\ 1\ 0)^T$. Hence it yields $v_4 = \sum_{i=1}^{1} \alpha \cdot 0 = 0$. In any steady state, the rates of production and degradation of S_3 must equal.

Example 5-9

For the running example, the entry in the last row of the kernel matrix, Eq. (5-78), is always zero. Hence, in steady state the rate of reaction v_8 must always vanish.

If all basis vectors contain the same entries for a set of rows, this indicates an unbranched reaction path. In each steady state, the net rate of all respective reactions is equal.

Example 5-10

Consider the reaction scheme

$$\xrightarrow{v_1} S_1 \xleftrightarrow{v_2} S_2 \xleftrightarrow{v_3} S_3 \xrightarrow{v_4} \ . \qquad\qquad \text{(with } v_6 \text{ up from } S_2, \ v_5 \text{ down from } S_1)$$

(5-79)

The system comprises $r = 6$ reactions. The stoichiometric matrix reads

$$N = \begin{pmatrix} 1 & -1 & 0 & 0 & -1 & 0 \\ 0 & 1 & -1 & 0 & 0 & 0 \\ 0 & 0 & 1 & -1 & 0 & 1 \end{pmatrix} \text{ with } Rank\, N = 3.$$ Thus the kernel matrix is spanned

by three basis vectors, e.g., $k_1 = (1\ 1\ 1\ 0\ 0\ -1)^T$, $k_2 = (1\ 0\ 0\ 0\ 1\ 0)^T$, and
$k_3 = (-1\ -1\ -1\ -1\ 0\ 0)^T$. The entries for the second and third reactions are always equal; thus, in any steady state the fluxes through reactions 2 and 3 must be equal.

Example 5-11

In the glycolysis model, the entries for the third, fourth, and fifth reactions are equal for each column of the kernel matrix (Eq. (5-78)). Therefore, reactions 3–5 constitute an unbranched pathway. In steady state, they must have equal rates.

Up to now, we have not been concerned about (ir)reversibility of reactions in the network. If a certain reaction is considered irreversible, this has no consequences for the stoichiometric matrix N but rather for the kernel K. The set of vectors belonging to K is restricted by the condition that some values may not become negative (or positive, depending on the definition of flux direction). If in Example 5-9 reaction 4 is considered irreversible, then the columns of K must not contain a negative entry in the fourth row. Choosing $k_3 = (a\ a\ a\ a\ 0\ 0)^T$ with $a > 0$ fulfills this condition.

5.2.3
Elementary Flux Modes and Extreme Pathways

The definition of the term "pathway" in a metabolic network is not straightforward. A descriptive definition of a pathway is a set of subsequent reactions that are in each case linked by common metabolites. Typical examples include glycolysis or amino acid synthesis. More detailed inspection of metabolic maps such as the Boehringer map (Michal 1999) shows that metabolism is highly interconnected. Pathways that have been known for a long time from biochemical experience are hard to recognize. It is even harder to discover new pathways, e.g., in metabolic maps that have been reconstructed from sequence data for bacteria.

This problem has been elaborated in the concept of *elementary flux modes* (Heinrich and Schuster 1996; Pfeiffer et al. 1999; Schilling et al. 1999; Schuster et al. 1999, 2000, 2002). Here, the stoichiometry of a metabolic network is investigated to find out which direct routes are possible that lead from one external metabolite to another external metabolite. The approach takes into account that some reactions are reversible, while others are irreversible.

A flux mode *M* is set of flux vectors that represent such direct routes through the metabolic networks. In mathematical terms it is defined as the set

$$M = \{v \in R^r \mid v = \lambda v^*, \lambda > 0\}, \tag{5-80}$$

where v^* is an r-dimensional vector (unequal to the null vector) fulfilling two conditions: (1) steady state, i.e., Eq. (72), and (2) sign restriction, i.e., the flux directions in v^* fulfill the prescribed irreversibility relations.

A flux mode *M* comprising *v* is called reversible if the set *M'* comprising $-v$ is also a flux mode. A flux mode is an elementary flux mode if it uses a minimal set of reactions and cannot be further decomposed, i.e., the vector *v* cannot be represented as a nonnegative linear combination of two vectors that fulfill conditions (1) and (2) but contain more zero entries than *v*. The number of elementary flux modes is equal to or higher than the number of basis vectors of the null space.

Example 5-12

The systems A and B differ by the (ir)reversibility of reaction 2.

A
$$S_0 \xleftrightarrow{v_1} S_1 \xleftrightarrow{v_2} 2S_2 \xleftrightarrow{v_3} S_4$$
$$\uparrow v_4$$
$$S_3$$

B
$$S_0 \xleftrightarrow{v_1} S_1 \xrightarrow{v_2} 2S_2 \xleftrightarrow{v_3} S_4 \tag{5-81}$$
$$\uparrow v_4$$
$$S_3$$

The elementary flux modes connect the external metabolites S_0 and S_3, S_0 and S_4, or S_3 and S_4. For case A and case B, they read

$$v^A = \begin{pmatrix} 1 \\ 1 \\ 1 \\ 0 \end{pmatrix}, \begin{pmatrix} 1 \\ 0 \\ 0 \\ 1 \end{pmatrix}, \begin{pmatrix} 0 \\ -1 \\ -1 \\ 1 \end{pmatrix}, \begin{pmatrix} -1 \\ -1 \\ -1 \\ 0 \end{pmatrix}, \begin{pmatrix} -1 \\ 0 \\ 0 \\ -1 \end{pmatrix}, \begin{pmatrix} 0 \\ 1 \\ 1 \\ -1 \end{pmatrix} \text{ and } v^B = \begin{pmatrix} 1 \\ 1 \\ 1 \\ 0 \end{pmatrix}, \begin{pmatrix} 1 \\ 0 \\ 0 \\ 1 \end{pmatrix}, \begin{pmatrix} -1 \\ 0 \\ 0 \\ -1 \end{pmatrix}, \begin{pmatrix} 0 \\ 1 \\ 1 \\ -1 \end{pmatrix}.$$
$$\tag{5-82}$$

The possible routes are illustrated in Fig. 5.8.

The set of elementary flux modes is uniquely defined. Pfeiffer et al. (1999) have developed the software Metatool to calculate the elementary flux modes for metabolic networks.

Elementary Flux Modes

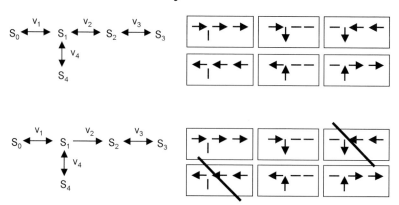

Fig. 5.8 Schematic representation of elementary flux modes for the reaction network depicted in Eq. (5-81).

The concept of *extreme pathways* (Schilling et al. 2000; Schilling and Palsson 2000; Wiback and Palsson 2002) is analogous to the concept of elementary flux modes, but here all reactions are constrained by flux directionality, while the concept of elementary flux modes allows for reversible reactions. To achieve this, reversible reactions are broken down into their forward and backward components. This way, the set of extreme pathways is a subset of the set of elementary flux modes and the extreme pathways are systemically independent.

Elementary flux modes can be used to understand the range of metabolic pathways in a network, to test a set of enzymes for production of a desired product and detect non-redundant pathways, to reconstruct metabolism from annotated genome sequences and analyze the effect of enzyme deficiency, to reduce drug effects, and to identify drug targets.

5.2.4
Flux Balance Analysis

Flux balance analysis (FBA) (Varma and Palsson 1994a, 1994b; Edwards and Palsson 2000a, 2000b; Ramakrishna et al. 2001) investigates the theoretical capabilities and operative modes of metabolism by involving further constraints in the stoichiometric analysis. The first constraint is set by the assumption of a steady state (Eqs. (5-72) and (5-73)). The second constraint is of a thermodynamic nature, respecting the irreversibility of reactions as considered in the concept of extreme pathways. The third constraint may result from the limited capacity of enzymes for metabolite conversion. For example, in the case of a Michaelis-Menten-type enzyme (Eq. (5-32)), the reaction rate is limited by the maximal rate, i.e., $0 \leq v \leq V_{max}$. In general, the constraints imposed on the magnitude of individual metabolic fluxes read

$$\alpha_i \leq v_i \leq \beta_i .$$

$$(5-83)$$

Further constraints may be imposed by biomass composition or other external conditions. The constraints confine the steady-state fluxes to a feasible set but usually do not yield a unique solution. The determination of a particular metabolic flux distribution has been formulated as a linear programming problem. The idea is to maximize an objective function Z that is subject to the stoichiometric and capacity constraints:

$$Z = \sum_{i=1}^{r} c_i v_i \rightarrow \textbf{max}.$$

(5-84)

where c_i represents weights for the individual rates. Examples of such objective functions are maximization of ATP production, minimization of nutrient uptake, maximal yield of a desired product, maximal growth rate, or a combination thereof.

Example 5-13

Maximization of ATP consumption in our running example (Example 5-1) necessitates

$$Z = v_1 + v_2 + v_4 - v_6 + v_7 + v_8 \rightarrow \textbf{max}$$

(5-85)

under the conditions of Eq. (5-78) and the maximal rates given in Example 5-1.

5.2.5
Conservation Relations: Null Space of N^T

If a substance is neither added to nor removed from the reaction system (neither produced nor degraded), its total concentration remains constant. This also holds if it interacts with other compounds by forming complexes. We have seen already as an example the constancy of the total enzyme concentration (Eq. (5-29)) when deriving the Michaelis-Menten rate equation. This was based on the assumption that enzyme production and degradation take place on a much larger timescale than the catalyzed reaction.

For the mathematical derivation of the conservation relations (Heinrich and Schuster 1996), we consider a matrix G fulfilling

$$GN = 0.$$

(5-86)

Due to Eq. (5-68) it follows that

$$G\dot{S} = GNv = 0.$$

(5-87)

Integrating this equation leads directly to the conservation relations

$$GS = const.$$

(5-88)

The number of independent rows of G is equal to $n - Rank\ N$, where n is the number of metabolites in the system. G^T is the kernel matrix of N^T; hence it has properties similar to those of K. Matrix G can also be found using the Gauss algorithm. It is not unique, but every linear combination of its rows is again a valid solution. It exists a simplest representation $G = (G_0 \quad I_{n-Rank\ N})$. Finding this representation may be helpful for simple statement of conservation relations, but this may necessitate renumbering and reordering of metabolite concentrations (see below).

Example 5-14

Consider a set of two reactions comprising a kinase and a phosphatase reaction:

$$\text{ATP} \underset{v_2}{\overset{v_1}{\rightleftharpoons}} \text{ADP} . \tag{5-89}$$

The metabolite concentration vector reads $S = (ATP\ ADP)^T$, and the stoichiometric matrix is $N = \begin{pmatrix} -1 & 1 \\ 1 & -1 \end{pmatrix}$, yielding $G = (1\ 1)$. From the condition $GS = const.$ follows $ATP + ADP = const.$ Thus we have a conservation of adenine nucleotides in this system. The actual values of $ATP + ADP$ must be determined from the initial conditions.

Example 5-15

For the glycolysis model with the stoichiometric matrix given in Eq. (5-71), the only possible representation of the conservation matrix is given by multiples of

$$G = (0\ \ 0\ \ 0\ \ 1\ \ 1\ \ 1). \tag{5-90}$$

This means that again the sum of concentrations of adenine nucleotide-containing substances remains constant ($AMP + ADP + ATP = const.$).

Importantly, conservation relations can be used to simplify the system of differential equations $\dot{S} = Nv$ describing the dynamics of our reaction system. The idea is to eliminate linearly dependent differential equations and to replace them by appropriate algebraic equations. Below, the procedure is explained systematically (Reder 1988).

First we have to reorder the rows in the stoichiometric matrix N as well as in the concentration vector S such that a set of independent rows is on top and the dependent rows are at the bottom. Then the matrix N is split into the independent part N^0 and the dependent part N', and a link matrix L is introduced in the following way:

$$N = \begin{pmatrix} N^0 \\ N' \end{pmatrix} = L N^0 = \begin{pmatrix} I_{Rank\ N} \\ L' \end{pmatrix} N^0 . \tag{5-91}$$

$I_{Rank\,N}$ is the identity matrix of size $Rank\,N$. The differential equation system may be rewritten accordingly

$$\dot{S} = \begin{pmatrix} \dot{S}_{indep} \\ \dot{S}_{dep} \end{pmatrix} = \begin{pmatrix} I_{Rank\,N} \\ L' \end{pmatrix} N^0 v, \tag{5-92}$$

and the dependent concentrations fulfill

$$\dot{S}_{dep} = L' \cdot \dot{S}_{indep}. \tag{5-93}$$

Integration leads to

$$S_{dep} = L' \cdot S_{indep} + const. \tag{5-94}$$

This relation is fulfilled during the entire time course. Thus we may replace the original system by a reduced differential equation system

$$\dot{S}_{indep} = N^0 v \tag{5-95}$$

supplemented with the set of algebraic equations (Eq. (5-94)).

Example 5-16

For the reaction system

$$\xrightarrow{v_1} S_1 \underset{S_3 \quad S_4}{\overset{v_2}{\rightleftharpoons}} S_2 \xleftarrow{v_3} , \tag{5-96}$$

the stoichiometric matrix, the reduced stoichiometric matrix, and the link matrix read

$$N = \begin{pmatrix} 1 & -1 & 0 & 0 \\ 0 & 1 & -1 & 0 \\ 0 & -1 & 0 & -1 \\ 0 & 1 & 0 & -1 \end{pmatrix}, \; N^0 = \begin{pmatrix} 1 & -1 & 0 & 0 \\ 0 & 1 & -1 & 0 \\ 0 & -1 & 0 & 1 \end{pmatrix}, \; L = \begin{pmatrix} 1 & 0 & 0 \\ 0 & 1 & 0 \\ 0 & 0 & 1 \\ 0 & 0 & -1 \end{pmatrix}, \; L' = (0 \; 0 \; -1).$$

The conservation relation $S_3 + S_4 = const.$ is expressed by $G = (0 \; 0 \; 1 \; 1)$. The ODE system

$$\dot{S}_1 = v_1 - v_2$$
$$\dot{S}_2 = v_2 - v_3$$
$$\dot{S}_3 = v_4 - v_2$$
$$\dot{S}_4 = v_2 - v_4$$

can be replaced by the differential-algebraic system

$$\dot{S}_1 = v_1 - v_2$$

$$\dot{S}_2 = v_2 - v_3$$
$$\dot{S}_3 = v_4 - v_2$$
$$S_3 + S_4 = const.$$

which has one differential equation less.

5.2.6
Compartments and Transport across Membranes

Eukaryotic cells contain a variety of organelles, e.g., the nucleus, mitochondria, or vacuoles, that are separated by membranes. Reaction pathways may cross the compartment boundaries. If a substance, say malate, occurs in two different compartments, e.g., in the cytosol and in mitochondria, the respective concentrations can be assigned to two different variables, c_{malate}^{mito} and $c_{malate}^{cytosol}$ (see Figure 5.9). Transport across the membrane has to be considered formally as a reaction with rate v. It is important to note that both compartments have different volumes, V^{mito} and $V^{cytosol}$. Thus transport of a certain amount of malate from one compartment into the other changes the concentrations by a different amount:

$$V^{mito} \cdot \frac{d}{dt} c_{malat}^{mito} = v \quad \text{and} \quad V^{cytosol} \cdot \frac{d}{dt} c_{malat}^{cytosol} = -v, \tag{5-97}$$

where $V \cdot c$ denotes the substance amount in moles.

5.2.7
Characteristic Times

An important feature of metabolism is the wide range of timescales in which cellular processes may occur. Some modifications may happen within seconds, while other processes take hours or even longer. Even on the level of enzymatic reactions, we may find large differences in the time they need to respond to changes. For the metabolic reactions the time regime is characterized by the kinetic constants. We will present different quantitative measures for their temporal description.

A time constant for the isolated first-order reaction

$$A \underset{k_-}{\overset{k_+}{\rightleftharpoons}} B \tag{5-98}$$

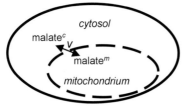

Fig. 5.9 Metabolites may be present in different organelles of the cell, e.g., malate is present in cytosol and mitochondrion. In this case it is appropriate to consider two compartments and assign malate in the different compartments two different species (malate^c, malate^m)

can be derived simply in the following way. Assume that the reaction is in equilibrium with $A = A_0$, $B = B_0$ determined by the temperature T. A small increase of T leads to a perturbation of the equilibrium, a concentration shift $x(t) = A_0 - A(t)$, and eventually a new equilibrium: $A = A_n$, $B = B_n$. Due to the mass action law, during relaxation it holds that

$$\frac{d(B_n - x)}{dt} = k_+(A_n + x) - k_-(B_n - x). \tag{5-99}$$

In the new equilibrium, the concentration changes vanish

$$\frac{dB_n}{dt} = k_+ A_n - k_- B_n = 0 \tag{5-100}$$

and it results in

$$-\frac{dx}{dt} = (k_+ + k_-)x. \tag{5-101}$$

Integration leads to

$$x = x_0 \, e^{-(k_+ + k_-)t}. \tag{5-102}$$

The initial shift of x at $t = 0$ is given by

$$x_0 = A_0 - A_n. \tag{5-103}$$

Setting

$$\frac{1}{\tau} = k_+ + k_- \tag{5-104}$$

determines τ as the *relaxation time* for the decrease of x from its initial value to the $1/e$-fold value. It results in

$$x = (A_0 - A_n) e^{-t/\tau}. \tag{5-105}$$

The relaxation time as introduced in Eqs. (5-104) and (5-105) concerns concentration changes. In general, one can distinguish between time constants for reaction rates and time constants for the change of concentrations.

A more general definition of a time constant for reactions is given by Higgins (1965). The *response time* is defined as

$$\tau_j = \left(\sum_i (n_{ij}) \frac{\partial v_j}{\partial S_i} \right)^{-1}. \tag{5-106}$$

This definition is applicable to reactions with more than one substrate or product and even with nonlinear rate expressions. For example, the response time for the reaction

$$A+B \; \rightleftharpoons \; C+D \tag{5-107}$$

is given by

$$\tau = (k_+(A+B) + k_-(C+D))^{-1}. \tag{5-108}$$

Time constants for metabolite concentrations have been defined in different ways. Reich and Sel'kov (1975), considered the *turnover time*, i.e., the time that is necessary to convert a metabolite pool once:

$$\tau_i^{turn} = \frac{S_i}{\sum\limits_{j=1}^{r} \left(n_{ij}^- v_j^+ + n_{ij}^+ v_j^- \right)}. \tag{5-109}$$

To this end, every reaction is split into a forward (v_j^+) and a backward (v_j^-) reaction with $v_j = v_j^+ - v_j^-$. Accordingly, the stoichiometric coefficients of substance S_i are assigned to the individual reaction directions (n_{ij}^+, n_{ij}^-).

Assume that we have an "empty" pathway, i.e., a pathway that consists of a set of enzymes but has no metabolites available. At once, the first substrate is added. Following Easterby (1973, 1981), the *transition time* describes the time necessary to build up the intermediate pools. It is a measure of the time it takes to reach steady-state concentrations. For each intermediate it holds that

$$\tau_i = \frac{S_i^{SS}}{J}, \tag{5-110}$$

where S_i^{SS} and J denote concentration and flux in the final steady state. The transition time of the complete pathway is the sum of the transition time of all intermediates, $\tau = \sum\limits_{i=1}^{n} \tau_i$.

A measure for the time necessary to return to a steady state after a small perturbation is the transition time according to Heinrich and Rapoport (1975). Let $\delta(t) = S(t) - \bar{S}$ be the deviation from steady-state concentrations. Then the transition time is defined as

$$\tau = \frac{\int\limits_0^\infty t \cdot \delta(t)\, dt}{\int\limits_0^\infty \delta(t)\, dt}. \tag{5-111}$$

This definition is applicable if $\delta(t)$ vanishes asymptotically for large t.

Llorens and et al. (1999) have introduced a more general definition. Let f denote a function such as a flux or a concentration that shall be analyzed after perturbation. The characteristic time can be calculated in analogy to center of mass as

$$T = \frac{\int_0^\infty t \cdot \left| \frac{df}{dx} \right| dt}{\int_0^\infty \left| \frac{df}{dx} \right| dt} . \tag{5-112}$$

This definition may be applied even for oscillating response to the perturbation.

As an example, the characteristic times for Gluc6P, Fruc6P, and Fruc1,6P$_2$ in the running example are given in Tab. 5.4. Whatever definition we apply, characteristic times may differ by orders of magnitude for reactions or concentrations in realistic reaction networks.

5.2.8
Approximations Based on Timescale Separation

Differing timescales in reaction networks allow for reducing the systems in terms of reducing the number of differential equations (and replacing them by algebraic equations). This is implicitly based on the assumption that we choose to consider a window of the timescale while neglecting faster or slower processes. Assume that we consider a process that takes place within minutes. Variables that are changed by faster processes (say within seconds) reach a quasi-steady state after a short transitional period. Variables that are changed by slower processes (processes proceeding within years, e. g., seasonal changes) may be considered as constant. A common example for neglecting slow processes in metabolic modeling is to assume that enzyme concentrations are constant. Their production and degradation is considered to be much slower than the reactions they catalyze. Two types of approximations are used: quasi-steady-state approximations and quasi-equilibrium approximations. A more general mathematical consideration of the effect of timescale separation is given in Heinrich and Schuster (1996).

5.2.8.1   The Quasi-steady-state Approximation
Consider a complex system of processes, e. g., a reaction network. If a metabolite participates in a very fast process (compared to the other processes), it may approach a steady state very quickly. After this transitional period, its concentration S may be

Tab. 5.4 Characteristic times (in min) for the metabolites of the running example. For the meaning of the quantities, see text.

	τ_i (Eq. (5-110))	τ (Eq. (5-111))	T (Eq. (5-112))
Gluc6P	0.0855	0.0724	0.0890
Fruc6P	0.0096	0.0171	0.0583
Fruc1,6P$_2$	0.1095	0.1653	0.1657

considered as constant, i.e. $\dot{S} = 0$. Since this variable is still involved in the complex system, this state is considered as quasi-steady state. The condition $\dot{S} = 0$ allows one to replace the differential equation for the change of S by an algebraic equation describing how S depends on the other variables of the system.

Example 5-17

Assume a pathway consisting of faster and slower reactions

$$P \xrightarrow{k_1} S_1 \underset{\text{fast}}{\xrightarrow{k_2}} S_2 \xrightarrow{k_3}$$

(5-113)

described by the differential equation system

$$\frac{dS_1}{dt} = Pk_1 - S_1 k_2$$

$$\frac{dS_2}{dt} = S_1 k_2 - S_2 k_3 \,.$$

(5-114)

If the second reaction is fast, i.e., $k_2 \gg k_1, k_3$, we may assume a quasi-steady state for S_1:

$$\frac{dS_1}{dt} = 0 \,.$$

(5-115)

This enables us to calculate the concentration of S_1 and to simplify the differential equation system. Now it comprises only one differential equation and one algebraic expression:

$$S_1 = \frac{Pk_1}{k_2}$$

(5-116)

$$\frac{dS_2}{dt} = Pk_1 - S_2 k_3 \,.$$

(5-117)

In Fig. 5.10, one can see that the introduced simplification describes the real behavior sufficiently well after an initial period.

5.2.8.2 Quasi-equilibrium Approximation

We again assume a coupling of slow and fast processes. The pathway is supposed to contain two substrates that can be converted rapidly and reversibly one into the other, such as the hexoses glucose-6-phosphate and fructose-6-phosphate in glycolysis. After a short transition period, their concentrations reach equilibrium. In mathematical terms, the differential equation for the concentration change of one of the substrates may be replaced by an algebraic expression for the concentration ratios in equilibrium. Since both substrates are still involved in the larger network, this is again only a quasi-equilibrium.

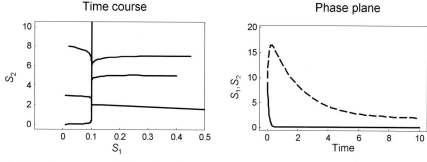

Fig. 5.10 Time course and phase plane for the reaction system presented in Eq. (5-113). Parameter values $k_1 = 1$, $k_2 = 10$, $k_3 = 0.5$. Initial conditions for the time course $S_1(0) = S_2(0) = 10$. It is obvious that S_1 reaches the quasi-steady state very quickly compared to the S_2. Trajectories in the phase plane are shown for different initial conditions.

Example 5-18

The pathway

$$\text{P} \xrightarrow{k_1} \text{S}_1 \underset{k_{-2}}{\overset{k_{+2}}{\rightleftharpoons}} \text{S}_2 \xrightarrow{k_3}$$

(5-118)

is described by the differential equation system

$$\frac{dS_1}{dt} = Pk_1 - S_1 k_{+2} + S_2 k_{-2}$$

$$\frac{dS_2}{dt} = S_1 k_{+2} - S_2 k_{-2} - S_2 k_3 \,.$$

(5-119)

The conversion is much faster than the other reactions, i.e., $k_{+2}, k_{-2} \gg k_1, k_3$. After a short period of time, it holds that

$$\frac{S_2}{S_1} \simeq \frac{k_{+2}}{k_{-2}} = q_2 \,,$$

(5-120)

where q_2 is the equilibrium constant of the second reaction. The second reaction operates close to equilibrium, although a non-vanishing flux ($v_2 \neq 0$) may pass this reaction. We may sum up the concentrations of S_1 and S_2, and it holds that

$$\frac{d(S_1 + S_2)}{dt} = \frac{d(1/q_2 + 1) S_2}{dt} = Pk_1 - S_2 k_3 \,.$$

(5-121)

The simplified equation system consists of a differential equation and an algebraic equation

$$\frac{dS_2}{dt} = \frac{q_2\,(Pk_1 - S_2k_3)}{1 + q_2} \tag{5-122}$$

$$S_1 = \frac{S_2}{q_2}. \tag{5-123}$$

Symbolically, the reaction scheme reduces to

$$P \xrightarrow{k_1} S_1 + S_2 \xrightarrow{k_3} . \tag{5-124}$$

As demonstrated, both types of approximations reduce the number of ODEs in the mathematical model by replacing some of them by algebraic equations. Applying these approximations systematically leads to skeleton models of the considered metabolic pathway, which preserve important features of the general models but are easier to analyze and perceive.

5.3
Metabolic Control Analysis

Metabolic control analysis (MCA) is a powerful quantitative and qualitative framework for studying the relationship between steady-state properties of a network of biochemical reactions and the properties of the individual reactions. It investigates the sensitivity of steady-state properties of the network to small parameter changes. MCA is a useful tool for theoretical and experimental analysis of control and regulation in cellular systems.

MCA was independently founded by two different groups in the 1970s (Kacser and Burns 1973; Heinrich and Rapoport 1974) and was further developed by different groups (e.g., Heinrich et al. 1977; Van Dam et al. 1977; Fell 1979, 1992; Kohen et al. 1983; Kholodenko 1984; Fell and Sauro 1985; Hofmeyr et al. 1986; Sauro et al. 1987; Westerhoff et al. 1987; Westerhoff and van Dam 1987; Cornish-Bowden 1989; Hofmeyr 1989, 1995; Small and Fell 1990; Cascante et al. 1991, 1995, 2002; Heinrich and Reder 1991; Kahn and Westerhoff 1991; Kholodenko et al. 1992, 1995 a, 1995 b, 1998; Hofer and Heinrich 1993; Kholodenko and Westerhoff 1993, 1994; Snoep et al. 1994; Bier et al. 1996; Heinrich and Schuster 1996, 1998; Hofmeyr and Cornish-Bowden 1996; Thomas and Fell 1996; Schuster and Westerhoff 1999; and Bruggeman et al. 2002–to mention only some of the work). A milestone in formalization was provided by Reder (1988). Originally intended for metabolic networks, MCA now also has applications for signaling pathways, gene expression models, and hierarchical networks (Kholodenko et al. 2000; Hofmeyr and Westerhoff 2001; Bruggeman et al. 2002; Westerhoff et al. 2002; Liebermeister et al. 2004).

Metabolic networks are very complex systems that are highly regulated and exhibit interactions such as feedback inhibition or common substrates for distant reactions. Many mechanisms and regulatory properties of isolated enzymatic reactions are known. The development of MCA was motivated by a series of questions like the following: Can their properties or their behavior in the metabolic network be predicted from the knowledge about isolated reactions? Which individual steps control a flux or a steady-state concentration? Is there a rate-limiting step? Which effectors or modifications have the most prominent effect on the reaction rate? In biotechnological production processes, it is of interest which enzyme(s) are to be activated in order to increase the rate of synthesis of a desired metabolite. There are also related problems in health care. For example, concerning metabolic disorders such as overproduction of a metabolite, which reactions should be modified in order to downregulate this metabolite while perturbing the rest of the metabolism as weakly as possible?

In metabolic networks, the steady-state variables, i.e., the fluxes and the metabolite concentrations, are controlled by parameters such as enzyme concentrations, kinetic constants (e. g., Michaelis constants and maximal activities), and other model-specific parameters. The relations between steady-state variables and kinetic parameters are usually nonlinear. Up to now, no general theory exists that predicts the effect of large parameter changes in a network. The approach presented here is basically restricted to small parameter changes. Mathematically, the system is linearized at steady state, which yields exact results if the parameter changes are infinitesimally small.

We will first define a set of mathematical expressions that are useful to quantify control. Later we will show the relations between these functions and their application for prediction of reaction network behavior.

5.3.1
The Coefficients of Control Analysis

Biochemical reaction systems are networks of metabolites connected by chemical reactions. Their behavior is determined by the properties of their components – the individual reactions and their kinetics – as well as by the network structure – the involvement of compounds in different reactions or, in short, the stoichiometry. Hence, the effect of a perturbation exerted at a reaction in this network will depend on both the local properties of this reaction and the embedding of this reaction in the global network.

Let $y(x)$ denote a quantity that depends on another quantity y. The effect of the change Δx on y is expressed in terms of coefficients:

$$c_x^y = \left(\frac{x}{y} \frac{\Delta y}{\Delta x} \right)_{\Delta x \to 0}. \tag{5-125}$$

In practical applications, Δx might be identified, e. g., with one percent change of x and Δy with the percentage change of y. The pre-factor x/y is a normalization factor that makes the coefficient independent of units and the magnitude of x and y. In the limiting case $\Delta x \to 0$, the coefficient defined in Eq. (5-125) can be written as

$$c_x^y = \frac{x}{y} \frac{\partial y}{\partial x}, \qquad (5\text{-}126)$$

which is mathematically equivalent to

$$c_x^y = \frac{\partial \ln y}{\partial \ln x}. \qquad (5\text{-}127)$$

Two distinct types of coefficients, local and global coefficients, reflect the relations among local and global changes. Elasticity coefficients (sensitivities) are local coefficients pertaining to individual reactions. They can be calculated in any given state. Control coefficients and response coefficients are global quantities. They refer to a given steady state of the entire system. After a perturbation of y, the relaxation of x to a new steady state is considered.

The general form of the coefficients in control analysis as defined in Eq. (5-126) contains the normalization x/y. The normalization has the advantage that we get rid of units and can compare, e.g., fluxes belonging to different branches of a network. The drawback of the normalization is that x/y is not defined as soon as $y = 0$, which may happen for certain parameter combinations. In those cases it is favorable to work with non-normalized coefficients. Throughout this chapter we will usually consider normalized quantities. If we use non-normalized coefficients, they are flagged as ^{non}c. In general, the use of one or the other type of coefficient is also a matter of the personal choice of the modeler.

A graphical representation of changes reflected in the different coefficients is shown in Fig. 5.11.

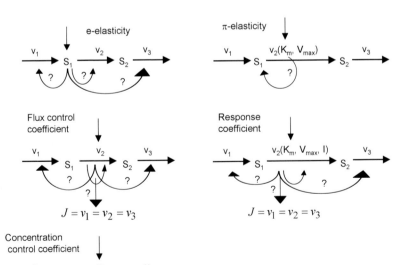

Fig. 5.11 Schematic representation of perturbation and effects quantified by different coefficients of metabolic control analysis.

5.3.1.1 The Elasticity Coefficients

An elasticity coefficient quantifies the sensitivity of a reaction rate to the change of a concentration or a parameter. It measures the direct effect on the reaction velocity, while the rest of the network is kept fixed. The sensitivity of the rate v_k of a reaction to the change of the concentration S_i of a metabolite is calculated by the ε-elasticity:

$$\varepsilon_i^k = \frac{S_i}{v_k} \frac{\partial v_k}{\partial S_i}. \tag{5-128}$$

While the ε-elasticity involves the derivative with respect to a variable, the metabolite concentration, the π-elasticity

$$\pi_m^k = \frac{p_m}{v_k} \frac{\partial v_k}{\partial p_m} \tag{5-129}$$

is defined with respect to parameters p_m such as kinetic constants, concentrations of enzymes, or external metabolites.

Example 5-19

In the glycolysis model, the rate of reaction 1 depends on the ATP concentration. The sensitivity is given by the elasticity

$$\varepsilon_{ATP}^1 = \frac{ATP}{v_1} \frac{\partial v_1}{\partial ATP}. \tag{5-130}$$

Since Eq. (5-2) defines the dependency of v_1 on the ATP concentration, it is easy to calculate that

$$\varepsilon_{ATP}^1 = \frac{ATP}{v_1} \frac{\partial}{\partial ATP} \left(\frac{V_{max,1} ATP}{K_{ATP,1} + ATP} \right) = \frac{ATP}{v_1} \frac{V_{max,1}(K_{ATP,1} + ATP) - V_{max,1} ATP}{(K_{ATP,1} + ATP)^2} =$$

$$= \frac{ATP}{K_{ATP,1} + ATP}. \tag{5-131}$$

The elasticities of all (other) rates with respect to any metabolite concentration can be calculated similarly. Whenever the rate does not depend directly on a concentration (like v_1 and AMP), the elasticity is zero.

Example 5-20

Typical values of elasticity coefficients will be explained for an isolated reaction transforming substrate S into product P. The reaction is catalyzed by enzyme E with the inhibitor I and the activator A as depicted below:

$$S \xrightarrow[\substack{\uparrow \\ I \\ A}]{\substack{E \\ \downarrow}} P . \tag{5-132}$$

Usually, the elasticity coefficients for metabolite concentrations are in the following range:

$$\varepsilon_S^v = \frac{\partial \ln v}{\partial \ln S} > 0 \quad \text{and} \quad \varepsilon_P^v = \frac{\partial \ln v}{\partial \ln P} \le 0 . \tag{5-133}$$

In most cases, the rate increases with the concentration of the substrate (compare, e.g., Eq. (5-131)) and decreases with the concentration of the product. An exception from $\varepsilon_S^v > 0$ occurs with substrate inhibition (Eq. (5-44)), where the elasticity will become negative for $S > S_{opt}$. The relation $\varepsilon_P^v = 0$ holds if the reaction is either irreversible or the product concentration is kept fixed at zero by external mechanisms. The elasticity coefficients with respect to effectors I or A should obey

$$\varepsilon_A^v = \frac{\partial \ln v}{\partial \ln A} > 0 \quad \text{and} \quad \varepsilon_I^v = \frac{\partial \ln v}{\partial \ln I} < 0 , \tag{5-134}$$

since this is essentially what the notions activator and inhibitor mean.

For the most kinetic types, the reaction rate v is proportional to the enzyme concentration E. For example, E is a multiplicative factor in the mass action rate law (Eq. (5-12)) as well as in the maximal rate of the Michelis-Menten rate law (Eq. (5-33)). Therefore, it holds that

$$\varepsilon_E^v = \frac{\partial \ln v}{\partial \ln E} = 1 . \tag{5-135}$$

More complicated interactions between enzymes and substrates, such as metabolic channeling (direct transfer of the metabolite from one enzyme to the next without release to the medium), may lead to exceptions to this rule.

5.3.1.2 Control Coefficients

When defining control coefficients, we refer to a stable steady state of the metabolic system characterized by steady-state concentrations $S = S(p)$ and steady-state fluxes $J = v(S(p), p)$. Any sufficiently small perturbation of an individual reaction rate by a parameter change, $v_k \rightarrow v_k + \Delta v_k$, drives the system to a new steady state in close proximity with $J \rightarrow J + \Delta J$ and $S \rightarrow S + \Delta S$. A measure for the change of fluxes and concentrations are the control coefficients.

Example 5-21

Consider the glycolysis model in the running example. We may ask, what is the impact of a change in the rate of ATP consumption, reaction 7, on the steady flux through the upper glycolysis, i.e., through reaction 1 or through reactions 3, 4, and 5? Or, what is the effect of an acceleration of the rate of reaction 3 on the concentrations of ATP or of Fruc6P? We cannot calculate these effects directly as we did for the elasticities in Example 5-19.

The flux-control coefficient for the control of rate v_k over flux J_j is defined as

$$C_k^j = \frac{v_k}{J_j} \frac{\partial J_j}{\partial v_k}, \tag{5-136}$$

while the concentration-control coefficient of concentration S_i with respect to v_k reads

$$C_k^i = \frac{v_k}{S_i} \frac{\partial S_i}{\partial v_k}. \tag{5-137}$$

The control coefficients quantify the control that a certain reaction v_k exerts on the steady-state flux J or on the steady state concentration S_i, respectively.

It should be noted that the rate change, Δv_k, is caused by the change of a parameter p_k that has a direct effect solely on v_k. Thus it holds that

$$\frac{\partial v_k}{\partial p_k} \neq 0 \quad \text{and} \quad \frac{\partial v_l}{\partial p_k} = 0 \ (l \neq k). \tag{5-138}$$

Example 5-22

In the glycolysis model, the Michaelis constant of ATP in reaction 1, $K_{ATP,1}$, is a parameter that directly influences only reaction 1.

Such a parameter might be the enzyme concentration, a kinetic constant, or the concentration of a specific inhibitor or effector. Hence, the definition of the flux-control coefficients *in extenso* is

$$C_k^j = \frac{v_k}{J_j} \frac{\partial J_j / \partial p_k}{\partial v_k / \partial p_k}. \tag{5-139}$$

As long as Eq. (5-138) holds, the value of the control coefficient does not depend on the choice of the perturbed parameter.

5.3.1.3 Response Coefficients

The steady state is determined by the values of the parameters. A third type of coefficient expresses the direct dependence of steady-state variables on parameters. The response coefficients are defined as

$$R_m^j = \frac{p_m}{J_j}\frac{\partial J_j}{\partial p_m} \quad \text{and} \quad R_m^i = \frac{p_m}{S_i}\frac{\partial S_i}{\partial p_m}, \tag{5-140}$$

where the first coefficient expresses the response of the flux to a parameter perturbation while the latter describes the response of a steady-state concentration.

Example 5-23

What is the influence of a perturbation of the Michaelis constant of ATP in reaction 1, $K_{ATP,1}$, on the steady-state flux of reaction 6 or on the concentration of Fruc1,6P$_2$?

5.3.1.4 Matrix Representation of the Coefficients

Control, response, and elasticity coefficients are defined with respect to all rates, steady-state concentrations, fluxes, or parameters in the metabolic system and in the respective model. They can be arranged in matrices:

$$C^J = \left\{C_k^j\right\}, C^S = \left\{C_k^i\right\}, R^J = \left\{R_m^j\right\}, R^S = \left\{R_m^i\right\}, \varepsilon = \left\{\varepsilon_i^k\right\}, \pi = \left\{\pi_m^k\right\}. \tag{5-141}$$

Matrix representation can also be chosen for the response coefficients as well as for all types of non-normalized coefficients. The arrangement in matrices allows applying of matrix algebra in control analysis. In particular, the matrices of normalized control coefficients can be calculated from the matrices of non-normalized control coefficient as follows:

$$C^J = (dg\,J)^{-1} \cdot {}^{non}C^J \cdot dg\,J$$

$$C^S = (dg\,S)^{-1} \cdot {}^{non}C^J \cdot dg\,J$$

$$R^J = (dg\,J)^{-1} \cdot {}^{non}R^J \cdot dg\,p$$

$$R^S = (dg\,S)^{-1} \cdot {}^{non}R^S \cdot dg\,p$$

$$\varepsilon = (dg\,J)^{-1} \cdot {}^{non}\varepsilon \cdot dg\,S$$

$$R^S = (dg\,S)^{-1} \cdot {}^{non}R^S \cdot dg\,p. \tag{5-142}$$

The symbol dg stands for the diagonal matrix, e.g., $dg\,J = \begin{pmatrix} J_1 & 0 & 0 \\ 0 & J_2 & 0 \\ 0 & 0 & J_r \end{pmatrix}$.

5.3.2

The Theorems of Metabolic Control Theory

We are interested in calculating the control coefficients for a system under investigation. Usually, the steady-state fluxes or concentrations cannot be expressed explicitly as a function of the reaction rates. Therefore, flux- and concentration-control coefficients cannot simply be determined by taking the respective derivatives, as we did for the elasticity coefficients in Example 5-19.

Fortunately, the work with control coefficients is eased by of a set of theorems. The first type of theorem, the summation theorems, makes a statement about the total control over a flux or a steady-state concentration. The second type of theorem, the connectivity theorems, relates the control coefficients to the elasticity coefficients. Both types of theorems together with dependency information encoded in the stoichiometric matrix contain enough information to calculate all control coefficients as function of the elasticities.

We will first introduce the theorems and then present a hypothetical perturbation experiment to illustrate the summation theorem. Finally, the theorems will be mathematically derived.

5.3.2.1 The Summation Theorems

The summation theorems make a statement about the total control over a certain steady-state flux or concentration. The flux-control coefficients fulfill

$$\sum_{k=1}^{r} C_{v_k}^{J_j} = 1 , \qquad (5\text{-}143)$$

where r is the number of reactions. The flux-control coefficients of a metabolic network for one steady-state flux sum up to 1. This means that all enzymatic reactions can share the control over this flux. For the concentration-control coefficients, we have

$$\sum_{k=1}^{r} C_{v_k}^{S_i} = 0 . \qquad (5\text{-}144)$$

The control coefficients of a metabolic network for one steady-state concentration are balanced. This means again that the enzymatic reactions can share the control over this concentration, but some exert a negative control while others exert a positive control. Both relations can also be expressed in matrix formulation. For the flux-control coefficients, we have

$$\boldsymbol{C}^J \cdot \boldsymbol{1} = \boldsymbol{1} , \qquad (5\text{-}145)$$

and for the concentration control coefficients, we have

$$\boldsymbol{C}^S \cdot \boldsymbol{1} = \boldsymbol{0} . \qquad (5\text{-}146)$$

The symbols 1 and 0 denote column vectors with r rows containing as entries only ones or zeros, respectively.

The summation theorems for the non-normalized control coefficients read

$$^{non}C^J \cdot K = K \tag{5-147}$$

and

$$^{non}C^S \cdot K = 0. \tag{5-148}$$

A more intuitive derivation of the summation theorems is given in the following example according to Kacer and Burns (1973).

Example 5-24

The summation theorem for flux-control coefficients can be derived using a thought experiment. Consider the unbranched pathway

$$P_0 \xrightarrow{v_1} S_1 \xleftrightarrow{v_2} S_2 \xrightarrow{v_3} P_3. \tag{5-149}$$

What happens to steady-state fluxes and metabolite concentrations if we perform a directed experimental manipulation of all three reactions leading to the same fractional change α of all three rates?

$$\frac{\delta v_1}{v_1} = \frac{\delta v_2}{v_2} = \frac{\delta v_3}{v_3} = \alpha. \tag{5-150}$$

The flux must increase to the same extent:

$$\frac{\delta J}{J} = \alpha. \tag{5-151}$$

But since producing and degrading reactions increase to the same amount, the concentrations of the metabolites remain constant

$$\frac{\delta S_1}{S_1} = \frac{\delta S_2}{S_2} = 0. \tag{5-152}$$

The combined effect of all changes in local rates on the system variables S_1, S_2, and J can be written as the sum of all individual effects caused by the local rate changes. For the flux it holds that

$$\frac{\delta J}{J} = C_1^J \frac{\delta v_1}{v_1} + C_2^J \frac{\delta v_2}{v_2} + C_3^J \frac{\delta v_3}{v_3}. \tag{5-153}$$

Using Eqs. (5-155) and (5-156), it follows that

$$\alpha = \alpha \left(C_1^J + C_2^J + C_3^J \right), \tag{5-154}$$

and, therefore, it holds that

$$1 = C_1^J + C_2^J + C_3^J. \tag{5-155}$$

This is just a special case of Eq. (143). In the same way, for the change of concentration S_1, we obtain

$$\frac{\delta S_1}{S_1} = C_1^{S_1} \frac{\delta v_1}{v_1} + C_2^{S_1} \frac{\delta v_2}{v_2} + C_3^{S_1} \frac{\delta v_3}{v_3}. \tag{5-156}$$

By means of Eqs. (5-155) and (5-152), we find

$$0 = C_1^{S_1} + C_2^{S_1} + C_3^{S_1}. \tag{5-157}$$

A similar result holds for the change of concentration S_2:

$$0 = C_1^{S_2} + C_2^{S_2} + C_3^{S_2}. \tag{5-158}$$

Although shown here only for a special case, these properties hold in general for systems without conservation relations. The general derivation is given in Section 5.3.2.3.

5.3.2.2 The Connectivity Theorems
Flux-control coefficients and elasticity coefficients are related by the expression

$$\sum_{k=1}^{r} C_{v_k}^{J_j} \varepsilon_{S_i}^{v_k} = 0. \tag{5-159}$$

Note that the sum runs over all rates v_k. Considering the concentration S_i of a fixed metabolite and a fixed flux J_j, each term contains the elasticity $\varepsilon_{S_i}^{v_k}$ describing the direct influence of a change of S_i on the rates v_k and the control coefficient expressing the control of v_k over J_j.

The connectivity theorem between concentration-control coefficients and elasticity coefficients reads

$$\sum_{k=1}^{r} C_{v_k}^{S_h} \varepsilon_{S_i}^{v_k} = -\delta_{hi}. \tag{5-160}$$

Again, the sum runs over all rates v_k, while S_h and S_i are the concentrations of two fixed metabolites. The symbol $\delta_{hi} = \begin{cases} 0, & \text{if } h \neq i \\ 1, & \text{if } h = i \end{cases}$ is the so-called Kronecker symbol.

In matrix formulation, the connectivity theorems read

$$\boldsymbol{C}^J \cdot \boldsymbol{\varepsilon} = \boldsymbol{0} \tag{5-161}$$

and

$$C^S \cdot \varepsilon = -I \tag{5-162}$$

where I denotes the identity matrix of size $n \times n$. For non-normalized coefficients, it holds that

$$^{non}C^J \cdot {}^{non}\varepsilon \cdot L = 0 \tag{5-163}$$

and

$$^{non}C^S \cdot \varepsilon \cdot L = -L \tag{5-164}$$

where L is the link matrix that expresses the relation between independent and dependent rows in the stoichiometric matrix (Eq. (5-91)). A very comprehensive representation of both summation and connectivity theorems for non-normalized coefficients is given by the following equation:

$$\begin{pmatrix} {}^{non}C^J \\ {}^{non}C^S \end{pmatrix} \cdot \begin{pmatrix} K & \varepsilon L \end{pmatrix} = \begin{pmatrix} K & 0 \\ 0 & -L \end{pmatrix}. \tag{5-165}$$

As mentioned above, the summation and connectivity theorems together with the structural information of the stoichiometric matrix are sufficient to calculate the control coefficients for a metabolic network as function of the elasticities. This shall be illustrated for a small network in the next example.

Example 5-25

To calculate the control coefficients, we study the following reaction system:

$$P_0 \xrightarrow{v_1} S_1 \xrightarrow{v_2} P_2 . \tag{5-166}$$

The flux-control coefficients obey the theorems

$$C_1^J + C_2^J = 1 \quad \text{and} \quad C_1^J \varepsilon_S^1 + C_2^J \varepsilon_S^2 = 0, \tag{5-167}$$

which can be solved for the control coefficients

$$C_1^J = \frac{\varepsilon_S^2}{\varepsilon_S^2 - \varepsilon_S^1} \quad \text{and} \quad C_2^J = \frac{-\varepsilon_S^1}{\varepsilon_S^2 - \varepsilon_S^1} . \tag{5-168}$$

Since usually $\varepsilon_S^1 < 0$ and $\varepsilon_S^2 > 0$ (see Example 5-20), both control coefficients assume positive values $C_1^J > 0$ and $C_2^J > 0$. This means that both reactions exert a positive control over the steady-state flux and that acceleration of any of them leads to increase of J, which is in accordance with common intuition.

The concentration control coefficients fulfill

$$C_1^S + C_2^S = 0 \quad \text{and} \quad C_1^S \varepsilon_S^1 + C_2^S \varepsilon_S^2 = -1,$$

(5-169)

which yields

$$C_1^S = \frac{1}{\varepsilon_S^2 - \varepsilon_S^1} \quad \text{and} \quad C_2^J = \frac{-1}{\varepsilon_S^2 - \varepsilon_S^1} .$$

(5-170)

With $\varepsilon_S^1 < 0$ and $\varepsilon_S^2 > 0$, we get $C_1^S > 0$ and $C_2^S < 0$, i.e., increase of the first reaction causes a rise in the steady-state concentration of S, while acceleration of the second reaction leads to the opposite.

5.3.2.3 Derivation of Matrix Expressions for Control Coefficients

After having introduced the theorems of metabolic control analysis, we will derive expressions for the control coefficients in matrix form. These expressions are suited for calculating the coefficients even for large-scale models. We start from the steady-state condition

$$Nv(S(p), p) = 0.$$

(5-171)

Implicit differentiation with respect to the parameter vector p yields

$$N \frac{\partial v}{\partial S} \frac{\partial S}{\partial p} + N \frac{\partial v}{\partial p} = 0.$$

(5-172)

Since we have chosen reaction-specific parameters for perturbation, the matrix of non-normalized parameter elasticities contains nonzero entries in the main diagonal and zeros elsewhere (compare Eq. (5-138)).

$$\frac{\partial v}{\partial p} = \begin{pmatrix} \dfrac{\partial v_1}{\partial p_1} & 0 & 0 \\ 0 & \dfrac{\partial v_2}{\partial p_2} & 0 \\ & \cdots & \\ 0 & 0 & \dfrac{\partial v_r}{\partial p_r} \end{pmatrix} .$$

(5-173)

Therefore, this matrix is regular and has an inverse. Furthermore, we consider the following Jacobian matrix:

$$M = N \frac{\partial v}{\partial S} .$$

(5-174)

The Jacobian matrix M is a regular matrix if the system is asymptotically stable and contains no conservation relations. The case with conservation relations is considered below. Here, we may pre-multiply Eq. (5-172) by the inverse of M and rearrange to get

$$\frac{\partial S}{\partial p} = -\left(N\frac{\partial v}{\partial S}\right)^{-1} N\frac{\partial v}{\partial p} = -M^{-1} N\frac{\partial v}{\partial p} \equiv {}^{non}R^{S} \, . \tag{5-175}$$

As indicated, $\partial S/\partial p$ is the matrix of non-normalized response coefficients for concentrations. Post-multiplication by the inverse of the non-normalized parameter elasticity matrix gives us

$$\frac{\partial S}{\partial p}\left(\frac{\partial v}{\partial p}\right)^{-1} = -\left(N\frac{\partial v}{\partial S}\right)^{-1} N = {}^{non}C^{S} \, . \tag{5-176}$$

This is the matrix of non-normalized concentration-control coefficients. The right (middle) side contains no parameters. This means that the control coefficients do not depend on the particular choice of parameters to exert the perturbation as long as Eq. (5-138) is fulfilled. The control coefficients are dependent on the structure of the network, represented by the stoichiometric matrix N, and on the kinetics of the individual reactions, represented by the non-normalized elasticity matrix $\partial v/\partial S$.

The implicit differentiation of

$$J = v\left(S\left(p\right), p\right) \tag{5-177}$$

with respect to the parameter vector p leads to

$$\frac{\partial J}{\partial p} = \frac{\partial v}{\partial p} + \frac{\partial v}{\partial S}\frac{\partial S}{\partial p} = \left(I - \frac{\partial v}{\partial S}\left(N\frac{\partial v}{\partial S}\right)^{-1} N\right)\frac{\partial v}{\partial p} \equiv {}^{non}R^{J} \, . \tag{5-178}$$

This yields, after some rearrangement, an expression for the non-normalized flux-control coefficients:

$$\frac{\partial J}{\partial p}\left(\frac{\partial v}{\partial p}\right)^{-1} = I - \frac{\partial v}{\partial S}\left(N\frac{\partial v}{\partial S}\right)^{-1} N = {}^{non}C^{J} \, . \tag{5-179}$$

The normalized control coefficients are (by use of Eq. (5-142))

$$C^{J} = I - \left(dgJ\right)^{-1}\left(\frac{\partial v}{\partial S}\left(N\frac{\partial v}{\partial S}\right)^{-1} N\right)\left(dgJ\right) \tag{5-180}$$

and

$$C^{S} = -\left(dgS\right)^{-1}\left(\left(N\frac{\partial v}{\partial S}\right)^{-1} N\right)\left(dgJ\right) \, . \tag{5-181}$$

These equations can easily be implemented for numerical calculation of control coefficients or used for analytical computation (see Example 5-26). They are also suited for derivation of the theorems of MCA. The summation theorems for the control coefficients follow from Eq. (5-180) or Eq. (5-181) by, respectively, post-multiplying with the vector 1 (the row vector containing only 1's) and consideration of the relations $(dg\mathbf{J}) \cdot 1 = \mathbf{J}$ and $N\mathbf{J} = 0$. The connectivity theorems result from post-multiplying Eq. (5-180) or Eq. (5-181) with the elasticity matrix $\varepsilon = (dg\mathbf{J})^{-1} \cdot \dfrac{\partial v}{\partial S} \cdot dg\mathbf{S}$, and using that multiplication of a matrix with its inverse yields the identity matrix $\mathbf{I}$ of respective type.

If the reaction system involves conservation relations, we eliminate dependent variables as explained in Section 5.2.5. In this case the non-normalized coefficients read

$$^{non}\mathbf{C}^J = \mathbf{I} - \frac{\partial v}{\partial S} L \left(N^0 \frac{\partial v}{\partial S} \right)^{-1} N^0 \tag{5-182}$$

$$^{non}\mathbf{C}^S = -L \left(N^0 \frac{\partial v}{\partial S} \right)^{-1} N^0 \tag{5-183}$$

and the normalized control coefficients are obtained by applying Eq. (5-142).

Example 5-26

Consider the simple reaction system of Example 5-25 and let the rate equations be $v_1 = k_1 P_0 - k_{-1} S_1$ and $v_2 = k_2 S_1 - k_{-2} P_2$. Then, the steady-state condition $J = v_1 = v_2$ results in

$$J = \frac{k_1 k_2 P_0 - k_{-1} k_{-2} P_2}{k_{-1} + k_2} \tag{5-184}$$

and

$$S_1 = \frac{k_1 P_0 + k_{-2} P_2}{k_{-1} + k_2}. \tag{5-185}$$

The stoichiometric matrix is $N = (1\ -1)$ and the non-normalized elasticity coefficients read

$$\frac{\partial v}{\partial S} = \begin{pmatrix} \dfrac{\partial v_1}{\partial S_1} \\[2mm] \dfrac{\partial v_2}{\partial S_1} \end{pmatrix} = \begin{pmatrix} -k_{-1} \\ k_2 \end{pmatrix}. \tag{5-186}$$

Introducing these expressions into Eq. (5-180) yields

$$C^J = \left(\begin{array}{cc} \dfrac{k_1 k_2 P_0 - k_{-1} k_{-2} P_2}{k_{-1} + k_2} & 0 \\ 0 & \dfrac{k_1 k_2 P_0 - k_{-1} k_{-2} P_2}{k_{-1} + k_2} \end{array} \right)^{-1}$$

$$\left(\left(\begin{array}{cc} 1 & 0 \\ 0 & 1 \end{array} \right) - \left(\begin{array}{c} -k_{-1} \\ k_2 \end{array} \right) \left((1 \;\; -1) \left(\begin{array}{c} -k_{-1} \\ k_2 \end{array} \right) \right)^{-1} (1 \;\; -1) \right) (dgJ) \tag{5-187}$$

$$= \left(\begin{array}{cc} \dfrac{k_1 k_2 P_0 - k_{-1} k_{-2} P_2}{k_{-1} + k_2} & 0 \\ 0 & \dfrac{k_1 k_2 P_0 - k_{-1} k_{-2} P_2}{k_{-1} + k_2} \end{array} \right)^{-1} \left(\dfrac{1}{k_{-1} + k_2} \left(\begin{array}{cc} k_2 & k_{-1} \\ k_2 & k_{-1} \end{array} \right) \right) (dgJ)$$

$$= \dfrac{1}{k_{-1} + k_2} \left(\begin{array}{cc} k_2 & k_{-1} \\ k_2 & k_{-1} \end{array} \right)$$

meaning that the flux-control coefficients are $C_1^J = \dfrac{k_2}{k_{-1} + k_2}$, $C_2^J = \dfrac{k_{-1}}{k_{-1} + k_2}$. For the concentration-control coefficients we have

$$C^S = -\left(\dfrac{k_1 P_0 + k_{-2} P_2}{k_{-1} + k_2} \right)^{-1} \left(\left((1 \;\; -1) \left(\begin{array}{c} -k_{-1} \\ k_2 \end{array} \right) \right)^{-1} (1 \;\; -1) \right) (dgJ) \tag{5-188}$$

$$= -\left(\dfrac{k_1 P_0 + k_{-2} P_2}{k_{-1} + k_2} \right)^{-1} \left(\dfrac{-1}{k_{-1} + k_2} (1 \;\; -1) \right)$$

$$\left(\begin{array}{cc} \dfrac{k_1 k_2 P_0 - k_{-1} k_{-2} P_2}{k_{-1} + k_2} & 0 \\ 0 & \dfrac{k_1 k_2 P_0 - k_{-1} k_{-2} P_2}{k_{-1} + k_2} \end{array} \right)$$

$$= \dfrac{(k_1 k_2 P_0 - k_{-1} k_{-2} P_2)}{(k_{-1} + k_2) \cdot (k_1 P0 + k_{-2} P_2)} (1 \;\; -1)$$

or

$$C_1^S = \dfrac{k_1 k_2 P_0 - k_{-1} k_{-2} P_2}{(k_{-1} + k_2) \cdot (k_1 P_0 + k_{-2} P_2)}, \quad C_2^S = \dfrac{-(k_1 k_2 P_0 - k_{-1} k_{-2} P_2)}{(k_{-1} + k_2) \cdot (k_1 P_0 + k_{-2} P_2)} \tag{5-189}$$

To investigate the implications of control distribution, we will now analyze the control pattern in an unbranched pathway

$$P_0 \overset{v_1}{\longleftrightarrow} S_1 \overset{v_2}{\longleftrightarrow} S_2 \cdots S_{r-1} \overset{v_r}{\longleftrightarrow} P_r \tag{5-190}$$

with linear kinetics $v_i = k_i S_{i-1} - k_{-i} S_i$ (with $S_0 = P_0$, $S_r = P_r$) and equilibrium constants $q_i = k_i/k_{-i}$. In this case, one can calculate an analytical expression for the steady-state flux

$$J = \frac{P_0 \prod\limits_{j=1}^{r} q_j - P_r}{\sum\limits_{l=1}^{r} \frac{1}{k_l} \prod\limits_{m=l}^{r} q_m},$$ (5-191)

as well as an analytical expression for the flux control coefficients

$$C_i^J = \frac{\frac{1}{k_i} \prod\limits_{j=i}^{r} q_j}{\sum\limits_{l=1}^{r} \frac{1}{k_l} \prod\limits_{m=l}^{r} q_m}.$$ (5-192)

Let us consider two very general cases. First, assume that all reactions have the same individual kinetics, $k_+ = k_i$, $k_- = k_{-i}$ for $i = 1, ..., r$, and that for the equilibrium constants, which are also equal, it holds that $q = k_+/k_- > 1$. In this case the ratio of two subsequent flux-control coefficients is

$$\frac{C_i^J}{C_{i+1}^J} = \frac{k_{i+1}}{k_i} q_i = q > 1.$$ (5-193)

Hence, the control coefficients of the preceding reactions are bigger than the control coefficients of the succeeding reactions, or flux-control coefficients are higher in the beginning of a chain than in the end. This conforms to the frequent observation that flux control resides in the upper part of an unbranched reaction pathway.

Now assume that the individual rate constants might be different but that all equilibrium constants are equal to 1, $q_i = 1$ for $i = 1, ..., r$. This implies that $k_i = k_{-i}$. Furthermore, Eq. (5-192) simplifies to

$$C_i^J = \frac{\frac{1}{k_i}}{\sum\limits_{l=1}^{r} \frac{1}{k_l}}$$

Now consider the relaxation time $\tau_i = 1/(k_i + k_{-i})$ (compare Section 5.2.7) as a measure of the rate of an enzyme. The flux-control coefficient reads

$$C_i^J = \frac{\tau_i}{\tau_1 + \tau_2 + ... + \tau_r}.$$ (5-194)

This expression helps to elucidate two aspects of metabolic control. First, all enzymes participate in the control since all enzymes have a relaxation time. No one enzyme has all the control or determines the flux through the pathway alone. Second, slow enzymes with a higher relaxation time exert in general more control than fast enzymes with a short relaxation time.

The predictive power of flux-control coefficients for directed changes of flux is illustrated in the following example.

Example 5-27

Assume that we can manipulate the pathway by changing the enzyme concentration in a predefined way. We would like to explore the effect of the perturbation of the individual enzymes. For a linear pathway of the type of Eq. (5-190) consisting of four consecutive reactions with $v_i = E_i(k_i S_{i-1} - k_{-i} S_i)$, we will calculate the flux-control coefficients. For $i = 1, ..., 4$, it shall hold that (1) all enzyme concentrations $E_i = 1$, (2) the rate constants $k_i = 2$, $k_{-i} = 1$, and (3) the concentrations of the external reactants $P_0 = P_4 = 1$. The resulting flux is $J = 1$ and the flux-control coefficients are $C^J = (0.533\ 0.267\ 0.133\ 0.067)^T$ according to Eq. (5-180).

If we now slightly perturb the first enzyme, perhaps by performing a percentage change of its concentration, i.e., $E_1 \rightarrow E_1 + 1\%$, then Eq. (5-125) implies that the flux increases as $J \rightarrow J + C_1^J \cdot 1\%$. In fact, the flux in the new steady state is $J^{E_1 \rightarrow 1.01 \cdot E_1} = 1.00531$. Increasing E_2, E_3, or E_4 by one percent leads to flux values of 1.00265, 1.00132, and 1.00066, respectively.

A strong perturbation would not yield similar effects. Assume that we can manipulate the system at will and can double the total amount of enzyme in the system. If we keep E_2 to E_4 constant but change $E_1 \rightarrow 5 E_1$, the resulting flux is $J^{E_1 \rightarrow 5 \cdot E_1} = 1.7441$. Changing instead $E_4 \rightarrow 5 E_4$ yields $J^{E_4 \rightarrow 5 \cdot E_4} = 1.0563$, a lower flux increase. Equal distribution of changes to all enzymes $E_i \rightarrow 2 E_i$, $i = 1, ..., 4$ results in $J^{E_i \rightarrow 2 \cdot E_i} = 2$. The maximal value for the flux $J^{max} = 2.2871$ is obtained for the optimal distribution of enzyme concentration to the individual reactions, which is $E_1 = 3.124$, $E_2 = 2.209$, $E_3 = 1.562$, $E_4 = 1.105$ (see Chapter 12). Changes in enzyme concentrations and their effects on flux control are illustrated in Fig. 5.12

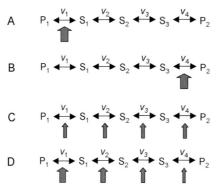
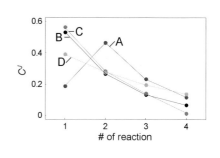

Fig. 5.12 Effect of enzyme concentration change on steady-state flux and on flux-control coefficients in an unbranched pathway consisting of four reactions. In the reference state, all enzymes have the concentration 1 (in arbitrary units), the control distribution is the same as in case (c), and the steady-state flux is $J = 1$. (a) Change of $E_1 \rightarrow 5 E_1$ while keeping the other enzyme concentrations constant results in a remarkable drop of control of the first enzyme. The resulting flux is $J^{E_1 \rightarrow 5 \cdot E_1} = 1.7441$. (b) The change $E_4 \rightarrow 5 E_4$ corresponds to $J^{E_4 \rightarrow 5 \cdot E_4} = 1.0563$. There is only slight change of control distribution. (c) Equal enzyme concentrations with $E_i \rightarrow 2 E_i$, $i = 1, ..., 4$ result in $J^{E_i \rightarrow 2 \cdot E_i} = 2$. (d) Optimal distribution of enzyme concentration $E_1 = 3.124$, $E_2 = 2.209$, $E_3 = 1.562$, $E_4 = 1.105$ resulting in the maximal steady-state flux $J^{max} = 2.2871$.

5.3.3
Extensions of Metabolic Control Analysis

5.3.3.1 Control Analysis for Variables other than Fluxes and Concentrations

Control coefficients are defined as the ratio of fractional changes in the system's variables at steady state to fractional changes in the biochemical activity that causes the change. The concept of control analysis can also be applied to other relevant variables of the system besides fluxes and concentrations (Schuster 1996). Such variables can be the transition time (Section 5.2.7), free energy differences (Section 5.1.2, Westerhoff and van Dam 1987), growth rate (Kacser and Beeby 1984; Dykhuizen et al. 1987), and others. Let X be a vector of generalized state variables and Y a vector of generalized response variables. State variables X characterize the state of the system, which is not necessarily the steady state. Response variables $Y = Y(X,p)$ can be calculated in terms of the state variables X and the parameters p. The reaction rates v are also considered as functions of X and p, $v = v(X,p)$. The matrix of non-normalized control coefficients can be expressed as

$$
{}^{non}C^{Y} = \frac{dY}{dp}\left(\frac{\partial v}{\partial p}\right)^{-1},
\tag{5-195}
$$

and for the matrix of normalized control coefficients, it holds that

$$
C^{Y} = (dgY)^{-1}\frac{dY}{dp}\left(\frac{\partial v}{\partial p}\right)^{-1}(dgv).
\tag{5-196}
$$

In Eqs. (5-195) and (5-196), the total derivative dY/dp has been used since not only the direct effect of p on Y but also the indirect effect via X must be taken into account. Schuster (1996) showed that the coefficients defined in Eq. (5-195) obey a unified summation theorem,

$$
{}^{non}C^{Y}K = \frac{\partial Y}{\partial p}\left(\frac{\partial v}{\partial p}\right)^{-1}K,
\tag{5-197}
$$

as well as a unified connectivity theorem,

$$
{}^{non}C^{Y}\frac{\partial v}{\partial X}\frac{\partial X}{\partial X_a} = \left[\frac{\partial Y}{\partial p}\left(\frac{\partial v}{\partial p}\right)^{-1}\frac{\partial v}{\partial X} - \frac{\partial Y}{\partial X}\right]\frac{\partial X}{\partial X_a},
\tag{5-198}
$$

where X_a is a subvector of X containing only independent variables (compare Chapter 5, Section 5.2.5).

Example 5-28

In a metabolic system with conservation relations such as the conservation $ATP + ADP = const.$ considered in Example 5-14, it could be of interest to interpret experimental results in terms of the concentration ratio $X_1 = ATP/ADP$. The vector $X = (ATP/ADP, \quad ATP + ADP)^T$ can formally replace the concentration vector $S = (ATP \quad ADP)^T$. The coefficients expressing the control of reaction k over the concentration ratio can be expressed in terms of the concentration control coefficients

$$^{non}C_k^{ATP/ADP} = \frac{\partial (ATP/ADP)}{\partial v_k} = \frac{1}{ADP}\,^{non}C_k^{ATP} - \frac{ATP}{ADP^2}\,^{non}C_k^{ADP}. \qquad (5\text{-}199)$$

Since $ATP + ADP = const.$, it holds that $^{non}C_k^{ATP} = -^{non}C_k^{ADP}$, and therefore,

$$^{non}C_k^{ATP/ADP} = \frac{(ATP/ADP)}{ADP^2}\,^{non}C_k^{ATP}. \qquad (5\text{-}200)$$

Coefficients for the control of molar free energy differences were defined by Westerhoff and Van Dam (Westerhoff et al. 1987). In non-normalized form, they read

$$^{non}C_k^{\Delta G_i} = \frac{\partial \Delta G_i}{\partial v_k} \qquad (5\text{-}201)$$

and obey the following summation and connectivity theorems:

$$\sum_{k=1}^r {}^{non}C_k^{\Delta G_i} \cdot J_k = 0 \qquad (5\text{-}202)$$

$$\sum_{k=1}^r {}^{non}C_k^{\Delta G_i} \cdot \varepsilon_{\Delta G_j}^k = -\delta_{ij}. \qquad (5\text{-}203)$$

The quantity $\varepsilon_{\Delta G_j}^k$ denotes the elasticity of reaction rate v_k with respect to the free energy difference of reaction j, and $\delta_{ij} = \begin{cases} 1, & \text{if } i = j \\ 0, & \text{if } i \neq j \end{cases}$ is the Kronecker symbol.

It may also be of interest to study the control over characteristic times of the reaction network. For unbranched reaction sequences like the one presented in Eq. (5-190), the control coefficient for the transition time τ_i of metabolite S_i (given in Eq. (5-109)) can be defined as

$$C_k^{\tau_i} = \frac{v_k}{\tau_i} \frac{\partial \tau_i}{\partial v_k}. \qquad (5\text{-}204)$$

Their properties have been investigated by Easterby, Melendez-Hevia, Schuster, and others (Easterby 1981, 1990; Melendez-Hevia et al. 1990; Schuster 1996). The following simple relation holds:

$$C_k^{\tau_i} = C_k^{S_i} - C_k^J . \tag{5-205}$$

The summation theorem reads

$$\sum_{i=1}^{r} C_k^{\tau_i} = -1 . \tag{5-206}$$

This implies that the activation of all enzymes by the same fractional amount reduces the transition time by the same factor. The connectivity theorem for pathways without conservation relations reads

$$\sum_{i=1}^{r} C_k^{\tau_i} \cdot \varepsilon_j^k = -\delta_{ij} . \tag{5-207}$$

5.3.3.2 Time-dependent Control Coefficients
Time-dependent control coefficients have been introduced for the case that the steady state is not reached within a reasonable time (Heinrich and Reder 1991). They are given as

$$^{non}C^J(t) = I + \frac{\partial v}{\partial S} \left(exp \left(tN \frac{\partial v}{\partial S} \right) - I \right) \left(N \frac{\partial v}{\partial S} \right)^{-1} N \tag{5-208}$$

and

$$^{non}C^S(t) = \left(exp \left(tN \frac{\partial v}{\partial S} \right) - I \right) \left(N \frac{\partial v}{\partial S} \right)^{-1} N . \tag{5-209}$$

The matrices $^{non}C^J(t)$ and $^{non}C^S(t)$ are time-dependent operators that transform the initial perturbation of the reaction rates into flux and concentration variations at time t. Consideration of relaxation processes does not change the summation relationships

$$^{non}C^J(t) \cdot K = K$$

$$^{non}C^S(t) \cdot K = 0 \tag{5-210}$$

but affects the connectivity relationships

$$^{non}C^J(t) \frac{\partial v}{\partial S} L = \frac{\partial v}{\partial S} L \cdot exp \left(tN \frac{\partial v}{\partial S} \right)$$

$$^{non}C^S(t) \frac{\partial v}{\partial S} L = L \left(exp \left(tN \frac{\partial v}{\partial S} \right) - I \right) \tag{5-211}$$

(Heinrich and Reder 1991). An extension of metabolic control analysis to non-steady-state trajectories is presented by Ingalls and Sauro (2003).

5.3.3.3 Spatially Heterogeneous and Time-varying Cellular Reaction Networks

Peletier et al. (2003) took into account that during signaling processes the assumption of spatial homogeneity (Eq. (5-10)) does not necessarily hold. Instead, the concentrations of activated proteins show temporally changing spatial gradients. These gradients are due to protein diffusion from the receptor to the place of action. They play an important role in the transmission of the respective signal. To tackle this problem, protein concentrations S_i are considered as functions of time and space. They may change due to occurrence of biochemical reactions with the rates v_j or due to diffusion with the diffusion constant D_i. The evolution of concentrations is given by the balance equations (Katchalsky and Curran 1965)

$$\frac{\partial S_i}{\partial t} - D_i \, \Delta S_i = \sum_{j=1}^{r} n_{ij} \, v_j \,, \tag{5-212}$$

where r is the number of reactions, $\Delta = \dfrac{\partial^2}{\partial x_1^2} + \dfrac{\partial^2}{\partial x_2^2} + \dfrac{\partial^2}{\partial x_3^2}$ is the Laplacian operator, and $x_1, ..., x_3$ are the spatial Cartesian coordinates.

In addition to reaction and diffusion, molecules may be transported across system boundaries (the plasma membrane or membranes of organelles) with a flux f_i. The quantity L denotes a characteristic length of the cell (e. g., the diameter) that may change due to cell swelling or growth. For modulation of these quantities around a reference state, dimensionless parameters α are introduced, such that

$$v_j \to \alpha_{vj} \cdot v_j, \quad D_i \to \alpha_{Di} \cdot D_i, \quad f_i \to \alpha_{fi} \cdot f_i, \quad \text{and} \quad L \to \alpha_L \cdot L. \tag{5-213}$$

The parameters α assume the value 1 at the reference state. The control over a steady-state variable q is expressed by the control coefficients

$$C_{v_j}^q = \frac{\partial \ln q}{\partial \ln \alpha_{vj}}, \quad C_{D_i}^q = \frac{\partial \ln q}{\partial \ln \alpha_{Di}}, \quad C_{f_i}^q = \frac{\partial \ln q}{\partial \ln \alpha_{fi}}, \quad \text{and} \quad C_L^q = \frac{\partial \ln q}{\partial \ln \alpha_L}, \tag{5-214}$$

i. e., by the ratio of the fractional change in q caused by the fractional change in α. For systems with transport processes and a non-homogeneous distribution of concentrations, the generalized summation theorem for the steady-state flux takes the form

$$\sum_{j=1}^{r} C_{v_j}^J + \sum_{i=1}^{n} C_{D_i}^J + \sum_{i=1}^{n} C_{f_i}^J = 1 \,, \tag{5-215}$$

i. e., the total control of 1 on any steady-state flux is shared by all diffusion, reaction, and transport processes.

A further extension of this concept takes into account a dependence on changing conditions in space or time. The space conditions may modify due to cell growth or shrinkage. The dependence of the system on time may be given if initial conditions alter with time. In an analogue way, as in Eq. (5-213), time t is rescaled according to

$t \to \alpha_t \cdot \tau$. The generalization of the summation theorem for flux-control coefficients for systems that depend on time reads

$$-C_t^{J(\tau)} + \sum_{j=1}^{r} C_{v_j}^{J(\tau)} + \sum_{i=1}^{n} C_{D_i}^{J(\tau)} + \sum_{i=1}^{n} C_{f_i}^{J(\tau)} = 1 . \qquad (5\text{-}216)$$

For control over concentrations, the following summation theorem holds:

$$-C_t^{S_k} + \sum_{j=1}^{r} C_{v_j}^{S_k} + \sum_{i=1}^{n} C_{D_i}^{S_k} + \sum_{i=1}^{n} C_{f_i}^{S_k} = 0 , \qquad (5\text{-}217)$$

where S_k is the concentration depending on space and time. The control exerted by cell size is reflected in two further summation theorems, namely, for fluxes:

$$2 \sum_{i=1}^{n} C_{D_i}^{J(t)} + \sum_{i=1}^{n} C_{f_i}^{J(t)} + C_L^{J(\tau)} = 1 . \qquad (5\text{-}218)$$

For control over concentrations, the following summation theorem holds:

$$2 \sum_{i=1}^{n} C_{D_i}^{S_k} + \sum_{i=1}^{n} C_{f_i}^{S_k} + C_L^{S_k} = 0 . \qquad (5\text{-}219)$$

The theorems introduced by Peletier et al. (2003) are well suited for application in signaling networks.

Suggested Further Reading

Schellenberger 1989; Kuby 1991; Fell 1992, 1997; Heinrich and Schuster 1996; Cornish-Bowden 2004.

References

BIER, M., TEUSINK, B., KHOLODENKO, B.N. and WESTERHOFF, H.V. Control analysis of glycolytic oscillations (1996) Biophys. Chem. *62*, 15–24.

BRIGGS, G.E. and HALDANE, J.B.S. A note on the kinetics of enzyme action (1925) Biochem. J. *19*, 338–339.

BROWN, A.J. Enzyme action (1902) J. Chem. Soc. *81*, 373–386.

BRUGGEMAN, F.J., WESTERHOFF, H.V., HOEK, J.B. and KHOLODENKO, B.N. Modular response analysis of cellular regulatory networks (2002) J. Theor. Biol. *218*, 507–20.

CASCANTE, M., TORRES, N.V., FRANCO, R., MELEN-DEZ-HEVIA, E. and CANELA, E.I. Control analysis of transition times. Extension of analysis and matrix method (1991) Mol. Cell. Biochem. *101*, 83–91.

CASCANTE, M., MELENDEZ-HEVIA, E., KHOLO-DENKO, B., SICILIA, J. and KACSER, H. Control analysis of transit time for free and enzyme-bound metabolites: physiological and evolutionary significance of metabolic response times (1995) Biochem. J. *308 (Pt 3)*, 895–9.

CASCANTE, M., BOROS, L.G., COMIN-ANDUIX, B., DE ATAURI, P., CENTELLES, J.J. and LEE, P.W. Metabolic control analysis in drug discovery and disease (2002) Nat. Biotechnol. *20*, 243–9.

CORNISH-BOWDEN, A. Metabolic control therapy and biochemical systems theory: different objectives, different assumptions, different results (1989) J. Theor. Biol. *136*, 365–77.

CORNISH-BOWDEN, A. Fundamentals of enzyme kinetics, 3rd edition (2004), Portland Press, London.

DYKHUIZEN, D.E., DEAN, A.M. and HARTL, D.L. Metabolic flux and fitness (1987) Genetics *115*, 25–31.

EADIE, G.S. The inhibition of cholinesterase by physostigmine and prostigmine (1942) J. Biol. Chem. *146*, 85–93.

EASTERBY, J.S. Coupled enzyme assays: a general expression for the transient (1973) Biochim. Biophys. Acta *293*, 552–8.

EASTERBY, J.S. A generalized theory of the transition time for sequential enzyme reactions (1981) Biochem. J. *199*, 155–61.

EASTERBY, J.S. Integration of temporal analysis and control analysis of metabolic systems (1990) Biochem. J. *269*, 255–9.

EDWARDS, J.S. and PALSSON, B.O. The *Escherichia coli* MG1655 in silico metabolic genotype: its definition, characteristics, and capabilities (2000 a) Proc. Natl. Acad. Sci. USA *97*, 5528–33.

EDWARDS, J.S. and PALSSON, B.O. Metabolic flux balance analysis and the in silico analysis of *Escherichia coli* K-12 gene deletions (2000 b) BMC Bioinformatics *1*, 1.

FELL, D.A. Theoretical studies of the control of adenosine 3:5-cyclic monophosphate by the high- and low-Km phosphodiesterases (Proceedings) (1979) Biochem. Soc. Trans. *7*, 1039–40.

FELL, D.A. Metabolic control analysis: a survey of its theoretical and experimental development (1992) Biochem. J. *286 (Pt 2)*, 313–30.

FELL, D. Understanding the control of metabolism (1997) 1st edition, K. Snell, ed. Portland Press, London, Miami.

FELL, D.A. and SAURO, H.M. Metabolic control and its analysis. Additional relationships between elasticities and control coefficients (1985) Eur. J. Biochem. *148*, 555–61.

GLANSDORFF, P. and PRIGOGINE, I. Thermodynamic theory of structure, stability and fluctuations (1971) Wiley-Interscience, London.

GULDBERG, C.M. and WAAGE, P. Über die chemische Affinität (1879) J. Prakt. Chem. *19*, 69.

HALDANE, J.B.S. Enzymes (1930) Longmans, Green and Co., London.

HANES, C.S. Studies on plant amylases. I. The effect of starch concentration upon the velocity of hydrolysis by the amylase of germinated barley (1932) Biochem. J. *26*, 1406–1421.

HAYNIE, D.T. Biological thermodynamics (2001) Cambridge University Press, Cambridge.

HEINRICH, R. and RAPOPORT, T.A. A linear steady-state treatment of enzymatic chains. General properties, control and effector strength (1974) Eur. J. Biochem. *42*, 89–95.

HEINRICH, R. and RAPOPORT, T.A. Mathematical analysis of multienzyme systems. II. Steady state and transient control (1975) Biosystems *7*, 136.

HEINRICH, R. and REDER, C. Metabolic control analysis of relaxation processes (1991) J. Theor. Biol. *151*, 343–350.

HEINRICH, R. and SCHUSTER, S. The regulation of cellular systems (1996) Chapman & Hall, New York.

HEINRICH, R. and SCHUSTER, S. The modelling of metabolic systems. Structure, control and optimality (1998) Biosystems *47*, 61–77.

HEINRICH, R., RAPOPORT, S.M. and RAPOPORT, T.A. Metabolic regulation and mathematical models (1977) Prog. Biophys. Mol. Biol. *32*, 1–82.

HIGGINS, J. Dynamics and control in cellular reactions (1965) in B. Chance, R. W. Estabrook and J. R. Williamson, eds. Control of the energy metabolism. Academic Press, New York, pp 13–46.

HILL, A.V. The possible effects of the aggregation of the molecules of hemoglobin on its dissociation curves (1910) J. Physiol. *40*, iv-vii.

HILL, A.V. The combinations of hemoglobin with oxygen and with carbonmonoxide (1913) Biochem. J. *7*, 471–480.

HOFER, T. and HEINRICH, R. A second-order approach to metabolic control analysis (1993) J. Theor. Biol. *164*, 85–102.

HOFMEYR, J.H. Control-pattern analysis of metabolic pathways. Flux and concentration control in linear pathways (1989) Eur. J. Biochem. *186*, 343–54.

HOFMEYR, J.H. Metabolic regulation: a control analytic perspective (1995) J. Bioenerg. Biomembr. *27*, 479–90.

HOFMEYR, J.H. and CORNISH-BOWDEN, A. Co-response analysis: a new experimental strategy for metabolic control analysis (1996) J. Theor. Biol. *182*, 371–80.

HOFMEYR, J.H. and WESTERHOFF, H.V. Building the cellular puzzle: control in multi-level reaction networks (2001) J. Theor. Biol. *208*, 261–85.

HOFMEYR, J.H., KACSER, H. and VAN DER MERWE, K.J. Metabolic control analysis of moiety-conserved cycles (1986) Eur. J. Biochem. *155*, 631–41.

HYNNE, F., DANO, S. and SORENSEN, P.G. Full-scale model of glycolysis in *Saccharomyces cerevisiae* (2001) Biophys. Chem. *94*, 121–63.

INGALLS, B.P. and SAURO, H.M. Sensitivity analysis of stoichiometric networks: an extension of metabolic control analysis to non-steady state trajectories (2003) J. Theor. Biol. *222*, 23–36.

KACSER, H. and BEEBY, R. Evolution of catalytic proteins or on the origin of enzyme species by means of natural selection (1984) J. Mol. Evol. *20*, 38–51.

KACSER, H. and BURNS, J.A. The control of flux (1973) Symp. Soc. Exp. Biol. *27*, 65–104.

KAHN, D. and WESTERHOFF, H.V. Control theory of regulatory cascades (1991) J. Theor. Biol. *153*, 255–85.

KATCHALSKY, A. and CURRAN, P.F. Nonequilibrium thermodynamics in biophysics (1965) Harvard University Press, Cambridge, M.A.

KHOLODENKO, B.N. Control of mitochondrial oxidative phosphorylation (1984) J. Theor. Biol. *107*, 179–88.

KHOLODENKO, B.N. and WESTERHOFF, H.V. Metabolic channelling and control of the flux (1993) FEBS Lett. *320*, 71–4.

KHOLODENKO, B.N. and WESTERHOFF, H.V. Control theory of one enzyme (1994) Biochim. Biophys. Acta *1208*, 294–305.

KHOLODENKO, B.N., LYUBAREV, A.E. and KURGANOV, B.I. Control of the metabolic flux in a system with high enzyme concentrations and moiety-conserved cycles. The sum of the flux control coefficients can drop significantly below unity (1992) Eur. J. Biochem. *210*, 147–53.

KHOLODENKO, B.N., CASCANTE, M. and WESTERHOFF, H.V. Control theory of metabolic channelling (1995 a) Mol. Cell. Biochem. *143*, 151–68.

KHOLODENKO, B.N., SCHUSTER, S., ROHWER, J.M., CASCANTE, M. and WESTERHOFF, H.V. Composite control of cell function: metabolic pathways behaving as single control units (1995 b) FEBS Lett. *368*, 1–4.

KHOLODENKO, B.N., SCHUSTER, S., GARCIA, J., WESTERHOFF, H.V. and CASCANTE, M. Control analysis of metabolic systems involving quasi-equilibrium reactions (1998) Biochim. Biophys. Acta *1379*, 337–52.

KHOLODENKO, B.N., BROWN, G.C. and HOEK, J.B. Diffusion control of protein phosphorylation in signal transduction pathways (2000) Biochem. J. *350 Pt 3*, 901–7.

KOHEN, E., KOHEN, C., HIRSCHBERG, J.G., WOUTERS, A.W., THORELL, B., WESTERHOFF, H.V. and CHARYULU, K.K. Metabolic control and compartmentation in single living cells (1983) Cell. Biochem. Funct. *1*, 3–16.

KOSHLAND, D.E., JR., NEMETHY, G. and FILMER, D. Comparison of experimental binding data and theoretical models in proteins containing subunits (1966) Biochemistry *5*, 365–85.

KUBY, S.A. A study of enzymes. I. Enzyme catalysis, kinetics, and substrate binding (1991) CRC Press, Boca Raton, FL.

LEHNINGER, A.L. Biochemistry, 2nd edition, (1975), New York, Worth, p 397.

LIEBERMEISTER, W., KLIPP, E., SCHUSTER, S. and HEINRICH, R. A theory of optimal differential gene expression (2004) Biosystems, in press.

LINEWEAVER, H. and BURK, D. The determination of enzyme dissociation constants (1934) J. Am. Chem. Soc. 56, 658–660.

LLORENS, M., NUNO, J.C., RODRIGUEZ, Y., MELENDEZ-HEVIA, E. and MONTERO, F. Generalization of the theory of transition times in metabolic pathways: a geometrical approach (1999) Biophys. J. 77, 23–36.

MELENDEZ-HEVIA, E., TORRES, N.V., SICILIA, J. and KACSER, H. Control analysis of transition times in metabolic systems (1990) Biochem. J. 265 195–202.

MICHAELIS, L. and MENTEN, M.L. Kinetik der Invertinwirkung (1913) Biochem. Z. 49, 333–369.

MICHAL, G. Biochemical pathways (1999) Spektrum Akademischer Verlag, Heidelberg.

MONOD, J., WYMAN, J. and CHANGEUX, J.P. On the nature of allosteric transitions: A plausible model (1965) J. Mol. Biol. 12, 88–118.

PELETIER, M.A., WESTERHOFF, H.V. and KHOLO-DENKO, B.N. Control of spatially heterogeneous and time-varying cellular reaction networks: a new summation law (2003) J. Theor. Biol. 225, 477–87.

PFEIFFER, T., SANCHEZ-VALDENEBRO, I., NUNO, J.C., MONTERO, F. and SCHUSTER, S. METATOOL: for studying metabolic networks (1999) Bioinformatics 15, 251–7.

RAMAKRISHNA, R., EDWARDS, J.S., McCULLOCH, A. and PALSSON, B.O. Flux-balance analysis of mitochondrial energy metabolism: consequences of systemic stoichiometric constraints (2001) Am. J. Physiol. Regul. Integr. Comp. Physiol. 280, R695–704.

REDER, C. Metabolic control theory: a structural approach (1988) J. Theor. Biol. 135, 175–201.

REICH, J.G. and SEL'KOV, E.E. Time hierarchy, equilibrium and non-equilibrium in metabolic systems (1975) Biosystems 7, 39–50.

SAURO, H.M., SMALL, J.R. and FELL, D.A. Metabolic control and its analysis. Extensions to the theory and matrix method (1987) Eur. J. Biochem. 165, 215–21.

SCHELLENBERGER, A. (ed.) Enzymkatalyse (1989) VEB Gustav Fischer Verlag, Jena.

SCHILLING, C.H. and PALSSON, B.O. Assessment of the metabolic capabilities of *Haemophilus influenzae* Rd through a genome-scale pathway analysis (2000) J. Theor. Biol. 203, 249–83.

SCHILLING, C.H., SCHUSTER, S., PALSSON, B.O. and HEINRICH, R. Metabolic pathway analysis: Basic concepts and scientific applications in the post-genomic era (1999) Biotechnol. Prog. 15, 296–303.

SCHILLING, C.H., LETSCHER, D. and PALSSON, B.O. Theory for the systemic definition of metabolic pathways and their use in interpreting metabolic function from a pathway-oriented perspective (2000) J. Theor. Biol. 203, 229–48.

SCHUSTER, S. Control analysis in terms of generalized variables characterizing metabolic systems (1996) J. Theor. Biol. 182, 259–68.

SCHUSTER, S. and WESTERHOFF, H.V. Modular control analysis of slipping enzymes (1999) Biosystems 49, 1–15.

SCHUSTER, S., DANDEKAR, T. and FELL, D.A. Detection of elementary flux modes in biochemical networks: a promising tool for pathway analysis and metabolic engineering (1999) Trends Biotechnol. 17, 53–60.

SCHUSTER, S., FELL, D.A. and DANDEKAR, T. A general definition of metabolic pathways useful for systematic organization and analysis of complex metabolic networks (2000) Nat. Biotechnol. 18, 326–32.

SCHUSTER, S., HILGETAG, C., WOODS, J.H. and FELL, D.A. Reaction routes in biochemical reaction systems: algebraic properties, validated calculation procedure and example from nucleotide metabolism (2002) J. Math. Biol. 45, 153–81.

SMALL, J.R. and FELL, D.A. Metabolic control analysis. Sensitivity of control coefficients to elasticities (1990) Eur. J. Biochem. 191, 413–20.

SNOEP, J.L. and OLIVIER, B.G. Java Web Simulation (JWS); a web based database of kinetic models (2002) Mol. Biol. Rep. 29, 259–63.

SNOEP, J.L., JENSEN, P.R., GROENEVELD, P., MOLENAAR, D., KHOLODENKO, B.N. and WESTERHOFF, H.V. How to determine control of growth rate in a chemostat. Using metabolic control analysis to resolve the paradox (1994) Biochem. Mol. Biol. Int. 33, 1023–32.

THOMAS, S. and FELL, D.A. Design of metabolic control for large flux changes (1996) J Theor Biol 182, 285–98.

VAN DAM, K., WIECHMANN, A.H., WESTERHOFF, H.V. and HELLINGWERF, K.J. Proton gradients across energy-transducing membranes (1977) Biochem. Soc. Trans. *5*, 28–9.

VARMA, A. and PALSSON, B.O. Metabolic flux balancing: basic concepts, scientific and practical use. (1994a) Biotechnology *12*, 994–998.

VARMA, A. and PALSSON, B.O. Stoichiometric flux balance models quantitatively predict growth and metabolic by-product secretion in wild-type *Escherichia coli* W3110 (1994b) Appl. Environ. Microbiol. *60*, 3724–31.

WEGSCHEIDER, R. Über simultane Gleichgewichte und die Beziehungen zwischen Thermodynamik und Reaktionskinetik homogener Systeme (1902) Z. Phys. Chem. *39*, 257–303.

WESTERHOFF, H.V. and VAN DAM, K. Thermodynamics and control of biological free-energy transduction. (1987) Elsevier, Amsterdam.

WESTERHOFF, H.V., PLOMP, P.J., GROEN, A.K. and WANDERS, R.J. Thermodynamics of the control of metabolism (1987) Cell. Biophys. *11*, 239–67.

WESTERHOFF, H.V., GETZ, W.M., BRUGGEMAN, F., HOFMEYR, J.H., ROHWER, J.M. and SNOEP, J.L. ECA: control in ecosystems (2002) Mol. Biol. Rep. *29*, 113–7.

WIBACK, S.J. and PALSSON, B.O. Extreme pathway analysis of human red blood cell metabolism (2002) Biophys. J. *83*, 808–18.

6
Signal Transduction

Introduction

Throughout intercellular communication or cellular stress response, the cell senses extracellular signals. They are commuted to intracellular signals and sequences of reactions. Different external changes or events may stimulate signaling. Typical signals are hormones, pheromones, heat, cold, light, osmotic pressure, and appearance or concentration change of substances such as glucose, K^+, Ca^+, or cAMP.

On a molecular level, signaling involves the same type of processes as metabolism: production or degradation of substances, molecular modifications (mainly phosphorylation, but also methylation and acetylation), and activation or inhibition of reactions. From a modeling point of view, there are some important differences between signaling and metabolism. First, signaling pathways serve for information processing and transfer of information, while metabolism provides mainly mass transfer. Second, the metabolic network is determined by the present set of enzymes catalyzing the reactions. Signaling pathways involve compounds of different types, and they may form highly organized complexes and may assemble dynamically upon occurrence of the signal. Third, the quantity of converted material is high in metabolism (amounts are usually given in concentrations on the order of µM or mM) compared to the number of molecules involved in signaling processes (the typical abundance of proteins in signal cascades is on the order of 10 to 10^4 molecules per cell). Finally, the different amounts of components have an effect on the concentration ratio of catalysts and substrates. In metabolism this ratio is usually low; the enzyme concentration is much lower than the substrate concentration, which gives rise to the quasi-steady-state assumption used in Michaelis-Menten kinetics (Chapter 5, Section 5.1). In signaling processes, amounts of catalysts and their substrates are frequently in the same order of magnitude.

Modeling of the dynamic behavior of signaling pathways is often not straightforward. Knowledge about components of the pathway and their interaction is still limited and incomplete. The interpretation of experimental data is context- and knowledge-dependent. Furthermore, the effect of a signal often changes the state of the whole cell, and this implies difficulties for determination of system limits. But in many cases we may apply the same tools as introduced in Chapter 5.

Systems Biology in Practice. Concepts, Implementation and Application.
E. Klipp, R. Herwig, A. Kowald, C. Wierling, H. Lehrach
Copyright © 2005 WILEY-VCH Verlag GmbH & Co. KGaA, Weinheim
ISBN: 3-527-31078-9

6.1
Function and Structure of Intra- and Intercellular Communication

Cells have a broad spectrum of receiving and processing signals; therefore, not all of them can be considered here. A typical sequence of events in signaling pathways is shown in Fig. 6.1 and proceeds as follows. The "signal" (a substance acting as a ligand or a physical stimulus) approaches the cell surface. Cells have developed two different modes of importing a signal. First, the stimulus may penetrate the cell membrane and bind to a respective receptor in the cell interior. Another possibility is that the signal is perceived by a transmembrane receptor. If the target of the signal is a receptor, it does not cross the membrane. Instead, the receptor changes its own state from susceptible to active and then triggers subsequent processes within the cell. The active receptor stimulates an internal signaling cascade. This cascade frequently includes a series of changes in protein phosphorylation states. The sequence of state changes crosses the nuclear membrane. Eventually, a transcription factor is activated or deactivated. The transcription factor changes its binding properties to regulatory regions on the DNA upstream of a set of genes, and the transcription rate of these genes is altered (typically increased). Either the newly produced proteins or the changes in protein concentration cause the actual response of the cell to the signal. In addition to this downstream program, signaling path-

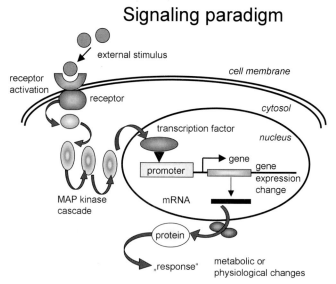

Fig. 6.1 Visualization of the signaling paradigm (for description, see text). The receptor is stimulated by a ligand or another kind of signal, and it changes its own state from susceptible to active. The active receptor initiates the internal signaling cascade, including a series of protein phosphorylation state changes. Subsequently, tran- scription factors are activated or deactivated. The transcription factors regulate the transcription rate of a set of genes. The absolute amount or the relative changes in protein concentrations alter the state of the cell and trigger the actual response to the signal.

Signaling Pathways in Baker's Yeast

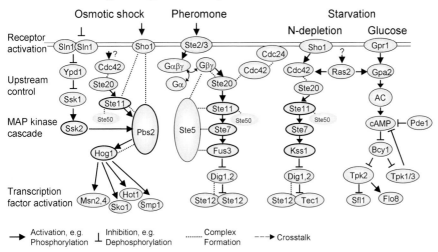

| Activation, e.g.
→ Phosphorylation | Inhibition, e.g.
⊥ Dephosphorylation | ⋯⋯ Complex
Formation | ---→ Crosstalk |

Fig. 6.2 Overview of signaling pathways in yeast: HOG pathway activated by osmotic shock, pheromone pathway activated by a pheromone from cells of opposite mating type, and pseudohyphal growth pathway stimulated by starvation conditions. In each case, the signal interacts with the receptor. The receptor activates a cascade of intracellular processes including complex formations, phosphorylations, and transport steps. A MAP kinase cascade is a particular part of many signaling pathways; its components are indicated by bold border. Eventually, transcription factors are activated that regulate the expression of a set of genes. Besides the indicated connections, further interactions of components are possible. For example, crosstalk may occur, i.e., the activation of the downstream part of one pathway by a component of another pathway. This is supported by the frequent incidence of proteins like Ste11 in the scheme.

ways are regulated by a number of control mechanisms including feedback and feed-forward modulation.

This is the typical picture; however, many pathways may work in a completely different manner. As an example, an overview of signaling pathways that are stimulated in yeast stress response is given in Fig. 6.2.

6.2
Receptor-Ligand Interactions

Many receptors are transmembrane proteins; they receive the signal and transmit it. Upon signal sensing, they change their conformation (see Fig. 6.3). In the active form they are able to initiate a downstream process within the cell. The simplest concept of the interaction between receptor R and ligand L is reversible binding to form the active complex LR:

$$L + R \leftrightarrow LR .$$ (6-1)

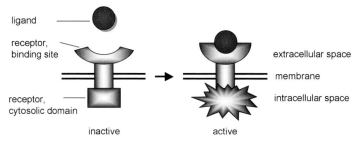

ligand

receptor, binding site

extracellular space

membrane

receptor, cytosolic domain

intracellular space

inactive

active

Fig. 6.3 Schematic representation of receptor activation.

The dissociation constant is calculated as

$$K_D = \frac{L \cdot R}{LR} . \tag{6-2}$$

Typical values for K_D are 10^{-12} M ... 10^{-6} M.

Cells have the ability to regulate the number and the activity of specific receptors, e. g., in order to weaken the signal transmission during long-term stimulation. Balancing production and degradation regulates the number of receptors. Phosphorylation of serine/threonine or tyrosine residues of the cytosolic domain by protein kinases mainly regulates the activity. Hence, a more realistic scenario for ligand-receptor interaction is depicted in Fig. 6.4.

We assume that the receptor is present in the inactive state R_i or the susceptible state R_s. The susceptible form can interact with the ligand to form the active state R_a. The inactive or susceptible form is produced from precursors (v_{pi}, v_{ps}), and all three forms may be degraded (v_{di}, v_{ds}, v_{da}). The rates of production and degradation processes, as well as the equilibria between the different states, might be influenced by the cell state, e. g., by the cell cycle stage. In general, the dynamics of this scenario can be described by the following set of differential equations:

$$\frac{d}{dt} R_i = v_{pi} - v_{di} - v_{is} + v_{si} + v_{ai}$$

$$\frac{d}{dt} R_s = v_{ps} - v_{ds} + v_{is} - v_{si} - v_{sa} + v_{as}$$

$$\frac{d}{dt} R_a = -v_{da} + v_{sa} - v_{as} - v_{ai} . \tag{6-3}$$

For the production terms, we may assume either constant values or (as mentioned above) rates that depend on the actual cell state. The degradation terms might be assumed to be linearly dependent on the concentration of their substrates $(v_{d*} = k_{d*} \cdot R_*)$. This may also be a first guess for the state changes of the receptor (e. g., $v_{is} = k_{is} \cdot R_i$). The receptor activation is dependent on the ligand concentration

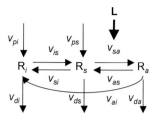

Fig. 6.4 Schematic representation of processes involved in receptor activation by a ligand. L = ligand, R_i = inactive receptor, R_s = susceptible receptor, R_a = active receptor. v_{p*} = production steps, v_{d*} = degradation steps, other steps = transition between inactive, susceptible, and active state of receptor.

(or any other value related to the signal). A linear approximation of the respective rate is $v_{sa} = k_{sa} \cdot R_s \cdot L$. If the receptor is a dimer or oligomer, it might be sensible to include this information into the rate expression as $v_{sa} = k_{sa} \cdot R_s \cdot \dfrac{K_b \cdot L^n}{1 + K_b \cdot L^n}$, where K_b denotes the binding constant and n the Hill coefficient (Chapter 5, Eq. (5-58)).

Example 6-1

An experimentally confirmed example for the activation of receptor and G protein of the pheromone pathway has been presented by Yi and colleagues (2003) for the binding of the pheromone α-factor to the receptor Ste2 in yeast. Concerning the receptor activation dynamics, they report a susceptible and an active form of the receptor, but no inactive form ($R_i = 0$, $v_{*i} = v_{i*} = 0$). The remaining rates are determined as follows:

$$v_{ps} = k_{ps}$$

$$v_{ds} = k_{ds} \cdot R_s$$

$$v_{da} = k_{da} \cdot R_a$$

$$v_{sa} = k_{sa} \cdot R_s \cdot L$$

$$v_{as} = k_{as} \cdot R_a , \tag{6-4}$$

with the following values for the rate constants: $k_{ps} = 4$ (molecules per cell) s^{-1}, $k_{ds} = 4 \cdot 10^{-4}\,s^{-1}$, $k_{da} = 4 \cdot 10^{-3}\,s^{-1}$, $k_{sa} = 2 \cdot 10^6\,M^{-1}s^{-1}$, and $k_{as} = 1 \cdot 10^{-2}\,s^{-1}$. The time course of receptor activation is depicted in Fig. 6.5.

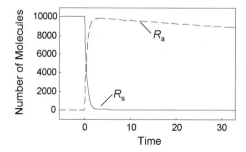

Fig. 6.5 Time course of active (solid line) and susceptible (dashed line) receptor after stimulation with 1 μM α-factor at $t = 0$. The total number of receptors is 10,000. The concentration of the active receptor increases immediately and then declines slowly, while the susceptible receptor is effectively reduced to zero.

6.3
Structural Components of Signaling Pathways

Signaling pathways constitute often highly complex networks, but it has been discovered that they are frequently composed of typical building blocks. These components include Ras proteins, G protein cycles, phosphorelay systems, and MAP kinase cascades. In this chapter we will discuss their general composition and function as well as modeling approaches.

6.3.1
G Proteins

G proteins are essential parts of many signaling pathways. The reason for their name is that they bind the guanine nucleotides GDP and GTP. They are heterotrimers, i.e., they consist of three different subunits. G proteins are associated to cell surface receptors with a heptahelical transmembrane structure, the so-called G protein–coupled receptors (GPCR). Signal transduction cascades involving (1) such a transmembrane surface receptor, (2) an associated G protein, and (3) an intracellular effector that produces a second messenger play an important role in cellular communication and are well studied (Neer 1995; Dohlman 2002). In humans, such G protein–coupled receptors mediate responses to light, flavors, odors, numerous hormones, neurotransmitters, and other signals (Blumer and Thorner 1991; Dohlman et al. 1991; Buck 2000). In unicellular eukaryotes, receptors of this type mediate signals that affect such basic processes as cell division, cell-cell fusion (mating), morphogenesis, and chemotaxis (Blumer and Thorner 1991; Banuett 1998; Dohlman et al. 1998; Wang and Heitman 1999).

The cycle of G protein activation and inactivation is shown in Fig. 6.6. When GDP is bound, the G protein α subunit (Gα) is associated with the G protein βγ heterodimer (Gβγ) and is inactive. Agonist binding to a receptor promotes guanine nucleotide exchange; Gα releases GDP, binds GTP, and dissociates from Gβγ. The dissociated subunits Gα or Gβγ, or both, are then free to activate target proteins (downstream effectors), which initiates signaling. When GTP is hydrolyzed, the subunits

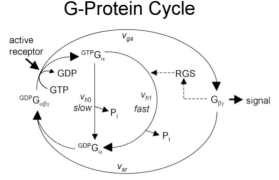

Fig. 6.6 Activation cycle of G protein. Without activation, the heterotrimeric G protein is bound to GPD. Upon activation by the activated receptor, an exchange of GDP with GTP occurs and the G protein is divided into GTP-bound Gα and the heterodimer Gβγ. Gα-bound GTP is hydrolyzed, either slowly in reaction v_{h0} or fast in reaction v_{h1}, supported by the RGS protein. GDP-bound Gα can reassociate with Gβγ (reaction v_{sr}).

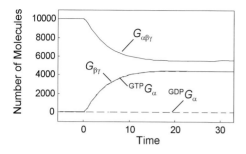

Fig. 6.7 Time course of G protein activation. The total number of molecules is 10,000. The concentration of GDP-bound Gα is low for the whole period due to fast complex formation with the heterodimer Gβγ.

are able to re-associate. Gβγ antagonizes receptor action by inhibiting guanine nucleotide exchange. RGS (regulator of G protein signaling) proteins bind to Gα, stimulate GTP hydrolysis, and thereby reverse G protein activation. This general scheme can also be applied to the regulation of small monomeric Ras-like GTPases, such as Rho. In this case, the receptor, Gβγ, and RGS are replaced by GEF and GAP (see Section 6.3.2).

Direct targets include different types of effectors, such as adenylyl cyclase, phospholipase C, exchange factors for small GTPases, some calcium and potassium channels, plasma membrane Na^+/H^+ exchangers, and certain protein kinases (Neer 1995; Offermanns 2000; Dohlman and Thorner 2001; Meigs et al. 2001). Typically, these effectors produce second messengers or other biochemical changes that lead to stimulation of a protein kinase or a protein kinase cascade (or, as mentioned, are themselves a protein kinase). Signaling persists until GTP is hydrolyzed to GDP and the Gα and Gβγ subunits re-associate, completing the cycle of activation. The strength of the G protein–initiated signal depends on (1) the rate of nucleotide exchange, (2) the rate of spontaneous GTP hydrolysis, (3) the rate of RGS-supported GTP hydrolysis, and (4) the rate of subunit re-association. RGS proteins act as GTPase-activating proteins (GAPs) for a variety of different Gα classes and thereby shorten the lifetime of the activated state of a G protein and contribute to signal desensitization. Furthermore, they may contain additional modular domains with signaling functions and contribute to diversity and complexity of the cellular signaling networks (Dohlman and Thorner 1997; Siderovski et al. 1999; Burchett 2000; Ross and Wilkie 2000).

Example 6-2

The model of the heterotrimeric G protein cycle of the yeast pheromone pathway was already mentioned in Example 6-1 and is linked to the receptor activation model via the concentration of the active receptor. The G protein cycle model comprises two ODEs and two algebraic equations for the mass conservation of the subunits Gα and Gβγ. This gives

$$\frac{d}{dt} G_{\alpha\beta\gamma} = -v_{ga} + v_{sr}$$

$$\frac{d}{dt} G_\alpha GTP = v_{ga} - v_{h0} - v_{h1}$$

$$G_t = G_{\alpha\beta\gamma} + G_\alpha GTP + G_\alpha GDP$$

$$G_{total} = G_{\alpha\beta\gamma} + G_{\beta\gamma}. \tag{6-5}$$

The rate equations for the G protein activation, v_{ga}, the hydrolysis of $G_\alpha GTP$, v_{h0} and v_{h1}, and the subunit re-association, v_{sr}, follow simple mass action kinetics:

$$v_{ga} = k_{ga} \cdot R_a \cdot G_{\alpha\beta\gamma}$$

$$v_{hi} = k_{hi} \cdot G_\alpha GTP, i = 0,1$$

$$v_{sr} = k_{sr} \cdot G_{\beta\gamma} \cdot G_\alpha GDP. \tag{6-6}$$

The parameters are $k_{ga} = 1 \cdot 10^{-5}$ (molecules per cell)$^{-1}$ s^{-1}, $k_{h0} = 0.004$ s^{-1}, $k_{h1} = 0.11$ s^{-1}, and $k_{sr} = 1$ (molecules per cell)$^{-1}$ s^{-1}. Fig. 6.7 shows the respective simulation. Note that in the original work two different yeast strains have been considered. For the strains with a constantly active RGS ($SST2^+$) or with a deletion of RGS ($sst2\Delta$), the rate constants k_{h1} and k_{h0} have been set to zero, respectively.

6.3.2
Ras Proteins

Small G proteins are monomeric G proteins with molecular weight of 20–40 kDa. Like heterotrimeric G proteins, their activity depends on the binding of GTP. More than 100 small G proteins have been identified. They belong to five families: Ras, Rho, Rab, Ran, and Arf. They regulate a wide variety of cell functions as biological timers that initiate and terminate specific cell functions and determine the periods of time (Takai et al. 2001).

Ras proteins cycle between active and inactive states (Fig. 6.8). The transition form GDP-bound to GTP-bound states is catalyzed by a guanine nucleotide exchange factor (GEF), which induces exchange between the bound GDP and the cellular GTP. The reverse process is facilitated by a GTPase-activating protein (GAP), which induces hydrolysis of the bound GTP (Schmidt and Hall 2002).

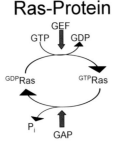

Fig. 6.8 The Ras activation cycle. GEF supports the transition from GDP-bound to GTP-bound states to activate Ras, while GAP induces hydrolysis of the bound GTP, resulting in Ras deactivation.

Mutations of the *Ras* proto-oncogenes (H-*Ras*, N-*Ras*, K-*Ras*) are found in many human tumors. Most of these mutations result in the abolishment of normal GTPase activity of Ras. The Ras mutants can still bind to GAP, but they cannot catalyze GTP hydrolysis. Therefore, they stay active for a long time.

6.3.3
Phosphorelay Systems

Most phosphorylation events in signaling pathways take place under consumption of ATP. Phosphorelay (or phosphotransfer) systems employ another mechanism: after an initial phosphorylation using ATP (or another phosphate donor), the phosphate group is transferred directly from one protein to the next without further consumption of ATP (or external donation of phosphate). Examples are the bacterial phosphoenolpyruvate:carbohydrate phosphotransferase (Postma et al. 1989, 1993; Rohwer et al. 2000; Francke et al. 2003), the two-component system of *E. coli*, or the Sln1 pathway involved in osmoresponse of yeast (Klipp et al. 2004).

Figure 6.9 shows a scheme of a phosphorelay system from the high osmolarity glycerol (HOG) signaling pathway in yeast. This pathway is organized as follows (Hohmann 2002). It involves the transmembrane protein Sln1, which is present as a dimer. Under normal conditions, the pathway is active, since Sln1 continuously autophosphorylates at a histidine residue, Sln1H-P, under consumption of ATP. Subsequently, this phosphate group is transferred to an aspartate group of Sln1 (resulting in Sln1A-P), then to a histidine residue of Ypd1, and finally to an aspartate residue of Ssk1. Ssk1 is continuously dephosphorylated by a phosphatase. Without stress, the proteins are present mainly in their phosphorylated form. The pathway is blocked by an increase in the external osmolarity and a concomitant loss of turgor pressure in the cell. The phosphorylation of Sln1 stops, the pathway runs out of transferable phosphate groups, and the concentration of Ssk1 rises. This constitutes the downstream signal.

Phosphorelay-System

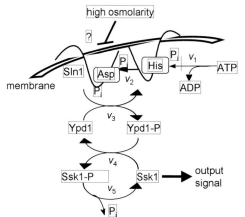

Fig. 6.9 Schematic representation of a phosphorelay system. (a) Phosphorelay system belonging to the Sln1-branch of the HOG pathway in yeast. (b) General scheme of phosphorylation and dephosphorylation.

The temporal behavior of the Sln1-phosphorelay module in yeast can be described with the following set of ODEs.

$$\frac{d}{dt} Sln1 = -k_1 \cdot Sln1 + k_3 \cdot Sln1A\text{-}P \cdot Ypd1$$

$$\frac{d}{dt} Sln1H\text{-}P = k_1 \cdot Sln1 - k_2 Sln1H\text{-}P$$

$$\frac{d}{dt} Sln1A\text{-}P = k_2 \cdot Sln1H\text{-}P - k_3 \cdot Sln1A\text{-}P \cdot Ypd1$$

$$\frac{d}{dt} Ypd1 = k_4 \cdot Ypd1\text{-}P \cdot Ssk1 - k_3 \cdot Sln1A\text{-}P \cdot Ypd1$$

$$\frac{d}{dt} Ypd1\text{-}P = -k_4 \cdot Ypd1\text{-}P \cdot Ssk1 + k_3 \cdot Sln1A\text{-}P \cdot Ypd1$$

$$\frac{d}{dt} Ssk1 = k_5 \cdot Ssk1\text{-}P - k_4 \cdot Ypd1\text{-}P \cdot Ssk1$$

$$\frac{d}{dt} Ssk1\text{-}P = -k_5 \cdot Ssk1\text{-}P + k_4 \cdot Ypd1\text{-}P \cdot Ssk1 . \tag{6-7}$$

For the ordinary differential equation (ODE) system in Eq. (6-7), the following conservation relations hold:

$$Sln1_{total} = Sln1 + Sln1H\text{-}P + Sln1A\text{-}P$$

$$Ypd1_{total} = Ypd1 + Ypd1\text{-}P$$

$$Ssk1_{total} = Ssk1 + Ssk1\text{-}P . \tag{6-8}$$

The existence of conservation relations is in agreement with the assumption that production and degradation of the proteins occur on a larger timescale than the phosphorylation events.

The temporal behavior of the Sln1 phosphorelay system is represented for an external stimulus of 200 s. Before the stimulus, the concentrations of Sln1, Ypd1, and Ssk1 are at low levels. After stimulation, they increase one after the other up to a maximal level that is determined by the total concentration of each protein. After removal of stimulus, all three concentrations return quickly to their initial values.

It is often discussed whether the low number of molecules involved in signaling cascades justifies stochastic rather than deterministic modeling of temporal behavior. We can use the phosphorelay model to compare deterministic and stochastic simulations. Figure 6.10 also shows simulations using the Next Reaction Method, which is based on the Gillespie algorithm (see Chapter 3). Curves in the upper panel show one simulation for low total molecule numbers per species, and in the lower panel one simulation for the experimentally determined number of molecules per cell is shown (Ghaemmaghami et al. 2003). In both cases, the median for a multi-

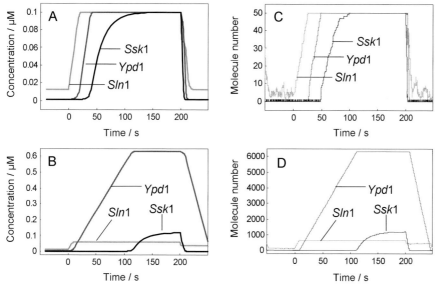

Fig. 6.10 Time course of the phosphorelay system after stimulation for 200 s. The results for deterministic simulation (panels A and B) and for stochastic simulation (panels C and D) are shown. Parameter values for all cases: $k1 = 0.4\ s^{-1}$, $k2 = 1\ s^{-1}$, $k3 = 50\ \mu M^{-1}\ s^{-1}$; $k4 = 50\ \mu M^{-1}\ s^{-1}$; $k5 = 0.5\ s^{-1}$. Total concentrations in the deterministic simulation: panel A: $Sln1_{total} = 0.1\ \mu M$, $Ypd1_{total} = 0.1\ \mu M$, $Ssk1_{total} = 0.1\ \mu M$; panel B: $Sln1_{total} = 0.06\ \mu M$, $Ypd1_{total} = 0.62\ \mu M$, $Ssk1_{total} = 0.12\ \mu M$. Total molecule numbers for stochastic simulation: panel C: $Sln1_{total}$: 50, $Ypd1_{total}$: 50, $Ssk1_{total}$: 50; panel D: $Sln1_{total}$: 656, $Ypd1_{total}$: 6300, $Ssk1_{total}$: 1200.

tude of simulations (not shown) tends towards the deterministic solution. For low molecule numbers, the stochastic curves show pronounced variance before onset and after conclusion of stress, but extremely low variance during stress. It is obvious that the switch from phosphorylated to non-phosphorylated states follows a strong order from one level to the next. While the deterministic simulation pretends a uniform behavior, the stochastic simulation typifies the individual behavior of different cells. For higher molecule numbers (here: realistic numbers), both simulation types are equally informative.

6.3.4
MAP Kinase Cascades

Mitogen-activated protein kinases (MAPKs) are a family of serine/threonine kinases that transduce signals from the cell membrane to the nucleus in response to a wide range of stimuli. Independent or coupled kinase cascades participate in many different intracellular signaling pathways that control a spectrum of cellular processes, including cell growth, differentiation, transformation, and apoptosis. MAPK cascades are widely involved in eukaryotic signal transduction, and these pathways are conserved from yeast to mammals.

A general scheme of a MAPK cascade is depicted in Fig. 6.11. This pathway consists of several levels (usually three), where the activated kinase at each level phosphorylates the kinase at the next level down the cascade. The MAP kinase (MAPK) is at the terminal level of the cascade. It is activated by the MAPK kinase (MAPKK) by phosphorylation of two sites: conserved threonine and tyrosine residues. The MAPKK is itself phosphorylated at serine and threonine residues by the MAPKK kinase (MAPKKK). Several mechanisms are known to activate MAPKKKs by phosphorylation of a tyrosine residue. In some cases the upstream kinase may be considered a MAPKKK kinase (MAPKKKK). Dephosphorylation of either residue is thought to inactivate the kinases, and mutants lacking either residue are almost inactive. At each cascade level, protein phosphatases can inactivate the corresponding kinase, although in some cases it is a matter of debate whether this reaction is performed by an independent protein or by the kinase itself as autodephosphorylation. Ubiquitin-dependent degradation of phosphorylated proteins is also reported.

Although they are conserved through species, elements of the MAPK cascade were given different names in various studied systems. Some examples are represented in Tab. 6.1 (see also Wilkinson and Millar 2000).

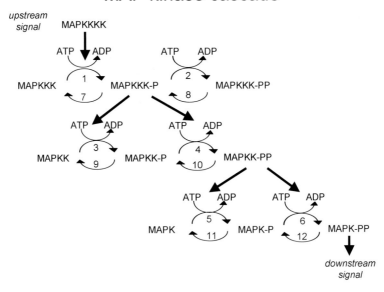

MAP kinase cascade

Fig. 6.11 Schematic representation of the MAP kinase cascade. An upstream signal (often by a further kinase called MAP kinase kinase kinase kinase) causes phosphorylation of the MAPKKK. The phosphorylated MAPKKK in turn phosphorylates the protein at the next level. Dephosphorylation is assumed to occur continuously by phosphatases or autodephosphorylation.

Tab. 6.1 Names of the components of MAP kinase pathways in different organisms and different pathways.

Organism	Budding yeast		Xensopus oocytes	Human, cell cycle regulation		
	HOG pathway	Pheromone pathway			p38 pathway	JNK pathway
MAPKKK	Ssk2/Ssk22	Ste11	Mos	Rafs (c-, A- and B-),	Tak1	MEKKs
MAPKK	Pbs2	Ste7	MEK1	MEK1/2	MKK3/6	MKK4/7
MAPK	Hog1	Fus3	p42 MAPK	ERK1/2	p38	JNK1/2

In the following we will present typical modeling approaches and then discuss functional properties of signaling cascades. The dynamics of a MAPK cascade may be represented by the following ODE system:

$$\frac{d}{dt}MAPKKK = -v_1 + v_7$$

$$\frac{d}{dt}MAPKKK\text{-}P = v_1 - v_7 - v_2 + v_8$$

$$\frac{d}{dt}MAPKKK\text{-}P_2 = v_2 - v_8 \tag{6-9}$$

$$\frac{d}{dt}MAPKK = -v_3 + v_9$$

$$\frac{d}{dt}MAPKK\text{-}P = v_3 - v_9 - v_4 + v_{10}$$

$$\frac{d}{dt}MAPKK\text{-}P_2 = v_4 - v_{10} \tag{6-10}$$

$$\frac{d}{dt}MAPK = -v_5 + v_{11}$$

$$\frac{d}{dt}MAPK\text{-}P = v_5 - v_{11} - v_6 + v_{12}$$

$$\frac{d}{dt}MAPK\text{-}P_2 = v_6 - v_{12} . \tag{6-11}$$

Please note that it is not clear whether MAPKKK-P$_2$ and v_2, v_8 exist at all. In this case their value may be simply set to zero.

The variables in the ODE system fulfill a set of moiety conservation relations, irrespective of the concrete choice of expression for the rates $v_1 ... v_{12}$. It holds that

$$MAPKKK_{total} = MAPKKK + MAPKKK\text{-}P + MAPKKK\text{-}P_2 \tag{6-12}$$

$$MAPKK_{total} = MAPKK + MAPKK\text{-}P + MAPKK\text{-}P_2 \tag{6-13}$$

$$MAPK_{total} = MAPK + MAPK\text{-}P + MAPK\text{-}P_2 \, . \tag{6-14}$$

The conservation relations reflect that we do not consider production or degradation of the involved proteins in this model. This is justified by the supposition that protein production and degradation take place on a different timescale than signal transduction.

The choice of the expressions for the rates is a matter of the elaborateness of experimental knowledge and of modeling taste. We will discuss different possibilities here. Assuming only mass action results in linear and bilinear expression such as

$$v_1 = k_1 \cdot MAPKKK \cdot MAPKKKK \tag{6-15}$$

$$v_7 = k_7 \cdot MAPKKK\text{-}P \, . \tag{6-16}$$

The kinetic constants k_i are first-order $(i \geq 7)$ and second-order $(i \leq 6)$ rate constants.

In these expressions, the concentrations of the donor and acceptor of the transferred phosphate group, ATP and ADP, are not explicitly considered but are included in the rate constants k_1 and k_7. Considering ATP and ADP explicitly results in

$$v_1 = k_1 \cdot MAPKKK \cdot MAPKKKK \cdot ATP \tag{6-17}$$

$$v_7 = k_7 \cdot MAPKKK\text{-}P \, . \tag{6-18}$$

In addition, we have to be concerned about the ATP-ADP balance and add three more differential equations:

$$\frac{d}{dt} ATP = -\sum_{i=1}^{6} v_i + v_x$$

$$\frac{d}{dt} ADP = \sum_{i=1}^{6} v_i + v_x$$

$$\frac{d}{dt} P = -\sum_{i=7}^{12} v_i + v_x \, . \tag{6-19}$$

Here we find two more conservation relations: the conservation of adenine nucleotides, $ATP + ADP = const.$, and the conservation of phosphate groups:

$$MAPKKK\text{-}P + 2 \cdot MAPKKK\text{-}P_2 + MAPKK\text{-}P + 2 \cdot MAPKK\text{-}P_2$$
$$+ MAPK\text{-}P + 2 \cdot MAPK\text{-}P_2 + 3 \cdot ATP + 2 \cdot ADP + P = const. \tag{6-20}$$

One may take into account that enzymes catalyze all steps (e. g., Huang and Ferrell 1996) and therefore consider Michaelis-Menten kinetics for the individual steps

(e. g., Kholodenko 2000). Taking again the first and seventh reactions as examples for kinase and phosphatase steps, we get

$$v_1 = k_1 \cdot MAPKKKK \frac{MAPKKK}{K_{m1} + MAPKKK} \tag{6-21}$$

$$v_7 = \frac{V_{max7} \cdot MAPKKK\text{-}P}{K_{m7} + MAPKKK\text{-}P} , \tag{6-22}$$

where k_1 is a first-order rate constant, K_{m1} and K_{m7} are Michaelis constants, and V_{max7} denotes a maximal enzyme rate. Reported values for Michaelis constants are 15 nM (Kholodenko 2000), 46 nM and 159 nM (Force et al. 1994), and 300 nM (Huang and Ferrell 1996). For maximal rates, values of about 0.75 nM $\cdot$ s^{-1} (Kholodenko 2000) are used in models.

The performance of MAPK cascades, i. e., their ability to amplify the signal and to notably enhance the concentration of the double-phosphorylated MAPK and the speed of activation, depends crucially on the kinetic constants of the kinases, k_+, and phosphatases, k_-, and, moreover, on their ratio (see Fig. 6.12). If the ratio k_+/k_- is low (phosphatases stronger than kinases), then the amplification is high, but at very low absolute concentrations of phosphorylated MAPK. High values of k_+/k_- ensure

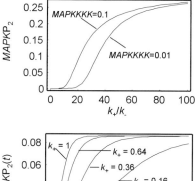

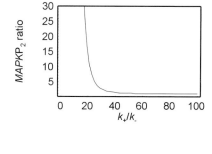

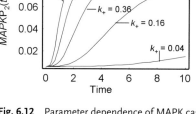

Fig. 6.12 Parameter dependence of MAPK cascade performance. In the upper row steady-state simulations are shown for changing values of rate constants for kinases, k_+, and phosphatases, k_- (in arbitrary units). Left panel: Absolute values of the output signal *MAPK-PP* depending on the input signal (high: *MAPKKKK* = 0.1 or low: *MAPKKKK* = 0.01) for varying ratio of k_+/k_-. Right panel: ratio of the output signal for high versus low input signal (*MAPKKKK* = 0.1 or *MAPKKKK* = 0.01) for varying ratio of k_+/k_-. Lower row, left panel: time course of MAPK activation for different values of k_+ and a ratio $k_+/k_- = 20$.

high absolute concentrations of MAPK-P$_2$, but with negligible amplification. High values of both k_+ and k_- ensure fast activation of downstream targets.

Frequently, the proteins of MAPK cascades interact with scaffold proteins. In this case, a reversible assembly of oligomeric protein complexes that include both enzymatic proteins and proteins without known enzymatic activity precedes the signal transduction. These non-enzymatic components can serve as scaffolds or anchors to the plasma membrane and regulate the efficiency, specificity, and localization of the signaling pathway.

6.3.5
Jak-Stat Pathways

Jak-Stat pathways play an important role in regulating immune responses and cellular homeostasis in human health and disease (Kisseleva et al. 2002; Schindler 2002). They are activated by cytokines, a large family of extracellular ligands. The family of structurally and functionally conserved receptors involves four Jaks and seven Stats. As is the case for many types of receptor families, downstream signaling entails tyrosine phosphorylation. Stat stands for "signal transducer and activator of transcription", because this class of proteins functions as both signal transducer and transcription activator. They are inactive as a monomer, and activation involves phosphorylation and dimerization.

A mathematical model of the Jak-Stat pathway presented by Swamaye and colleagues (2003) presupposes the binding of the ligand (here, the hormone Epo) to the receptor (EpoR), which results in phosphorylation of Jak2 and of the cytoplasmatic domain of EpoR. The model involves the recruitment of monomeric Stat5 ($x_1 = Stat5$) to the phosphorylated and thereby activated receptor, EpoR$_A$. Upon receptor recruitment, monomeric Stat5 is tyrosine-phosphorylated ($x_2 = Stat5$-P). It dimerizes in a second step to yield x_3 and migrates in the third step to the nucleus (x_4), where it binds to the promoter of target genes. After it has fulfilled its job, it is dephosphorylated and exported to the cytoplasm (fourth step). Using simple mass action kinetics for the four steps indicated in Fig. 6.13, the respective ODE system reads:

$$\frac{dx_1}{dt} = -k_1 x_1 \, EpoR_A + 2k_4 x_4^\tau$$

$$\frac{dx_2}{dt} = -k_2 x_2^2 + k_1 x_1 \, EpoR_A$$

$$\frac{dx_3}{dt} = -k_3 x_3 + \frac{1}{2} k_2 x_2^2$$

$$\frac{dx_4}{dt} = -k_4 x_4^\tau + k_3 x_3 . \tag{6-23}$$

The parameter τ represents the time Stat5 molecules have to reside in the nucleus with $x_4^\tau = x_4 (t - \tau)$. This model has been used to show that recycling of Stat5 mole-

Jak-Stat pathway

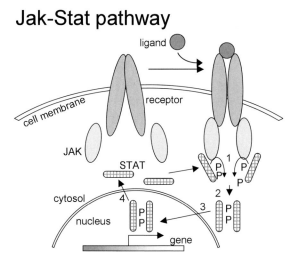

ligand

receptor

cell membrane

JAK

STAT

cytosol

nucleus

gene

Fig. 6.13 The Jak-Stat signaling pathway. Upon ligand binding, receptor-associated Jaks become activated and mediate phosphorylation of specific receptor tyrosine residues. This leads to the recruitment of specific Stats, which are then also tyrosine-phosphorylated. Activated Stats are released from the receptor, dimerize, translocate to the nucleus, and bind to enhancers.

cules is an important event in the activation cycle and is necessary to explain experimental data.

6.4
Signaling: Dynamic and Regulatory Features

A nice overview of dynamic and regulatory features of modules of signaling pathways is given by Tyson et al. (2003). In line with this work, we show here the behavior of simple motifs of signaling pathways. We will also present measures for the characterization of the dynamics of components of signaling pathways.

6.4.1
Simple Motifs

Here, we consider motifs of many signaling networks, which stand symbolically for the action pairs of protein synthesis and degradation or phosphorylation and dephosphorylation. The shape of response curves depends on network structure and respective implementation in mathematical expression. A set of the simplest motifs as well as their implementation and respective behavior are represented in Tab. 6.2.

The dynamics of such a network depends on the concentrations of the signal S and the responder R

$$\frac{dR}{dt} = f(S, R).$$ (6-24)

with S = signal strength (e. g., mRNA concentration) and R = response magnitude (e. g., protein concentration), as well as on the individual kinetics. Assuming linear

Tab. 6.2 Simple signaling motifs, their kinetic implementation, and characterization of behavior.

Scheme	Kinetic	Steady state	Response
Linear S ⋮ $\rightarrow R \longrightarrow$	Linear $\dfrac{dR}{dt} = k_0 + k_1 S - k_2 R$	$R^{ss} = \dfrac{k_0 + k_1 S}{k_2}$	Linear
	Michaelis-Menten $\dfrac{dR}{dt} = \dfrac{V_1 S}{K_{m1} + S} - \dfrac{V_2 R}{K_{m2} + R}$	$R^{ss} = \dfrac{V_1 K_{m2} S}{V_2 K_{m1} + S(V_2 - V_1)}$	Hyperbolic
One loop S ↓ $R_0 \; R$ ⤸	Linear $\dfrac{dR}{dt} = k_1 S(R_t - R) - k_2 R$ $R + R_0 = R_{total}$	$R^{ss} = \dfrac{R_{total} k_1 S}{k_2 + k_1 S}$	Hyperbolic
	Michaelis-Menten $\dfrac{dR}{dt} = \dfrac{k_1 S(R_{total} - R)}{K_{m1} + R_{total} - R} - \dfrac{k_2 R}{K_{m2} + R}$ $R + R_0 = R_{total}$	$R^{ss} = R_{total} \cdot G\left(k_1 S, k_2, \dfrac{K_{m1}}{R_{total}}, \dfrac{K_{m2}}{R_{total}}\right)$	Sigmoid
Two loops S $R_0 \; R_1 \; R$	Linear $\dfrac{dR}{dt} = k_3 S R_1 - k_4 R$ $\dfrac{dR_1}{dt} = k_1 S R_0 - (k_2 + k_3 S)R_1 + k_4 R$ $R + R_0 = R_{total}$	$R^{ss} = \dfrac{R_{total} k_1 k_3 S^2}{k_2 k_4 + k_1 S k_4 + k_1 k_3 S^2}$	Sigmoid

kinetics for all steps of the linear mechanism in Tab. 6.2 leads to a linear response in terms of steady-state values (R^{ss} = steady-state values). Figure 6.14 shows the dependencies of steady-state concentrations on the signal strength. Assuming Michaelis-Menten kinetics implies a hyperbolic response. On the other hand, a hyperbolic response can be caused by the network structure. Consider the one-loop mechanism depicted in Tab. 6.2. Consideration of the conservation relation for the different forms of R ($R + R_0 = R_{total}$) and the assumption of linear kinetics cause a hyperbolic response. Description of the one-loop mechanism with Michaelis-Menten kinetics gives rise to a switch-like sigmoidal response curve based on a quadratic solution for steady state (only the following solution applies for $0 < R < R_{total}$). The function G with

$$G(u, v, J, K) = \dfrac{2uK}{v - u + vJ + uK + \sqrt{(v - u + vJ + uK)^2 - 4(v - u)uK}} \tag{6-25}$$

used in Tab. 6.2 is the so-called Goldbeter-Koshland function (Goldbeter and Koshland 1981, 1984), which is frequently applied in modeling switch-like behavior.

All three types of response (linear, hyperbolic, sigmoidal) are gradual, i.e., the response increases continuously with signal strength, and reversible, i.e., the steady-

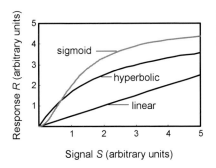

Fig. 6.14   Signal-response curves for different signaling motifs. Shown are linear, hyperbolic, and sigmoid curves.

state value depends only on the actual value of the signal but not on its history (whether it was increased or decreased); moreover, the response is switched off (downregulated) if there is no more signal S. The response of these motifs directly transmits what the signal stipulates. There is no intrinsic stimulation or downregulation.

6.4.2
Adaptation Motif

Combination of a simple linear response element with a second signaling pathway yields perfectly adapted signal-response curves. This results in the following effect: although the signaling pathway exhibits a transient response to changes in signal strength, its steady-state response R^{ss} is independent of S. Tyson and colleagues (2003) called them *sniffer* due to their similarity to the sense of smell.

$$\frac{dR}{dt} = k_1 S - k_2 X \cdot R \qquad \text{with} \qquad R^{ss} = \frac{k_1 k_4}{k_2 k_3}$$

$$\frac{dX}{dt} = k_3 S - k_4 X \qquad\qquad X^{ss} = \frac{k_3 S}{k_4} . \qquad\qquad (6\text{-}26)$$

The time course is represented in Fig. 6.15.

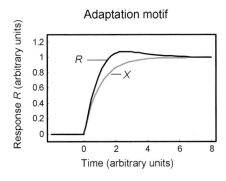

Fig. 6.15   Temporal profile of the adaptation motif.

6.4.3
Negative Feedback

Among the various regulatory features of signaling pathways, negative feedback has attracted outstanding interest. It also plays an important role in metabolic pathways, e.g., in amino acid synthesis pathways, where a negative feedback signal from the amino acid at the end to the precursors at the beginning of the pathway prevents an overproduction of this amino acid. The implementation of the feedback and the respective dynamic behavior show a wide variation. In Chapter 7 we will show how feedback can bring about limit cycle–type oscillations in cell cycle models. In signaling pathways, negative feedback may cause an adjustment of the response or damped oscillations (Section 7.1.1.3).

Example 6-3

Some possible effects of negative feedback are illustrated in Fig. 6.16 for an unbranched chain of six reactions, as depicted in Eq. (5-190), in which the rate expressions are $v_i = S_{i-1}k_i$ for $i = 1, ..., 6$. Feedback inhibition of the first reaction by the j-th metabolite is implemented as $v_1 = S_1 k_1 / (1 + S_j K_I)$.

In the absence of feedback, the metabolite concentrations reach a steady state after a short transition period. If the second metabolite inhibits the first reaction, one may observe an overshooting of the concentration of the first metabolite. In the case of a long-ranging feedback, oscillations can occur. In the given example, damped oscillations result from the inhibition of the first reaction by the last metabolite.

6.4.4
Quantitative Measures for Properties of Signaling Pathways

To characterize the dynamic behavior of signaling pathways in a quantitative way, Heinrich and colleagues (2002) introduced three measures. Let $X_i(t)$ be the time-dependent concentration of the kinase i. The signaling time τ_i describes the average time to activate the kinase i. The signal duration ϑ_i gives the average time during which the kinase i remains activated. The signal amplitude S_i is a measure of the average concentration of activated kinase i. The following definitions have been introduced. The quantity

$$I_i = \int_0^\infty X_i(t)dt \tag{6-27}$$

is the total amount of active kinase i generated during the signaling period, i.e., the integrated response of X_i (the area covered by a plot $X_i(t)$ versus time). Further measures are

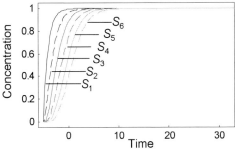

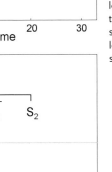

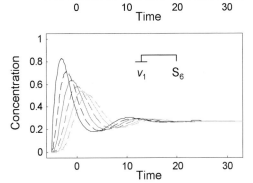

Fig. 6.16 Effect of negative feedback on the dynamics of a simple unbranched reaction scheme. Upper panel: no feedback. All substrate concentrations reach asymptotically a high, constant level. Center: Feedback from the second metabolite on first reaction. The substrate concentrations approach a constant but remarkably lower level. Lower panel: Feedback from the last metabolite on first reaction. The substrate concentrations approach a lower level than without feedback and show damped oscillations.

$$T_i = \int\limits_0^\infty t \cdot X_i(t)dt \tag{6-28}$$

$$Q_i = \int\limits_0^\infty t^2 \cdot X_i(t)dt. \tag{6-29}$$

The signaling time can now be defined as

$$\tau_i = T_i/I_i, \tag{6-30}$$

i.e., as the average of time, analogous to mean value of a statistical distribution. Note that other definitions for characteristic times have been introduced in Chapter 5 (Section 5.2.6). The signal duration

$$\vartheta_i = \sqrt{Q_i/I_i - \tau_i^2} \tag{6-31}$$

gives a measure of how extended the signaling response is around the mean time (compatible to standard deviation). The signal amplitude is defined as

$$A_i = I_i/(2\vartheta_i).$$ (6-32)

In a geometric representation, this is the height of a rectangle whose length is $2\vartheta_i$ and whose area equals the area under the curve $X_i(t)$.

Example 6-4

For the model of the phosphorelay system presented in Section 6.3.3, the characteristic quantities are given in Tab. 6.3. How these measures relate to the actual time course is shown for Ssk1 in Fig. 6.17.

Tab. 6.3 Dynamic characteristics of the phosphorelay system.

Protein Signal amplitude (A μM^{-1})	Characteristic time (τ s^{-1})	Signal duration (ϑ s^{-1})
Sln1	109.182	57.693	0.151
Ypd1	116.283	51.325	0.170

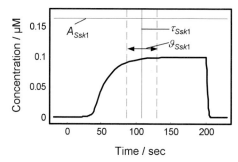

Fig. 6.17 Representation of characteristic measures for the output signal of the phosphorelay system, Ssk1. The horizontal line indicates the calculated signal amplitude, the solid vertical line marks the characteristic time, and the dotted vertical lines cover the signaling time.

References

BANUETT, F. Signalling in the yeasts: an informational cascade with links to the filamentous fungi (1998) Microbiol. Mol. Biol. Rev. *62*, 249–74

BLUMER, K.J. and THORNER, J. Receptor-G protein signaling in yeast (1991) Annu. Rev. Physiol. *53*, 37–57

BUCK, L.B. The molecular architecture of odor and pheromone sensing in mammals (2000) Cell *100*, 611–8

BURCHETT, S.A. Regulators of G protein signaling: a bestiary of modular protein binding domains (2000) J. Neurochem. *75*, 1335–51

DOHLMAN, H.G. G proteins and pheromone signaling (2002) Annu. Rev. Physiol. *64*, 129–52

DOHLMAN, H.G. and THORNER, J. RGS proteins and signaling by heterotrimeric G proteins (1997) J. Biol. Chem. *272*, 3871–4

DOHLMAN, H.G. and THORNER, J.W. Regulation of G protein-initiated signal transduction in yeast: paradigms and principles (2001) Annu. Rev. Biochem. *70*, 703–54

DOHLMAN, H.G., THORNER, J., CARON, M.G. and LEFKOWITZ, R.J. Model systems for the study of seven-transmembrane-segment receptors (1991) Annu. Rev. Biochem. *60*, 653–88

DOHLMAN, H.G., SONG, J., APANOVITCH, D.M., DiBELLO, P.R. and GILLEN, K.M. Regulation of G protein signalling in yeast (1998) Semin. Cell. Dev. Biol. *9*, 135–41

FORCE, T., BONVENTRE, J.V., HEIDECKER, G., RAPP, U., AVRUCH, J. and KYRIAKIS, J.M. Enzymatic characteristics of the c-Raf-1 protein kinase (1994) Proc. Natl. Acad. Sci. U S A *91*, 1270–4

FRANCKE, C., POSTMA, P.W., WESTERHOFF, H.V., BLOM, J.G. and PELETIER, M.A. Why the phosphotransferase system of *Escherichia coli* escapes diffusion limitation (2003) Biophys. J. *85*, 612–22

GHAEMMAGHAMI, S., HUH, W.K., BOWER, K., HOWSON, R.W., BELLE, A., DEPHOURE, N., O'SHEA, E.K. and WEISSMAN, J.S. Global analysis of protein expression in yeast (2003) Nature *425*, 737–41

GOLDBETER, A. and KOSHLAND, D.E., JR. An amplified sensitivity arising from covalent modification in biological systems (1981) Proc. Natl. Acad. Sci. USA *78*, 6840–4

GOLDBETER, A. and KOSHLAND, D.E., JR. Ultrasensitivity in biochemical systems controlled by covalent modification. Interplay between zero-order and multistep effects (1984) J. Biol. Chem. *259*, 14441–7

HEINRICH, R., NEEL, B.G. and RAPOPORT, T.A. Mathematical models of protein kinase signal transduction (2002) Mol. Cell. *9*, 957–70

HOHMANN, S. Osmotic stress signaling and osmoadaptation in yeasts (2002) Microbiol. Mol. Biol. Rev. *66*, 300–72

HUANG, C.Y. and FERRELL, J.E., JR. Ultrasensitivity in the mitogen-activated protein kinase cascade (1996) Proc. Natl. Acad. Sci. USA *93*, 10078–83

KHOLODENKO, B.N. Negative feedback and ultrasensitivity can bring about oscillations in the mitogen-activated protein kinase cascades (2000) Eur. J. Biochem. *267*, 1583–8

KISSELEVA, T., BHATTACHARYA, S., BRAUNSTEIN, J. and SCHINDLER, C.W. Signaling through the JAK/STAT pathway, recent advances and future challenges (2002) Gene *285*, 1–24

KLIPP, E., NORDLANDER, B., KRUEGER, R., GENNEMARK, P. and HOHMANN, S. The dynamic response of yeast cells to osmotic shock – a systems biology approach (2004) submitted

MEIGS, T.E., FIELDS, T.A., McKEE, D.D. and CASEY, P.J. Interaction of Galpha 12 and Galpha 13 with the cytoplasmic domain of cadherin provides a mechanism for beta -catenin release (2001) Proc. Natl. Acad. Sci. USA *98*, 519–24

NEER, E.J. Heterotrimeric G proteins: organizers of transmembrane signals (1995) Cell *80*, 249–57

OFFERMANNS, S. Mammalian G-protein function in vivo: new insights through altered gene expression (2000) Rev. Physiol. Biochem. Pharmacol. *140*, 63–133

POSTMA, P.W., BROEKHUIZEN, C.P. and GEERSE, R.H. The role of the PEP: carbohydrate phosphotransferase system in the regulation of bacterial metabolism (1989) FEMS Microbiol. Rev. *5*, 69–80

POSTMA, P.W., LENGELER, J.W. and JACOBSON, G.R. Phosphoenolpyruvate:carbohydrate phosphotransferase systems of bacteria (1993) Microbiol. Rev. *57*, 543–94

ROHWER, J.M., MEADOW, N.D., ROSEMAN, S., WESTERHOFF, H.V. and POSTMA, P.W. Understanding glucose transport by the bacterial phosphoenolpyruvate:glucose phosphotransferase system on the basis of kinetic measurements in vitro (2000) J. Biol. Chem. *275*, 34909–21

Ross, E.M. and Wilkie, T.M. GTPase-activating proteins for heterotrimeric G proteins: regulators of G protein signaling (RGS) and RGS-like proteins (2000) Annu. Rev. Biochem. *69*, 795–827

Schindler, C.W. Series introduction. JAK-STAT signaling in human disease (2002) J. Clin. Invest. *109*, 1133–7

Schmidt, A. and Hall, A. Guanine nucleotide exchange factors for Rho GTPases: turning on the switch (2002) Genes Dev. *16*, 1587–609

Siderovski, D.P., Strockbine, B. and Behe, C.I. Whither goest the RGS proteins? (1999) Crit. Rev. Biochem. Mol. Biol. *34*, 215–51

Swameye, I., Muller, T.G., Timmer, J., Sandra, O. and Klingmuller, U. Identification of nucleocytoplasmic cycling as a remote sensor in cellular signaling by databased modeling (2003) Proc. Natl. Acad. Sci. USA *100*, 1028–33

Takai, Y., Sasaki, T. and Matozaki, T. Small GTP-binding proteins (2001) Physiol. Rev. *81*, 153–208

Tyson, J.J., Chen, K.C. and Novak, B. Sniffers, buzzers, toggles and blinkers: dynamics of regulatory and signaling pathways in the cell (2003) Curr. Opin. Cell. Biol. *15*, 221–31

Wang, P. and Heitman, J. Signal transduction cascades regulating mating, filamentation, and virulence in *Cryptococcus neoformans* (1999) Curr. Opin. Microbiol. *2*, 358–62

Wilkinson, M.G. and Millar, J.B. Control of the eukaryotic cell cycle by MAP kinase signaling pathways (2000) Faseb J *14*, 2147–57

Yi, T.M., Kitano, H. and Simon, M.I. A quantitative characterization of the yeast heterotrimeric G protein cycle (2003) Proc. Natl. Acad. Sci. USA *100*, 10764–9

7
Selected Biological Processes

Introduction

Biological processes that are of special interest for systems biology are those that contain many reactions forming a complex system or that have the potential to interact and influence many other processes. In this chapter we will take a closer look at three selected processes that fulfill these requirements, namely, biological oscillations, the cell cycle, and the aging process. Oscillations represent a ubiquitous phenomenon in biology that often drives other complex and important functions of the organism. An example of such a central periodic function is the cell cycle, which dominates many aspects of cellular biochemistry. Furthermore, modifications to critical components of the cell cycle can lead to diseases such as cancer or Alzheimer's disease. The final example, aging, is a complex phenomenon that affects practically all components of an organism and becomes ever more important as the average life span of the world population increases. Because of space limitations we restricted ourselves to the mentioned examples, but of course there are other candidates (for instance, development or the immune system) that in principle would fit into this section.

7.1
Biological Oscillations

Periodic changes of biochemical and biophysical quantities are a universal phenomenon in living systems. Examples from everyday experience are the pulse of the heart, spontaneous respiration, the circadian rhythm, cycles of ovulation in mammals, or the annual flowering of trees. Well studied are calcium waves (Goldbeter et al. 1990; Bootman et al. 2001a, 2001b), oscillations in neuronal signals (Rabinovich and Abarbanel 1998), oscillations in cyclic AMP in the slime mold *Dictyostelium discoideum* (Roos et al. 1977; Halloy et al. 1998; Nanjundiah 1998), the periodic conversion of sugar to alcohol (glycolysis) in anaerobic yeast cultures (Chance et al. 1964; Ghosh and Chance 1964; Sel'kov 1968), the circadian rhythm (Smaaland 1996; Turek 1998), and the cell cycle (Tyson 1991; Tyson et al. 1995; Novak et al. 1999; Mori and Johnson 2000; Tyson and Novak 2001). Periodic patterns can be a function

Systems Biology in Practice. Concepts, Implementation and Application.
E. Klipp, R. Herwig, A. Kowald, C. Wierling, H. Lehrach
Copyright © 2005 WILEY-VCH Verlag GmbH & Co. KGaA, Weinheim
ISBN: 3-527-31078-9

of time (glycolytic oscillations), space (striping in *Drosophila melanogaster* embryos), or both (*D. discoideum*, calcium waves, neuronal oscillations), depending on the mechanism of the oscillator. The oscillation periods may cover ranges from milliseconds to years. Some oscillations are initiated externally, while others have intrinsic causes. Many cellular oscillations are associated with the regulation of enzyme activity, receptor function, transport processes, or gene expression in an autocatalytic manner or by positive or negative feedback and feed-forward loops. Other cases of oscillations arise from the regulation of ionic conductances in electrically excitable cells.

Temporarily changing patterns are observed in different complexity. Types of behavior include simple periodic oscillations, complex periodicity with several maxima per period, and even irregular and aperiodic behavior, owing to the appearance of chaos. In the following sections we will introduce the Higgins-Sel'kov oscillator as a classical example of oscillations caused by positive feedback and a model of a multiply regulated biochemical system as an example of more complex oscillatory patterns. Coupled oscillators are presented to illustrate that oscillations in individual cells are sometimes hidden on the population level and therefore are hard to measure experimentally.

7.1.1
Glycolytic Oscillations: The Higgins-Sel'kov Oscillator

The product-activated enzyme reaction is a simple model with two variables for periodic oscillations of the limit-cycle type. The most intensively studied example is the positive feedback exerted by ADP on the enzyme phosphofructokinase I (PFK I). It is believed to cause the oscillations observed in glycolysis in yeast and muscles. The dynamic behavior of this model system was first studied by Higgins (1964) and Sel'kov (1968) and later by many others (e.g., Goldbeter and Lefever 1972; Sel'kov 1975).

The two-variable model takes into account the allosteric regulation of the enzyme PFK I and the autocatalytic effect exerted by the product. For a large range of parameter values, it exhibits a stable steady state, but beyond a critical parameter value, the system becomes instable and evolves towards a stable limit cycle. Then, it shows sustained oscillations.

$$\xrightarrow{v_0} S \xrightarrow{v_1} P \xrightarrow{v_2} . \qquad (7\text{-}1)$$

The temporal behavior of the concentrations of substrate S and product P can be described by the following ODEs:

$$\frac{dS}{dt} = v_0 - Sk_1 \cdot r(P)$$

$$\frac{dP}{dt} = Sk_1 \cdot r(P) - Pk_2 . \qquad (7\text{-}2)$$

The supply rate of S, v_0, is positive. The parameters k_1, k_2 are mass-action rate constants. The function $r(P)$ represents the autocatalytic effect of the product P on its own production. The simplest expression for this function is

$$r(P) = P^2 , \tag{7-3}$$

yielding

$$\frac{dS}{dt} = v_0 - SP^2 k_1 = f(S, P)$$

$$\frac{dP}{dt} = SP^2 k_1 - Pk_2 = g(S, P) . \tag{7-4}$$

The dynamic behavior of this system is represented in Fig. 7.1 for a set of parameters that gives rise to oscillations. Figure 7.1a shows the values of the variables as function of time. Further information about the dynamics of the system can be in-

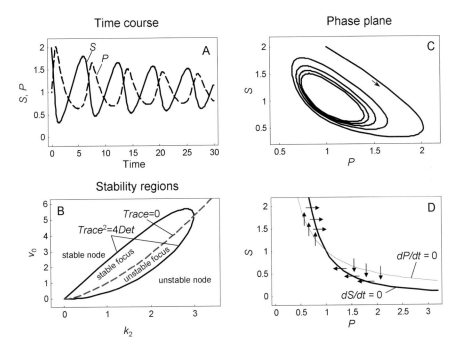

Fig. 7.1 Higgins-Sel'kov oscillator. The dynamic behavior of the ODE system in Eq. (7-4) is presented for the following choice of parameters: $v_0 = 1$, $k_1 = 1$, $k_2 = 1.00001$, $S(0) = 2$, and $P(0) = 1$ in arbitrary units. (a) Time course of the solution. (b) Stability regions for fixed values of $k_1 = 1$ and varying values of v_0 and k_2.

(c) Phase plane representation of the trajectory of the solution. (d) Representation of nullclines $dS/dt = 0$ (black line) and $dP/dt = 0$ (gray line) in the phase plane. Arrows indicate the direction of a trajectory that crosses the nullcline at the respective point.

ferred by inspection of the phase plane. Figure 7.1c shows the trajectory for a given set of parameters and initial conditions in a plot of S versus P, using the time as parameter. The nullclines, i. e., the lines for $dS/dt = f = 0$ or $dP/dt = g = 0$, respectively, are shown in Fig. 7.1d. These lines must always be crossed by the trajectories in a horizontal (for $f = 0$) or vertical (for $g = 0$) manner, respectively, as indicated by the little arrows. The sign of g determines the direction of the arrow for the nullcline $f = 0$ at a certain point, and *vice versa*.

The steady state of the equation system in Eq. (7-4) is unique and is determined by

$$\bar{S} = \frac{k_2^2}{k_1\, v_0}\,, \bar{P} = \frac{v_0}{k_2}\,.$$ (7-5)

The stability of the steady state can be analyzed by inspection of the Jacobian matrix (Chapter 3.2),

$$J = \begin{pmatrix} -\bar{P}^2 k_1 & -2\,\bar{S}\bar{P}\,k_1 \\ \bar{P}^2 k_1 & 2\,\bar{S}\bar{P}\,k_1 - k_2 \end{pmatrix} = \begin{pmatrix} -v_0^2 \dfrac{k_1}{k_2^2} & -2\,k_2 \\ v_0^2 \dfrac{k_1}{k_2^2} & k_2 \end{pmatrix}.$$ (7-6)

The character of the steady state is given by the determinant and the trace of the Jacobian matrix. The determinant reads

$$Det J = v_0^2 \frac{k_1}{k_2^2}\,.$$ (7-7)

Since $v_0 > 0$, the determinant is always positive. However, the trace

$$Trace J = -v_0^2 \frac{k_1}{k_2^2} + k_2$$ (7-8)

changes its sign at

$$v_0^2 = \frac{k_2^3}{k_1}\,.$$ (7-9)

This surface separates stable from unstable steady states in the parameter space. Further critical values can be found by the condition $(Trace J)^2 = 4\, Det J$ (Section 3.2.3) separating nodes from foci. This condition is fulfilled at

$$v_0^4 \frac{k_1^2}{k_2^4} - 6\, v_0^2 \frac{k_1}{k_2} + k_2^2 = 0\,.$$ (7-10)

At the transition from the region of stable focus $((Trace J)^2 < 4\, Det, Trace J < 0)$ to the region of instable focus $((Trace J)^2 < 4\, Det, Trace J > 0)$, limit cycles arise. The change in the stability and character of the steady state with changing parameters is called a bifurcation. This special type of bifurcation, where the eigenvalues of the Jacobian matrix are purely imaginary, is called a Hopf bifurcation (Hopf 1942). The stability regions are represented in Fig. 7.1 b.

It should be noted that the different types of dynamics occur upon changes in the system parameters. It is convenient to keep some of the parameters constant and to follow the change of one parameter, in order to observe the regions of various behaviors. If, for example, k_1 and v_0 are kept constant, then the value of the kinetic constant of product degradation, k_2, is an indicator for the dynamic behavior and can mark the point of the Hopf bifurcation.

7.1.2
Other Modes of Behavior

In biological systems, dynamics have been observed that are more complex than just simple oscillation with fixed amplitudes and frequencies. An example of this type of dynamic behavior is a system of two product-activated enzyme reactions that are coupled in series.

$$\xrightarrow{v_0} S \xrightarrow{v_1} P_1 \xrightarrow{v_2} P_2 \xrightarrow{v_3} . \tag{7-11}$$

The system involves three variables: the substrate S and the products P_1 and P_2. S is produced, the two enzymes E_1 and E_2 transform S into P_1 and P_1 into P_2, respectively, and P_2 is degraded. Their respective products activate both allosteric enzymes. Thus we now have two positive feedback loops. Each of the reactions may show instability as discussed above.

Decroly and Goldbeter (1982) investigated intensively the possible modes of behavior of this system, assuming that the kinetics of both enzymes obeys Monod kinetics (Chapter 5, Eqs. (5-60) and (5-61)). The respective equation system reads

$$\frac{dS}{dt} = \frac{v_0}{K_{m1}} - \sigma_1 \cdot \frac{S(1+S)(1+P_1)^2}{L_1 + (1+S)^2 (1+P_1)^2}$$

$$\frac{dP_1}{dt} = q_1 \cdot \sigma_1 \cdot \frac{S(1+S)(1+P_1)^2}{L_1 + (1+S)^2(1+P_1)^2} - \sigma_2 \cdot \frac{P_1(1+d \cdot P_1)(1+P_2)^2}{L_2 + (1+d \cdot P_1)^2(1+P_2)^2}$$

$$\frac{dP_2}{dt} = q_2 \cdot \sigma_2 \cdot \frac{P_1(1+d \cdot P_1)(1+P_2)^2}{L_2 + (1+d \cdot P_1)^2(1+P_2)^2} - k_3 P_2, \tag{7-12}$$

where K_{m1} is the Michealis constant for the substrate, σ_i is the maximal activity, L_i is the allosteric constant of enzyme i, and q_i and d are ratios of Michaelis constants. In the investigation of the dynamic behavior, all parameters are kept fixed except for the rate constant k_3 for the degradation of P_2. It could be shown that for increasing values of k_3 the system may assume (1) a stable steady state; (2) a limit cycle with simple oscillations; (3) coexistence of a stable state and a limit cycle; (4) birhythmicity, i.e., coexistence of two limit cycles that are reached depending on the initial values; (5) complex periodic oscillations; (6) a strange attractor associated with chaos; and (7) a folded limit cycle with complex but periodic oscillations. Examples of complex periodic behavior and chaos are shown in Fig. 7.2.

7.1.3
Coupling of Oscillators

In yeast cell suspensions, the dynamics of glycolysis are usually studied on a population level by monitoring mean concentrations. In this way, one obtains only limited information about the behavior of single cells. A series of experiments has shown that individual cells also must show oscillations (e.g., Richard et al. 1996). When these oscillations are synchronized, they can be observed on the population level. The absence of oscillations on the population level may be due to the absence of oscillations on the individual level or due to the fact that cells oscillate out of phase and only the mean values are measured.

Synchronization of oscillations is mediated by a coupling compound, which is shared by all cells of the suspension. For glycolytic oscillations, ethanol, pyruvate, and acetaldehyde have been proposed as coupling metabolites, the latter being the most probable.

Wolf and Heinrich (1997) employed the Higgins-Sel'kov oscillator to explain basic features of coupled oscillators. Consider for N cells the situation shown in Fig. 7.3a. The dynamics is described by the following equation system:

$$\frac{dS_i}{dt} = v_0 - S_i P_i^2$$

$$\frac{dP_i}{dt} = S_i P_i^2 - P_i k_2 - k_3(P_i - C)$$

$$\frac{dC}{dt} = \frac{k_3 \varphi}{N}\left(\sum_{i=1}^{N} P_i - N \cdot C\right), \tag{7-13}$$

where C is the extracellular concentration of the coupling metabolite, N is the number of cells, φ denotes the ratio of intracellular and extracellular volume, and k_3 is the effective rate constant for the transmembrane diffusion of the coupling compound. All cells are assumed to be identical.

It is easy to see that the equation system in Eq. (7-13) for N coupled cells has a unique steady state for all cells identical to the steady state derived for an isolated cell (Eq. (7-5)) with $\bar{P} = \bar{C}$. This steady state is stable in certain regions of the parameter space. At the boundary of this region, Hopf bifurcations lead to synchronous or asynchronous oscillations. Here, the solution of the characteristic equation (Eq. (3-29)) yields a pair of purely imaginary eigenvalues. In the vicinity of the bifurcation points, two typical types of behavior may occur: synchronous oscillations and regular asynchronous oscillations (see Fig. 7.3). Synchronous oscillations for cell po-

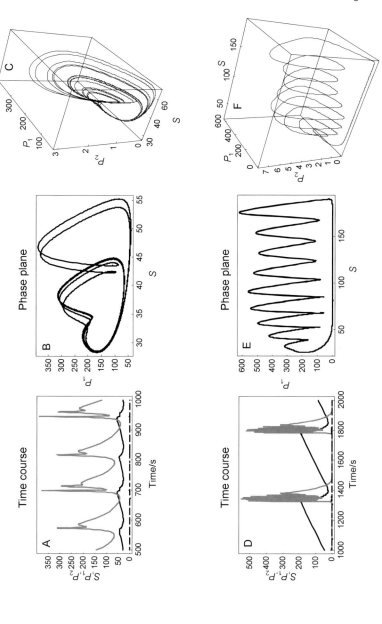

Fig. 7.2 Decroly-Goldbeter model. The model depicted in Eqs. (11) and (12) shows interesting patterns of temporal self-organization. The upper panels show behavior associated with chaos, and the lower panels show trajectories for complex periodic behavior. (a, d) Time courses. (b, e) Phase planes for S and P_1. (c, f) Trajectories in the space spanned by all three concentrations. Parameters: $v_0/K_{m1} = 0.5$ s^{-1}, $\sigma_1 = \sigma_2 = 10$ s^{-1}, $q_1 = 50$, $q_2 = 0.02$, $L_1 = 5 \cdot 10^8$, $L_2 = 100$. (a–c): $k_3 = 2.032$ s^{-1}, $d = 0.00001$, (d–f): $k_3 = 2.5$ s^{-1}, $d = 0.0001$.

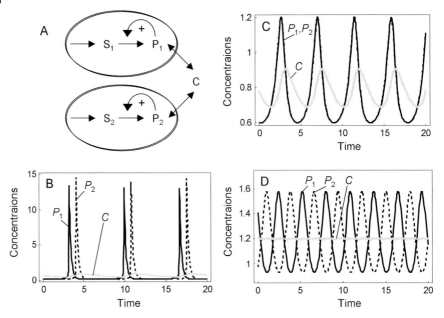

Fig. 7.3 Dynamics of coupled oscillators according to the model of Wolf and Heinrich (1997). (a) Schematic representation of two oscillators. The metabolites S_1 and P_1 occur in a compartment (cell) that is different from the compartment containing the metabolites S_2 and P_2. The metabolite C is the coupling compound that is present in both cells and in the extracellular space. (b–d) Time course simulations with parameter values $v_0 = 3$, $\varphi = 0.2$. (b) Asynchronous oscillations, parameter values: $k_2 = 4.3$, $k_3 = 1$, (c) Synchronous oscillations, parameter values: $k_2 = 3.84$, $k_3 = 3.2$. The coupling compound C oscillates with the same frequency. (d) Regular asynchronous oscillations, parameter values: $k_2 = 2.5$, $k_3 = 1$. Oscillations of the coupling compound practically disappeared, i.e., the amplitudes are very small. All parameters are given in arbitrary units.

pulations can even be experimentally observed. Regular asynchronous oscillations are hidden; upon concentration measurements for cell populations, they result in constant concentration values at the level of the mean for all cells. Two experiments demonstrate the character of both types of oscillations. Upon mixing of two cell populations that are synchronized internally but exhibit a phase shift of 180° with respect to each other, the oscillations are initially strongly damped but reappear after a while (Richard et al. 1996). This means that both populations synchronize within a time that depends on the strength of the coupling parameter k_3. The hidden oscillations in the case of regular asynchronous oscillations can be made visible by increasing or decreasing the concentration of the coupling substance in a pulse-like manner. Far from the area of Hopf bifurcation, other modes of behavior may occur, e.g., non-regular oscillations.

7.1.4

Sustained Oscillations in Signaling Cascades

Sustained oscillations are an emerging property of ultrasensitive cascades with negative feedback, as there is always a range of kinetic constants in which oscillatory behavior is observed. To analyze this feature, Kholodenko (2000) employed a numerical analysis of the dynamics of the MAPK cascades as illustrated in Fig. 6.11 with the dynamics described in the equation systems (Eqs. (6-9)–(6-11)) with Michaelis-Menten kinetics of the individual reaction steps (Eqs. (6-21) and (6-22)). In addition, a feedback from the MAPK-P$_2$ to the first reaction is considered that changes the rate equation of the first reaction to

$$v_1 = V_{m1} \cdot MAPKKKK \frac{MAPKKK}{(K_1 + MAPKKK)} \cdot \frac{1}{\left(1 + \left(\frac{MAPK\text{-}P_2}{K_I}\right)^n\right)}, \tag{7-14}$$

where K_1 is the Michealis constant for MAPKKK, V_{m1} is the maximal reaction rate, and K_I is the dissociation constant for MAPK-P$_2$ with respect to MAPKKKK. Negative feedback can bring about oscillations in the kinase activities. Following the activation of the initial kinase and a subsequent activation of the terminal cascade kinase, a strong negative feedback can in some cases be operational in turning off the activation of a cascade. In other cases, implementation of a strong negative feedback may have the effect that the system steady state loses its stability. Since there is no other stable state, the phosphorylation level of cascade kinases starts to oscillate in a sustained manner. This dramatic change in the system's dynamic behavior is again a Hopf bifurcation.

The time course of the active and inactive forms of the MAPK cascade kinases is shown in Fig. 7.4 for an abrupt increase in the input stimulus (i.e., active MAPKKKK concentration) at time point zero. At low basal stimulus, the kinases of the cascade remained predominantly in the inactive forms, and the corresponding

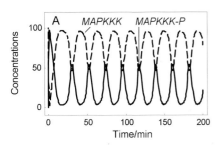
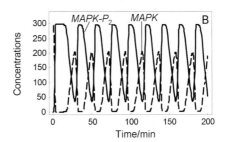

Fig. 7.4 Sustained oscillations in MAPK concentrations according to the model of Kholodenko (2000). (a) Oscillations of *MAPKKK* (b) Oscillations of *MAPK*   Parameters $V_{m1} = 2.5, V_{m2} = 0.25,$ $V_{m3} = V_{m4} = V_{m7} = V_{m_8} = 0.025, V_{m5} = V_{m6} = 0.75, V_{m9} = V_{m10} = 0.5,$ (in s^{-1} and nM s^{-1}, respectively) $K_{m1} = 1,$, $K_{m2} = 8, K_{mi} = 15$ $(i = 3,$ ..., 10) (in nM), $n = 1, K_I = 9.$

steady state (off state) is stable. A high stimulus switches the kinases into the active forms (on state), but this state is instable. The cascade kinases do not remain phosphorylated for a prolonged period of time. Due to the negative feedback from MAPK-P$_2$, the rate of activating phosphorylation of MAPKKK decreases with an increase in MAPK-P$_2$. As the phosphatase continues to operate, the rate of MAPKKK-P dephosphorylation begins to exceed the phosphorylation rate and the concentration of MAPKKK-P decreases. A decrease in the MAPKKK-P causes the kinase activity down the cascade (MAPKK) to drop. Finally, the concentration of MAPK-P$_2$ decreases, and a new oscillation cycle begins. The amplitude of oscillation in the concentrations of the active biphosphorylated MAPK-P$_2$ and inactive MAPK can be large. The period of oscillation is about 20 min, but it depends on the choice of kinetic parameters. Importantly, the oscillations appear to be stable to changes in the initial distribution of active and inactive kinase forms. Whether oscillations can occur at all under conditions of negative feedback depends (1) on the saturation of kinases and phosphatases, i.e., on the ratio between their total concentrations and their K_m values, and (2) on the strength of the negative feedback. Tendentially it holds that the stronger the feedback, the more likely oscillations are.

7.2
Cell Cycle

The eukaryotic cell cycle is the repeated sequence of events accompanying the division of a cell into daughter cells (Johnson and Walker 1999). It includes two main sections: the doubling of the genome (DNA) and all other cell components in the S phase (synthesis phase) and halving of the genome during the M phase (mitosis). The periods between the M and S phases are the gap or growth phases G$_1$ and G$_2$ (Fig. 2.13). Passage through the eukaryotic cell cycle is strictly regulated by the periodic synthesis and destruction of cyclins that bind and activate cyclin-dependent kinases (CDKs). The notion "kinase" expresses that their function is phosphorylation of proteins with controlling functions. Cyclin-dependent kinase inhibitors (CKI) also play important roles in cell cycle control by coordinating internal and external signals and impeding proliferation at several key checkpoints.

The general scheme of the cell cycle is conserved from yeast to mammals. The levels of cyclins rise and fall during the stages of the cell cycle. The levels of CDKs appear to remain constant during the cell cycle, but the individual molecules are either unbound or bound to cyclins. In budding yeast, one CDK (Cdc28) and nine different cyclins (Cln1 to Cln3, Clb1 to Clb6) that seem to be at least partially redundant are found. In contrast, mammals employ a variety of different cyclins and CDKs. Cyclins include a G1 cyclin (cyclin D), S-phase cyclins (A and E), and mitotic cyclins (A and B). Mammals have nine different CDKs (referred to as CDK1–CDK9) that are important in different phases of the cell cycle. The anaphase-promoting complex (APC) triggers the events leading to destruction of the cohesions, thus allowing the sister chromatids to separate and degrade the mitotic cyclins.

7.2.1
Steps in the Cycle

Let us take a course through the mammalian cell cycle starting in the G1 phase. As the level of G_1 cyclins rises, they bind to their CDKs and signal the cell to prepare the chromosomes for replication. When the level of S phase–promoting factor (SPF) rises, which includes cyclin A bound to CDK2, it enters the nucleus and prepares the cell to duplicate its DNA (and its centrosomes). As DNA replication continues, cyclin E is destroyed, and the level of mitotic cyclins begins to increase (in G_2). The M phase–promoting factor (the complex of mitotic cyclins with the M-phase CDK) initiates (1) assembly of the mitotic spindle, (2) breakdown of the nuclear envelope, and (3) condensation of the chromosomes. These events take the cell to metaphase of mitosis. At this point, the M phase–promoting factor activates the APC, which allows the sister chromatids at the metaphase plate to separate and move to the poles (anaphase), thereby completing mitosis. APC destroys the mitotic cyclins by coupling them to ubiquitin, which targets them for destruction by proteasomes. APC turns on the synthesis of G_1 cyclin for the next turn of the cycle and it degrades geminin, a protein that keeps the freshly synthesized DNA in the S phase from being re-replicated before mitosis.

A number of checkpoints ensure that all processes connected with cell cycle progression and DNA doubling and separation occur correctly. At these checkpoints, the cell cycle can be aborted or arrested. They involve checks on completion of the S phase, on DNA damage, and on failure of spindle behavior. If the damage is irreparable, apoptosis is triggered. An important checkpoint in G_1 has been identified in both yeast and mammalian cells. Referred to as "start" in yeast and as "restriction point" in mammalian cells, this is the point at which the cell becomes committed to DNA replication and completing a cell cycle (Hartwell 1974; Hartwell et al. 1974; Pardee 1974; Nurse 1975). All the checkpoints require the services of complexes of proteins. Mutations in the genes encoding some of these proteins have been associated with cancer. These genes are regarded as oncogenes. Failures in checkpoints permit the cell to continue dividing despite damage to its integrity. Understanding how the proteins interact to regulate the cell cycle became increasingly important to researchers and clinicians when it was discovered that many of the genes that encode cell cycle regulatory activities are targets for alterations that underlie the development of cancer. Several therapeutic agents, such as DNA-damaging drugs, microtubule inhibitors, antimetabolites, and topoisomerase inhibitors, take advantage of this disruption in normal cell cycle regulation to target checkpoint controls and ultimately induce growth arrest or apoptosis of neoplastic cells.

For the presentation of modeling approaches, we will focus on the yeast cell cycle since intensive experimental and computational studies have been carried out using different types of yeast as model organisms. Mathematical models of the cell cycle can be used to tackle, for example, the following relevant problems.

1. The cell seems to monitor the volume ratio of nucleus and cytoplasm and to trigger cell division at a characteristic ratio. During oogenesis, this ratio is abnormally

small (the cells accumulate maternal cytoplasm), while after fertilization cells divide without cell growth. How is the dependence on the ratio regulated?
2. Cancer cells represent a failure in cell cycle regulation. Which proteins or protein complexes are essential for checkpoint examination?
3. What causes the oscillatory behavior of the compounds involved in the cell cycle?

7.2.2
Minimal Cascade Model of a Mitotic Oscillator

One of the first genes to be identified as being an important regulator of the cell cycle in yeast was *cdc2/cdc28* (Nurse and Bissett 1981), where *cdc2* refers to fission yeast and *cdc28* to budding yeast. Activation of the *cdc2/cdc28* kinase requires association with a regulatory subunit referred to as a cyclin.

A minimal model for the mitotic oscillator involving a cyclin and the Cdc2 kinase has been presented by Goldbeter (1991). It covers the cascade of post-translational modifications that modulate the activity of Cdc2 kinase during cell cycle. In the first cycle of the bicyclic cascade model, the cyclin promotes the activation of the Cdc2 kinase by reversible dephosphorylation, and in the second cycle, the Cdc2 kinase activates a cyclin protease by reversible phosphorylation. The model was used to test the hypothesis that cell cycle oscillations may arise from a negative feedback loop, i.e., the cyclin activates the Cdc2 kinase while the Cdc2 kinase triggers the degradation of the cyclin.

The minimal cascade model is represented in Fig. 7.5. It involves only two main actors, cyclin and cyclin-dependent kinase. Cyclin is synthesized at constant rate, v_i, and triggers the transformation of inactive (M+) into active (M) Cdc2 kinase by enhancing the rate of a phosphatase, v_1. A kinase with rate v_2 reverts this modification. In the lower cycle, the Cdc2 kinase phosphorylates a protease (v_3) shifting it from the inactive (X+) to the active (X) form. The activation of the cyclin protease is reverted by a further phosphatase with rate v_4. The dynamics is governed by the ODE system

$$\frac{dC}{dt} = v_i - v_d \frac{X \cdot C}{K_{md} + C} - k_d C$$

$$\frac{dM}{dt} = \frac{V_{m1} \cdot (1 - M)}{K_{m1} + (1 - M)} - \frac{V_{m2} \cdot M}{K_{m2} + M}$$

$$\frac{dX}{dt} = \frac{V_{m3} \cdot (1 - X)}{K_{m3} + (1 - X)} - \frac{V_{m4} \cdot X}{K_{m4} + X}, \tag{7-15}$$

where C denotes the cyclin concentration; M and X represent the fractional concentrations of active Cdc2 kinase and active cyclin protease, and $(1 - M)$ and $(1 - X)$ are the fractions of inactive kinase and phosphatase, respectively. K_m values are Michaelis constants. $V_{m1} = V_1 C/(K_{mc} + C)$ and $V_{m3} = V_3 \cdot M$ are effective maximal rates (compare Section 5.1.3). Note that the differential equations for the changes of M and X are modeled with the so-called Goldbeter-Koshland switch (compare Section 6.4).

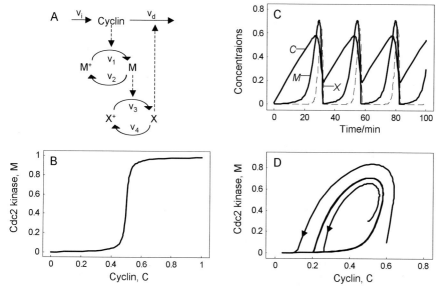

Fig. 7.5 Goldbeter's minimal model of the mitotic oscillator. (a) Illustration of the model comprising cyclin production and degradation, phosphorylation and dephosphorylation of Cdc2 kinase, and phosphorylation and dephosphorylation of the cyclin protease (see text). (b) Threshold-type dependence of the fractional concentration of active Cdc2 kinase on the cyclin concentration. (c) Time courses of cyclin (*C*), active Cdc2 kinase (*M*), and active cyclin protease (*X*) exhibiting oscillations according to the equation system in Eq. (7-15). (d) Limit cycle behavior, represented for the variables *C* and *M*. Parameter values: $K_{mi} = 0.05$ ($i = 1, ..., 4$), $K_{mc} = 0.5$, $k_d = 0.01$, $v_i = 0.025$, $v_d = 0.25$, $V_{m1} = 3$, $V_{m2} = 1.5$, $V_{m3} = 1$, $V_{m4} = 0.5$. Initial conditions in (b): $C(0) = M(0) = X(0) = 0.01$, and in (c): $X(0) = 0.01$. Units: µM and min^{-1}.

This model involves only Michaelis-Menten type kinetics, but no form of positive cooperativity. It can be used to test whether oscillations can arise solely as a result of the negative feedback provided by the Cdc2-induced cyclin degradation and of the threshold and time delay involved in the cascade. The time delay is implemented by considering post-translational modifications (phosphorylation/dephosphorylation cycles v_1/v_2 and v_3/v_4). For certain parameters they lead to a threshold in the dependence of steady-state values for *M* on *C* and for *X* on *M* (Fig. 7.5 b). Provided that this threshold exists, the evolution of the bicyclic cascade proceeds in a periodic manner (Fig. 7.5 c). Starting from low initial cyclin concentration, this value accumulates at a constant rate, while *M* and *X* stay low. As soon as *C* crosses the activation threshold, *M* rises. If *M* crosses the threshold, *X* starts to increase sharply. *X* in turn accelerates cyclin degradation and consequently, *C*, *M*, and *X* drop rapidly. The resulting oscillations are of the limit cycle type. The respective limit cycle is shown in phase plane representation in Fig. 7.5 d.

7.2.3
Models of Budding Yeast Cell Cycle

Tyson, Novak, and colleagues have developed a series of models describing the cell cycle of budding yeast in detail (Tyson et al. 1996; Novak et al. 1999; Chen et al. 2000, 2004). These comprehensive models employ a set of assumptions that are summarized in the following.

The cell cycle is an alternating sequence of the transition from the G_1 phase to the S/M phase, called "Start", and the transition from S/M to G_1, called "Finish". An overview is given in Fig. 7.6.

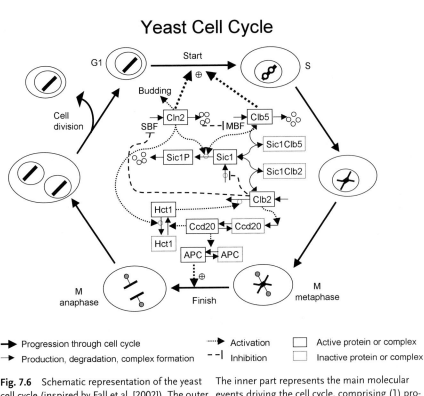

Fig. 7.6 Schematic representation of the yeast cell cycle (inspired by Fall et al. [2002]). The outer ring represents the cellular events. Beginning with cell division, the G_1 phase follows. The cells possess a single set of chromosomes (shown as one black line). At Start, the cell goes into the S phase and replicates the DNA (two black lines). The sister chromatids are initially kept together by proteins. During the M phase they are aligned, attached to the spindle body, and segregated to different parts of the cell. The cycle closes with formation of two new daughter cells. The inner part represents the main molecular events driving the cell cycle, comprising (1) protein production and degradation, (2) phosphorylation and dephosphorylation, and (3) complex formation and disintegration. For sake of clarity, CDK Cdc28 is not shown. The Start is initiated by activation of CDK by cyclins Cln2 and Clb5. The CDK activity is responsible for progression through the S and M phases. At Finish, the proteolytic activity coordinated by APC destroys the cyclins and thereby renders the CDK inactive.

The CDK (Cdc28) forms complexes with the cyclins Cln1 to Cln3 and Clb1 to Clb6, and these complexes control the major cell cycle events in budding yeast cells. The complexes Cln1-2/Cdc28 control budding, the complex Cln3/Cdc28 governs the executing of the checkpoint Start, Clb5–6/Cdc28 ensures timely DNA replication, Clb3-4/Cdc28 assists DNA replication and spindle formation, and Clb1-2/Cdc28 is necessary for completion of mitosis.

The cyclin-CDK complexes are in turn regulated by synthesis and degradation of cyclins and by the Clb-dependent kinase inhibitor (CKI) Sic1. The expression of the gene for Cln2 is controlled by the transcription factor SBF, and the expression of the gene for Clb5 is controlled by the transcription factor MBF. Both transcription factors are regulated by CDKs. All cyclins are degraded by proteasomes following ubiquitination. APC is one of the complexes triggering ubiquitination of cyclins.

For the implementation of these processes in a mathematical model, the following points are important. Activation of cyclins and cyclin-dependent kinases occurs in principle by the negative feedback loop presented in Goldbeter's minimal model (see Section 7.2.1). Furthermore, the cells exhibit exponential growth. For the dynamics of the cell mass M, it holds that $dM/dt = \mu M$. At the instance of cell division, M is replaced by $M/2$. In some cases uneven division is considered. Cell growth implies adaptation of the negative feedback model to growing cells.

The transitions Start and Finish characterize the wild-type cell cycle. At Start, the transcription factor SBF is turned on and the levels of the cyclins Cln2 and Clb5 increase. They form complexes with Cdc28. The boost in Cln2/Cdc28 has three main consequences: it initiates bud formation, it phosphorylates the CKI Sic1 promoting its disappearance, and it inactivates Hct1, which in conjunction with APC is responsible for Clb2 degradation in the G_1 phase. Hence, DNA synthesis takes place and the bud emerges. Subsequently, the level of Clb2 increases and the spindle starts to form. Clb2/Cdc28 inactivates SBF and Cln2 decreases. Inactivation of MBF causes Clb5 to decrease. Clb2/Cdc28 induces progression through mitosis. Cdc20 and Hct1, which target proteins to APC for ubiquitination, regulate the metaphase-anaphase transition. Cdc20 has several tasks in the anaphase. Furthermore, it activates Hct1, promoting degradation of Clb2, and it activates the transcription factor of Sic1. Thus, at Finish, Clb2 is destroyed and Sic1 reappears.

The dynamics of some key players in the cell cycle according to the model given in Chen et al. (2000) is shown in Fig. 7.7 for two successive cycles. At Start, Cln2 and

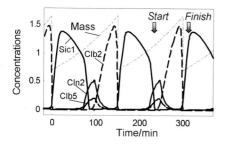

Fig. 7.7 Temporal behavior of some key players during two successive rounds of the yeast cell cycle. The dotted line indicates the cell mass that halves after every cell division. The levels of Cln2, Clb2$_{total}$, Clb5$_{total}$, and Sic1$_{total}$ are simulated according to the model presented by Chen et al. (2000).

Clb5 levels rise and Sic1 is degraded, while at Finish, Clb2 vanishes and Sic1 is newly produced.

7.3
Aging

Aging is a complex biological process that affects practically all components of an organism. It is difficult to give a good definition of aging that holds for all organisms, but for populations a very useful description is that aging consists of all those processes that lead to a monotonic increase of mortality with time. Humans, for instance, have a yearly mortality of roughly 0.1% at age 20, but of about 10% at 80 years of age!

There are two different aspects of the aging process that need to be understood. First, there is the question of *why* the aging process has evolved. A process that leads to an increase of mortality reduces the average life span of the organism and thus reduces the number of offspring the organism can have. This, however, should lead directly to a reduction of evolutionary fitness. It is therefore not trivial to understand why such a biological trait should have evolved in practically all higher organisms.

The second important question is of course *how* the actual biochemical mechanism works that leads to the gradual functional decline. Unfortunately, the evolutionary models do not predict specific mechanisms that might be involved in aging. As a consequence a large number of mechanistic models have been proposed. A review of the available literature showed that more than 300 different mechanistic theories exist (Medvedev 1990). Figure 7.8 shows a small sample of the most popular mechanistic theories. The spatial arrangement of the diagram aims to reflect connections between the theories. For example, oxygen radicals can damage DNA, leading to somatic mutations, or damage mitochondrial membranes and DNA, leading to defective mitochondria. Radical reactions with cytoplasmic or mitochondrial proteins or membranes can also lead to the accumulation of indestructible waste products. And finally, reactions of radicals with macromolecules can lead to the formation of cross-links that impair their biological functioning.

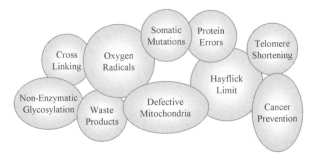

Fig. 7.8 Small selection of the large number of mechanistic theories of aging. The topology of the diagram is intended to reflect overlap and points of interaction between different theories.

It is therefore clear that this chapter cannot be a comprehensive treatment of the aging process. Instead, we will discuss selected models. In Section 7.3.1 we will study a model that deals with the evolution of the aging process, and in Section 7.3.2 we look at a model that deals with damage to mitochondria.

7.3.1
Evolution of the Aging Process

It is not immediately obvious why organisms should grow old and die. What is the selective advantage of this trait? And if aging is advantageous, why do different species have such widely differing life spans?

The first attempt to explain the evolution of aging was made by Weismann (1891). He proposed that aging is beneficial by removing crippled and worn-out individuals from the population and thus making space and resources available for the next generation. This type of reasoning is very similar to suggestions such as the prevention of overcrowding or the acceleration of evolution by decreasing the generation time.

These ideas suggest that aging itself confers a selective advantage and that the evolution of genes that bring life to an end is an adaptive response to selective forces. All these theories have in common that they rely on group selection, the selection of a trait that is beneficial for the group but detrimental to the individual. However, group selection works only under very special circumstances such as small patch size and low migration rates (Maynard Smith 1976). A second major argument against adaptive theories is the empirically found paucity of old individuals in natural populations. Extrinsic mortality in natural populations is so high that only very few individuals survive long enough to be killed by intrinsic mortality. But if intrinsic mortality, which is caused by the aging process, is not the main cause of death under natural conditions, it is difficult to see how aging could have evolved for the purpose of removing animals from the population.

The weaknesses of adaptive theories have been recognized for some time, and newer theories are no longer based on group selection but rather on the "declining force of natural selection" with time. This important concept is based on the fact that even in the absence of aging, individuals in a population are always at risk of death due to accidents, predators, and diseases. For a given cohort this leads to an exponential decline over time in the fraction of individuals that are still alive. Events (e.g., biochemical processes) that occur only in chronologically old individuals will therefore affect only a small proportion of the whole population. The later the onset of the events, the smaller the involved fraction of the population is.

Medawar (1952) was the first to present a theory for the evolution of the aging process based on this idea. His "mutation-accumulation" theory states that aging might be caused by an accumulation of deleterious genes that are expressed only late in life. Because of the declining force of natural selection, only a small part of the population would be affected by this type of mutation and the resulting selection pressure to remove them would only be very weak. Mutations with a small selection pressure to be removed can persist in a mutation-selection balance and thus explain the emergence of an aging phenotype.

Another theory of this kind is the "antagonistic pleiotropy" theory (Williams 1957). Genes that affect two or more traits are called pleiotropic genes, and effects that increase fitness through one trait at the expense of a reduced fitness of another trait are antagonistic. Now consider a gene that improves the reproductive success of younger organisms at the expense of the survival of older individuals. Because of the declining force of natural selection, such a gene will be favored by selection and aging will occur as a side effect of the antagonistic pleiotropy property of this gene. Possible candidate genes might be found in males and females. Prostate cancer appears frequently in males at advanced ages, but it can be prevented by administration of female hormones or castration. It seems to be a consequence of long-term exposure to testosterone, which is necessary for male sexual, and thus reproductive, success. In older females osteoporosis is mediated by estrogens that are essential for reproduction in younger women. In both cases, gene effects that are beneficial at younger ages have negative consequences later in life.

Genes that trade long-term survival against short-term benefit are probably the strongest candidates to explain the aging process. A specific version of this hypothesis that connects evolutionary concepts with molecular mechanisms is the "disposable soma" theory (Kirkwood and Holliday 1986; Kirkwood and Rose 1991). The theory realizes that organisms have a finite energy budget (food resources) that must be distributed among different tasks like growth, maintenance, and reproduction. Energy spent for one task is not available for another. Organisms have to solve this optimal resource allocation problem such that evolutionary fitness is maximized. On the basis of quite general assumptions, a mathematical model can be constructed that describes the relationship between investment in maintenance and fitness. We will have a closer look at this model as an example how to formulate a mathematical description of such a qualitative idea.

To get started we need a mathematical concept of fitness. A standard measure that is often used in population genetics is the intrinsic rate of natural increase, r, (also called the Malthusian parameter), which can be calculated by numerically solving the Euler-Lotka equation (Eq. (7-16)). To calculate r for a given genotype, the survivorship function, $l(t)$, and the fertility function, $m(t)$, have to be known. $l(t)$ denotes the probability that an individual survives to age t and $m(t)$ is the expected number of offspring produced by an individual of age t.

$$\int_0^\infty e^{-r \cdot t} \cdot l(t) \cdot m(t) \, dt = 1 . \tag{7-16}$$

If the value of r that solves this equation is negative, it implies a shrinking population; if it is positive, the population grows. Thus, the larger r is, the higher the fitness is. An exact derivation of the Euler-Lotka equation is outside the scope of this chapter but can be found in Maynard Smith (1989) or Stearns (1992). Investment in somatic maintenance and repair will affect both survivorship and fertility, and the question remains whether there is an optimal level of maintenance that maximizes fitness. Unfortunately, the precise physiological tradeoffs are unknown, so we have to develop some qualitative relationship. In many species mortality increases exponentially according to the Gompertz-Makeham equation (Eq. (7-17)) (Makeham 1867). μ_0, β, and γ represent basal vulnerability, actuarial aging rate, and age-independent environmental mortality, respectively.

$$\mu(t) = \mu_0 \cdot e^{\beta t} + \gamma. \tag{7-17}$$

Mortality and survivorship are connected via the relation $dl/dt = -\mu(t) \cdot l(t)$. By solving this equation we obtain an expression for $l(t)$ that depends on two factors that are influenced by the level of maintenance, μ_0 and β (Eq. (7-18)). We now define the variable ρ to be the fraction of resources that are allocated for maintenance and repair, $\rho = 0$ corresponding to zero repair and $\rho = 1$ corresponding to the maximum that is physiologically possible. We also make the assumption that above a critical level of repair, ρ^*, damage does not accumulate and the organism has reached a non-aging state. The rationale for this postulation is the idea that aging is caused by the accumulation of some kind of damage and that by investing more in repair, the accumulation rate is slowed down until finally the incidence rate is equal to the removal rate, in which case the physiological steady state can be maintained indefinitely. The modifications to μ_0 (Eq. (7-19) and β (Eq. (7-20)) are only one way to implement the desired tradeoff (decreasing μ_0 and β with increasing ρ), but in qualitative models like this, the principle results are often very robust with regard to the exact mathematical expression used.

$$l(t) = e^{(1-e^{\beta t}) \cdot \mu_0/\beta + \gamma t}, \tag{7-18}$$

$$\mu_0 = \mu_{min}/\rho, \tag{7-19}$$

$$\beta = \beta_0 \left(\frac{\rho^*}{\rho} - 1 \right) \qquad \rho \le \rho^*$$

$$\beta = 0 \qquad \rho > \rho^*. \tag{7-20}$$

The level of maintenance also influences fertility, $m(t)$. It is assumed that the age at maturation, a, will increase with rising ρ and that the initial reproductive rate, f, is a decreasing function of ρ. It is also assumed that fertility declines due to age-related deterioration with the same Gompertzian rate term as survivorship. From these conditions equations can be derived for fertility (Eq. (7-21)), age at maturation (Eq. (7-22)), and initial reproductive rate (Eq. (7-23)).

$$m(t) = f \cdot e^{(e^{\beta a} - e^{\beta t}) \cdot \mu_0/\beta}, \tag{7-21}$$

$$a = a_0/(1 - \rho), \tag{7-22}$$

$$f = f_{max} \cdot (1 - \rho). \tag{7-23}$$

Now we have all the information necessary to solve the Euler-Lotka equation for different values of repair, ρ (Fig. 7.9). The calculations confirm that an optimal level

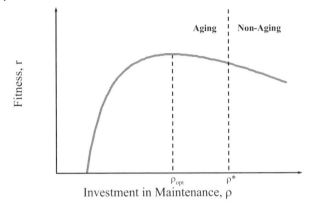

Fig. 7.9 The disposable soma theory predicts that the optimal investment in maintenance is always less than what would be required to achieve a non-aging state. The exact position of this optimum (which maximizes fitness) depends on the environmental risk a species is exposed to over evolutionary times. Organisms living in a niche with heavy external mortality should invest less in maintenance than do organisms that are exposed to little external mortality.

of maintenance, ρ_{opt}, exists, which results in a maximal fitness. Depending on the ecological niche (represented by environmental mortality, γ), the optimal amount of maintenance varies. In a risky environment the optimum is shifted towards lower maintenance, and a niche with low external mortality selects for individuals with a relatively high investment in maintenance.

This fits quite nicely with biological data. Species like mice or rabbits live in a high-risk environment, and, as predicted, they invest heavily in offspring but have little left for maintenance. Consequently, their aging rate is high and their life expectancy is low (even under risk-free laboratory conditions). Humans or elephants, by contrast, inhabit a low-risk environment, expend fewer resources for offspring, and invest more in repair. Especially instructive are birds, which live two to three times as long as mammals of comparable body weight. Again, this long life span can be predicted by the enormous reduction of external mortality that accompanies the ability to fly and thus escape predators or starvation.

Another important result of the model is that the optimal level of maintenance and repair is always below the critical level, ρ^*, that is required for the evolution of a non-aging organism. This result can also be understood intuitively. Since all species have an external mortality that is above zero, they have a finite life expectancy, even without aging. This means that even though it might be physiological possible to have such an efficient repair system that damage does not accumulate with time, resulting in a potentially immortal organism, this never results in a maximal fitness value. Only in the limit of $\gamma = 0$ does ρ_{opt} approach ρ^*.

Although the disposable soma theory is very successful in explaining the evolution of the aging process, it unfortunately does not predict which specific molecular damage accumulates or which repair systems are the most important. All possible mechanisms that somehow influence the steady state of the cell are viable candidates.

Indeed, this can be taken as an argument that many types of damage accumulate with time and that many types of repair processes contribute to the rate of aging. Under those conditions it is not fruitful to study individual biochemical mechanisms in isolation, but rather as a network of connected processes. The investigation of the aging process is thus a prime candidate for a systems biological approach.

7.3.2
Accumulation of Defective Mitochondria

Figure 7.8 shows that defective mitochondria play a prominent role in one of the most favored theories regarding the biochemical mechanism of the aging process. Mitochondria are not only the powerhouses of the cell, generating the majority of the cellular ATP, but also are the main producers of reactive oxygen species (ROS). These reactive molecules damage proteins, membranes, and the mitochondrial DNA (mtDNA). The mitochondrial theory of aging is based on the fact that damage to the mtDNA impairs the genes responsible for ATP production but not those involved in the replication of the mtDNA, because they are located in the nucleus. Thus ROS-induced damage to the mitochondria could turn a symbiont into a parasite, leading to a progressive decline in the cellular energy supply. Experimental findings of the past few years have confirmed that in aging post-mitotic cells there is indeed a clonal accumulation of defective mitochondria with time (Brierley et al. 1998; Khrapko et al. 1999). This means that a single mutant appeared and expanded clonally, out-competing the wild-type population. The actual molecular mechanism of this accumulation, however, remains unclear, since it is difficult to see how energy-starved mutant mitochondria can grow faster than wild-type organelles.

A possible solution to this problem rests on the fact that mitochondria, like proteins, have a certain turnover rate. Newly synthesized mitochondria typically exist within the cell only for a period of two to four weeks, after which they are degraded (Huemer et al. 1971; Menzies and Gold 1971). Mitochondrial mutants can therefore accumulate in a population either by increasing their division rate or by lowering their rate of degradation. Therefore, it has been suggested that damaged mitochondria accumulate because they have a slower degradation rate (de Grey 1997). If it is furthermore assumed that defective organelles actually grow more slowly than wild type (Kowald and Kirkwood 2000), this would explain clonal expansion and avoids the energy paradox that arises if defective mitochondria are required to have a faster proliferation rate. The idea is that individual mitochondria are targeted for turnover in accordance with the level of oxidative damage to their inner mitochondrial membrane. The more the membrane is damaged, the sooner the mitochondrion is destroyed. Defective mitochondria have decreased respiratory activity, and it is therefore assumed that they inflict less oxidative damage to their membranes than do wild-type mitochondria.

In the following sections we give an overview of this model, which has been called "survival of the slowest" (SOS) hypothesis. For pedagogical purposes we will place more emphasize on the development of the differential equations than on the actual simulation results.

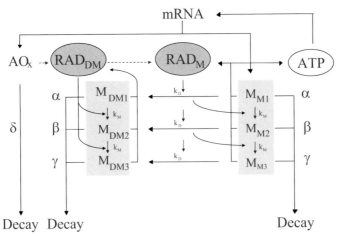

Fig. 7.10 Reactions described by the survival of the slowest model. Two main classes of mitochondria are considered, with and without DNA damage (M_{DM}, M_M). These are further divided into subclasses containing little, medium, and much membrane damage. The different classes of mitochondria produce different amounts of ROS, which cause the transition of mitochondria from one damage class to another. Finally, the mitochondria are degraded with a rate constant that is proportional to the amount of membrane damage. Further details are given in the text.

Figure 7.10 gives an overview of the model, which separates the mitochondrial population into two major classes, intact mitochondria with no damage to their DNA (M_{Mi}) and defective organelles that have acquired some form of mtDNA damage (M_{DMi}). Furthermore, mitochondria also accumulate damage to their membranes and a further subdivision is therefore necessary. Both major classes are divided into three additional groups based on the amount of membrane damage. M_{M1} and M_{DM1} stand for mitochondria with no or only slight damage to their membranes, M_{M2} and M_{DM2} contain a medium amount of damage, and M_{M3} and M_{DM3} contain a large amount of damaged membranes. Mitochondrial turnover is proportional to the level of membrane damage, so the relation $\gamma > \beta > \alpha$ holds for the decay rates. RAD_M represents the radical concentration in intact mitochondria, and RAD_{DM} represents the level in damaged mitochondria. RAD_M can interact with the membranes of intact mitochondria with a rate k_M, shifting mitochondria into a higher membrane damage class, or it can damage the mitochondrial DNA (with a rate k_D), converting intact mitochondria into defective ones. Once mitochondria have suffered DNA damage, further reactions with radicals (now RAD_{DM}) can only increase the amount of membrane damage. Finally, the model contains a generic antioxidant species (AO_x) that destroys radicals. The main reason for including such a species in the model is to provide a sink for radicals, which otherwise would increase without limit.

The model consists of nine ordinary differential equations describing the time course of the different molecular species. Six equations are needed for the various types of mitochondria, one for the level of antioxidants, one for the ATP level, and one for the amount of radicals. Although the model contains different radical levels for damaged and intact mitochondria, it turns out that under certain assumptions those values can be calculated from one equation (see Section 7.3.2.2).

7.3.2.1 Synthesis Rates

Mitochondria are continually being turned over, which means that new mitochondria must be synthesized to balance degradation. It is assumed that the synthesis rate is controlled by the cellular energy level. A low ATP concentration stimulates mitochondrial growth, while a high concentration diminishes it. This is known as product inhibition. The mathematical expression used to simulate this behavior is given by Eq. (7-24).

$$\frac{k_1}{1 + \left(\dfrac{ATP}{ATP_c}\right)^n} \cdot \tag{7-24}$$

This artificial promoter has been used successfully in other models (Kowald and Kirkwood 1994, 1996) and is also employed here. Depending on the amount of ATP, it results in a value between zero and k_1, which can be interpreted as the activity of this promoter. If ATP is equal to ATP_c, the promoter control parameter, activity is reduced to 50%. The constant n determines how sensitive the promoter is to deviations of the energy level from ATP_c.

Although mitochondria contain their own genetic material, they cannot be treated as self-replicating entities because the genes coding for the overwhelming majority of their proteins are located in the nucleus and these proteins have to be imported from the cytoplasm. Therefore, the synthesis rate is not proportional to the number of existing mitochondria but has a fixed upper limit, k_1.

Equation (24) is further modified to take account of the fact that the synthesis of macromolecules requires energy and that the synthesis rate is proportional to the ATP concentration in the cell. Hence the expression is multiplied by $ATP/(ATP+ATP_c)$. This construct has the attractive property that new mitochondria are produced only if energy levels are low, but that biosynthesis works best with a high-energy charge.

The resulting expression describes the total number of new mitochondria that are synthesized per time interval, but it does not specify to which class they belong. If all classes of mitochondria were to grow at the same rate, the total number would simply have to be distributed proportionally between the six different classes. However, because of the assumed growth disadvantage of defective mitochondria, the contributions to the different classes have to be weighted. All mitochondria with DNA damage have the same growth disadvantage, GDF, because their oxidative phosphorylation is nonfunctional. GDF is the factor by which the growth rate is reduced compared to intact mitochondria. The same growth disadvantage is assumed for mitochondria with intact DNA but with the highest amount of membrane damage (M_{M3}). For mitochondria with intact DNA and a medium amount of damage (M_{M2}), the growth disadvantage is assumed to be $(1+GDF)/2$. Taking these considerations into account, the fraction of the total number of new mitochondria that belongs to a given damage class is given by

$$\frac{1}{M_{M1} + \dfrac{2}{GDF+1} \cdot M_{M2} + \dfrac{1}{GDF} \cdot (M_{M3} + M_{DM1} + M_{DM2} + M_{DM3})} \cdot X, \qquad (7\text{-}25)$$

where X specifies mitochondria of the given damage class. In the case of intact mitochondria, $X = M_{M1}$, for intact mitochondria with a medium amount of membrane damage, $X = 2/GDF + 1 \cdot M_{M2}$, and for all other classes, $X = M/GDF$.

7.3.2.2 Radical Levels

Figure 7.10 shows that the model includes two different radical pools. Rad_M is the number of radicals in a single intact mitochondrion and Rad_{DM} is the number of radicals in a mitochondrion that suffered damaged to its DNA. It is assumed that radicals are generated at a fixed rate and that their removal is proportional to the existing amount of radicals. The equations can therefore be written as

$$\frac{dRad_M}{dt} = k_R - f \cdot Rad_M \qquad (7\text{-}26)$$

and

$$\frac{dRad_{DM}}{dt} = RDF \cdot k_R - f \cdot Rad_{DM}, \qquad (7\text{-}27)$$

where k_R is the rate of radical production of intact mitochondria and it is assumed that the production rate of defective mitochondria is increased by a factor RDF, the radical difference factor. In the complete model, f is a function that depends on the amount of antioxidants per mitochondrion (see Eq. (7-38)), but for any instant of time it is identical for Eqs. (7-26) and (7-27). These equations can be solved analytically, and if $Rad_M(t=0) = Rad_{DM}(t=0) = 0$, it holds that $Rad_{DM}/Rad_M = RDF$. Therefore, only one equation is necessary to describe the time course of radicals in this model.

7.3.2.3 Dilution of Membrane Damage

An important aspect of the SOS hypothesis is that fast mitochondrial growth acts as a rejuvenation mechanism because it dilutes membrane damage. When newly synthesized components are incorporated into the mitochondrial membrane, the preexisting level of membrane damage is reduced and the new damage level, NDL, is the result of mixing existing membrane components with the new ones. If, for example, the amount of new membrane components is equal to the existing ones, NDL is 50%. This can be formalized and it holds that for all mitochondria with a growth disadvantage of GDF (M_{DM1}, M_{DM2}, M_{DM3}, M_{M3})

$$NDL = \frac{M_{DM}}{S \cdot \dfrac{M_{DM}}{GDF} + M_{DM}} = \frac{GDF}{S + GDF}, \qquad (7\text{-}28)$$

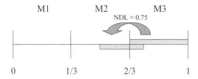

Fig. 7.11 Mitochondrial growth dilutes membrane damage. The incorporation of new proteins and lipids into existing mitochondrial membranes leads to a reduction in the level of membrane damage. The maximum amount of membrane damage is defined as 1, and mitochondria are assigned to one of three classes (M_1, M_2, M_3), depending on the degree of damage. The new damage level (NDL) can be calculated according to Eq. (7-28) and the diagram shows how this affects mitochondria that were originally in M_3.

where S is the total amount of newly synthesized mitochondria as defined by Eq. (7-40) (see below). In this model, we used three different classes to group the amount of membrane damage into low, medium, and high. If NDL is, for instance, 75 %, we need to know how this affects the number of mitochondria in the three damage classes. This situation is depicted in Fig. 7.11. The minimal amount of membrane damage is zero and the maximum amount is defined as one. The different damage classes are represented by dividing the range 0–1 into three equal segments. Under the assumption that the membrane damage is evenly distributed between 2/3 and 1 (upper gray box), a 25 % reduction ($NDL = 0.75$) means that the new distribution of membrane damage is given by the lower gray box ranging from 0.5 to 0.75. From this diagram we can now calculate the fraction of mitochondria leaving M_3 (valid for $NDL > 2/3$):

$$\frac{2/3 - 2/3\ NDL}{1/3\ NDL} = 2\ \frac{S}{GDF} . \tag{7-29}$$

Of course, not only do some mitochondria leave M_3 and enter M_2, but also some mitochondria that were originally in M_2 become shifted to M_1. Following the same line of reasoning as above, this fraction turns out to be (valid for $NDL > 1/2$)

$$\frac{1/3 - 1/3\ NDL}{1/3\ NDL} = \frac{S}{GDF} . \tag{7-30}$$

The calculation of NDL is slightly different for $M_{M2,}$ which has a growth disadvantage of $(GDF + 1)/2$. Here $NDL_{M_{M2}} = \dfrac{GDF + 1}{2\,S + GDF + 1}$ and the fraction leaving M_{M2} is $\dfrac{2\,S}{GDF + 1}$. We do not need to be concerned about M_{M1}, since their membrane status cannot improve.

7.3.2.4 The Equations

From the assumptions and details given in the previous sections, the differential equations of the model can be developed. Although the equations might in some respects have been written in a more compact way, we chose this representation to improve clarity. The different terms of Eqs. (7-31)–(7-36) describe the consequences of growth and radical damage on the numbers of mitochondria in the various classes. To illustrate this, consider Eq. (7-31), which describes the time course of intact mitochondria with little membrane damage (M_{M1}). The first term defines the increase of M_{M1} caused by synthesis of new mitochondria. The next term describes the fraction of mitochondria belonging to M_{M2}, which are converted into M_{M1} because of the membrane damage dilution effect (see previous section). The last term summarizes all processes leading to a loss of M_{M1}, i.e., decay (with rate constant α) and acquisition of further membrane (k_M) or DNA damage (k_D). Similar terms exist in the other equations such as in Eq. (7-35) for M_{DM2}. The individual expressions describe loss and gain caused by the damage dilution process, increase through M_{M2} that suffered DNA damage and M_{DM1} that acquired further membrane damage, and finally the loss caused by degradation and membrane damage. In some of these terms, the expression $RDF \cdot Rad_M$ appears. This reflects the fact that the amount of radicals in damaged mitochondria can be calculated from Rad_M by multiplication with the factor RDF.

Equation (7-37) for the antioxidants consists of just two expressions describing synthesis and degradation. Synthesis is controlled by the ATP level and the antioxidant promoter. As for mitochondria, it is assumed that a low level of ATP diminishes the protein synthesis rate.

In the model it is assumed that the removal of radicals, Eq. (7-38), depends on the amount of antioxidants per mitochondrion. Although this is a reasonable assumption, other possibilities, such as elimination depending on the total amount of antioxidants, exist. In a qualitative model like this, the exact molecular details of the modeled reactions are often not known, and thus neither way of modeling would be wrong. If in doubt, both versions should be implemented and the simulation results compared.

Regarding the generation of energy, Eq. (7-39), it is assumed that ATP production is directly proportional to the proposed growth disadvantage. This means that M_{M2} generates half of the energy of M_{M1} and that all other types of mitochondria do not contribute to the cellular energy production. The model incorporates three energy-consuming processes: the synthesis of mitochondria, the synthesis of antioxidants, and a fixed amount k_{EC} that represents all other energy-consuming processes of the cell that are not explicitly included in the model.

$$\frac{dM_{M1}}{dt} = S \cdot M_{M1} + \frac{2S}{GDF + 1} \cdot M_{M2} - (\alpha + (k_M + k_D)Rad_M) \cdot M_{M1} \qquad (7\text{-}31)$$

$$\frac{dM_{M2}}{dt} = -\frac{2S}{GDF + 1} \cdot M_{M2} + \frac{2S}{GDF} \cdot M_{M3} + k_M Rad_M \cdot M_{M1}$$
$$- (\beta + (k_M + k_D)Rad_M) \cdot M_{M2} \qquad (7\text{-}32)$$

$$\frac{dM_{M3}}{dt} = -\frac{2S}{GDF} \cdot M_{M3} + k_M Rad_M \cdot M_{M2} - (\gamma + k_D Rad_M) \cdot M_{M3} \qquad (7\text{-}33)$$

$$\frac{dM_{DM1}}{dt} = \frac{S}{GDF} \cdot (M_{DM1} + M_{DM2}) + k_D Rad_M \cdot M_{M1} - (\alpha + k_M \cdot RDF \cdot Rad_M) \cdot M_{DM1}$$
$$(7\text{-}34)$$

$$\frac{dM_{DM2}}{dt} = -\frac{S}{GDF} \cdot M_{DM2} + \frac{2S}{GDF} \cdot M_{DM3} + k_D Rad_M \cdot M_{M2} + k_M \cdot RDF \cdot Rad_M \cdot M_{DM1}$$
$$- (\beta + k_M \cdot RDF \cdot Rad_M) \cdot M_{DM2} \tag{7-35}$$

$$\frac{dM_{DM3}}{dt} = -\frac{2S}{GDF} \cdot M_{DM3} + k_D Rad_M \cdot M_{M3} + k_M \cdot RDF \cdot Rad_M \cdot M_{DM2} - \gamma \cdot M_{DM3} \tag{7-36}$$

$$\frac{dAOx}{dt} = \frac{ATP}{ATP + ATP_c} \cdot$$
$$\frac{k_2}{1 + \left(\dfrac{PAOx}{Rad_M(M_{M1} + M_{M2} + M_{M3}) + RDF \cdot Rad_M(M_{DM1} + M_{DM2} + M_{DM3})} \right)^3} - \delta AOx \tag{7-37}$$

$$\frac{dRad_M}{dt} = k_R - k_3 \frac{AOx \cdot Rad_M}{M_{M1} + M_{M2} + M_{M3} + M_{DM1} + M_{DM2} + M_{DM3}} \tag{7-38}$$

$$\frac{dATP}{dt} = k_{ATP} \cdot M_{M1} + \frac{1}{2} k_{ATP} \cdot M_{M2} - \frac{ATP}{ATP + ATP_c} \cdot$$
$$\left(\frac{k_{EM} k_1}{1 + \left(\dfrac{ATP}{ATP_c} \right)^3} + k_{EC} + \right.$$
$$\left. \frac{k_{EP} k_2}{1 + \left(\dfrac{PAOx}{Rad_M(M_{M1} + M_{M2} + M_{M3}) + RDF \cdot Rad_M(M_{DM1} + M_{DM2} + M_{DM3})} \right)^3} \right) \tag{7-39}$$

$$S = \frac{ATP}{ATP + ATP_c} \cdot \frac{k_1}{1 + \left(\dfrac{ATP}{ATP_c} \right)^3} \cdot$$
$$\frac{1}{M_{M1} + \dfrac{2}{GDF + 1} \cdot M_{M2} + \dfrac{1}{GDF} \cdot (M_{M3} + M_{DM1} + M_{DM2} + M_{DM3})} \cdot \tag{7-40}$$

7.3.2.5 Choice of Parameters and Simulation Results

The numerical values of the model parameters can have a large influence on the dynamic behavior of the model. Ideally, all parameters used by the model would have a clear biochemical representation and all parameters would be measured experimentally, so that these values can be used directly for the numerical simulation. Unfortunately, this situation only rarely applies. Often a biological process that in reality consists of several reactions is collapsed into a single reaction because the details are either unknown or of no importance for the current model. An example is the generic antioxidant (AOx) that is used in this model to represent all cellular antioxidant reactions. Clearly, the parameters controlling the synthesis, degradation, or activity of AOx have no direct presentation in reality. In this case an educated guess has to be made to choose initial parameter settings. Additionally, a parameter scan should be performed to see whether the model behavior depends critically on the chosen numerical values. The other reason that exact numerical values cannot be used is of course that they have not yet been measured (or cannot be measured for technical reasons). GDF, RDF, k_M, k_D, k_1, and k_2 are examples of such parameters. A qualitative model can cope with uncertain parameters by varying those parameters over a possible range of values to see if this leads to a qualitative change in the model predictions (e. g., loss of stable steady state, appearance of oscillations, drastic changes in timescale). Quantitative models that seek to predict or reproduce experimental data as closely as possible can try to estimate the unknown parameters by fitting the model to experimental measurements. This, however, depends on the availability of such data.

The following table lists the parameters of the SOS model together with the standard values used for the numerical simulations and a short description.

Name	Value	Description
α	0.01 d^{-1}	Decay rate for mitochondria with little membrane damage (M_{M1}, M_{DM1}). The resulting half-life is 70 days. The values of α, β, and γ are based on the data of Huemer et al. (1971) and Menzies and Gold (1971).
β	0.05 d^{-1}	Decay rate for mitochondria with medium membrane damage (M_{M2}, M_{DM2}). The resulting half-life is 14 days.
γ	0.1 d^{-1}	Decay rate for mitochondria with much membrane damage (M_{M3}, M_{DM3}). The resulting half-life is 7 days.
δ	0.693 d^{-1}	Decay rate for antioxidants. The resulting half-life is 1 day.
RDF	0.2	Factor specifying how much fewer radicals are generated by mutant mitochondria than by intact ones.
GDF	5	Factor specifying the growth rate difference between intact and mutant mitochondria.
k_M	0.003 d^{-1}	Constant controlling the rate of membrane damage accumulation.
k_D	0.003 d^{-1}	Constant controlling the rate of mtDNA damage accumulation.
k_1	100 d^{-1}	Maximum number of mitochondria synthesized per day.
k_2	100 d^{-1}	Maximum number of antioxidants synthesized per day.
k_3	7000 d^{-1}	Rate of radical removal by antioxidants in units of 10^6. This value is based on work of Rotilio et al. (1972) concerning superoxide dismutase.
k_{EM}	400	Molecules of ATP needed for the synthesis of a mitochondrion in units of 10^6. It is assumed that the main costs are synthesizing lipids and proteins in the membrane and the proteins of the matrix. To calculate these costs, the following assumptions have been made. A mitochondrion is a rod-like structure 0.5 μm in diameter and 1 μm long. The matrix consists of 18% proteins with an average weight of 40,000 Da. The membrane consists of 75% protein, which is equivalent to 25 lipid molecules per protein. The diameter of a lipid is approximately 1.5 nm and 5.5 nm for a protein. Finally, 800 molecules of ATP are required to synthesize one protein and 15 molecules to synthesize one lipid. These assumptions are based on the data of Alberts et al. (1994) and Stryer (1988).
k_{EP}	0.0008	Molecules of ATP needed for the synthesis of one antioxidant protein in units of 10^6. A size of 400 amino acids is assumed.

Name	Value	Description
k_{EC}	10^6 d^{-1}	Amount of ATP consumed per day per cell in units of 10^6. This value is calculated under the assumptions that the specific metabolic rate for humans is 0.25 mL of O_2 per g/h (Adelman et al. 1988), that six molecules of ATP are generated from each molecule of oxygen, and that the cell volume is 1000 μm³.
k_R	900 d^{-1}	Radicals produced by genetically intact mitochondria per day in units of 10^6. It is assumed that 10^6 radicals are generated per second per cell (Joenje et al. 1985) and that the cell has a mitochondrial population of approximately 100.
k_{ATP}	1200 d^{-1}	ATP produced per day by a functional mitochondrion (M_{M1}) in units of 10^6.
ATP_c	100	Promoter control parameter for the synthesis of mitochondria. If the ATP level is equal to ATP_c, the promoter is 50% repressed.
PAO_x	1	Promoter control parameter for the synthesis of antioxidants. If the radical level is equal to PAO_x, the promoter is 50% activated.

After all of the efforts to develop the equations for the model of the SOS hypothesis Fig. 7.12 finally shows some numerical results that have been obtained by solving the set of coupled ODEs with Mathematica (see Section 14.1.1). For the simulation shown on the left side, the standard values of the decay rates α, β, and γ were used and the system quickly reached a stable steady state. The simulation on the right side investigates how the resulting steady-state values are influenced by changes in the turnover rate. For convenience, the turnover rate is shown here in multiples of the standard turnover rate. This means that the time course shown in Fig. 7.12a approaches the steady-state values corresponding to a turnover rate of one

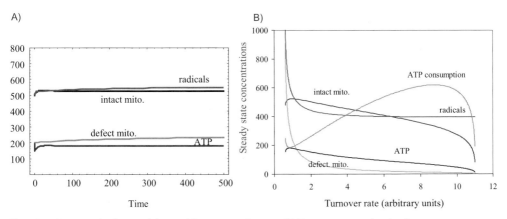

Fig. 7.12 Numerical solution of the model equations. To display all variables in one diagram, appropriate scaling factors have been applied to the different variables. (a) For this calculation, the standard values for the mitochondrial turnover rates α, β, and γ were used. In this case, the population quickly reaches a stable steady state. (b) Parameter scan showing how a variation of the turnover rate (in multiples of the standard values) affects the steady-state levels. The important conclusion is that a turnover rate that is either too low (<0.6) or too high (>11) leads to an unstable system.

in Fig. 7.12 b. If the turnover rate is too low (<0.6) or too high (>11), the system has no stable steady state, which means that the mitochondrial population will finally break down. If the turnover rate is too high, mitochondria are degraded faster than they can be synthesized by the cellular machinery. But, if the turnover rate is too low, mitochondria have a much longer time to accumulate damage, because now the half-life of the organelles is substantially increased. This additional burden also leads to a collapse of the system.

With such a complex model as we have developed here, there are of course many more simulations possible. It is especially possible to investigate the consequences of cell division on the stability of the mitochondrial population. However, for further details, the reader is referred to Kowald and Kirkwood (1999, 2000).

References

ADELMAN, R., SAUL, R.L. and AMES, B.N. Oxidative damage to DNA: Relation to species metabolic rate and life span (1988) Proc. Natl. Acad. Sci. USA *85*, 2706–2708.

ALBERTS, B., BRAY, D., LEWIS, J., RAFF, M., ROBERTS, K. and WATSON, J.D. Molecular biology of the cell. (1994) 3rd Edition, Garland Publishing, Inc.

BOOTMAN, M.D., COLLINS, T.J., PEPPIATT, C.M., PROTHERO, L.S., MACKENZIE, L., DE SMET, P., TRAVERS, M., TOVEY, S.C., SEO, J.T., BERRIDGE, M.J., CICCOLINI, F. and LIPP, P. Calcium signalling: an overview (2001 a) Semin. Cell Dev. Biol. *12*, 3–10.

BOOTMAN, M.D., LIPP, P. and BERRIDGE, M.J. The organisation and functions of local Ca(2+) signals (2001 b) J. Cell Sci. *114*, 2213–22.

BRIERLEY, E.J., JOHNSON, M.A., LIGHTOWLERS, R.N., JAMES, O.F.W. and TURNBULL, D.M. Role of mitochondrial DNA mutations in human aging: Implications for the central nervous system and muscle (1998) Ann. Neurology *43*, 217–223.

CHANCE, B., GHOSH, A., HIGGINS, J.J. and MAITRA, P.K. Cyclic and Oscillatory Responses of Metabolic Pathways Involving Chemical Feedback and Their Computer Representations (1964) Ann. NY Acad. Sci. *115*, 1010–24.

CHEN, K.C., CSIKASZ-NAGY, A., GYORFFY, B., VAL, J., NOVAK, B. and TYSON, J.J. Kinetic analysis of a molecular model of the budding yeast cell cycle (2000) Mol. Biol. Cell. *11*, 369–91.

CHEN, K.C., CALZONE, L., CSIKASZ-NAGY, A., CROSS, F.R., NOVAK, B. and TYSON, J.J. Integrative analysis of cell cycle control in budding yeast (2004) Mol. Biol. Cell. *15*, 3841–62.

DE GREY, A.D.N.J. A proposed refinement of the mitochondrial free radical theory of aging (1997) BioEssays *19*, 161–166.

DECROLY, O. and GOLDBETER, A. Birhythmicity, chaos, and other patterns of temporal self-organization in a multiply regulated biochemical system (1982) Proc. Natl. Acad. Sci. USA *79*, 6917–21.

GHOSH, A. and CHANCE, B. Oscillations of glycolytic intermediates in yeast cells (1964) Biochem. Biophys. Res. Commun. *16*, 174–81.

GOLDBETER, A. A minimal cascade model for the mitotic oscillator involving cyclin and cdc2 kinase (1991) Proc. Natl. Acad. Sci. USA *88*, 9107–11.

GOLDBETER, A. and LEFEVER, R. Dissipative structures for an allosteric model. Application to glycolytic oscillations (1972) Biophys. J. *12*, 1302–15.

GOLDBETER, A., DUPONT, G. and BERRIDGE, M.J. Minimal model for signal-induced Ca2+ oscillations and for their frequency encoding through protein phosphorylation (1990) Proc. Natl. Acad. Sci. USA *87*, 1461–5.

HALLOY, J., LAUZERAL, J. and GOLDBETER, A. Modeling oscillations and waves of cAMP in Dictyostelium discoideum cells (1998) Biophys. Chem. *72*, 9–19.

HARTWELL, L.H. Saccharomyces cerevisiae cell cycle (1974) Bacteriol. Rev. *38*, 164–98.

HARTWELL, L.H., CULOTTI, J., PRINGLE, J.R. and REID, B.J. Genetic control of the cell division cycle in yeast (1974) Science *183*, 46–51.

HIGGINS, J. A chemical mechanism for oscillation of glycolytic intermediates in yeast cells (1964) Proc. Natl. Acad. Sci. USA *51*, 989–94.

HOPF, E. Abzweigung einer periodischen Lösung von einer stationären Lösung eines Differentialgleichungssystems (1942) Ber. Math. Phys. Kl. Sächs. Akad. Wiss. *94*, 3–22.

HUEMER, R.P., LEE, K.D., REEVES, A.E. and BICKERT, C. Mitochondrial studies in senescent mice – II. Specific activity, bouyant density, and turnover of mitochondrial DNA (1971) Experimental Gerontology *6*, 327–334.

JOENJE, H., GILLE, J.J.P., OOSTRA, A.B. and VAN DER VALK, P. Some characteristics of hyperoxia-adapted HeLa cells. (1985) Laboratory Investigation *52*, 420–428.

JOHNSON, D.G. and WALKER, C.L. Cyclins and cell cycle checkpoints (1999) Annu. Rev. Pharmacol. Toxicol. *39*, 295–312.

KHOLODENKO, B.N. Negative feedback and ultrasensitivity can bring about oscillations in the mitogen-activated protein kinase cascades (2000) Eur. J. Biochem. *267*, 1583–8.

KHRAPKO, K., BODYAK, N., THILLY, W.G., van ORSOUW, N.J., ZHANG, X., COLLER, H.A., PERLS, T.T., UPTON, M., VIJG, J. and WEI, J.Y. Cell by cell scanning of whole mitochondrial genomes in aged human heart reveals a significant fraction of myocytes with clonally expanded deletions (1999) Nucleic Acids Res. *27*, 2434–2441.

KIRKWOOD, T.B.L. and HOLLIDAY, R. Ageing as a consequence of natural selection. (1986) In: K. J. Collins, ed. The biology of human ageing. Cambridge University Press, pp 1–15.

KIRKWOOD, T.B.L. and ROSE, M.R. Evolution of senescence: Late survival sacrificed for reproduction. (1991) Philos. Trans. R Soc., London B *332*, 15–24.

KOWALD, A. and KIRKWOOD, T.B.L. Towards a network theory of ageing: a model combining the free radical theory and the protein error theory. (1994) J. Theor. Biol. *168*, 75–94.

KOWALD, A. and KIRKWOOD, T.B.L. A network theory of ageing: the interactions of defective mitochondria, aberrant proteins, free radicals and scavengers in the ageing process. (1996) Mutation Research *316*, 209–236.

KOWALD, A. and KIRKWOOD, T.B.L. Modeling the role of mitochondrial mutations in cellular aging (1999) Journal of Anti-Aging Medicine *2*, 243–253.

KOWALD, A. and KIRKWOOD, T.B.L. Accumulation of defective mitochondria through delayed degradation of damaged organelles and

its possible role in the ageing of post-mitotic and dividing cells (2000) J. Theor. Biol. *202*, 145–160.

MAKEHAM, W.H. On the law of mortality (1867) J. Inst. Actuaries *13*, 325–358.

MAYNARD SMITH, J. Group selection (1976) Quarterly Review of Biology *51*, 277–283.

MAYNARD SMITH, J. Evolutionary genetics (1989) Oxford University Press, Oxford.

MEDAWAR, P.B. An unsolved problem of biology (1952) H.K. Lewis, London.

MEDVEDEV, Z.A. An attempt at a rational classification of theories of ageing. (1990) Biological Reviews *65*, 375–398.

MENZIES, R.A. and GOLD, P.H. The turnover of mitochondria in a variety of tissues of young adult and aged rats. (1971) J. Biol. Chem. *246*, 2425–2429.

MORI, T. and JOHNSON, C.H. Circadian control of cell division in unicellular organisms (2000) Prog. Cell Cycle Res. *4*, 185–92.

NANJUNDIAH, V. Cyclic AMP oscillations in Dictyostelium discoideum: models and observations (1998) Biophys. Chem. *72*, 1–8.

NOVAK, B., TOTH, A., CSIKASZ-NAGY, A., GYORFFY, B., TYSON, J.J. and NASMYTH, K. Finishing the cell cycle (1999) J. Theor. Biol. *199*, 223–33.

NURSE, P. Genetic control of cell size at cell division in yeast (1975) Nature *256*, 547–51.

NURSE, P. and BISSETT, Y. Gene required in G1 for commitment to cell cycle and in G2 for control of mitosis in fission yeast (1981) Nature *292*, 558–60.

PARDEE, A.B. A restriction point for control of normal animal cell proliferation (1974) Proc. Natl. Acad. Sci. USA *71*, 1286–90.

RABINOVICH, M.I. and ABARBANEL, H.D. The role of chaos in neural systems (1998) Neuroscience *87*, 5–14.

RICHARD, P., BAKKER, B.M., TEUSINK, B., VAN DAM, K. and WESTERHOFF, H.V. Acetaldehyde mediates the synchronization of sustained glycolytic oscillations in populations of yeast cells (1996) Eur. J. Biochem. *235*, 238–41.

ROOS, W., SCHEIDEGGER, C. and GERISH, G. Adenylate cyclase activity oscillations as signals for cell aggregation in Dictyostelium discoideum (1977) Nature *266*, 259–61.

ROTILIO, G., BRAY, R.C. and FIELDEN, E.M. A pulse radiolysis study of superoxide dismutase (1972) Biochimica et Biophysica Acta *268*, 605–609.

Sel'kov, E.E. Self-oscillations in glycolysis.
1. A simple kinetic model (1968) Eur. J. Biochem. *4*, 79–86.

Sel'kov, E.E. Stabilization of energy charge, generation of oscillations and multiple steady states in energy metabolism as a result of purely stoichiometric regulation (1975) Eur. J. Biochem. *59*, 151–7.

Smaaland, R. Circadian rhythm of cell division (1996) Prog. Cell Cycle Res. *2*, 241–66.

Stearns, S.C. The evolution of life histories (1992) Oxford University Press, Oxford.

Stryer, L. Biochemistry (1988) 3rd Edition, W.H. Freeman and Company, New York.

Turek, F.W. Circadian rhythms (1998) Horm. Res. *49*, 109–13.

Tyson, J.J. Modeling the cell division cycle: cdc2 and cyclin interactions (1991) Proc. Natl. Acad. Sci. USA *88*, 7328–32.

Tyson, J.J. and Novak, B. Regulation of the eukaryotic cell cycle: molecular antagonism, hysteresis, and irreversible transitions (2001) J. Theor. Biol. *210*, 249–63.

Tyson, J.J., Novak, B., Chen, K. and Val, J. Checkpoints in the cell cycle from a modeler's perspective (1995) Prog. Cell Cycle Res. *1*, 1–8.

Tyson, J.J., Novak, B., Odell, G.M., Chen, K. and Thron, C.D. Chemical kinetic theory: understanding cell-cycle regulation (1996) Trends Biochem. Sci. *21*, 89–96.

Weismann, A. Essays upon heredity and kindred biological problems. (1891) 2nd Edition, Clarendon Press, Oxford.

Williams, G.C. Pleiotropy, natural selection and the evolution of senescence (1957) Evolution *11*, 398–411.

Wolf, J. and Heinrich, R. Dynamics of two-component biochemical systems in interacting cells; synchronization and desynchronization of oscillations and multiple steady states (1997) Biosystems *43*, 1–24.

8
Modeling of Gene Expression

Introduction

The expression of genes, which is a highly regulated process in eukaryotic as well as in prokaryotic cells, has a profound impact on the ability of the cells to maintain vitality, perform cell division, and respond to environmental changes or stimuli. In theoretical modeling of gene expression, two diverse approaches have been developed. On the one hand, the expression of one or a few genes has been described on the level of transcription or translation by detailed mathematical models that include the binding of transcription factors and RNA polymerases to DNA, the effect of specific inhibitors or activators, the formation of various stages of maturation of mRNA or proteins, and the regulation by internal feedback loops or external regulators. The basis of this type of modeling is knowledge or hypotheses about the processes and interactions taking place during gene expression. Like most types of kinetic modeling, it often lacks specific kinetic parameters for the individual processes under consideration. On the other hand, the expression changes of thousands of genes are analyzed in parallel over time with DNA arrays. Gene expression profiles (expression levels at different time points) and gene expression patterns (comparison of expression values of different genes under different experimental conditions) are used to search for clusters and motifs and, eventually, to deduce functional correlations. Based on this information, reverse engineering methods seek to reconstruct the underlying regulatory networks (Section 9.6). While these approaches largely neglect the highly complex regulatory machinery behind the emergence of detectable mRNA involving the action of proteins and other regulatory molecules, they cover a large fraction or almost all genes of a cell – compared to the first approach, which can deal only with a few genes.

In this chapter we describe the basic steps of gene expression (Section 8.1). A fundamental step is the regulation of transcription through transcription factors that bind to DNA motifs upstream of the transcription start point. Section 8.2 introduces computational methods for the detection of binding sites that determine such transcription factor binding to the DNA. Section 8.3 covers the detailed modeling of basic processes of eukaryotic gene expression, and Section 8.4 discusses the regulation of gene expression in prokaryotes in the context of the operon concept.

Systems Biology in Practice. Concepts, Implementation and Application.
E. Klipp, R. Herwig, A. Kowald, C. Wierling, H. Lehrach
Copyright © 2005 WILEY-VCH Verlag GmbH & Co. KGaA, Weinheim
ISBN: 3-527-31078-9

8.1
Modules of Gene Expression

In the following section, we will outline a general view of the processes representing gene expression, from the activation of transcriptional regulators to the synthesis of a functional protein (Orphanides and Reinberg 2002; Proudfoot et al. 2002; Reed and Hurt 2002).

Hundreds of different cell types exist and fulfill specific roles in the organism. Each cell type theoretically contains information on the same set of genes; however, only a proportion of these genes is expressed, determining the specific role of cells of this type. Gene expression in eukaryotes is controlled at six different steps, which determine the diversity and specification of the organism (Alberts et al. 2002):

1. Transcriptional control: when and how often a gene is transcribed.
2. RNA processing control: how the RNA transcript is spliced.
3. RNA transport and localization control: which mRNAs in the nucleus are exported to cytosol and where in the cytosol they are localized.
4. Translation control: which mRNAs in the cytosol are translated by ribosomes.
5. mRNA degradation control: which mRNAs in the cytosol are destabilized.
6. Protein activity control: determines activation, inhibition, compartmentalization, and degrading of the translated protein.

Each step is complex and has been studied extensively in isolation. The process is typically modeled with a linear structure of more or less independent modules where the output of the previous module is the input for the current module.

The expression level of the majority of genes is controlled by transcription factors. Transcription factors are proteins that bind to DNA regulatory sequences upstream of the site at which transcription is initiated. Various regulatory pathways control their activities (see Chapter 6). More than 5% of human genes encode transcription factors (Tupler et al. 2001). Once activated, transcription factors bind to gene regulatory elements and, through interactions with other components of the transcription machinery, promote access to DNA and facilitate the recruitment of the RNA polymerase enzymes to the transcriptional start site.

In eukaryotes, there are three RNA polymerases, namely, RNAP I, II, and III. RNAP II catalyzes the transcription of protein-coding genes and is responsible for the synthesis of mRNAs and certain small nuclear RNAs, while the others are responsible for generating primarily tRNAs (RNAP III) and ribosomal RNAs (RNAP I) (Allison et al. 1985).

The RNAP II enzyme itself is unable to initiate promoter-dependent transcription in the absence of complementing factors. It needs to be supplemented by so-called general transcription factors (GTFs) (Orphanides et al. 1996). RNAP II together with these GTFs and the DNA template form the pre-initiation complex, and the assembly of this complex is nucleated by binding of TBP (a component of TFIID) to the "TATA box" (Woychik and Hampsey 2002). The TATA box is a core promoter (or minimal promoter) that directs transcriptional initiation at a short distance (about

30 bp downstream). Soon after RNAP II initiates transcription, the nascent RNA is modified by the addition of a cap structure at its 5' end. This cap serves initially to protect the new transcript from attack by nucleases and later serves as a binding site for proteins involved in export of the mature mRNA into the cytoplasm and its translation into protein.

The start of RNA synthesis catalyzed by RNAP II is the transcription initiation. During transcription elongation, the polymerase moves along the gene sequence from the 5' to the 3' end and extends the transcript. The transition between these early transcriptional events, initiation and elongation, seems to be coordinated by the capping process. A family of elongation factors then regulates the elongation phase (Uptain et al. 1997). Upon reaching the end of a gene, RNAP II stops transcription (termination), the newly RNA is cleaved (cleavage), and a polyadenosine (poly(A)) tail is added to the 3' end of the transcript (polyadenylation). The resulting pre-mRNA contains coding sequences in the gene (exons) that are divided by long non-coding sequences (introns). These introns are removed by pre-mRNA splicing.

Transcription, i.e., the transfer of information from DNA to RNA, and translation, i.e., the transfer of information from RNA to protein, are spatially separated in eukaryotes by the nuclear membrane; transcription occurs in the nucleus, whereas translation is a cytoplasmic event. For this reason, processed mRNAs must be transported from the nucleus to the cytoplasm before translation can occur. The bidirectional transport of macromolecules between nucleus and cytoplasm occurs through protein-covered pores in the nuclear membrane. The export of mRNA is mediated by factors that interact with proteins of the nuclear pores and bind to mRNA molecules in the nucleus and direct them into the cytoplasm. Translation of mRNA into protein takes place on ribosomes, i.e., large ribonucleoprotein complexes, and follows principles similar to those of transcription. Important for the translation process is the presence of transfer RNA molecules (tRNAs), which deliver the correct amino acid to the currently considered nucleotide triplet. tRNAs have a common characteristic secondary structure and are bound to the mRNA by means of anticodons complementary to the triplet for which they carry the appropriate amino acid. Subsequently, tRNAs are recruited and the polypeptide is synthesized until the first stop codon is present. The first step is the location of the start codon in conjunction with subunits of the ribosome triggered by translational initiation factors. Subsequent phases are elongation and termination. The nascent polypeptide chain then undergoes folding and often post-translational chemical modifications to generate the final active protein (cf. Section 2.4).

8.2
Promoter Identification

Transcriptional control is very important in gene expression, which makes biological sense since the cell invests energy to synthesize products and this energy should not be wasted through subsequent termination of the activity of these products. Gene transcription is controlled by RNAP II and it depends on the presence of several additional proteins in order to transcribe the gene in the proper cellular context. In eukaryotes, gene expression requires a complex regulatory region that defines the transcription start point and controls the initiation of transcription, i.e., the promoter. Several algorithms are available that try to identify promoters for specific genes. Some of these algorithms are discussed in this section.

8.2.1
General Promoter Structure

Promoter prediction algorithms implicitly assume a specific model for a typical promoter. The general structure of an RNAP II promoter is described in Fig. 8.1a. The typical promoter is composed of three levels of regulatory sequence signals. The first level contains sequence motifs that enable the binding of specific transcription factors. The next level is the combination of binding sites to promoter modules that jointly act as functional units. The third level consists of the complete promoter that modulates gene transcription depending on cell type, tissue type, developmental stage, or activation by signaling pathways.

The promoter must contain binding sites for the GTFs, such as the TATA box. These proximate regulatory motifs constitute the core promoter that is able to bind the preinitiation complex and to determine the exact transcription start site. The core promoter needs additional regulatory motifs at varying distances from the transcriptional start point, the regulatory binding sites (transcription factor–binding sites, TFBSs). These sites can be situated nearby or kilobases away from the core promoter.

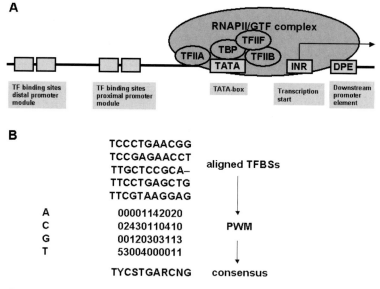

Fig. 8.1 (a) General structure of a eukaryotic gene promoter. (b) Example of a positional weight matrix and a consensus sequence derived from different transcription factor–binding sites.

Transcription initiation can be viewed as a process involving successive formation of protein complexes. In the first step, transcription factors bind to upstream promoter and enhancer sequence motifs and form a multiprotein complex. In the next step, this complex recruits the RNAP II/GTF complex to the core promoter and the transcription start site. This is done through protein-protein interactions either directly or by adaptor proteins (Ptashne and Gann 1997). The full complex then starts the transcription process.

The core promoter is located in the direct neighborhood of the transcription start site (approximately 30 bp). The core promoter is the best-characterized part of the promoter and is defined as a set of binding sites sufficient for the assembly of the RNAP II/GTF complex and for specifying transcriptional initiation. Several types of core promoters are known (Berg and von Hippel 1987):

1. TATA box: If TBP is present in the RNAP II/GTF complex, then this protein binds to the sequence motif and the transcription starts approximately 30 bp downstream.
2. TATA-less: No TATA box is present. The start site is determined by a sequence motif INR (initiator region) surrounding the start site (Smale 1994).
3. A combination of both INR and TATA box
4. Null promoter: Neither of the two sequence motifs is present. Transcription initiation is based solely on upstream (or downstream) promoter elements (Novina and Roy 1997).
5. In some cases, a downstream promoter element (DPE) exists in addition to INR, and both elements are able to specify the transcription start site (Burke and Kadonga 1997).

Whereas the core promoter determines the transcription start site, this function cannot explain how genes whose protein products are needed in parallel are co-regulated, e.g., from genes that are located on different chromosomes. Thus, additional regulatory elements are necessary that meet the requirement of higher flexibility and coordinated gene expression.

Typically a few hundred base pairs upstream of the core promoter is the proximate promoter module, which contains TFBSs for proteins responsible for the modulation of the transcription. The corresponding factors can influence the binding of the core promoter components or the chromatin structure (or both). Furthermore, a promoter can contain a distal promoter module (on the order of kilobases apart from the transcription start site). Although these modules cannot act as promoters on their own, they are able to enhance or suppress the activity of transcription up to orders of magnitude (enhancer or silencer). Enhancer and silencer often exhibit a tissue-specific activity. Like the transcription factors binding to the proximate module of the promoter, the factors binding to the distal module influence gene expression by interactions with the factors in the RNAP II/GTF complex or by changing the chromatin structure. There is no clear boundary for the promoter in the 5′ direction, and the common explanation for interactions with distal factors to the transcription apparatus is given by the formation of large loops in the DNA. The function of a promoter is to increase or repress the transcription from the core promoter (basal transcription). Thus, any given gene will have a specific regulatory region determined by the binding sites of the transcription factors that ensure that the gene is transcribed in the appropriate cell type and at the proper point in development. The transcriptional activation is determined not only by the presence of the binding sites but also through the availability of the corresponding transcription factors. These transcription factors are themselves subjected to regulation and activation, e.g., through signaling pathways, and the whole process can entail complex procedures such as transcriptional cascades and feedback control loops (Pedersen et al. 1999).

8.2.2
Sequence-based Prediction of Promoter Elements

This section discusses promoter prediction algorithms that incorporate solely the genome sequence. As described in the previous section, promoters are complex and diverse, which makes promoter prediction a difficult task. Early reviews on promoter recognition programs can be found in Fickett and Hatzigeorgiou (1997) and Stormo (2000); a more recent review on algorithms for promoter prediction can be found in Werner (2003).

The modeling of gene transcription regulation follows its combinatorial nature, starting from the detection of individual binding sites (5–25 bp in length), moving to the detection of specific combinations of binding sites, so-called composite regulatory elements (Kel et al. 1995), and finally to the detection of the promoter.

The detection of individual binding sites is the first level in that process. TFBSs have high sequence variability, which distinguishes them, for example, from restriction sites, i.e., the recognition sequences of a restriction enzyme. Whereas restriction sites are almost exact in the sense that sites varying by only a single mismatch will be cut less well by orders of magnitude, transcription factor binding can tolerate high sequence variability of the TFBSs (Stormo 2000). This variation makes biological sense in that it allows a higher flexibility of the regulatory system and assigns the promoters different activity levels.

In order to meet this flexibility, known TFBSs for the same transcription factor that may vary slightly are often represented by a consensus sequence that is close to each single motif according to some criterion. There is a tradeoff in the consensus sequences between the number of mismatches that are allowed and the precision of the representation and thus a tradeoff between the specificity and the sensitivity of the algorithms. A consensus sequence is typically denoted in the IUPAC code to describe ambiguities in nucleotide composition (Fig. 8.1 b).

An alternative to consensus sequences is the use of positional weight matrices (PWM). A PWM is a matrix representation of a TFBS, with rows representing one of the bases, "A," "C," "G," and "T," and columns representing the position within the motif (Fig. 8.1 b). Each entry in the matrix corresponds to a numerical value indicating the confidence for the specific base at that position. The PWM approach is somewhat more general than the consensus sequence approach in the sense that each consensus can be represented by a PWM (for example, through frequency counts across the aligned motifs) such that the same set of sites can be matched but not vice versa (Stormo 2000). The calculation of the matrix elements can be performed in different ways. Stormo et al. (1982) applied a neural network learning algorithm to determine the weights of a PWM to distinguish known sites from non-sites in a training sample of E. coli sequences. Afterwards they predicted new sequences using the calculated weights. Berg and von Hippel (1987) used thermodynamic considerations to compute the weights of a PWM. They showed that the logarithms of the base frequencies should be proportional to the binding energy contribution of the bases, assuming an equal distribution of base pairs through the genome. The most comprehensive collection of PWMs can be found in the TRANSFAC database.

Recognition of composite regulatory elements has been proposed in order to meet the combinatorial nature of gene regulation, e.g., of two transcription factors that interact with each other in gene regulation. Here, statistical approaches have been made to reveal common pairs from DNA sequences. For example, Kel et al. (1999) developed a method that employs pairs of weight matrices for two corresponding transcription factors. The method takes into account the matching distances of the matrices on the DNA sequence and the mutual orientation and combines this with binding energy considerations. A number of examples of composite regulatory elements have been collected in the TRANSCompel database (Kel-Margoulis et al. 2002).

The general principle of promoter recognition methods is based on the strategy to determine a promoter model by features that are trained on a set of known promoter and non-promoter sequences. These features are subsequently used to search for an unknown number of promoters in a contiguous DNA sequence. The methods are distinguished from each other by the way the features are determined. Typically, they fall into two groups. The first group uses the pure sequence composition and is based on scoring moving sequence windows, whereas the second group employs prediction based on the detection of motifs from the core promoter element such as TATA box or INR.

The first group of algorithms can be exemplified by the PromFind method described in Hutchinson (1996). This method is based on the idea of discriminative counts of sequence groups. PromFind uses the frequency of heptamers in coding and non-coding sequences trained on sequences of 300 bp in length. Discrimination is based on the following measure:

$$d_i(s) = \frac{f(s)}{f(s) + f_i(s)}, \quad i = 1, 2. \tag{8-1}$$

Here, $f(s)$ denotes the frequency of heptamer s in the promoter sequences and $f_i(s)$ corresponds to the frequency of the heptamer in the training sample ($i = 1$: non-coding, $i = 2$: coding). For each sequence in a window of size 300 bp, the two measures are calculated and the window with the best score is returned. Another way of computing discriminative counts is employed in PromoterInspector developed by Scherf et al. (2000).

The second group of algorithms uses biological sequence features from the core promoter. Prestridge (1995) combined several of those patterns. The hit ratio of known TFBSs within promoters and non-promoters is used as an indicator for the identification of a promoter. The combined ratio scores of all TFBSs in a certain sequence window are used to build a scoring profile. This profile combined with a weight matrix for TATA boxes is used for predicting the transcription start site. Other methods model the core promoter with artificial neural networks (Reese 2001), ensembles of multi-layer perceptrons for binding sites or Hidden Markov models.

A list of some promoter recognition programs is found in the following table:

Program	*Web location*	*Reference*
FunSiteP	http://compel.bionet.nsc.ru/FunSite/fsp.html	Kondrakhin et al. (1995)
PomoterInspector	http://www.genomatix.de/cgi-bin/ promoterinspector/promoterinspector.pl	Scherf et al. (2000)
PromoterScan	http://bimas.dcrt.nih.gov/molbio/proscan	Prestridge (1995)
NNNP	http://www.fruitfly.org/seq_tools/promoter.html	Reese (2001)
PromFind	http://iubio.bio.indiana.edu/soft/molbio/mswin/ mswin-or-dos/profin11.exe	Hutchinson (1996)
TSSG/TSSW	http://www.softberry.com	Solovyev and Salamov (1997)
FirstEF	http://rulai.cshl.org/tools/FirstEF	Davuluri et al. (2001)

8.2.3
Approaches that Incorporate Additional Information

Since it has been shown that the error rates of the promoter prediction programs are fairly unsatisfactory (Fickett and Hatzigeorgiou 1997), new developments are trying to incorporate additional information as a backup when predicting TFBSs. A first class of approaches combines binding site prediction with gene expression data derived from DNA arrays. The widespread use of DNA arrays (cf. Chapter 9) has given rise to the following general program: (1) identify co-expression groups by clustering or other statistical methods and (2) search in the upstream regions of the grouped genes for common regulatory motifs. This approach was utilized for the first time by Tavazoie et al. (1999) for identifying novel regulatory networks in *Saccharomyces cerevisiae*. The authors used a K-means clustering algorithm to identify groups of co-regulated genes. They identified common sequence motifs in the upstream sequences of the genes and identified 18 motifs in 12 clusters that were highly over-represented within their own cluster and absent in the others, thus indicating the existence of different regulation patterns.

This and other studies (Pilpel et al. 2001) have demonstrated that genes that are co-expressed across multiple experimental conditions underlie common regulatory mechanisms and thus share common TFBSs in their promoters. Although these results are promising, methods that work well in yeast are difficult to extend to higher eukaryotes. This is mainly due to the fact that in yeast regulatory sequences are fairly proximal to the transcription start site, whereas in higher eukaryotes these sequences can be located many kilobases on either side of the coding region. A recent approach to human data has been published (Elkon et al. 2003). Here, the authors used DNA array data and human genome sequence data to identify putative regulatory elements that control the transcriptional program of the human cell cycle. They identified several transcription factors (such as E2F, NF-Y, and CREB) whose regulatory sequences were enriched in cell cycle–regulated genes and assigned these factors to certain phases of the cell cycle.

A second class of approaches uses comparative sequence analysis from upstream sequences of orthologous genes through different organisms (Wassermann et al. 2000). These authors investigated skeletal muscle–specific transcription factors and found that their binding sites are highly conserved in human and mouse DNA sequences. The general observation of conserved non-coding regions throughout different organisms has given rise to a number of recent developments that incorporate cross-species analysis of promoter elements. For example, Dieterich et al. (2003) have developed a comparative approach to human and mouse regulatory regions and built up a database of so-called conserved non-coding sequences (CORG, http://corg.molgen.mpg.de/).

A combination of these two approaches has been applied to the detection and experimental verification of a novel cis-regulatory element involved in the heat shock response in C. elegans (Thakurta et al. 2002). The authors identified co-regulated genes with DNA arrays and investigated the upstream regions of these genes for putative binding sites by pattern recognition algorithms. In the case of either significant over-representation or cross-species conservation, they build biological assays of the regulatory motifs using GFP reporter transgenes.

Additional sequence information is also sometimes incorporated in promoter identification, in particular the identification of CpG islands. It has been reported that these CpG islands correlate with promoters in vertebrates so that their features are used in the computational process. By definition (Gardiner-Garden and Frommer 1987) CpG islands are genomic regions that (1) are longer than 200 bp, (2) have nucleotide frequencies of C and G in that region greater than 50%, and (3) have CpG dinucleotide frequency in that region higher than 0.6 of that expected from mononucleotide frequencies.

Despite all these developments, the recognition and identification of promoter elements remain error prone due to the highly complex nature of eukaryotic gene regulation. Future approaches thus will have to incorporate additional information to a much larger extent than is currently done.

8.3
Modeling Specific Processes in Eukaryotic Gene Expression

We want to know which genes are expressed, to what level, and where and when in order to comprehend the functioning of organisms at the molecular level. A network of interactions among DNA, RNA, proteins, and other molecules realizes the regulation of gene expression. This network involves many components. There is forward flow of information from gene to mRNA to protein according to the dogma of molecular biology. Moreover, positive and negative feedback loops and information exchange with signaling pathways and energy metabolism ensure the appropriate regulation of the expression according to the actual state of the cell and its environment.

Modeling of gene expression is an example of a scientific field where one may obtain results with different techniques. The dynamics or the results of gene expression have been mathematically described with Boolean networks, Bayesian networks, directed graphs, ordinary and partial differential equation systems, stochastic equations, and rule-based formalisms.

Although understanding of the regulation of large groups of genes, of the emergence of complex patterns of gene expression, and of relations with inter- and intracellular communication is still a scientific challenge, many insights have already been gained from the modeling of particular processes or of the regulation of individual sets of genes.

8.3.1
One Example, Different Approaches

In the following sections we will present an overview of modeling approaches and the scientific questions that can be tackled with different techniques. For the sake of clarity, we will use only examples with a low number of components (genes and proteins), although the presented approaches can also be applied to larger systems.

The example presented in Fig. 8.2 contains four genes, a through d, which code for the proteins A through D. mRNA is not shown for sake of simplicity. The proteins A and B may form a heterodimer that activates the expression of gene c. Protein C inhibits the expression of genes b and d, which are in this way co-regulated. Protein D is necessary for the transcription of protein B.

8.3.1.1 Description with Ordinary Differential Equations
Gene expression can be mathematically described with systems of ordinary differential equations in the same way as dynamical systems in metabolism (Chapter 5), signaling (Chapter 6), and other cellular processes (Chapter 7). In general, one considers

$$\frac{dx_i}{dt} = f_i(x_1, .., x_n) \quad i = 1, ..., n. \tag{8-2}$$

The variables x_i represent the concentrations of mRNAs, proteins, or other molecules. The functions f_i comprise the rate equations that express the changes of x_i due to transcription, translation, or other individual processes. For details about how to specify the rate equations and how to analyze the resulting ODE systems, compare Sections 5.1, 5.2 and 3.2.

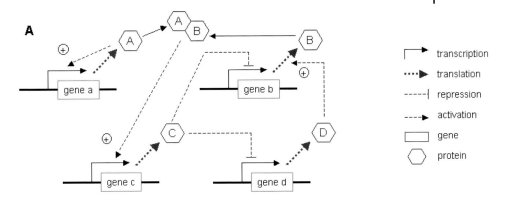

A

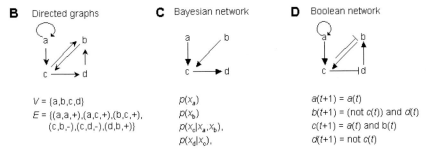

B Directed graphs

$V = \{a,b,c,d\}$
$E = \{(a,a,+),(a,c,+),(b,c,+),$
$(c,b,-),(c,d,-),(d,b,+)\}$

C Bayesian network

$p(x_a)$
$p(x_b)$
$p(x_c|x_a,x_b),$
$p(x_d|x_c),$

D Boolean network

$a(t+1) = a(t)$
$b(t+1) = (\text{not } c(t)) \text{ and } d(t)$
$c(t+1) = a(t) \text{ and } b(t)$
$d(t+1) = \text{not } c(t)$

Fig. 8.2 Gene regulatory network comprising four genes a–d. (a) Dependence of translation of genes a–d, the transcription of their mRNAs (not shown), and the influence of the respective proteins A–D. (b) Representation as directed graph. (c) Respective Bayesian network. Note that some interactions are neglected (inhibition of b by c, activation of b by d) in order to get a network without cycles. (d) The Boolean network.

Example 8-1

The dynamics of the system depicted in Fig. 8.2 can be described in several ways depending on the desired particularization. If we consider only the mRNA abundances a, b, c, and d, we get:

$$\frac{da}{dt} = f_a(a)$$

$$\frac{db}{dt} = f_b(b, c, d)$$

$$\frac{dc}{dt} = f_c(a, b, c)$$

$$\frac{dd}{dt} = f_d(c, d). \tag{8-3}$$

Specific expressions for the functions f, which consider the depicted regulatory interactions, could be the following:

$$f_a(a) = v_a - k_a \cdot a$$

$$f_b(b, c, d) = \frac{V_b \cdot d^{n_d}}{(K_b + d^{n_d})(K_{Ic} + c^{n_c})} - k_b \cdot b$$

$$f_c(a, b, c) = \frac{V_c \cdot (a \cdot b)^{n_{ab}}}{K_c + (a \cdot b)^{n_{ab}}} - k_c \cdot c$$

$$f_d(c, d) = \frac{V_d}{K_{Ic} + c^{n_c}} - k_d \cdot d. \tag{8-4}$$

Here, k_a, k_b, k_c, and k_d are the first-order rate constants of the degradation of a, b, c, and d, respectively. v_A denotes the constant rate of expression of gene a, and the Hill term $\frac{V_b \cdot d^{n_d}}{K_b + d^{n_d}}$ describes the formation of b activated by d with maximal rate V_b, dissociation constant K_b, and Hill coefficient n_d. The inhibition by c is expressed by the term $(K_{Ic} + c^{n_c})$. The formation of c is modeled with a Hill expression that points to a threshold of the formation of c depending on the concentrations of a and b. V_c and K_c are maximal rate and dissociation constant, respectively, and n_{ab} is the Hill coefficient. The production of d depends on the maximal rate V_d and on the inhibition by c. The dynamics for a certain choice of parameters is shown in Fig. 8.3.

The ODE formalism allows involving more details, e. g., the explicit consideration of the protein concentrations. Considering specifically the mRNA of gene b and protein B, we get

$$\frac{d}{dt} b = \frac{V_b}{(K_{Ic} + C^{n_c})} - k_b \cdot b$$

$$\frac{d}{dt} B = D \cdot \frac{V_B \cdot b}{K_B + b} - k_B \cdot B - k_{AB} \cdot A \cdot B. \tag{8-5}$$

This means that we can distinguish between the processes determining the velocity of translation (basic rate V_b and inhibition by protein C), transcription (dependence on mRNA concentration b and on the activator concentration D), and degradation or consumption on both levels (degradation of b and B and formation of complex AB).

The advantage of the description with ODE systems is that one can take into account detailed knowledge about gene regulatory mechanisms such as individual kinetics, individual interactions of proteins with proteins or proteins with mRNA, and so on. A profound disadvantage is the current lack of exactly this type of knowledge – the lack of kinetic constants due to measurement difficulties and uncertainties in the function of many proteins and their interactions.

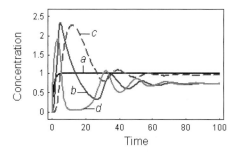

Fig. 8.3 Dynamics of the mRNA concentrations of the system presented in Example 8-1 according to Eq. (8-4). Parameters: $v_a = 1$, $k_a = 1, V_b = 1, K_b = 5, K_{lc} = 0.5, n_c = 4, k_b = 0.1$, $V_c = 1, K_c = 5, k_c = 0.1, V_d = 1, k_d = 1$. Initial conditions: $a(0) = b(0) = c(0) = d(0) = 0$.

The ODE formalism allows consideration of many specific aspects of gene regulation and cellular physiology. Time delay in gene regulation due to the involvement of many different and comparatively slow processes can be considered either by using delay differential equations or by considering all slow processes individually (see Section 8.3.2). Dilution of compounds due to cell growth is usually considered by adding a dilution term.

8.3.1.2 Representation of Gene Network as Directed and Undirected Graphs

A directed graph G is a tuple $\langle V, E \rangle$, where V denotes a set of vertices and E a set of edges (cf. Section 3.5). The vertices $i \in V$ correspond to the genes (or other components of the system) and the edges correspond to their regulatory interactions. An edge is a tuple $\langle i, j \rangle$ of vertices. It is directed if i and j can be assigned to the head and tail of the edge, respectively. The labels of edges or vertices may be expanded to contain information about the genes and their interactions. In a general way, one may express an edge as a tuple $\langle i, j, properties \rangle$. The entry *properties* can simply indicate whether j activates (+) or inhibits (–) i (Fig. 8.2b). The entry *properties* can also be a list of regulators and their influence on that specific edge, such as $\langle i, j, ((k, \text{activation}), (l, \text{inhibition as homodimeric protein})) \rangle$.

In principle, many databases that provide information about genetic regulation are organized as richly annotated directed graphs (e. g., Transfac, KEGG; see Chapter 13). Directed graphs are not suited to predict the dynamics of a network, but they may contain information that allows certain predictions about network properties:

- Tracing paths between genes yields the sequence of regulatory events, shows redundancy in the regulation, or indicates missing regulatory interactions (that are, for example, known from experiment).
- A cycle in the network may indicate feedback regulation.
- Comparison of gene regulatory networks of different organisms may reveal evolutionary relations and reveal targets for bioengineering and for pharmaceutical applications (Dandekar et al. 1999).
- The network complexity can be measured by the connectivity, i. e., the distribution and the average of the numbers of regulators per gene.

8.3.1.3 Bayesian Networks

A Bayesian network (see also Section 3.5.2.3) is based on the representation of the regulatory network as a directed acyclic graph $G = \langle V, E \rangle$. Again, the vertices $i \in V$ represent genes and edges denote regulatory interactions. Variables x_i belonging to the vertices i denote a property relevant to the regulation, e.g., the expression level of a gene or the amount of active protein. A conditional probability distribution $p(x_i | L(x_i))$ is defined for each x_i, where $L(x_i)$ are the parent variables belonging to the direct regulators of i. The directed graph G and the conditional distributions together specify a joint probability distribution $p(x)$ that determines the Bayesian network. The joint probability distribution can be decomposed into

$$p(x) = \prod_i p\left(x_i | L(x_i)\right). \tag{8-6}$$

The directed graph expresses dependencies of probabilities: the expression level of a gene represented by a child vertex depends on the expression levels of genes belonging to the parent vertices. Hence, it also implies conditional independencies $i(x_i; y | z)$, meaning that x_i is independent of the set of variables y given the set of variables z. Two graphs or Bayesian networks are equivalent if they imply the same set of independencies. In this case they can be considered as the same undirected graph, but with varying direction of edges. Equivalent graphs cannot be distinguished by observation of the variables x (Friedman et al. 2000).

Example 8-2

For the network given in Fig. 8.2c the conditional independence relations are $i(x_a; x_b)$ and $i(x_d; x_a, x_b | x_c)$. The joint probability distribution of the network is $p(x_a, x_b, x_c, x_d) = p(x_a) \cdot p(x_b) \cdot p(x_c | x_a, x_b) \cdot p(x_d | x_c)$.

Bayesian networks have been used to deduce gene regulatory networks from gene expression data. The aim is to find the network or equivalence class of networks that best explains the measured data. A problem is the determination of initial probability distributions.

8.3.1.4 Boolean Networks

In the Boolean network approach (see also Section 3.5.2.2 and Section 10.3.3 for Boolean rules), the expression level of each gene is assigned to a binary variable: a gene is considered to be either on (1) or off (0), i.e., it is transcribed or not. The states of the genes are updated simultaneously in discrete time steps. The new state can depend on the previous state of the same gene or other genes. These dependencies cause the Boolean network. The following termini are used: the N genes are the N nodes of the network, the k interactions regulating the expression of a certain gene are the k inputs of that node, and the binary expression value of each gene is its output. Since every node can be in one of two different states, a network of N genes can assume 2^N different states. An N-dimensional vector of variables can describe the state at time t. The value of each variable at time $t+1$ depends on the values of its inputs. It can be computed by means of the Boolean rules (see Section 10.3.3). For a node with k inputs, the number of possible Boolean rules is 2^{2^k}. Although a Boolean network is a very simplified representation of the gene regulatory network, it enables a first computation of gene expression dynamics.

Example 8-3

For the network presented in Fig. 8.2 d the following Boolean rules apply:

$a(t+1) = f_a(a(t)) = a(t)$ Rule 1 for $k = 1$

$b(t+1) = f_b(c(t), d(t)) = (\text{not } c(t)) \text{ and } d(t)$ Rule 2 for $k = 2$

$c(t+1) = f_c(a(t), b(t)) = a(t) \text{ and } b(t)$ Rule 2 for $k = 2$

$d(t+1) = f_d(c(t)) = (\text{not } c(t))$ Rule 0 for $k = 1$

The temporal behavior is determined by the sequence of states (a, b, c, d) given an initial state (compare also Section 10.3.3).
From Tab. 8.1 it is easy to see that this network has two different types of stationary behavior. If the initial state of a is 0, then the system evolves towards the steady state 0101, meaning that genes a and c are off, while genes b and d are on. If the initial state of a is 1, then the system evolves towards a cyclic behavior including the following sequence of states: $1000 \rightarrow 1001 \rightarrow 1101 \rightarrow 1111 \rightarrow 1010 \rightarrow 1000$.

Tab. 8.1 Successive states in the Boolean network.

$0000 \rightarrow 0001$	$1000 \rightarrow 1001$
$0001 \rightarrow 0101$	$1001 \rightarrow 1101$
$0010 \rightarrow 0000$	$1010 \rightarrow 1000$
$0011 \rightarrow 0000$	$1011 \rightarrow 1000$
$0100 \rightarrow 0001$	$1100 \rightarrow 1011$
$0101 \rightarrow 0101$	$1101 \rightarrow 1111$
$0110 \rightarrow 0000$	$1110 \rightarrow 1010$
$0111 \rightarrow 0000$	$1111 \rightarrow 1010$

The sequence of states given by the Boolean transitions represents the trajectory of the system. Since the number of states in the state space is finite, the number of possible transitions is also finite. Therefore, each trajectory will lead either to a steady state or to a state cycle. These states are called attractors. Transient states are those states that do not belong to an attractor. All states that lead to the same attractor constitute the basin of attraction.

Boolean networks have been used to explore general and global properties of large gene expression networks. Considering random networks (the number k of inputs per gene and the corresponding Boolean rules are chosen by chance), Kauffman (1991, 1993) has shown that the systems exhibit highly ordered dynamics for small k

and certain choices of rules. The expectation value of the median number of attractors is about $\sqrt{N}$, and the length of attractors is restricted to a value proportional to $\sqrt{N}$. Kauffman suggested the interpretation of the number of possible attractors as the number of possible cell types arising from the same gene type.

Example 8-4: Reverse engineering

Reverse engineering of Boolean networks aims to derive the Boolean interaction rules from time-dependent gene expression data. In Section 9.6 we discuss the REVEAL algorithm (Liang et al. 1999) that addresses this problem. We applied this algorithm to the model described in Fig. 8.2d. Expression data were generated using the ODE model of Example 8-1. The model constructed by REVEAL entails most of the rules with two steps ($k = 1$ and $k = 2$). Binarization of the time course concentration data yielded 54 different state transitions, out of which 21 corresponded to correct transitions. Pre-processing the state transitions after frequency of occurrence yielded a confidence value for each transition. If only the transitions with the highest confidence are considered, we end up with seven transitions, out of which six were correct:

State transition	t	t + 1	Confidence	Validity
1	0000	0001	1	True
2	1101	1111	0.5	True
3	1111	1110	0.625	False
4	1110	1010	0.5	True
5	1010	1000	0.3	True
6	1000	1001	1	True
7	1001	1101	0.5	True

The rules derived from this table are

$$a(t+1) = f_a(a(t)) = a(t)$$

$$b(t+1) = \tilde{f}_b(c(t), d(t)) = (c(t) \text{ and } d(t)) \text{ or } ((\text{not } c(t)) \text{ and } d(t))$$

$$c(t+1) = f_c(a(t), b(t)) = a(t) \text{ and } b(t)$$

$$d(t+1) = f_d(c(t)) = (\text{not } c(t))$$

The second rule, $\tilde{f}_b$, is partly wrong, whereas the others hold. The network was reconstructed within two steps of the algorithm.

The example illustrates several practical problems of reverse engineering Boolean networks:

1. Binarization is difficult and strongly influences the result. It is not quite clear from expression data what the level for binarization should be. Furthermore, the level should be determined gene-wise in order to distinguish low abundant from high abundant genes.

2. States are incomplete. In practice, most of the state transitions are missing after binarization. In our example, only seven out of 16 state transitions occur.
3. Availability of many time points is crucial. In order to filter correct states from false states, we have to screen many state transitions to get a stable result. In our example, we used 100 time points to reconstruct the network.
4. Time points should not be too close to each other. The selection of time points determines the granularity of the set of state transitions. It is a tradeoff between the detection of as many state transitions as possible and avoiding false-positive transitions. If two time points are too close together, the transition shows no changes since the binarization is a very rough threshold that does not detect small concentration changes. This will lead to many false-positive self-loops in the corresponding graph.

8.3.1.5 Gene Expression Modeling with Stochastic Equations

For gene expression processes, it can be argued that the assumptions of continuous and deterministic concentration changes employed in the description with ODEs are not valid. Each gene is present in only one, two, or a few copies. The number of transcription factor molecules is usually small (about a dozen or a few hundred), and even the abundance of mRNA molecules is often at the detection limit. Therefore, it is not certain whether the actors of the considered processes are actually present, and the character of the events becomes probabilistic. Furthermore, the involved processes can hardly be considered as continuous. For example, in transcription it takes a certain amount of time from the initiation until termination. The discrete and probabilistic character of processes is taken into account in stochastic modeling of gene regulation. In this approach the state variables are discrete molecule numbers x. The quantity $p(x, t)$ expresses the probability that there are x molecules of type x at time t. Consideration of the probability for all possible values of $x = 0, 1, 2, \ldots$ yields the probability distribution. Time evolution is given by the relation

$$p(x, t + \Delta t) = f\big(p(x, t)\big), \tag{8-7}$$

where the function f comprises all processes increasing or decreasing x occurring during the period Δt. Note that only simple reaction steps (formation of a molecule, complex formation, degradation) but no composed processes (like in Michaelis-Menten kinetics) can be regarded. The period Δt must be chosen so small that only one reaction step may occur in Δt. Equation (8-7) gives the probability of the system being in a certain state (having a certain number of molecules of a species) at a certain time. The simulation yields one realization of the system behavior, while another simulation run may yield another realization. Equation (8-7) is discrete in values of the state variables *and* in time. Taking the limit $\Delta t \to 0$ leads to the master equation that is discrete in state values but continuous in time:

$$\frac{\partial}{\partial t} p(x, t) = f\big(p(x, t)\big). \tag{8-8}$$

This equation gives the probability of the system being in a certain state at a certain time. This equation is usually hard to solve, both analytically and numerically. The Gillespie algorithm is a convenient alternative approach that is mathematically equivalent and employs repeated individual stochastic simulations (Gillespie 1977).

Example 8-5

The equation governing the behavior of mRNA a in the gene regulatory network shown in Fig. 8.2 is

$$p(a, t + \Delta t) = k_{a1} \cdot p(a-1, t) + k_{a2} \cdot p(a, t) - k_{a3} \cdot p(a, t) + k_{a4} \cdot p(a+1, t). \quad (8\text{-}9)$$

The term $k_{a1} \cdot p(a-1, t)$ expresses the probability that the number of molecules was $a-1$ at time t and that one molecule has been produced in Δt (due to transcription); $k_{a2} \cdot p(a, t)$ denotes the probability that the number a did not change at all during Δt; and the term $k_{a3} \cdot p(a, t)$ stands for the probability that the number of molecules was a at time t and that one molecule was degraded. Finally, $k_{a4} \cdot p(a+1, t)$ denotes the decrease of the molecule number from $a+1$ to a in period Δt due to degradation of one molecule.

The advantage of stochastic modeling is the explicit consideration of uncertainties due to the stochastic and discrete character of processes involving low molecule numbers. In some cases, experimentally observed behavior (switch between different states) could be explained with fluctuations that are inherent to stochastic modeling but not to differential equations. A problem common to stochastic equations and ODEs is the limited knowledge about appropriate kinetic parameters. Furthermore, the simulation of large systems demands computational power, especially for higher molecule numbers. Therefore, algorithms are developed to combine stochastic simulation for low-abundance species with deterministic simulations for high-concentration species.

8.3.2
Time Delay in Gene Regulation

An important issue in modeling gene expression is the fact that individual processes need a certain amount of time to be finished. For example, mature mRNA is not immediately available (not even in very small amounts) shortly after initiation of transcription. Different approaches have been employed to handle this problem, namely, the explicit consideration of numerous intermediate reaction steps or the incorporation of a discrete time delay.

Studying a system where a transcription factor, TF-A, activates its own transcription, Smolen and colleagues (1998, 1999) gave an example of a model with discrete time delay. For the mechanism (see Fig. 8.4), they consider that TF-A forms a phosphorylated homodimer that activates transcription by binding to an enhancer

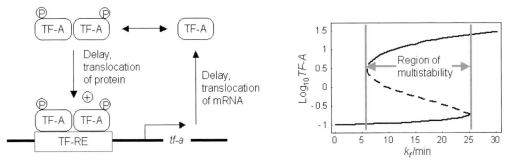

Fig. 8.4 TF-A dynamics with discrete time delay.

(TF-RE). Monomeric and dimeric TF-A are in rapid equilibrium. The transcription is described with saturation kinetics dependent on the concentration of dimeric TF-A with maximal rate k_f and dissociation constant K_D. Degradation of TF-A is modeled by applying mass action kinetics with rate constant k_d, and the basal production of TF-A has the rate R_{bas}.

Using these assumptions, the temporal behavior of TF-A is described by a single delay differential equation

$$\frac{d\,TF\text{-}A}{dt} = \left\{ \frac{k_f \cdot (TF\text{-}A)^2}{(TF\text{-}A)^2 + K_D} \right\}(t - \tau) - k_d \cdot TF\text{-}A + R_{bas}. \tag{8-10}$$

The steady-state solution of Eq. (8-10) shows a bistable behavior for a range of parameter values. There is one solution with low concentration of TF-A and a synthesis rate close to R_{bas} and one solution with high concentration, as shown in Fig. 8.4. Perturbations, exerted by transient changes in k_f, can lead to a switch between both states. The natural counterpart of these perturbations is changes in kinase or phosphatase activities caused by external signals.

An example for modeling time delay with several reaction steps is the model of GATA-3 transcriptional imprinting in Th2 lymphocytes by Höfer et al. (2002). The model describes the regulation of GATA-3 activity on the transcriptional and post-translational level. Transcription is enhanced by two transcription factors, Stat6 and NF-κB, and by autoactivation. Post-translational regulation involves phosphorylation, acetylation, and interaction with inhibitory proteins.

Starting with the synthesis of the primary transcript R_1, a series of conversions, including splicing and nuclear export of mRNA, produces the intermediary mRNA forms R_i ($i = 2, ..., m - 1$) and, eventually, the functional mRNA R_m, which is associated to ribosomes. The translated GATA-3 polypeptide chain, G_1, is also stepwise modified (intermediates G_j) to yield the active transcription factor G_n. The respective ODE system reads

$$\frac{dR_1}{dt} = v(G_n, t) - (k_1 + l_1) R_1$$

$$\frac{dR_i}{dt} = k_{i-1} R_{i-1} - (k_i + l_i) R_i \quad i = 2, ..., m$$

$$\frac{dG_1}{dt} = k_t R_m - \left(k_1' + l_1'\right) G_1$$

$$\frac{dG_j}{dt} = k_{j-1}' G_{j-1} - \left(k_j' + l_j'\right) G_j \quad j = 2, ..., m. \tag{8-11}$$

The k's and l's are first-order rate constants of conversion reactions and loss reactions, respectively. The function $v(G_n, t) = k_B + k_S \varepsilon(t) + k_G \dfrac{G_n^2}{(1 + G_n)^2}$ contains the term $\varepsilon(t) = \begin{cases} 0, t < 0 \\ e^{-t/T}, t \geq 0 \end{cases}$, expressing exponential decay of an external signal after time $t = 0$. The intention of the model was to demonstrate the coexistence of two expression states of GATA-3 depending on autoactivation. But it can also be used to demonstrate time delay. Figure 8.5 shows the effect of changing the number of intermediary mRNA species on the appearance of active GATA-3.

8.3.3
Modeling the Elongation of a Peptide Chain

The speed of translation as the second part of the gene expression process depends on the velocity of the elongation process. This, in turn, is dependent on the rate of the individual steps during growth of the nascent peptide chain and on the availability of the different types of tRNA bound amino acids.

A very general model accounting for the dynamics of protein expression in prokaryotes is given by (Drew 2001)

$$\frac{dmRNA}{dt} = -k_R \cdot R \cdot mRNA + \kappa_{N-1} \cdot mRNA_{N-1}$$

$$\frac{dmRNA_0}{dt} = -\kappa_1 \cdot a_1 \cdot mRNA_0 + k_R \cdot R \cdot mRNA$$

$$\frac{dmRNA_j}{dt} = -\kappa_{j+1} \cdot a_{j+1} \cdot mRNA_j + \kappa_R \cdot a_j \cdot mRNA_{j-1}, \quad j = 1..N \tag{8-12}$$

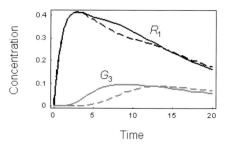

Fig. 8.5 Temporal behavior of mRNA species R_1 and active transcription factor G_n for different numbers of intermediary steps in transcription according to Eq. (8-11) Solid lines: three intermediary steps ($m = 3$), dashed lines: seven intermediary steps ($m = 7$). A higher number of intermediary steps leads to a later onset in the formation of transcription factor GATA-3. Parameters: $k_B = 0.001$, $k_G = 5$, $k_S = 0.5$, $T = 15$, $k_{i,j} = 1$ (all i, j), $l_{i,j} = 0$ (all i, j), except of $l_{m,n} = 1$, $n = 3$.

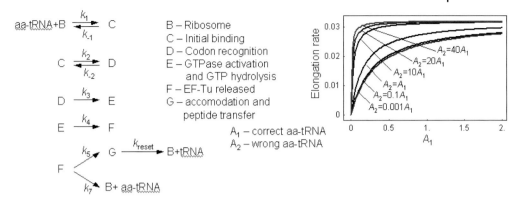

Fig. 8.6 Model for the elongation of a peptide chain according to Heyd and Drew. Left: Reaction steps involved in elongation. Right: Elongation rate for different ratios correct tRNA A_1 and wrong tRNA A_2.

where *mRNA* denotes the concentration of the messenger RNA, $mRNA_0$ is the concentration of mRNA-ribosome complex, and $mRNA_j$ is the concentration of mRNA-ribosome complex with a nascent peptide chain of length j attached. k_R is the rate constant for the mRNA-ribosome complex formation process and κ_j with $j = 1..N$ are the rate constants for the elongation steps.

The elongation step occurring at the ribosome can also be considered in more detail. In Fig. 8.6, the sequence of events during each elongation step is presented: (1) the binding of the tRNA, which is bound to an amino acid (aa) and in complex with the elongation factor Tu, to the ribosome; (2) recognition of the codon; (3) activation of a GTPase and GTP hydrolysis; (4) conformational change and release of the elongation factor Tu together with a proofreading for the correct amino acid; (5) either rejection of the wrong tRNA or accommodation of the correct tRNA; (6) formation of the peptide bond and resetting of the ribosome into a form ready for the next elongation step; (7) even the correct form of tRNA does not lead to the formation of a peptide bond in all cases. The kinetics of this mechanism depends partly on the nature of the tRNA. The process proceeds faster if the tRNA is the correct one that provides the amino acid to be next in the peptide sequence. The process shown in Fig. 8.6 can be described with a set of differential equations. Denoting the correct tRNA with A_1 and the wrong tRNA with A_2 leads to

$$\frac{dB}{dt} = -k_1 \cdot A_i \cdot B + k_{-1} \cdot C + k_r \cdot G + k_7 \cdot F \quad (i = 1, 2)$$

$$\frac{dC}{dt} = k_1 \cdot A_i \cdot B - k_{-1} \cdot C - k_2 \cdot C + k_{-2} \cdot D$$

$$\frac{dD}{dt} = k_2 \cdot C - k_{-2} \cdot D - k_3 \cdot D$$

$$\frac{dE}{dt} = k_3 \cdot D - k_4 \cdot E$$

$$\frac{dF}{dt} = k_4 \cdot E - k_5 \cdot F - k_7 \cdot F$$

$$\frac{dG}{dt} = k_5 \cdot F - k_r \cdot G . \qquad (8\text{-}13)$$

This model is suited to study the temporal behavior of peptide chain elongation. It can also be used to study the effect of tRNA supply. Figure 8.6 shows the dependence of the elongation rate from the ratio of correct and wrong tRNA. As can be expected, the lower the ratio of wrong tRNA, the higher the elongation rate is. If no correct tRNA is present, then no elongation occurs. With high concentrations of correct tRNA, the wrong tRNA is out-competed. Heyd and Drew (2003) studied a similar system with a stochastic approach, obtaining similar results.

8.4
Modeling the Regulation of Operons in *E. coli*

In this section we will discus the regulation of gene expression in prokaryotes in context of the operon concept. The operon concept suggests that genes are controlled by means of operons through a single feedback regulatory mechanism known as repression. An operon consists of a set of genes preceded by a small DNA segment (the operator), where repression takes place and mRNA-polymerase binds to initiate transcription. An operon is repressed when an active repressor molecule binds the operator, blocking it and preventing the binding of mRNA-polymerase. The term *operon* was introduced by Jacob et al. (1960) and had a deep impact on the biological sciences. Shortly after the implementation of the operon concept, Goodwin (1965) gave the first mathematical analysis of operon dynamics. Griffith performed a more complete analysis of simple repressible (negative feedback [Griffith 1968 a]) and inducible (positive feedback [Griffith 1968 b]) gene control networks. During the last four decades, models including more and more details of the dynamic behavior of operons have been presented along with various experimental data (Nicolis and Prigogine 1977; Santillan and Mackey 2001; Yildirim and Mackey 2003; Mackey et al. 2004).

8.4.1
Mechanism of the Lac Operon in *E. coli*

E. coli prefers glucose as energy source. Under all conditions it contains the enzymes necessary for the metabolism of glucose. If the cells are short of glucose they are able to utilize other sugars, e. g., lactose. However, cells grown on glucose-rich medium are unable to metabolize lactose immediately when they are exposed to a lactose-rich medium. Only after a certain lag time they can assimilate this sugar at a high rate. *E. coli* can sense the presence and concentrations of its nutrients. The con-

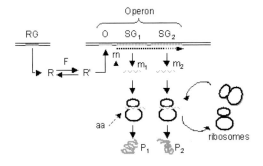

Fig. 8.7 The operon model of Jacob and Monod: the operon comprises the operator O and structural genes SG$_1$ and SG$_2$. The structural genes code for the mRNAs m1 and m2, which in turn are translated to the proteins P$_1$ and P$_2$. A regulatory gene, RG, provides the regulator R. The effector F catalyzes the transition of the regulator from the active to the inactive form (R and R'). R binds to the operator and prevents binding of the RNA polymerase. If the repressor is inactive, then transcription of the structural genes can occur.

centration of cyclic AMP (cAMP) decreases with increasing concentration of glucose, and a lack of glucose induces a rise in cAMP. Lactose is sensed in form of allolactose, an isomer formed by a reaction converting the 1–4 bond of lactose into a 1–6 bond.

The adequate response of cells on the availability of nutrients is due to regulatory processes in the cell, i. e., is due to the control of the synthesis of proteins. The chromosome of E. coli consists of only one circular DNA molecule containing genes for about 4000 proteins. The expression of many of these proteins is regulated depending on the intracellular concentration of certain metabolites. The *lac* operon is a transcription unit that ensures that the enzymes for the lactose metabolism are expressed only if lactose is in the medium and glucose is missing. The *lac* operon (see Fig. 8.7) contains a gene for a repressor protein R. In its active form, R binds to the operator, O, a specific DNA sequence of 21 base pairs. The operator sequence overlaps with the RNA polymerase–binding region, the promoter, of the following structural genes. These genes code for β-galactosidase (E), permease (M), and thiogalactoside transacetylase.

Jacob and Monod (Jacob et al. 1960) formulated a set of general assumptions for their model:

1. The primary product of structural genes is the messenger RNA. It is short-lived and brings information to the ribosomes. The second transcription takes place at the ribosomes, polypeptides are formed, and mRNA is destroyed. Ribosomes are reused.
2. mRNA synthesis is a sequential, oriented process that can start only on specific regions of the DNA, the operators. One operator may control the transcription of several subsequent structural genes, together denoted as operon or a unit of primary transcription.
3. Besides structural genes, there are also regulatory genes that code for a repressor. A repressor binds reversibly to a specific operator such that transcription initiation is blocked and protein synthesis is prevented.
4. The repressor R can specifically interact with small molecules, i. e., with the effectors F that change its activity.

$$R + F \leftrightarrow R' + F'. \tag{8-14}$$

In inducible systems only the R form associates with the operator. Interaction with the effector (here: inducer) inactivates the repressor and permits transcription. In repressible systems is the R' form is active. Transcription happens in absence of the effector (here: repressor).

The *lac* operon is controlled by four processes, which are detailed below: (1) the repression of the operator, (2) the derepression in the presence of lactose, (3) the promoter activation, and (4) the catabolite repression.

1. If the repressor binds to the operator sequence, the RNA polymerase cannot start the transcription of these neighboring genes. Since the binding of a regulator protein suppresses the transcription, this kind of genetic control is a negative regulation.
2. In the presence of lactose in the cell, a fraction of lactose is transformed by β-galactosidase into an inducer I (allolactose). The inducer binds to the repressor R and induces an allosteric conformational change; the repressor dissociates from the DNA and liberates the operator O. The transcription can start, and the genes are said to be derepressed. Consequently, the cells can produce the enzymes for the degradation of lactose only in the presence of lactose. The entry of lactose is facilitated by permease M, which is a positive feedback mechanism. The transport of lactose by permease is inhibited by glucose, an effect known as inducer exclusion.
3. The promoter of the *lac* operon is relatively weak and binds the RNA polymerase loosely. The activity of the polymerase can be enhanced by the action of a gene activator protein, which binds to a neighboring DNA sequence, enhances the contact with the polymerase, and increases the probability of a transcription start. This phenomenon is a positive regulation, since the presence of the activator leads to an increase in the transcription rate. Lack of glucose leads to an intracellular increase of cyclic AMP. The cAMP binds to the cAMP receptor protein, CRP, and causes a conformational change of this protein such that the whole complex can bind to the DNA near the *lac* promoter and enhances the transcription of the neighboring genes.
4. The remainder of the lactose and allolactose are hydrolyzed to galactose and glucose, which enter glycolysis and the Krebs cycle. If the concentration of glucose in the cell is high enough, then the concentration of cAMP decreases, it dissociates from CRP, and the transcription of the genes is significantly reduced. Glucose exerts in this way a negative feedback on its own formation.

In the case of the *lac* operon the lactose repressor protein (negative regulation) and the CRP (positive regulation) cooperate, yielding the observed gene expression pattern. This ensures that the cells can react on the nutrient supply without wasting energy on the expression of currently unnecessary genes.

8.4.2
The Model According to Griffith

This model (Griffith 1968a) considers the activation of the genes, the formation of mRNA, the synthesis of the enzymes permease and β-galactosidase, and the degradation of lactose. Permease supports the transport of lactose through the bacterial membrane. β-galactosidase isomerizes lactose to allolactose and catalyzes the cleavage of lactose to glucose and galactose.

Due to fluctuations, the genes G are rendered active even by trace amounts of allolactose (P).

$$G_{inactive} + mP \rightleftharpoons G_{active} .$$ (8-15)

The portion of active gene is given by $p = \dfrac{P^m}{k_{eq}^m + P^m}$. The concentration of mRNA (M) is determined by a basal production rate, M_0, and a degradation rate, $k_2 M$, as well as by the production from activated gene:

$$\frac{dM}{dt} = M_0 + k_1 \frac{P^m}{k_{eq}^m + P^m} - k_2 M .$$ (8-16)

The concentration changes of the enzymes permease (E_1) and β-galactosidase (E_2) are given by production from mRNA and degradation:

$$\frac{dE_1}{dt} = c_1 M - d_1 E_1$$

$$\frac{dE_2}{dt} = c_2 M - d_2 E_2 .$$ (8-17)

The uptake of lactose from the external ($_{ex}$) into the internal ($_{int}$) of the bacterial cell is mediated by permease (E_1), and the decay of lactose depends on β-galactosidase (E_2):

$$\frac{dLac_{ex}}{dt} = -\sigma_0 E_1 \frac{Lac_{ex}}{k_0 + Lac_{ex}}$$

$$\frac{dLac_{in}}{dt} = \sigma_0 E_1 \frac{Lac_{ex}}{k_0 + Lac_{ex}} - \sigma_1 E_2 \frac{Lac_{in}}{k_S + Lac_{in}} .$$ (8-18)

Allolactose is produced from lactose and converted to glucose and galactose:

$$\frac{dP}{dt} = \sigma_1 E_2 \frac{Lac_{in}}{k_S + Lac_{in}} - \sigma_2 E_2 \frac{P}{k_P + P} .$$ (8-19)

The equation system in Eqs. (8-16)–(8-19) has been simplified using the following assumptions: (1) the quasi-steady-state approximation (Section 5.2.7) applies for the concentration of mRNA; (2) the concentrations of the enzymes are equal, i.e., $E_1 = E_2$, as well as their rate constants of degradation, i.e., $d_1 = d_2$; and (3) there is no delay in the conversion of lactose into allolactose, expressed by $dLac_{in}/dt = 0$.

For the sake of simplicity, dimensionless variables are considered, i.e., $lac = Lac_{ex}/k_0$, $p = P/k_P$, $e = E/e_0$, and $\tau = t/t_0$. Taken together, this yields the final system of equations

$$\frac{de}{d\tau} = m_0 + \frac{p^m}{\kappa^m + p^m} - \varepsilon e$$

$$\frac{dp}{d\tau} = \mu e \left(\frac{lac}{1 + lac} - \lambda \frac{p}{1 + p} \right)$$

$$\frac{d\,lac}{d\tau} = -e \frac{lac}{1 + lac} , \tag{8-20}$$

with $e_0 = \dfrac{c_1 k_0 k_1}{\sigma_0 k_2}$, $t_0 = \dfrac{k_0}{\sigma_0 e_0}$, $\lambda = \dfrac{\sigma_2}{\sigma_0}$, $\mu = \dfrac{k_0}{k_p}$, $\kappa = \dfrac{k_{eq}}{k_p}$, $m_0 = \dfrac{M_0}{k_1}$, and $\varepsilon = t_0 d_1$.

The temporal behavior of this system for low and high external initial concentration of lactose is represented in Fig. 8.8.

For low initial concentration of *lac*, there is only a weak activation of gene expression, resulting in a low enzyme concentration. For high concentration of *lac*, the production of the enzyme is activated as long as its substrate – *lac* – is available.

8.4.3
The Model According to Nicolis and Prigogine

This model includes more details of the gene expression regulation than the model of Griffith. It comprises the action of the repressor, the inducer, and the subsequent enzyme synthesis. The corresponding chemical steps are represented in Fig. 8.9.

Reaction 1 describes the equilibrium between the inactive (R_i) and the active (R_a) form of the repressor. It should be noted that this is a fairly simplified scheme since

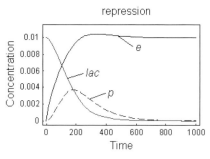
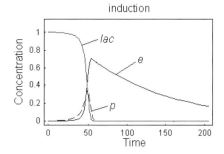

Fig. 8.8 Temporal behavior of compounds in the operon model of Griffith. Left: Adding of a low amount of lactose leads to very short activation of gene and a low amount of structural proteins. Right: A large amount of lactose stimulates gene expression strongly and provokes pronounced increase of structural proteins, which decays as soon as lactose is metabolized. Parameters: $\mu = \lambda = \kappa = 1$, $m_0 = 1$, $\varepsilon = 1$, $m = 1$. Initial conditions: $p(0) = 0$, $e(0) = 0$, $lac(0) = 0.01$ (A), $lac(0) = 1.0$ (B). Note different axes scaling.

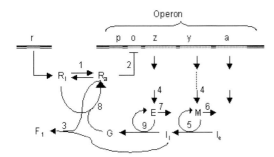

Fig. 8.9 The *lac* operon model of Nicolis and Prigogine. The structural genes z and y code for proteins E and M, and their expression is regulated by operon o. The repressor is encoded by gene r; active repressor R_a prevents transcription of the operon. In addition to the Griffith model, the uptake of inducer I catalyzed by protein M, the reaction of inducer to glucose catalyzed by protein E, and the catabolite repression exerted by glucose are considered.

the repressor is, in fact, an allosteric protein with four subunits. In reaction 2 the active form of the repressor binds reversibly to the free operator O_f and forms a complex O_c, which prevents the access of the RNA polymerase to the promoter. The presence of n_I molecules of the inducer I_i causes a conformational change of the active repressor to the form F_1, which dissociates from the operator in reaction 3. If the operator is free, the RNA polymerase can bind in reaction 4 to the promoter and transcribe the structural genes; η represents the amino acid pool. The permease facilitates the entry of inducer from the external medium (I_e) into the cell (I_i). This transport process (reaction 5) comprises many steps. An accumulation of I_i in the cell is possible if $k_5 \gg k_{-5}$. Reactions 6 and 7 represent the dilution of the enzymes in the cell. Besides stimulating the derepression of *lac* operon, the inducer (lactose/allolactose) is also metabolized to glucose under the action of enzyme E in reaction 9. Reaction 8 describes the catabolite repression. Glucose (G), which has been formed from lactose, has a stimulating effect on the formation of an active repressor. This reaction, like reaction 3, is cooperative. It should be kept in mind that all reactions represent complex phenomena, which involve several steps and could be described in much more detail.

For the system outlined, a set of ODEs describes the temporal behavior of the reactants. Assuming homogeneity in the extra- and intracellular medium, the influence of diffusion will be neglected. Inactive repressor R_i, amino acids η, and the repressor form F_1 are assumed to be in excess and are treated as constants.

$$\frac{dR_a}{dt} = k_1 R_i - k_{-1} R_a - k_2 R_a O_f + k_{-2} O_c - k_3 R_a I_i^{n_I} + k_{-3} F_1 + k_8 R_i G^{n_G} - k_{-8} R_a D$$

$$\frac{dO_f}{dt} = -k_2 R_a O_f + k_{-2} O_c$$

$$\frac{dE}{dt} = \eta k_4 O_f - k_7 E$$

$$\frac{dM}{dt} = \eta k_4 O_f - k_6 M$$

$$\frac{dI_i}{dt} = -n_I k_3 R_a I_i^{n_I} + n_I k_{-3} F_1 + k_5 I_e M - k_{-5} I_i M - k_9 I_i E$$

$$\frac{dG}{dt} = -n_G k_8 R_i G^{n_G} + n_G k_{-8} R_a D + k_9 I_i E . \tag{8-21}$$

The amount of total operator is conserved in the cell, which is why the set of equations in Eq. (8-21) has to be considered together with

$$O_f + O_c = \chi = const. \tag{8-22}$$

In the following, the steady-state characteristics and the time-dependent behavior of the model will be analyzed. Some of the quantities entering this model are known from experiments: R_a, F_1, χ, η, k_2, k_{-2}, k_3, k_{-3}, k_5, and k_{-5}. The stoichiometric coefficients in reactions 3 and 9 are chosen as $n_I = n_G = 2$. The remaining constants I_e, k_1, k_{-1}, k_4, k_6, k_7, k_8, k_{-8}, and k_9 are used as parameters in the numerical calculations.

The equation system can be simplified a bit by setting

$$k_{-8} = k_{-8} D$$
$$\mu = k_{-1} + k_{-8}$$
$$\tau = k_1 R_i + k_{-3} F_1 , \tag{8-23}$$

which leads to the following system of ODEs:

$$\frac{dR_a}{dt} = \tau - \mu R_a - k_2 R_a O_f + k_{-2}(\chi - O_f) - k_3 R_a I_i^2 + k_8 R_i G^2$$

$$\frac{dO_f}{dt} = -k_2 R_a O_f + k_{-2}(\chi - O_f)$$

$$\frac{dE}{dt} = \eta k_4 O_f - k_7 E$$

$$\frac{dM}{dt} = \eta k_4 O_f - k_6 M$$

$$\frac{dI_i}{dt} = -2 k_3 R_a I_i^2 + 2 k_{-3} F_1 + k_5 I_e M - k_{-5} I_i M - k_9 I_i E$$

$$\frac{dG}{dt} = -2 k_8 R_i G^2 + 2 k_{-8} R_a + k_9 I_i E . \tag{8-24}$$

Depending on the values of the parameters, the dynamic behavior of the equation system in Eq. (8-24) shows several interesting features, including "all-or-none" transitions and oscillations.

Neglecting the catabolite repression (reactions 8 and 9 or setting $k_8 = k_{-8} = k_9 = 0$), the steady state shows a sigmoid dependence of the concentration E on the external inducer I_e. The lower level is at 10^{-6}, the upper level at $3 \cdot 10^{-3}$, which corresponds to the experimentally determined value. This sigmoid switch can be interpreted as an all-or-none transition depending on the inducer concentration.

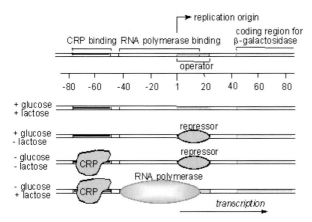

Fig. 8.10 Gene regulation via the *lac* operon. The upper scale shows
the binding sites for CRP and RNA polymerase as well as the operator and coding region on the DNA. In the lower part it is shown that
transcription can occur only if glucose is absent and lactose is present, since this is the only case when CRP and polymerase can bind
at the same time.

Note that the system has multiple steady states. Nicolis and Prigogine saw this in
accordance with the observation that in a medium with a certain inducer concentration, some cells are induced and other cells are not induced.

In the following, the dynamic behavior under catabolite repression is analyzed. Assuming a quasi-steady state for the active repressor R_a, the free operator O_f, and for
the enzymes E and M, one obtains for the time dependence of the glucose concentration G and of the internal inducer I_i:

$$\frac{dI_i}{dt} = -2\,k_3\,I_i^2\,\frac{(k_8\,R_i\,G^2 + \tau)}{(k_3\,I_i^2 + \mu)} + 2\,k_{-3}\,F_1 + \frac{(k_5\,I_e - (k_9 + k_{-5})\,I_i)\,k_{-2}\,\chi\,k_4\,\eta\,(k_3\,I_i^2 + \mu)}{k_7\,(k_2\,(k_8\,R_i\,G^2 + \tau) + k_{-2}(k_3\,I_i^2 + \mu))}$$

$$\frac{dG}{dt} = -2\,k_8\,R_i\,G^2 + \frac{2\,k_{-8}(k_8\,R_i\,G^2 + \tau)}{(k_3\,I_i^2 + \mu)} + \frac{k_9\,I_i\,k_{-2}\,\chi\,k_4\,\eta\,(k_3\,I_i^2 + \mu)}{k_7\,(k_2\,(k_8\,R_i\,G^2 + \tau) + k_{-2}\,(k_3\,I_i^2 + \mu))} \quad . \quad (8\text{-}25)$$

For this equation system, the steady state has been analyzed for fixed parameters
except for varying k_{-1}. The parameters are given in the legend of Fig. 8.11. Depending on the choice of k_{-1} the system may exhibit a stable focus only, a stable focus together with an unstable and a stable limit cycle, an unstable focus with a stable limit
cycle, or an unstable focus and a stable node.

For operons involved in amino acid synthesis (tryptophan, histidine, and phenylalanine operon), an additional control element has been demonstrated, the attenuator.
This is a DNA region between the promoter-operator region and the first structural
gene. At this place the transcription can be stopped, which permits fine-tuning of
the gene expression.

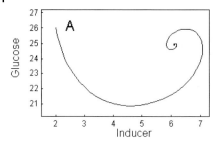
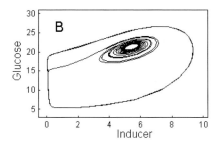

Fig. 8.11 Dynamics of the *lac* operon model according to Eq. (8-25) in phase plane representation. (a) Stable focus. (b) Unstable focus and stable limit cycle. Parameter values: $k_1 = 0.2$, $k_{-1} = 2$ (a), $k_{-1} = 0.008$ (b), $k_2 = 4 \cdot 10^5$, $k_{-2} = 0.03$, $k_3 = 0.2$, $k_{-3} = 60$, $k_4 = 1$, $k_5 = 0.6$, $k_{-5} = 0.006$, $k_6 = 3 \cdot 10^{-6}$, $k_7 = 3 \cdot 10^{-6}$, $k_8 = 0.03$, $k_{-8} = 1 \cdot 10^{-5}$, $k_9 = 5000$, $\eta = 0.005$, $\chi = 0.002002$, $r_i = 0.01$, $F_1 = 0.0001$, $I_E = 91100$.

More recent models of the regulation and the dynamics of operons (e.g., Yildirim and Mackey 2003) explicitly consider that different processes such as transcription initiation and translation do not occur immediately but need a certain amount of time to finish. To include this delay into the mathematical description, delay differential equations are employed. For example, the dynamics of mRNA is modeled as

$$\frac{dM}{dt} = \alpha_M \frac{1 + K_1 \cdot (e^{-\mu \tau_M} \cdot A(t - \tau_M))^n}{K + K_1 \cdot (e^{-\mu \tau_M} \cdot A(t - \tau_M))^n} + \Gamma_0 - (\gamma_M - \mu)M, \tag{8-26}$$

where Γ_0 is the spontaneous mRNA production rate, α_M is a rate constant, K and K_1 characterize equilibriums between repressor and allolactose or operator, γ_M is the rate constant of mRNA degradation, μ quantifies effective loss of mRNA due to dilution during growth, and τ_M is the time required to produce the mRNA. τ_M is given as 0.1 min.

References

ALBERTS, B., JOHNSON, A., LEWIS, J., RAFF, M., ROBERTS, K. and WALTER, P. Molecular biology of the cell (2002) 4th Edition Garland Science, New York.

ALLISON, L.A., MOYLE, M., SHALES, M. and INGLES, C.J. Extensive homology among the largest subunits of eukaryotic and prokaryotic RNA polymerases (1985) Cell 42, 599–610.

BERG, O.G. and VON HIPPEL, P.H. Selection of DNA binding sites by regulatory proteins. Statistical mechanical theory and application to operators and promoters (1987) J. Mol. Biol. 193, 723–750.

BURKE, T.W. and KADONGA, J.T. The downstream promoter element, DPE, is conserved from Drosophila to humans and is recognized by TAF-II60 of Drosophila (1997) Genes Dev. 11, 3020–3031.

DANDEKAR, T., SCHUSTER, S., SNEL, B., HUYNEN, M. and BORK, P. Pathway alignment: application to the comparative analysis of glycolytic enzymes (1999) Biochem. J. 343 Pt 1, 115–24.

DAVULURI, R.V., GROSSE, I. and ZHANG, M.Q. Computational identification of promoters and first exons in the human genome (2001) Nat. Genet. *29*, 412–7.

DIETERICH, C.,WANG, H., RATEITSCHAK, K., LUZ, H. and VINGRON, M. CORG: a database for COmparative Regulatory Genomics (2003) Nucleic Acids Res. *31*, 55–7.

DREW, D.A. A mathematical model for prokaryotic protein synthesis (2001) Bull. Math. Biol. *63*, 329–51.

ELKON, R., LINHART, C., SHARAN, R., SHAMIR, R. and SHILOH,Y. Genome-wide in silico identification of transcriptional regulatiors controlling the cell cycle in human cells (2003) Genome Res. *13*, 773–780.

FICKETT, J.W. and HATZIGEORGIOU, A.C. Eukaryotic promoter recognition (1997) Genome Res. *7*, 861–878.

FRIEDMAN, N., LINIAL, M., NACHMAN, I. and PE'ER, D. Using Bayesian networks to analyze expression data (2000) J. Comput. Biol. *7*, 601–20.

GARDINER-GARDEN, M. and FROMMER, M. CpG islands in vertebrate genomes (1987) J. Mol. Biol. *196*, 261–282.

GILLESPIE, D.T. Exact stochastic simulation of coupled chemical chemical reactions (1977) J. Phys. Chem. *81*, 2340–2361.

GOODWIN, B.C. Oscillatory behavior in enzymatic control processes (1965) Adv. Enzyme Regul. *3*, 425–38.

GRIFFITH, J.S. Mathematics of cellular control processes. I. Negative feedback to one gene (1968a) J. Theor. Biol. *20*, 202–8.

GRIFFITH, J.S. Mathematics of cellular control processes. II. Positive feedback to one gene (1968b) J. Theor. Biol. *20*, 209–16.

HEYD, A. and DREW, D.A. A mathematical model for elongation of a peptide chain (2003) Bull. Math. Biol. *65*, 1095–109.

HOFER,T., NATHANSEN, H., LOHNING, M., RADBRUCH, A. and HEINRICH, R. GATA-3 transcriptional imprinting in Th2 lymphocytes: a mathematical model (2002) Proc. Natl. Acad. Sci. USA *99*, 9364–8.

HUTCHINSON, G.B. The prediction of vertebrate promoter regions using differential hexamer frequency analysis (1996) CABIOS *12*, 391–398.

JACOB, F., PERRIN, D., SANCHEZ, C. and MONOD, J. [Operon: a group of genes with the expression coordinated by an operator] (1960) C. R. Hebd. Seances Acad. Sci. *250*, 1727–9.

KAUFFMAN, S.A. Antichaos and adaptation (1991) Sci. Am. *265*, 78–84.

KAUFFMAN, S.A. The origins of order: Self-organization and selection in evolution (1993) Oxford University Press, New York.

KEL, O.V., ROMASCHENKO, A.G., KEL, A.E., WINGENDER, E. and KOLCHANOV, N.A. A compilation of composite regulatory elements affecting gene transcription in vertebrates (1995) Nucleic Acids Res. *23*, 4097–103.

KEL, A., KEL-MARGOULIS, O., BABENKO,V. and WINGENDER, E. Recognition of NFATp/AP-1 composite elements within genes induced upon the activation of immune cells (1999) J Mol Biol *288*, 353–76.

KEL-MARGOULIS, O.V., KEL, A.E., REUTER, I., DEINEKO, I.V. and WINGENDER, E.TRANSCompel: a database on composite regulatory elements in eukaryotic genes (2002) Nucleic Acids Res. *30*, 332–4.

KONDRAKHIN,Y., KEL, A., KOLCHANOV, N., ROMASHENKO, A. and MILANESI, L. Eukaryotic promoter recognition by binding sites for transcription factors (1995) Comp. Appl. Biosc. *111*, 477–488.

LIANG, S., FUHRMAN, S. and SOMOGYI, R. REVEAL, a general reverse engineering algorithm for inference of genetic network architecture (1999) In: R. Altman et al., ed. Proceedings of the Pacific Symposium on Biocomputing 98. Singapore, pp 18–28.

MACKEY, M.C., SANTILLAN, M. and YILDIRIM, N. Modeling operon dynamics: the tryptophan and lactose operons as paradigms (2004) C. R. Biol. *327*, 211–24.

NICOLIS, G. and PRIGOGINE, I. Self-organization in non-equilibrium systems (1977) J. Wiley & Sons, New York.

NOVINA, C.D. and ROY, A.L. Core promoters and transcriptional control (1997) Trends Genet. *12*, 351–355.

ORPHANIDES, G. and REINBERG, D. A unified theory of gene expression (2002) Cell *108*, 439–51.

ORPHANIDES, G., LaGRANGE,T. and REINBERG, D. The general initiation factors of RNA polymerase II (1996) Genes Dev. *10*, 2657–2683.

PEDERSEN, A.G., BALDI, P., CHAUVIN,Y. and BRUNAK, S. The biology of eukaryotic promoter prediction – a review (1999) Comput. Chem. *1999* 191–207.

PILPEL,Y., SUDARSANAM, P. and CHURCH, G.M. Identifying regulatory networks by combinatorial analysis of promoter elements (2001) Nature Genet. *29*, 153–159.

PRESTRIDGE, D.S. Prediction of pol II promoter sequences using transcription factor binding sites (1995) J. Mol. Biol. *249*, 923–932.

PROUDFOOT, N.J., FURGER, A. and DYE, M.J. Integrating mRNA processing with transcription (2002) Cell *108*, 501–12.

PTASHNE, M. and GANN, A. Transcriptional activation by recruitment (1997) Nature *386*, 569–577.

REED, R. and HURT, E. A conserved mRNA export machinery coupled to pre-mRNA splicing (2002) Cell *108*, 523–31.

REESE, M.G. Application of a time-delay neural network to promoter annotation in the Drosophila melanogaster genome (2001) Comput. Chem. *26*, 51–6.

SANTILLAN, M. and MACKEY, M.C. Dynamic behavior in mathematical models of the tryptophan operon (2001) Chaos *11*, 261–268.

SCHERF, M., KLINGENHOFF, A. and WERNER, T. Highly specific localization of promoter regions in large genomic sequences by Promoter-Inspector: a novel context analysis approach (2000) J. Mol. Biol. *297*, 599–606.

SMALE, S.T. Core promoter architecture for eukaryotic protein-coding genes (1994) In: R. C. Conaway and J. W. Conaway, eds. Transcription: mechanisms and regulation. Raven Press, New York, pp 63–81.

SMOLEN, P., BAXTER, D.A. and BYRNE, J.H. Frequency selectivity, multistability, and oscillations emerge from models of genetic regulatory systems (1998) Am. J. Physiol. *274*, C531–42.

SMOLEN, P., BAXTER, D.A. and BYRNE, J.H. Effects of macromolecular transport and stochastic fluctuations on dynamics of genetic regulatory systems (1999) Am. J. Physiol. *277*, C777–90.

SOLOVYEV, V., and SALAMOV, A. (1997) The gene finder computer tools for analysis of human and model organisms genome sequences. In:

Proceedings of the 5th International Conference on Intelligent Systems for Molecular Biology, pp. 294–302.

STORMO, G.D. DNA binding sites: representation and discovery (2000) Bioinformatics *16*, 16–23.

STORMO, G.D., SCHNEIDER, T.D., GOLD, L. and EHRENFEUCHT, A. Use of the perceptron algorithm to distinguish translation initiation sites in E.coli (1982) Nucleic Acids Res. *10*, 2997–3012.

TAVAZOIE, S., HUGHES, J.D., CAMPBELL, M.J., CHO, R.J. and CHURCH, G.M. Systematic determination of genetic network architecture (1999) Nat. Genet. *22*, 281–5.

THAKURTA, D.G., PALOMAR, L., STORMO, G.D., TEDESCO, P., JOHNSON, T.E., WALKER, D.W., LITHGOW, G., KIM, S. and LINK, C.D. Identification of a novel cis-regulatory element involved in the heat shock response in C.elegans using microarray gene expression and computational methods (2002) Genome Res. *12*, 701–712.

TUPLER, R., PERINI, G. and GREEN, M.R. Expressing the human genome (2001) Nature *409*, 832–3.

UPTAIN, S.M., KANE, C.M. and CHAMBERLIN, M.J. Basic mechanisms of transcript elongation and its regulation (1997) Annu. Rev. Biochem. *66*, 117–72.

WASSERMANN, W.W., PALUMBO, M., THOMPSON, W., FICKETT, J.W. and LAWRENCE, C.E. Human-mouse genome comparisons to locate regulatory sites (2000) Nature Genet. *26*, 225–228.

WERNER, T. The state of the art of mammalian promoter recognition (2003) Briefings Bioinf. *4*, 22–30.

WOYCHIK, N.A. and HAMPSEY, M. The RNA polymerase II machinery: structure illuminates function (2002) Cell *108*, 453–463.

YILDIRIM, N. and MACKEY, M.C. Feedback regulation in the lactose operon: a mathematical modeling study and comparison with experimental data (2003) Biophys. J. *84*, 2841–51.

9
Analysis of Gene Expression Data

Introduction

The analysis of transcriptome data has become increasingly popular in the last decade due to the advent of new high-throughput technologies in genome research. In particular, DNA arrays have become the most prominent experimental technique to analyze gene expression data. An important component of systems biology is the analysis of those data and their validation in the context of other data for the identification of molecular markers and the development of wiring diagrams and organization of these markers into networks of interacting components.

9.1
Data Capture

A DNA array consists of a solid support that carries DNA sequences representing genes – the probes (cf. Chapter 4). In hybridization experiments with the target sample of labeled mRNAs and through subsequent data capture, a numerical value, the signal intensity, is assigned to each probe. It is assumed that this signal intensity is proportional to the number of molecules of the respective gene in the target sample. Changes in signal intensities are interpreted as concentration changes. It should be pointed out that the signal intensities are only crude estimators for the actual concentrations and that the interpretation as a concentration change is valid only if the intensity-concentration correspondence is approximately linear. Microarray measurements often show deviations from this assumption, such as saturation effects if, for example, the spot signals are above a limit that no longer allows the detection of concentration changes or other nonlinearities if the concentration of the gene is below the detection limit of a microarray.

9.1.1
DNA Array Platforms

DNA array platforms date back to the late 1980s when they were described for the first time as a tool to screen thousands of DNA sequences in parallel by a single hy-

Systems Biology in Practice. Concepts, Implementation and Application.
E. Klipp, R. Herwig, A. Kowald, C. Wierling, H. Lehrach
Copyright © 2005 WILEY-VCH Verlag GmbH & Co. KGaA, Weinheim
ISBN: 3-527-31078-9

bridization experiment (Poustka et al. 1986), using this, among other applications, to determine transcript levels for many genes in parallel. Since then, several array platforms have been developed and a vast number of studies have been conducted. The principle of these techniques is the same (cf. Chapter 4): large numbers of probes (typically on the order of 10,000) are immobilized on a solid surface and hybridization experiments with a complex pool of labeled RNAs are performed. After attaching to the reverse complementary sequence, the amount of bound labeled material is quantified by a scanning device and is transformed into a numerical value that reflects the abundance of the specific probe in the RNA pool. The different technologies differ in the material of the solid support, the labeling procedure, and the nature of the probes.

Historically, macroarrays were the first DNA array platform. This technique, developed in the late 1980s (Poustka et al. 1986; Lehrach et al. 1990; Lennon and Lehrach 1991), employs PCR products of cDNA clones that are immobilized on nylon filter membranes. The mRNA target material is labeled radioactively (^{33}P) by reverse transcription. cDNA macroarrays typically have a size of $8 \times 12 \text{ cm}^2$ to $22 \times 22 \text{ cm}^2$ and cover up to 80,000 different cDNAs. The bound radioactivity is detected using a phosphor imager. Multiple studies using this technique have been published (Gress et al. 1992, 1996; Granjeaud et al. 1996; Nguyen et al. 1996; Dickmeis et al. 2001; Kahlem et al. 2004).

Another platform is microarrays. Here, cDNA sequences are immobilized on glass surfaces and hybridizations are carried out with fluorescently labeled target material. Chips are small ($1.8 \times 1.8 \text{ cm}^2$) and allow the spotting of tens of thousands of different cDNA clones. cDNA microarrays are widely used in genome research (Schena et al. 1995, 1996; DeRisi et al. 1996, 1997; Spellman et al. 1998; Iyer et al. 1999; Bittner et al. 2000; Whitfield et al. 2002). A specific advantage of this technology is the fact that two RNA samples labeled with different dyes can be mixed within the same hybridization experiment (cf. Chapter 4). For example, the material of interest (tissue, time point, etc.) can be labeled with Cy3 dye and control material (tissue pool, reference time point) can be labeled with Cy5 dye (e.g., Amersham Pharmacia Biotech, Santa Clara, CA). The labeled RNAs of both reverse transcription steps can be mixed and bound to the immobilized gene probes. Afterwards, the bound fluorescence is detected by two scanning procedures, and two digital images are produced for the first and second dye labeling, respectively.

While the first two platforms are widely used in academic research, most commercially available DNA arrays are oligonucleotide chips, based on the spotting of long oligonucleotides that are synthesized separately (e.g., Agilent) or synthesized *in situ* using, e.g., a photolithographic procedure depositing approximately 10 million molecules per spot (Affymetrix). In the latter technology a set of approximately 20 different oligonucleotide probes is used to characterize a single gene. Slides are typically small ($1.28 \times 1.28 \text{ cm}^2$) and lengths of oligonucleotides vary according to the producer, e.g., 20–25 mers with Affymetrix (Lockhart et al. 1996; Wodicka et al. 1997; Lipshutz et al. 1999) or 60 mers with Agilent (Hughes et al. 2000, 2001) platforms. Target mRNA is labeled fluorescently and detection of the signals is performed with a scanning device.

Several studies have tried to compare data derived from cDNA and oligonucleotide chips and came to the conclusion that the correlation is rather poor (Kuo et al. 2002; Tan et al. 2003). This is a daunting problem that is due to the fact that although DNA arrays are widespread, there is a lack of standardization methods and standardized protocols among the different laboratories.

9.1.2
Image Analysis and Data Quality Control

Image analysis is the first bioinformatics module in the data analysis pipeline (Fig. 9.1). Here, the digital information stored after the scanning of the arrays is translated into a numerical value for each entity (cDNA, oligonucleotide) on the array. Commonly, image analysis is a two-step procedure. In the first step, a grid is found whose nodes describe the center positions of the entities, and in the second step the digital values for each entity are quantified in a particular pixel neighborhood around its center. Different commercial products for image analysis of microarrays are available, e.g., GenePix (Axon), ImaGene (BioDiscovery), Genespotter (MicroDiscovery), AIDA (Raytest), and Visual Grid (GPC Biotech). Furthermore, academic groups have developed their own software for microarray image analysis, e.g., ScanAlyze (Stanford University), FA (Max Planck Institute for Molecular Genetics), and UCSF Spot (University of California, San Francisco).

9.1.2.1   Grid Finding
Grid-finding procedures are mostly geometric operations (rotations, projections, etc.) of the pixel rows and columns. Grid finding is defined differently with different methods, but the essential steps are the same. The first step usually identifies the global borders of the originally rectangular grid. In a step-down procedure, smaller sub-grids are found, and finally the individual spot positions are identified (Fig. 9.2 a). Grid finding has to cope with many perturbations of the ideal grid of spot positions, such as irregular spaces between the blocks in which the spots are grouped and nonlinear transformations of the original rectangular array to the stored image. Due to spotting problems, sub-grids can be shifted against each other and spots can distort irregularly in each direction from the virtual ideal position.

Of course, there are many different parameters for finding grids, and thus image analysis programs show several variations. However, common basic steps of the grid-finding procedure are (1) pre-processing of the pixel values, (2) detection of the spotted area, and (3) spot finding. The purpose of the first step is to amplify the regular structure in the image through robustification of the signal-to-noise ratio, e.g., by shifting a theoretical spot mask across the image and assigning those pixels to grid-center positions that show the highest correlation between the spot mask and the actual pixel neighborhood. In the second step, a quadrilateral is fitted to mark the spotted region of the slide within the image. Several of the above programs require manual user interaction in this step. In the third step, each node of the grid is detected by mapping the quadrilateral to a unit square and detecting local maxima of the projections in the x- and y-directions of the pixel intensities (e.g., in FA).

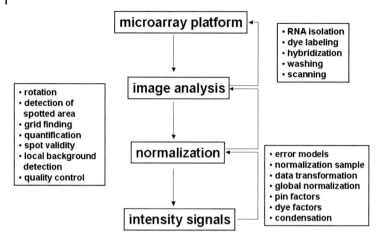

Fig. 9.1 Scheme of basic data capture modules consisting of the microarray platform, image analysis, and normalization. The entire process estimates for each gene the concentration in the target sample material by assigning a numerical value to the gene's representative on the array (probe). It is assumed that this process (gene concentration to probe signal) is approximately linear. The bioinformatics modules in this process model the factors of influences not inherent in the probe-target interactions and try to eliminate those influence factors for further analysis. Boxes describe the different tasks in detail.

9.1.2.2 Quantification of Signal Intensities

Once the center of the spot has been determined for each probe, a certain pixel area around that spot center is used to compute the signal intensity. Here, the resolution of the image is important as well as the scanner transfer function, i.e., the function that determines how the pixel was calculated from the electronic signals within the scanning device. Quantification is done in two distinct ways. Segmentation tries to distinguish foreground from background pixels (Jain et al. 2002) and to sum up all pixels for the actual signal and the background, respectively. Spot shape fitting tries to fit a particular probability distribution (cf. Section 3.1), e.g., a two-dimensional Gaussian spot shape around the spot center. Then the signal intensity is computed as a weighted sum of the pixel intensities and the fitted density. A reasonable fit can be achieved using the maximum-likelihood estimators of the probability distributional parameters (Steinfath et al. 2001). Not surprisingly, different strategies in spot quantification will lead to different results.

Image analysis methods can be grouped into three different classes: manual, semiautomated, and automated methods. Manual methods rely on the strong supervision of the user by requiring an initial guess on the spot positions. This can be realized by clicking the edges of the grid or by adjusting an ideal grid manually on the screen. Semiautomated methods require less interaction but still need prior information, e.g., the definition of the spotted area. Automated methods try to find the spot grid without user interaction. Simulation studies on systematically perturbed artificial images have shown that the data reproducibility increases with the grade of automation of the software (Wierling et al. 2002). However, for noisy images that show a very irregular structure, manual methods might be the best choice (Fig. 9.2 b).

9.1.2.3 Signal Validity

Signal validity has two tasks – the detection of spot artifacts (e. g., overshining of two spots, background artifacts, irregular spot forms, etc.) and judgment on the detection limit, i. e., whether the spot can reasonably be detected and thus if the gene is expressed in the tissue of interest or not. Spot artifacts are identified by applying morphological feature recognition criteria such as circularity, regularity of spot form, and background artifact detection methods. In the Affymetrix oligo-chip design, spot validity is often judged by comparison of the PM/MM (perfect-match/mismatch) pairs using a statistical test. Each gene is represented on the chip by a set of n oligonucleotides (~20mers) that are distributed across the gene sequence (PM_1, ..., PM_n). For each perfect match, PM_i, there is an oligonucleotide next to it, MM_i, with a central base pair mismatch in the original PM sequence (Fig. 9.2 c). This value serves as a local background for the probe. For each gene the perfect matches and the mismatches yield two series of values, PM_1, ..., PM_n and MM_1, ..., MM_n, and a Wilcoxon rank test can be calculated for the hypothesis that the two signal series are equal or not (cf. Section 3.4). If the P-value is low, this indicates that the signal series have significantly higher values than the mismatch signal series, and thus it is likely that the corresponding gene is expressed in the tissue. Conversely, if the P-value is not significant, then there is no great difference in PM and MM signals, and thus it is likely that the gene is not expressed. In order to calculate a single expression value to the probe, it has been assumed that the average of PM-MM differences is a good estimator for the expression of the corresponding gene:

$$y_i = \frac{1}{n} \sum_{j=1}^{n} (PM_{ij} - MM_{ij})$$

Here, y_i corresponds to the ith gene and PM_{ij} and MM_{ij} are the jth perfect-match and mismatch probe signals for gene i. This use of the mismatches for analysis has been criticized. It has been reported that the MM signals often interact with the transcript and thus produce high signal values (Chudin et al. 2001). This fact is known as cross-hybridization and is a severe practical problem. It has yielded to alternative computation of the local background, e. g., by evaluating local neighborhoods of low expressed probes (background zone weighting) (Draghici 2003).

In cDNA arrays, such types of significance tests for signal validity cannot be performed on the spot level because, most commonly, each cDNA is spotted only a small number of times so that there are not enough replicates for performing a test. Instead, this procedure can be carried out on the pixel level. Here, for each spot a local background area is defined, e. g., by separating foreground and background pixels by the segmentation procedure or by defining specific spot neighborhoods (corners, rings, etc.) as the local background. Alternatively, the signals can be compared on the spot level to a negative control sample. For example, several array designs incorporate empty positions on the array (i. e., no material was transferred). The scan-

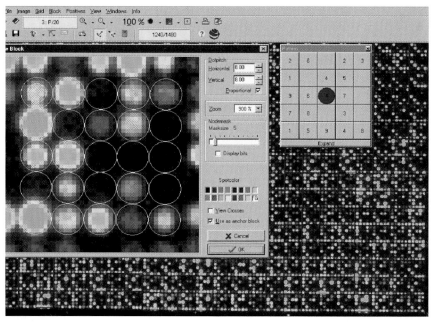

(a)

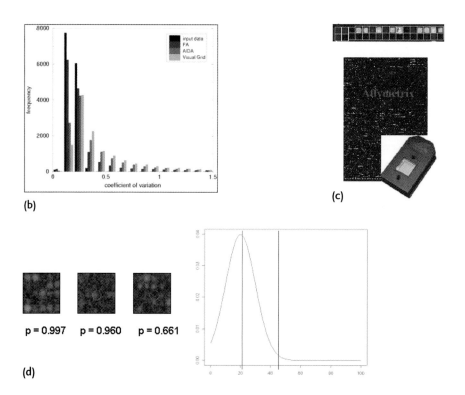

(b)

(c)

(d)

ning and image analysis will assign each such position a small intensity level that corresponds to the local background. For each regular spot, a certain probability can then be calculated that the spot is different from the negative sample (Fig. 9.2 d). This can be done by outlier criteria or by direct comparison to the negative sample (Kahlem et al. 2004).

Signal validity indices can be used as an additional qualifier for the expression ratio. Suppose we compare a gene's expression in two different conditions (A and B) and then we distinguish four cases (1 = signal is valid, 0 = signal is invalid):

A	B	Ratio	Interpretation	Possible marker
1	1	Valid	Gene expression is detectable in both conditions.	Yes
1	0	Invalid	Gene expression is detectable in condition A but not in B.	Yes
0	1	Invalid	Gene expression is detectable in condition B but not in A.	Yes
0	0	Invalid	Gene expression is not detectable in both conditions.	No

Probes belonging to the fourth case should be removed from further analysis since they represent genes that either are not expressed in both conditions or cannot be detected using the microarray procedure (possibly a very low number of molecules). This will occur fairly often in practice since only a part of the genes on the array will be actually activated in the tissue under analysis. The other three cases might reveal potential targets, but the expression ratio is meaningful only in the first case, where both conditions generate valid signals.

◄ **Fig. 9.2** Image analysis and data acquisition. (a) Visualization of individual sub-grid adjustment with Visual Grid (GPC Biotech AG). Spotting patterns show the geometry of the cDNAs organized in sub-grids. Local background can be assigned to each spot by defining specific neighborhoods. (b) Image analysis was performed with three image analysis programs classified by manual (green bars), semiautomated (red bars), and automated (blue bars) procedures on simulated data. The purpose of the simulation was to compare the reproducibility of the signals by replicated analysis of perturbed signals (CV value). The histogram shows the frequencies (y-axis) over the range of the CV (x-axis). (c) Affymetrix geometry employs successive printing of gene representatives (oligonucleotide probes). Approximately 20 different oligonucleotides that are spread across the gene sequence are immobilized (perfect matches), with each PM having a one-base-pair mismatch (MM) next to it that is an estimator for the local background. The pair PM-MM is called a probe pair. The whole set of PM-MM pairs for the same gene is called a probe set. After image analysis the feature values are condensed to a single value reflecting the gene's concentration in the target sample. (d) Spot validity can be judged by a negative control sample distributed on the array. After quantification a small, nonzero intensity is assigned to each of these empty spots, reflecting the amount of background signal on the array. Since these positions are spread uniformly over the array, the distribution of these signals reflects the distribution for signal noise for this experiment and is an indicator of whether signals are at the background level or reflect reliable expression levels. If the cumulative distribution function for the spot's signal is close to one (blue line), this indicates that the cDNA is expressed in the tissue, whereas low values reflect noise (red line). In practice cDNAs are considered "expressed" when their signal exceeds a proportion above 0.9, a threshold consistent with the limit of visual detection of the spots.

9.1.3
Pre-processing

The task of data pre-processing (or normalization) is the elimination of influence factors that are not due to the probe-target interaction, such as labeling effects (different dyes), background correction, pin effects (spotting characteristics), outlier detection (cross-hybridization of oligonucleotide-probes), etc. Many different algorithms and methods have been proposed to fulfill these tasks. Rather than listing these different methods, we will concentrate here on describing some common fundamental concepts. Data normalization has become a major research component in recent years, resulting in many different methods that claim specific merits. A review on normalization methods is given by Quackenbush (2002).

The purpose of pre-processing methods is to make signal values comparable across different experiments. This involves two steps: the selection of a set of probes (the normalization sample) and the calculation of numerical factors that are used to transform the signal values within each experiment (the normalization parameters). The selection of a normalization sample is commonly implicitly based on the assumption that the expression for the same probe in the normalization sample will not vary across experiments for biological reasons. Different methods have been proposed for that purpose, including (1) housekeeping genes, (2) selected probes whose mRNA is spiked to the labeled target sample in equal amounts, and (3) numerical methods to select a set of non-varying probes across the batch of experiments. While the first two cases involve additional biological material, the third is directly based on the probes of interest. Numerical methods try, for example, to calculate a maximal normalization sample by so-called maximal invariant sets, i.e., maximal sets of probes whose signals have the same rank order (compare Section 3.4) across all experiments under analysis, or by applying an iterative regression approach (Draghici 2003).

9.1.3.1 **Global Measures**
The weakest transformation of data is given by estimating global factors to eliminate multiplicative noise across arrays. A very robust procedure calculates the median signal of each array and determines a scaling factor that equalizes those medians. In the next step this scaling factor is applied to each individual signal to adjust the raw signals.

Alternatively, an iterative regression method can be applied to normalize the experimental batch. Assume we have two experiments; then, this algorithm reads as follows (compare Section 3.4.4):

1. Apply a simple linear regression fit of the data from the two experiments.
2. Calculate the residual.
3. Eliminate those probes that have residuals above a certain threshold.
4. Repeat steps 1–3 until the changes in residuals are below a certain threshold.

A batch of more than two experiments can be normalized with this approach by comparing each single experiment with a pre-selected experiment or with the *in silico* average across the entire batch. Global measures can be used for normalizing for overall influence factors that are approximately linear. Nonlinear and spatial effects (if present) are not addressed by these methods.

9.1.3.2 Linear Model Approaches

Linear model approaches have been used for cDNA arrays as well as for oligo chips. The most common approaches of normalization using linear models are the models of Kerr et al. (2000) and Li and Wong (2001).

A model for a spotted microarray developed by Kerr et al. (2000) defines several influence factors that contribute to artificial spot signals. The model reads

$$\log(y_{ijkl}) = b + a_i + d_j + v_k + g_l + ag_{il} + vg_{kl} + \varepsilon_{ijkl} \,. \tag{9-1}$$

This model (cf. Section 3.4.3) takes into account a global mean effect, b, the effect of the array i, and the effect of the dye j. v_k is the effect of variety k, i.e., the specific cDNA target sample, and g_l is the effect of gene l. ε_{ijkl} is the random error assumed to be Gaussian distributed with mean zero (compare Section 3.4.4). In a simpler model there are no interactions. In practice, for example, there will be interactions between gene and array effects, ag_{il}, or between gene and sample effects, vg_{kl}. This can then be solved with ANOVA methods incorporating interaction terms (Christensen 1996).

Li and Wong (2001) use a linear model approach for normalizing oligonucleotide chips (d-chip). Here, the model assumes that the intensity signal of a probe j increases linearly with the expression of the corresponding gene in the ith sample. Equations for mismatch oligonucleotides and perfect-match oligonucleotides are then given by

$$PM_{ij} = a_j + g_i v_j + g_i w_j + \varepsilon$$
$$M_{ij} = a_j + g_i v_j + \varepsilon \,. \tag{9-2}$$

Here, a_j is the background response for probe pair j, g_i is the expression of the ith gene, and v_j and w_j are the rates of increase for the mismatch and the perfect-match probe, respectively. The authors developed a software package for performing analysis and normalization of Affymetrix oligo chips that is available for academic research (www.dchip.org).

9.1.3.3 Nonlinear and Spatial Effects

Spotted cDNA microarrays commonly incorporate nonlinear and spatial effects due to different characteristics of the pins, the different dyes, and local distortions of the spots.

A very popular normalization method for eliminating the dye-effect is LOWESS (or LOESS), *locally weighted polynomial regression* (Cleveland 1979; Cleveland and Devlin 1983). LOWESS is applied to each experiment with two dyes separately. The data axis is screened with sliding windows and in each window a polynomial is fit (compare Section 3.4.4)

$$y = \beta_0 + \beta_1 x + \beta_2 x^2 + \dots \qquad (9\text{-}3)$$

Parameters of the LOWESS approach are the degree of the polynomial (usually 1 or 2) and the size of the window. The local polynomials fit to each subset of the data are almost always either linear or quadratic. Note that a zero-degree polynomial would correspond to a weighted moving average. LOWESS is based on the idea that any function can be well approximated in a small neighborhood by a low-order polynomial. High-degree polynomials would tend to overfit the data in each subset and are numerically unstable, making accurate computations difficult. At each point in the dataset, the polynomial is fit using weighted least squares, giving more weight to points near the point whose response is being estimated and less weight to points further away. This can be achieved by the standard weight function, such as

$$w(x) = \begin{cases} \left(1 - |x - x_i|^3\right)^3, & |x| < 1 . \\ 0, |x| \geq 1 \end{cases} \qquad (9\text{-}4)$$

Here x_i is the current data point. After fitting the polynomial in the current window, the window is moved and a new polynomial is fit. The value of the regression function for the point is then obtained by evaluating the local polynomial using the explanatory variable values for that data point. The LOWESS fit is complete after regression function values have been computed for each of the n data points. The final result is a smooth curve providing a model for the data. An additional user-defined smoothing parameter determines the proportion of data used in each fit. Large values of this parameter produce smooth fits. Typically smoothing parameters lie in the range 0.25 to 0.5 (Yang et al. 2002).

9.1.3.4 Other Approaches

There are many other approaches to DNA array data normalization. One class of such models employs variance stabilization (Durbin et al. 2002; Huber et al. 2002). These methods address the problem that gene expression measurements have an expression-dependent variance and try to overcome this situation by a data transformation that can stabilize the variance across the entire range of expression. The transformation step is usually connected with an error model for the data and a normalization method (such as regression). The most popular of these variance stabilizations is the log transformation. However, the log transformation is difficult for small expression values, which has led to the definition of alternative transformations.

A lot of the above-discussed normalization methods are included in the R statistical software package (www.r-project.org) and, particularly for microarray data evaluation, in the R software packages distributed by the Bioconductor project, an open-source and open-development software project to provide tools for microarray data analysis (www.bioconductor.org).

9.2
Fold-change Analysis

The analysis of fold changes is a central part of transcriptome analysis. Questions of interest are whether there are genes that can be identified as being differentially expressed when comparing two different conditions (e.g., a normal versus a disease condition).

9.2.1
Planning and Designing Experiments

Whereas early studies of fold-change analysis were based on the expression ratio of probes derived from the expression in a treatment and a control target sample, it has been a working standard to perform experimental repetitions and to base the identification of differentially expressed genes on statistical testing procedures (recall Section 3.4.3) judging the null hypothesis $H_0 : \mu_x = \mu_y$ versus the alternative $H_0 : \mu_x \neq \mu_y$ where μ_x, μ_y are the population means of the treatment and the control sample, respectively. However, the expression ratio still carries valuable information and is used as an indicator for the fold change. Strikingly, it is still very popular to present the expression ratio in published results without any estimate of the error, and studies that employ ratio error bounds are hard to find (for an exception, see (Kahlem et al. [2004]). It should be noted that the use of the fold change without estimates of the error bounds is of very limited value. For example, probes with low expression values in both conditions can have tremendous ratios, but these ratios are meaningless because they reflect only noise. A simple error calculation can be done as follows. Assume that we have replicate series for control and treatment series $x_1, ..., x_n$ and $y_1, ..., y_m$. A widely used error of the sample averages is the standard error of the mean

$$S_x = \sqrt{\frac{1}{(n-1)\,n} \sum_{i=1}^{n} (x_i - \bar{x})^2} \quad \text{and} \quad S_y = \sqrt{\frac{1}{(m-1)\,m} \sum_{i=1}^{m} (y_i - \bar{y})^2}. \tag{9-5}$$

The standard error of the ratio can then be calculated as

$$\frac{\bar{x}}{\bar{y}} \pm \frac{1}{\bar{y}^2} \sqrt{\bar{x}^2 S_y^2 + \bar{y}^2 S_x^2}. \tag{9-6}$$

An important question in the design of such an experiment is how many replicates should be used and what level of fold change can be detected. This, among other factors, is dependent on the experimental noise. Experimental observations indicate that an experimental noise of 15–25 % can be assumed in a typical microarray experiment. The experimental noise can be interpreted as the mean CV (compare Section 3.4.2) of replicated series of expression values of the probes. The dependence of the detectable fold change on the number of experimental repetitions and on the experimental error has been discussed in several papers (Herwig et al. 2001; Zien et al. 2003).

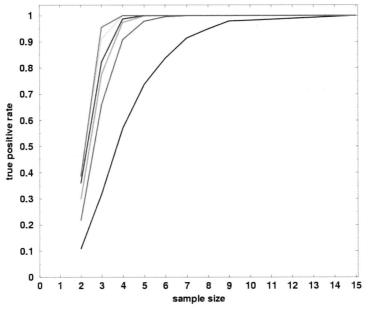

Fig. 9.3 Simulation of the dependency of fold-change detection on the sample size. Experimental error is assumed to be 20%, i.e., CV of replicated control and treatment series equals 0.2. Samples are drawn from Gaussian distributions with mean equal to 1 for the control series and mean equal to 1.5 (black), 2 (red), 2.5 (green), 3 (blue), 5 (yellow), and 10 (magenta) for the treatment samples, respectively, in order to simulate the fold changes. Sampling is repeated 1000 times and the proportion of true-positive test results (*P*<0.05) is plotted (y-axis) over the sample size (x-axis).

Figure 9.3 shows a simple simulation of this fact. Replicate series are sampled from a Gaussian distribution with mean $\mu = 1$ and $\sigma^2 = 0.04$ (i.e., $CV = 0.2$) for the control series. In order to simulate fold changes, the mean of the treatment series is changed, subsequently holding the CV constant (for example, $\mu = 2$ and $\sigma^2 = 0.16$ [i.e., CV = 0.2] if a fold change of factor two is simulated). Then, replicates are sampled from that distribution. A Welsh test is performed and it is marked whether the *P*-value is significant (<0.05) or not. The sampling is repeated 1000 times and the number of positive test results is denoted. The curves show the dependency of the true positive rate on the sample size. For example, a 1.5-fold change is detectable in only 32% of all cases when three repetitions are used. This number increases to 95% when eight replicates are used (black line). The simulation suggests that a fold-change analysis should be performed with at least four independent replicates.

The planning and design of experiments are tightly connected to normalization and pre-processing steps. For example, when a spotting device is used, pin effects should be measured by spotting different replicates on the same array with different pins. If two labeling dyes are used, then experimental replicates should incorporate dye swaps. Studies of experimental design for series of such types of microarray experiments can be found in Yang and Speed (2002).

9.2.2

Tests for Differential Expression

Let $x_1, ..., x_n$ and $y_1, ..., y_m$ be the independent samples derived from replicated measurements of the same probe across two conditions (treatment and control). Differential expression of the gene represented by the probe in the two conditions can be judged by the location tests introduced in Chapter 3 (Section 3.4). These tests can be used to assign to each single gene observation a P-value that judges the significance of the fold change, i.e., the significance of the rejection of the null hypothesis of equal population means. Here, it is notable that such a P-value is valid only if the distributional assumptions are valid. For example, if a t-test is applied to a single gene observation resulting in a P-value of 0.01, this value is true only if both series are Gaussian distributed and have equal variances. Furthermore, the test assumes that the replicates are independent of each other. Strikingly, there are many studies around that miss this fact entirely, for example, applying a Gaussian-based t-test without checking the validity of the distributional assumptions. Thus, replicates on the same array and replicates in different experiments should not be mixed since they have different characteristics and cannot be treated as independent replicates. Important issues of a test procedure are (1) whether the distributional assumptions are valid, (2) whether the replicates are independent of each other, (3) whether the number of replicates is sufficient to detect the fold change that you are interested in, and (4) whether outliers are removed from the samples. Most commonly, modifications of four different tests are applied in microarray data analysis: Student's t-test, Welch's test, Wilcoxon's rank sum test, and permutation tests. While the first two tests assume Gaussian-distributed data and that the P-values are calculated by a probability distribution, the latter two are nonparametric and the P-values are calculated with combinatorial arguments.

A permutation test (Lehmann 1979) has the following schema:

1. Choose a suitable test statistic, T, that reflects expression changes and calculate the value from the two signal series, $T = t_{obs}$.
2. Mix the two series and assign them to two groups of size n and m according to a random permutation, j, and calculate the test statistic, $T = t_j^{rand}$.
3. Repeat step 2 for all possible permutations or for a fixed number of K different permutations.
4. Calculate the P-value by counting how many random assignments result in a value of the test statistic as extreme or more extreme than the observed one divided by the total number of permutations, $p = \dfrac{\left|\left\{ j; \left| t_j^{rand} \right| \geq |t_{obs}| \right\}\right|}{K}$.

A suitable test statistic, T, could be, for example, the t-test statistic (compare Eq. (3-11) in Chapter 3) or the absolute difference of the group means $T(x_1, ..., x_n, y_1, ..., y_m) = |\bar{x} - \bar{y}|$.

Wilcoxon's rank sum test is based on the sum of ranks of the replicates from the treatment sample within the combined sample of $n+m$ values. This test (and other tests based on linear rank statistics such as the van der Waerden test) is preferable to the *t*-tests if the distributional assumptions cannot be proven to be Gaussian. Furthermore, for noisy data this test yields more robust results since it is less sensitive to outlier values (recall Example 3.26). It should further be noted that any rank-based method is invariant against strictly monotone transformations of the data such as a log transformation. For larger sample sizes, $n + m > 25$, we can approximate the *P*-value of the Wilcoxon rank test by the standard normal distribution (Eq. (3-12) in Chapter 3). However, most practical applications will be based on a rather smaller number of observations (sample sizes on the order of 3–12). Therefore, those *P*-values must be calculated exactly. This can be done using a recursive method (Herwig et al. 2001).

Let $w(z, n, m)$ be the number of possible rank orderings that result in a value of T equal to z. This number is a sum of the number of possible rank orderings of T that contain the highest rank, $m+n$, and those that do not, which can be described as

$$w(z, n, m) = w(z - (m + n), n - 1, m) + w(z, n, m - 1). \tag{9-7}$$

If *T* contains the highest rank, then we can describe this with the left part of the above sum and reduce the first sample by 1. If *T* does not contain the highest rank, then we can describe this with the right part of the sum and reduce the second sample by 1. The *P*-value of the observation, $T = t_{obs}$, can be derived by counting all combinations of rank orderings that yield a more extreme value of *T* divided by the total number of possible rank orderings, i.e.,

$$p = \frac{2 \sum\limits_{z \geq t_{obs}} w(z, n, m)}{\binom{n + m}{n}} \quad \text{if} \quad t_{obs} \geq E_{H_0}(T) \quad \text{and}$$

$$p = \frac{2 \sum\limits_{z \leq t_{obs}} w(z, n, m)}{\binom{n + m}{n}} \quad \text{if} \quad t_{obs} < E_{H_0}(T), \tag{9-8}$$

where $E_{H_0}(T)$ is the theoretical expectation of *T* under the null hypothesis that no expression difference is present (Lehmann 1979).

Example 9.1: Wilcoxon test revisited

Consider the case $n = m = 3$. There are $\binom{6}{3} = 20$ different possible rank orderings that lead to the following distribution of values of *T*:

T	6	7	8	9	10	11	12	13	14	15
Combinations	1	1	2	3	3	3	3	2	1	1

For example, if the three observations from the treatment sample have ranks 1, 3, and 5, this will lead to a value of $T = 9$. The theoretical expectation of T under the hypothesis that no expression difference is present is (compare Eq. (3-71) in Chapter 3) $E_{H_0}(T) = \dfrac{n(n+m+1)}{2} = 10.5$. Thus, the P-value of the observation according to Eq. (9-8) is $p = 2\,\dfrac{1+1+2+3}{20} = 0.7$ and the observation is not significant to reject the null hypothesis. It is clear that the distribution of T is symmetric around the expectation value. This example illustrates a disadvantage of the test: with small sample sizes, hardly any result will be significantly below the 0.05 level. This results from the combinatorial nature of the P-value computation in contrast to t-tests, where a theoretical probability distribution is assumed. However, for reasonable sample sizes the number of permutations increases rapidly. For example, there are 70, 720, and 12,870 possible combinations of rank orderings for sample sizes equal to 4, 6, and 8, respectively.

Example 9.2: Comparison of tests

In a microarray study incorporating approximately 15,000 different cDNAs and four independent hybridization experiments, we investigated the early differentiation event in human blastocysts, i.e., the formation of the trophectoderm and the inner cell mass. *HMBG1* is a specific gene of interest because it has been published as a potential "stemness" gene in human stem cell lines, i.e., a gene that is relevant for remaining pluripotency of cells. *HMBG1* is a member of the high-mobility group of transcription factor–encoding proteins that act primarily as architectural facilitators in the assembly of nucleoprotein complexes, e.g., the initiation of transcription factor target genes.

The four measurements for the trophectoderm and ICM, respectively, are

32,612, 46,741, 29,238, 32,671
and 49,966, 58,037, 94,785, 122,044.

P-values are 3.7E-02 for Student's t-test, 6.8E-02 for the Welch test, and 2.9E-02 for the Wilcoxon test. The ANOVA test results in a non-significant P-value. This example shows how a high variance (ICM sample) can mislead the Gaussian-based tests, whereas the rank-based test is fairly stable. Note that ranking separates the groups perfectly.

9.2.3
Multiple Testing

The single-gene analysis described above has a major statistical drawback. We cannot view each single test separately but have to take into account the fact that we perform thousands of tests in parallel (for each gene on the array). Thus, a global significance level of $\alpha = 0.05$, for example, performed with $n = 10{,}000$ cDNAs will imply a false-positive rate of 5%. This means that we must expect that 500 (!) individual tests are false-positive results and thus that many cDNAs are falsely identified as potential targets. Inclusion of such false positives in the further analysis steps can be extremely costly. Therefore, corrections for multiple testing are commonly applied to microarray studies that assure a global significance rate of 5%.

Let α_g be the global significance level and let α_s be the significance level at the single-gene level. It is clear that we cannot assure a global significance level α_g without adjusting the single-gene levels. For example, the probability of making the correct decision given that we reject the null hypothesis (i.e., the probability of selecting a truly differentially expressed gene) is

$$p_s = 1 - \alpha_s .$$

The probability of making the correct decision on the global level is the product of the probabilities on the individual levels:

$$p_g = (1 - \alpha_s)^n .$$

The probability of drawing the wrong conclusion in either of the n different tests is

$$P\,(wrong) = \alpha_g = 1 - (1 - \alpha_s)^n . \tag{9-9}$$

For example, if we have 100 different genes on the array and we set the gene-wise significance level to 0.05, we will have a probability of 0.994 of making a type I error. This is the so-called family-wise error rate (FWER) of the experiment, i.e., the global type I error rate. Multiple testing corrections try to adjust the single-gene level type I error rate in such a way that the global type I error rate will be below a given threshold. In practice, that means that the calculated P-values have to be corrected.

The most conservative correction is the Bonferroni correction. Here, we approximate Eq. (9-9) by the first terms of the binomial expansion, i.e.,

$$(1 - \alpha_s)^n = \sum_{i=0}^{n} \binom{n}{i}(-1)^{n-i}\alpha_s^i . \tag{9-10}$$

Thus, we rewrite

$$\alpha_g = 1 - \sum_{i=0}^{n} \binom{n}{i}(-\alpha_s)^i \approx n\,\alpha_s \Rightarrow \alpha_s = \frac{\alpha_g}{n} . \tag{9-11}$$

The Bonferroni correction of the single-gene level is the global level divided by the number of tests performed. This is far too conservative. For example, when using an array of $n = 10{,}000$ probes and an experiment FWER of 0.01, only those observations whose P-value is below 1.0e-06 would be judged as "significantly differentially expressed." Fairly few genes would meet this requirement. The result would therefore consist of many true negatives.

The Bonferroni correction is too strict in the sense that we apply the same significance level to all genes. Consider now the following stepwise procedure. For a given global significance level α_g, sort the probes in increasing order after their P-values are calculated on the single-gene basis. If $p_1 < \frac{\alpha_g}{n}$, then adjust the remaining $n-1$ P-values by comparing the next P-value $p_2 < \frac{\alpha_g}{n-1}$, etc. If m is the largest integer for which $p_m < \frac{\alpha_g}{n-m+1}$, then we call genes 1, ..., m significantly differentially expressed. This procedure is called Holm's stepwise correction, and it assures that the global significance level is valid. Although it is more flexible than the Bonferroni correction, it is still too strict for practical purposes.

A widely used method for adjusting P-values is the Westfall and Young step-down correction (Westfall and Young 1993). This procedure is essentially based on permutations of the data.

1. Perform $d = 1, ..., D$ permutations of the sample labels, and let p_i be the gene-wise P-value of the ith probe.
2. For each permutation, compute the P-value p_{id} from the dth permutation for the ith probe.
3. Adjust the P-value of probe i by $\tilde{p}_i = \frac{|\{d; min_i \ p_{id} \le p_i\}|}{D}$.

The advantage of this resampling method is that, unlike the approaches above, it takes data dependencies into account.

An alternative to controlling the FWER is the computation of the false discovery rate (FDR). The FDR is defined as the expected number of type I errors among the rejected hypotheses (Benjamini and Hochberg 1995). The procedure follows the following scheme:

1. As in the case of Holm's procedure, sort the probes in increasing order after their P-values are calculated on the single-gene basis. Select a level α_g for the FDR.
2. Let $j^* = max\{j; p_j \le j\alpha/n\}$.
3. Reject the hypotheses for $j = 1, ..., j^*$.

Recent variations of controlling the FDR with application to microarray data have been published (Tusher 2001; Storey and Tibshirani 2003).

The practical use of multiple testing is not entirely clear. Whereas on the one hand it is useful to select false-positive results from true-positive results, this will on the other hand discard a lot of potentially useful targets, and the experimentalist might lose important biological information.

9.2.4
ROC Curve Analysis

In Section 3.4, we introduced the basic types of errors of a statistical test procedure. If, in practice, a training sample is available (e.g., a set of gene probes known to be differentially expressed and a set of probes that is known to be unchanged), for each test result we can calculate the true- and false-positive rates. The performance of a specific test (normalization method, etc.) can then be displayed using a receiver operating characteristic (ROC) curve. The purpose and result of a ROC curve analysis is,

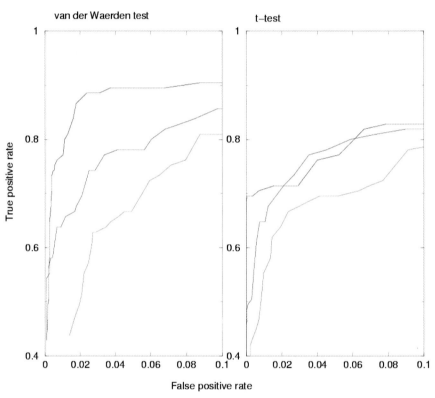

Fig. 9.4 ROC curve for visualizing performance of normalization methods and test procedures. Six independent hybridization experiments were performed with wild-type zebrafish embryos (control) and lihtium-treated embryos (treatment). The true-positive sample was identified by 105 cDNAs that were verified by an independent experimental technique (*in situ* hybridization); the false-positive sample was estimated by 2304 copies of an *Arabidopsis thaliana* cDNA whose complementary sequence was spiked to the treatment and control target samples, re-spectively. Left graph: The van der Waerden test is used for judging differential expression on three different normalization methods: global median normalization (black), variance stabilization (red), and linear regression (green). Right graph: Student's *t*-test is used for judging differential expression using the same normalization methods. ROC analysis reveals that the nonparametric test outperforms the Gaussian-based test and, furthermore, that the global normalization performs best with both test methods compared to the other methods.

for example, to evaluate several normalization and test procedures and to choose the best methods.

Figure 9.4 shows a typical example of a ROC curve analysis. Here, we map the false-positive rate (x-axis) and the true positive rate (y-axis) and compare the performance of three normalization procedures and two statistical tests on an experimental test set with known expression changes. Ideally, the ROC curve has an integral of one and is a straight line (no false positives, maximal sensitivity), and those procedures that give the highest overall integral are preferable. Alternatively, one might select a specific area of interest (for example, a false-positive rate below the experimental significance level) and choose the procedure that shows the highest performance in the selected area. Similar ROC curve analysis has been used to compare different normalization strategies (Irizarry et al. 2003).

9.2.5
Validation Methods

Typically, computationally selected targets will be verified by an independent experimental method. This method varies depending on the question of interest. For example, if one is interested in localizing gene expression, whole-mount *in situ* hybridizations are used to visualize changes in gene expression in a specific tissue (Fig. 9.5 a, b). The state-of-the art validation of array measurements is RT-PCR (compare Chapter 4). This is a very sensitive technique that allows the amplification of small quantities of a given mRNA that might be far below the detection limit of array measurements (Fig. 9.5 c).

Verification of the microarray results with RT-PCR typically yields a success rate of 80 %, meaning that 80 % of the predicted fold changes by microarrays can be verified by the independent measurements (Dickmeis et al. 2001; Kahlem et al. 2004).

9.3
Clustering Algorithms

Clustering algorithms are a general group of tools from multivariate explorative statistics. They are used to group data objects according to their pairwise similarity with respect to a set of characteristics measured on these objects. Clustering algorithms are widely used in order to identify co-regulated genes with microarray experiments. There is a simple assumption behind that strategy: the concept of "guilt by association." The rationale behind this concept is that those genes whose probes show a similar profile through a set of experimental conditions will share common regulatory rules. Thus, gene expression clusters are used to identify common functional characteristics of the genes.

Clustering algorithms are explorative statistical methods that group together genes with similar profiles and separate genes with dissimilar profiles, whereby similarity (or dissimilarity) is defined numerically by a real-valued pairwise (dis)similarity function. Considering p experiments that have been performed on n different gene probes on the array, the profile of gene i is a p-dimensional vector $x_i = (x_{i1}, ..., x_{ip})$ and a

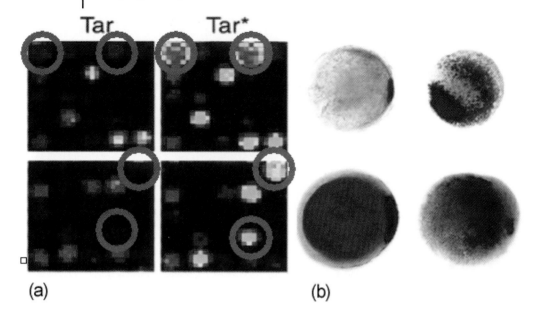

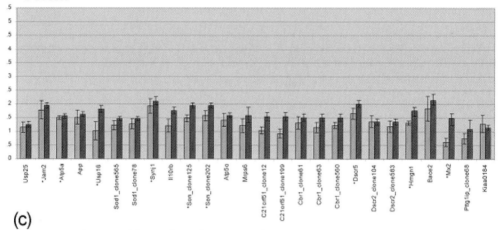

Fig. 9.5 Validation of array data. (a) Visual inspection of expression strength of two selected genes from a developmental study on zebrafish embryos (Dickmeis et al. 2001). Both cDNAs show a strong overexpression when comparing Tar*-injected target material with Tar wild-type. (b) *In situ* hybridizations verify the overexpression by localized gene expression. (c) Histogram showing the correlation between array and qPCR results for cortex brain tissue from control mice and TS65Dn mice (a mouse model for trisomy 21). Blue bars represent mean ratios of three independent array hybridizations, and red bars represent mean ratios of two independent qPCR experiments (Kahlem et al. 2004).

pairwise similarity measure can be any function $d : \Re_p \times \Re_p \rightarrow \Re$. Intuitively, one would prefer functions that reflect some kind of geometric distance such as the Euclidean distance, or more generally, the Minkowsky or l^q distances defined by

$$d_q(x_n, x_m) = \left(\sum_{i=1}^{p} |x_{ni} - x_{mi}|^q \right)^{\frac{1}{q}}.$$

(9-12)

Note that for $q = 1$ we have the Manhattan distance and for $q = 2$ we have the Euclidean distance. Another class of pairwise similarity measures is correlation measures such as Pearson's or Spearman's correlation coefficient (Section 3.4.2).

A practical problem occurs with missing values since there may be some measurements that yield an unreliable value for a given probe. However, one wants to keep the other reliable measurements of that probe and use its profile for further analysis. The fact that the profile now consists only of $p - 1$ values has to be taken into account. The treatment of missing values is a characteristic of the pairwise similarity measure. For example, one could try to estimate the distance of two vectors with missing values by the valid values. Assuming two vectors x_n, x_m, the squared Euclidean distance is given by $d_2^2(x_n, x_m) = \sum_{i=1}^{p} (x_{ni} - x_{mi})^2$ if both vectors have no missing values. If there are missing values, count the number of coordinate pairs that include at least one missing value, k, compute the distance on the remaining coordinate pairs, and estimate the distance by a multiplicative factor proportional to the amount of missing pairs, i.e., $d_2^2(x_n, x_m) = \dfrac{p}{p-k} \sum_i (x_{ni} - x_{mi})^2$. If, for example, half of the data are missing, the remaining distance is multiplied by 2. This and other adjustments for missing data can be found in the book of Jain and Dubes (1988).

Example 9.3: Data transformation

In practice, it might be useful to transform data prior to computing pairwise distances. Consider the profiles $x_1 = (100, 200, 300)$, $x_2 = (10, 20, 30)$ and $x_3 = (30, 20, 10)$. Euclidean distance will assign a higher similarity to the pair x_2, x_3 than to the pair x_1, x_2 because it takes into account only the geometric distance of the three data vectors. Correlation measures would assign a higher similarity to the pair x_1, x_2 than to the pair x_2, x_3 since they take into account whether the components of both vectors change in the same direction. For example, if these data were derived from a time series measurement, one would argue that both vectors x_1, x_2 increase with time (although on different levels of expression), whereas x_3 decreases with time. Therefore, in many applications it makes sense to transform the data vectors before calculating pairwise similarities. A straightforward geometric data transformation would be to divide each component x_j of a p-dimensional data vector $x = (x_1, ..., x_p)^T$ by its Euclidian norm, i.e., perform the transformation $\tilde{x}_j = \dfrac{x_j}{\|x\|}$. The resulting effect is that after transformation each data vector $\tilde{x}$ has a Euclidean norm of 1 and is mapped to the unit sphere.

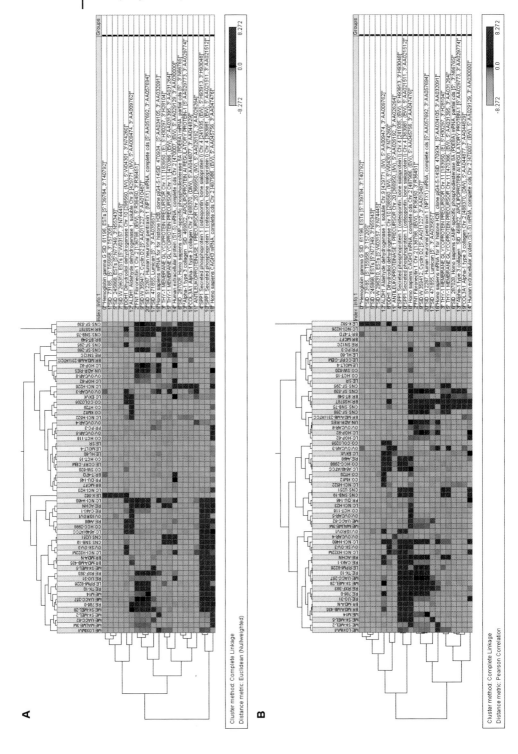

The choice of the similarity measure is important since it influences the output of the clustering algorithm. It should be adapted to the question of interest. Figure 9.6 shows two different clustering results using two different distances.

Two classes of clustering algorithms are commonly distinguished, namely, the hierarchical and partitioning methods (Jain and Dubes 1988; Mirkin 1996). In contrast to partitioning methods that try to find the "best" partition given a fixed number of clusters, hierarchical methods calculate a full series of partitions starting from n clusters, each of which contains one single data point, and ending with one cluster that contains all n data points (or vice versa); in each step of the procedure, two clusters are merged according to a pre-specified rule. In the following we describe the classical hierarchical algorithm and commonly used partitioning methods (self-organizing maps and K-means).

Not surprisingly, there are many other cluster algorithms used in the context of gene expression profiling, e. g., algorithms based on graph theoretic concepts (CAST [Ben-Dor et al. 1999], CLICK [Sharan and Shamir 2000], gene shaving [Hastie et al. 2000], and algorithms that are used in supervised classification approaches such as support vector machines [Brown et al. 1999]).

9.3.1
Hierarchical Clustering

Let $x_1, ..., x_n$ be the p-dimensional data points (expression profiles of n gene representatives across the p experiments). The process of hierarchical algorithms requires a dissimilarity measure, d, between pairs of clusters (related to a dissimilarity measure, $\tilde{d}$, between pairs of data points) and an update procedure for recalculation of the merged clusters. It then has the following scheme:

1. For $v = n$ start with the finest possible partition.
2. Calculate a new partition by joining two clusters that minimize d.
3. Update the distances of the remaining clusters and the joined cluster.
4. Stop if $v = 1$, i. e., all data points are in one cluster; otherwise, repeat steps 1–3. (9-13)

Several cluster dissimilarity measures are in use:

single linkage $\qquad d(C_k^{(v)}, C_l^{(v)}) = min_{x_i \in C_k^{(v)}, x_j \in C_l^{(v)}} \tilde{d}(x_i, x_j)$, $\qquad\qquad$ (9-14)

complete linkage $\qquad d(C_k^{(v)}, C_l^{(v)}) = max_{x_i \in C_k^{(v)}, x_j \in C_l^{(v)}} \tilde{d}(x_i, x_j)$, $\qquad\qquad$ (9-15)

◀ **Fig. 9.6** Influence of similarity measure on clustering. Two dendrograms of a subgroup of genes using the microarray expression data of Ross et al. (2000) were generated using hierarchical clustering with Euclidean distance (a) and Pearson correlation (b) as pairwise similarity measure. Although all other parameters are kept constant, results show differences in both gene and cancer cell line groupings. Clustering was performed with the J-Express Pro software package (Molmine, Bergen, Norway).

and average linkage $d(C_k^{(v)}, C_l^{(v)}) = \dfrac{1}{|C_k^{(v)}||C_l^{(v)}|} \displaystyle\sum_{x_i \in C_k^{(v)}, x_j \in C_l^{(v)}} \tilde{d}(x_i, x_j)$. (9-16)

Here, $C_i^{(v)}$, denotes the ith cluster at the vth iteration step ($i = k, l$). In the single-linkage procedure, the distance of two clusters is given by the minimal pairwise distance of the members of the one and the members of the other; in the complete-linkage procedure, the distance of two clusters is given by the maximal pairwise distance of the members of the one and the members of the other; and in the average-linkage procedure, the distance of two clusters is given by the pairwise distance of the arithmetic means of the clusters. In all three procedures, those two clusters that minimize the cluster distance over all possible pairs of clusters are merged.

Once two clusters have been merged to a new cluster, the distances to all other clusters must be recomputed. This is usually implemented using the following recursive formula:

$$d(C_m^{(v-1)}, C_k^{(v)} \cup C_l^{(v)}) = \alpha_k d(C_m^{(v)}, C_k^{(v)}) + \alpha_l d(C_m^{(v)}, C_l^{(v)}) + \beta d(C_k^{(v)}, C_l^{(v)}) +$$

$$\gamma |d(C_m^{(v)}, C_l^{(v)}) - d(C_m^{(v)}, C_k^{(v)})|. \quad (9\text{-}17)$$

where the parameters depend on the cluster distance measure. The parameters for the update procedure are summarized in the table below:

Method	a_i ($i = k, l$)	β	γ
Single linkage	0.5	0	−0.5
Complete linkage	0.5	0	0.5
Average linkage	$\dfrac{|C_i^{(v)}|}{|C_k^{(v)}| + |C_l^{(v)}|}$	0	0

The parameter β is 0 in these examples, but other update methods exist (e.g., the centroid and the Ward method) that incorporate a positive β.

Hierarchical methods have been applied in the context of clustering gene expression profiles (Eisen et al. 1998; Wen et al. 1998; Alon et al. 1999). They are memory intensive because all pairwise distances must be calculated and stored. Hierarchical methods suffer from the fact that they do not "repair" false joining of data points from previous steps; indeed, they follow a determined path for a given rule. Figure 9.7 displays this problem. In a recent study, Kahlem et al. (2004) studied the gene expression profiles of chromosome 21 mouse orthologs in nine different mouse tissues from a mouse model for trisomy 21 (TS65Dn mouse). Among genes predominantly active in the brain, they found *DSCAM*, a cell surface protein acting as an axon guidance receptor. A hierarchical clustering using average linkage as an update rule was performed, and the resulting dendrogram is displayed. This cluster is sig-

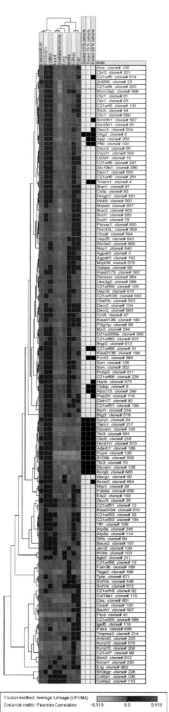

Fig. 9.7 Practical example of a dendrogram from nine different mouse tissues. For each cDNA the logarithm (base 2) of the ratio between the normalized intensity in the specific tissue and the average of intensities of this cDNA across the nine control tissues was calculated. Ratios are represented with a color gradient spanning from green (underexpressed) to red (overexpressed). Hierarchical clustering was performed with the average-linkage update rule and Pearson correlation as similarity measure (J-Express, Molmine, Bergen, Norway). Additionally, clones with the most similar expression profiles to *DSCAM* (with respect to the Pearson correlation) are displayed: 10%-closest (13 clones, left column), 15%-closest (20 clones, middle column), and 20%-closest (26 clones, right column). Note that in hierarchical clustering procedures, clones with similar expression profiles can be split to different parts of the dendrogram (e.g., *Olig2*) and *vice versa* (e.g., *Abcg1*).

nificantly non-random; however, several of the profiles numerically close to *DSCAM* are missing (black bars) due to false joining in previous steps.

Another problem with hierarchical clustering methods is that it may be difficult to decide on a representative member for each cluster, especially when using the single-linkage algorithm. In contrast, when a partitioning algorithm is used, the center of each cluster is a natural representation of the cluster's feature.

9.3.2
Self-organizing Maps (SOMs)

Clustering methods are implicitly used in the construction of self-organizing maps (SOMs), a method in the neural network framework introduced by Kohonen (1997). Kohonen's algorithm tries to find an illustrative display of n-dimensional data points in a given lattice, L, of points, usually in two or three dimensions such that the high-dimensional data structure (neighborhoods, topological ordering, clusters) is preserved and can be detected in this low-dimensional structure. The points $r_j \in L$ are called nodes (neurons). Each node r_j has a representation in the n-dimensional space of the data points; this representation is called reference vector, c_j (or weight vector of the neuron). Basically, there are two main steps repeated for each data vector for a number of iterations, on the order of tens of thousands iterations:

1. Randomly initialize the reference vector $c_j^{(1)}$ for each node.
2. For each iteration step $v + 1$ do the following:
    a. Randomly pick an input data vector x_{v+1}. Denote by $c_j^{(v)}$ the weight vector of the jth node at iteration v. The matching node is defined by
    $$c_{j_0}^{(v)} \in \arg\min\left\{d_2\left(x_{v+1}, c_j^{(v)}\right); j\right\},$$ where d_2 is defined in Eq. (9-12).
    b. Update the reference vector of the matching node and its neighbors by the update formula $c_j^{(v+1)} = c_j^{(v)} + \eta^{(v)} h_{j_0 j}^{(v)}\left(x_{v+1} - c_j^{(v)}\right)$.
3. Assign each data vector to the cluster with the most similar reference vector.

$0 < \eta^{(v)} < 1$ is called the learning function, which monotonically decreases with the number of iterations; $0 < h_{j_0 j}^{(v)} < 1$ is called the neighborhood function, which decreases monotonically with the distance of the nodes.

The main task of the neighborhood function is to provide learning, i.e., updating of the weights, not only for the best matching node but also for its neighbors. The task of the learning function is to shrink learning in time as iterations increase.

The result of Kohonen's algorithm is that units that are spatially close tend to develop similar weight vectors. Of course, the rate at which the neighborhood shrinks is critical. If the neighborhood is large and it shrinks slowly, the cluster centers will tend to stick close to the overall mean of all of the samples.

Commonly used neighborhood functions are $h_{j_0 j}^{(v)} = e^{-\frac{d_2(r_{j_0}, r_j)^2}{2\sigma^2(v)}}$ and

$$h_{j_0 j}^{(v)} = \begin{cases} 1, d_2(r_{j_0}, r_j) < \sigma(v) \\ 0, d_2(r_{j_0}, r_j) \geq \sigma(v) \end{cases},$$ where r_{j_0} is the matching node, r_j is the adapted node

whose reference vector is updated, and $\sigma^2(v)$ is the neighborhood radius that decreases with the number of iterations. Self-organizing maps have been used in the context of clustering gene expression profiles (Tamayo et al. 1999; Törönen et al. 1999).

9.3.3
K-means

K-means algorithms are a fast and large-scale-applicable clustering method. The main idea behind these techniques is the optimization of an objective function usually taken up as a function of the deviates between all patterns of the data points from their respective cluster centers. The most commonly used optimization is the minimization of the within-cluster sum of squared Euclidean distances utilizing an iterative scheme that starts with a random initialization of the cluster centers and then alters the clustering of the data to obtain a better value of the objective function.

K-means algorithms alternate between two steps until a stopping criterion is satisfied. These steps are a pairwise distance measure of the data vectors and the cluster centers related to the optimization criterion and an update procedure for the cluster centers.

In most cases, Euclidean distance has been used as pairwise similarity measure because of its computational simplicity. The cluster center at each iteration can be calculated in a straightforward manner by the arithmetic mean of the data vectors currently assigned to the cluster, which is known to minimize the within-cluster sum of squared Euclidean distances.

The original K-means algorithm reads as follows:

1. Start with an initial partition of the data points in K cluster with cluster centers $c_1^{(1)}, ..., c_K^{(1)}$ and let $W^{(1)}$ be the value of the initial objective function.
2. At the vth step of the iteration, assign each data point to the cluster with the lowest pairwise distance.
3. Recompute the cluster centers $c_1^{(v+1)}, ..., c_K^{(v+1)}$ by minimizing $W^{(v+1)}$.
4. If for all k, $\left| c_k^{(v)} - c_k^{(v+1)} \right| < \varepsilon$, stop; otherwise, return to step 2.
5. Assign each data vector to the nearest cluster center. $\hspace{2cm}$ (9-18)

If the pairwise distance is defined as the Euclidean distance, the algorithm minimizes the within-cluster sum of squares of the K clusters if the cluster centers at every iteration are recomputed as the arithmetic means of the respective data points. Other pairwise distance measures found in the literature (Jain and Dubes 1988) include l^1-metric (K-median clustering) and l_∞-metric (K-midranges clustering). A common criticism of K-means algorithms focuses on the fact that the number of centers has to be fixed from the beginning of the procedure. Furthermore, the results are highly dependent on the initialized set of centers. Alternative algorithms have been published that do not require one to determine the number of clusters in advance, and thus they overcome this criticism (MacQueen 1967; Herwig et al. 1999; Tavazoie et al. 1999).

A simple approach to refining the K-means algorithm employs two thresholding parameters (sequential K-means). The original idea dates back to MacQueen (1967). A parameter ρ controlling the distance within the clusters is used to define new cluster centers, and a parameter σ controlling the distance between cluster centers is used to merge cluster centers. The algorithm reads as follows:

1. Initialize K cluster centers $c_1^{(1)}, ..., c_K^{(1)}$.
2. Select a new data point x_i at the $v+1$th step.
3. Compute the distances to all cluster centers from the previous step $c_1^{(v)}, ..., c_K^{(v)}$. Let $w_1^{(v)}, ..., w_K^{(v)}$ be the weights of the clusters in that step, i.e., the number of data points already assigned to the cluster centers. If $\min\{d(c_j^{(v)}, x_i); j = 1, ..., K\} < \rho$, then (a) assign x_i to the cluster center with the minimal distance, $c_{j_0}^{(v)}$ and update the centroid and its weight by $w_{j_0}^{(v+1)} = w_{j_0}^{(v)} + 1$ and $c_{j_0}^{(v+1)} = \dfrac{w_{j_0}^{(v)} c_{j_0}^{(v)} + x_i}{w_{j_0}^{(v+1)}}$ and

(b) compute the distance of the updated center to each of the other cluster centers. While $\min\{d(c_j^{(v)}, c_{j_0}^{(v+1)}); j = 1, ..., K\} < \sigma$, merge the center with the minimal distance and update again according to (a). Repeat this step until for all centers $d(c_j^{(v)}, c_{j_0}^{(v+1)}) \geq \sigma$. If $\min\{d(c_j^{(v)}, x_i); j = 1, ..., K\} \geq \rho$, initialize a new cluster center by $c_{K+1}^{(v+1)} = x_i$ and $w_{K+1}^{(v+1)} = 1$.
4. Reclassify the data points.

The above algorithm iteratively allows one to join clusters that are similar to each other and to initialize new cluster centers in each step of the iteration; thus, it is a very flexible alternative. It should be pointed out that K-means algorithms are not very stable in their solutions, i.e., running the same algorithm with different parameters will lead to different results. Thus, this algorithm should not be applied only one time on the dataset but rather several times with several initializations of cluster centers. In a post-processing step the stable clusters can then be retrieved.

9.4
Validation of Gene Expression Data

9.4.1
Cluster Validation

Many clustering algorithms are currently available, each of which claims special merits and has some interpretation that makes it suitable for a class of applications. However, it is important to compare the output of cluster algorithms in order to decide which one gives best results for the current problem. For that purpose, cluster validation measures are used. In principle, two groups of measures can be separated: external and internal measures (Jain and Dubes 1988). External validation measures incorporate *a priori* knowledge on the clustering structure of the data, e.g., in simulation experiments when the true partition of the data is known or in real experiments when specific gene clusters are known. Typically, an external cluster validation measure is a numerical function that evaluates two different groupings of the same dataset. This is done by the following scheme. Assume that we have n p-dimensional data vectors $x_1, ..., x_n$; and that a clustering result generates a partition of this dataset in disjoint subsets. This is implicitly done with partitioning algorithms (cf. Section 9.3), whereas with hierarchical algorithms the dendrogram has to be cut in a suitable post-processing step. Each partition can be represented by a binary $n \times n$ partitioning matrix, $C = (c_{ij})$, with

$$c_{ij} = \begin{cases} 0, \text{ if data vectors } i \text{ and } j \text{ are not in the same cluster} \\ 1, \quad \text{ if data vectors } i \text{ and } j \text{ are in the same cluster} \end{cases}$$

Let C and T be two partitioning matrices computed from two different clustering algorithms. Then, most external indices are defined as numerical functions on the 2×2 contingency table

C/T	0	1	Total
0	n_{00}	n_{01}	$n_{0.}$
1	n_{10}	n_{11}	$n_{1.}$
Total	$n_{.0}$	$n_{.1}$	n^2

Here, n_{11} denotes the number of pairs that are in a common cluster in both partitions, and $n_{1.}$ and $n_{.1}$ are the marginals of the partition matrices T and C, respectively. Likewise, the other cell entries are defined. A commonly used index is for example the Jaccard coefficient,

$$J(T, C) = \frac{n_{11}}{n_{11} + n_{01} + n_{10}},$$

which measures the data pairs clustered together proportionally to the marginals. Other examples are Hubert's Γ statistic, the goodness-of-fit statistic, or measures based on information theory (Jain and Dubes 1988; Mirkin 1996; Herwig et al. 1999).

Internal validation measures compare the quality of the calculated clusters solely by the data itself. Indices of quality are topological concepts, e.g., compactness or isolation, that are computed by numerical functions, information theoretic concepts that quantify, e.g., high informative clusters, and variance concepts that quantify the overall variance explained by the cluster. A widely used topological measure is the Silhouette index (Rousseeuw 1984). Consider a clustering of n data vectors that results in K clusters, $S_1, ..., S_K$. For each data vector, x_i, we can calculate two topological values. Let S_l be the cluster that is assigned to x_i. Then, the compactness value describes the average distance of x_i to all other data points in the same cluster, i.e.,

$$a_i = \frac{1}{|S_l| - 1} \sum_{x_k \in S_l, k \neq i} d(x_i, x_k),$$

where d is a suitable distance measure. The isolation value describes the minimal average distance to all other clusters, i. e.,

$$b_i = \min \left\{ \frac{1}{|S_j|} \sum_{x_k \in S_j} d(x_i, x_k); j = 1, \ldots, K, j \neq l \right\}.$$

The compactness (isolation) of a cluster is defined as the average compactness (isolation) value of its cluster members. Apparently, clusters of high quality are compact and isolated. The Silhouette index combines compactness and isolation by

$$SI(x_i) = \frac{b_i - a_i}{\max \{a_i, b_i\}} . \tag{9-19}$$

The value of the Silhouette index is bound to the interval $[-1,1]$. Negative values indicate that this data vector should belong to a different cluster rather than the computed one.

Another approach in cluster validation is to calculate "figures of merit" (Yeung et al. 2001). Here, the predictive power of the clustering is quantified in a straightforward way by leaving out one of the p conditions from the gene expression matrix, clustering the gene expression profiles according to the remaining p–1 conditions, and calculating the mean deviation of the patterns of the data points and the respective cluster centroids according to the left-out condition.

Cluster validation is an important topic that has drawn insufficient attention in gene expression analysis. Currently, the situation is somewhat troublesome for the user of clustering software packages. On the one hand there is the choice between a multitude of sophisticated algorithms, algorithmic parameters, and visualization tools. However, each of these methods will generate a different result, contributing to the confusion and frustration of the user, and there are too few tools that validate and compare results and select the best one. Thus, future research will focus on the comparison and integration of different methods in order to reduce the bias of the individual methods.

9.4.2
Principal Component Analysis

Principal component analysis (PCA) is a statistical method to reduce dimensionality and to visualize high-dimensional data in two or three dimensions. Consider an nxp expression matrix X where rows correspond to genes and columns correspond to experiments. Thus, each gene is viewed as a data vector in the p-dimensional space. In general not all dimensions will contribute equally to the variation across the genes; therefore, we can hope to reduce the overall dimension to the central ones. The idea of PCA is to transform the coordinate system to a system whose axes display the maximal directions of variations of the data sample (Jolliffe 1986).

Figure 9.8a shows an example for $p = 2$. Here, essentially one dimension contains the variation of the sample and thus the dimensionality can be reduced to one after transforming the coordinate system appropriately.

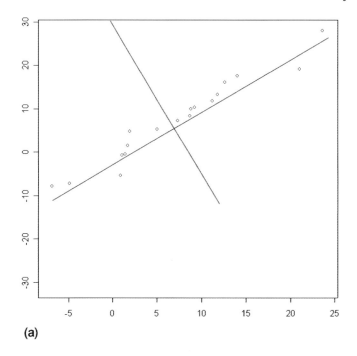

(a)

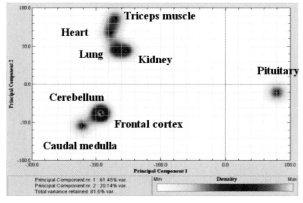

(b)

Fig. 9.8 PCA performance. (a) Two-dimensional example of dimension reduction. The scatterplot shows a high-correlated data sample that shows significant variation with respect to the coordinate axes. Applying PCA will replace the original axes by principal components centered at the mean data vector whose directions determine the data variation. In the new coordinate system, component 1 explains practically the complete data variation. (b) Practical example of visualization of eight bovine tissues. Gene expression was measured with DNA arrays and a subset of probes was preselected that separates these tissues appropriately. PCA allows the display using only two main directions and explaining 82 % of the variance. The analysis was generated with J-Express Pro (Molmine, Bergen, Norway).

Consider now more generally n p-dimensional data vectors $x_1, ..., x_n$ with component-wise mean vector $\bar{x}$. PCA is computed with a decomposition of the pxp-dimensional empirical covariance matrix of the sample (compare Eq. (3-64) in Chapter 3):

$$S = \frac{1}{n-1} \sum_{i=1}^{n} (x_i - \bar{x})(x_i - \bar{x})^T .$$ (9-20)

Since the matrix S is symmetric and positive semi-definite, there exist p nonnegative eigenvalues $\lambda_1 \geq ... \geq \lambda_p \geq 0$ (which we may assume to numerate in decreasing order, cf. Section 3.1.2). Let $r_1, ..., r_p$ be the corresponding eigenvectors, such that

$$r_j^T r_k = \begin{cases} 1, \text{ if } j = k \\ 0, \text{ if } j \neq k \end{cases}$$

$$S r_j = \lambda_j r_j .$$ (9-21)

If we denote with R the pxp-dimensional matrix whose columns are composed of the p eigenvectors from S, and if $\Lambda = \begin{pmatrix} \lambda_1 & 0 & 0 \\ 0 & \ddots & 0 \\ 0 & 0 & \lambda_p \end{pmatrix}$ denotes the pxp-dimensional diagonal matrix whose diagonal elements are the p eigenvalues, we get the decomposition

$$S = R\Lambda R^T .$$ (9-22)

Geometrically, the eigenvectors of S are the main axes of dispersion of the dataset $\{x_1, ..., x_n\}$. The dispersion is maximally high in the first principal component, second highest with the second principal component, etc. The dispersion in each principal component, i, equals $\sqrt{\lambda_i}$. Suppose now that an eigenvalue λ_k is close to zero. This means that there is not much variance along that principal component at all and that the kth coordinate of the vectors x_i is close to zero in the transformed coordinate system. Thus, this dimension does not contribute very much to the overall dispersion of the data and can be neglected without essential loss of information. Similarly, this holds for $j = k + 1, ..., p$, since we assumed the eigenvalues to be sorted in decreasing order. Thus, we have replaced the original p dimensions with $k - 1 < p$ dimensions that explain the relevant variance of the data sample.

An important question is how many principal components are needed to explain a sufficient amount of the data variance. Denote each vector by its coordinates $x_i = (x_{i1}, ..., x_{ip})^T$ and let $\bar{x}_j$ be the jth coordinate of the mean vector $\bar{x}$. A suitable measure for the total variance of the sample is the sum of the variances of the p coordinates given by

$$\sum_{j=1}^{p} \frac{1}{n-1} \sum_{i=1}^{n} (x_{ij} - \bar{x}_j)^2 = Trace(S) = \sum_{j=1}^{p} \lambda_j .$$ (9-23)

Thus, for each $k < p$ the relative amount of variance explained by the first k principal components is given by

$$\frac{\sum\limits_{j=1}^{k} \lambda_k}{\sum\limits_{j=1}^{p} \lambda_p} . \tag{9-24}$$

In gene expression analysis, PCA is widely used to reduce the gene expression matrix or its transpose matrix, the condition expression matrix, to two or three reductions. Equation (9-24) is widely used in practice to characterize the computed dimension reduction. If the amount of variance explained is high, then such a reduction makes some sense; otherwise, the dataset is too complex to visualize with PCA.

Example 9.4: PCA examples

Figure 9.8b shows a display after PCA for eight different bovine tissues that were screened with a cDNA array. Six hundred cDNAs were filtered from the total set of 20,000 cDNAs in order to represent the tissues in a suitable way. Criteria were fold changes between tissues and reliable expression differences. PCA shows that the brain regions (cortex, cerebellum) form a tissue cluster separated from the others. The selected first two principal components explain approximately 82% of the data variance, indicating that the visualization is meaningful.

9.4.3
Functional Categorization

The guilt-by-association concept so far has not been proven to hold generally. However, in many studies functional classification of specific clusters has been shown to be successful. Since more and more functional annotations are available for genes, e.g., through the Gene Ontology Consortium (2003), these annotations are used to validate clustering results. Here, we can use a simple statistical method to assign each cluster a significance P-value that judges whether it contains some untypical agglomeration of functional information (compare Section 13.1).

Consider a cluster of m genes, out of which k genes belong to a certain functional class and $m - k$ genes belong to different classes. Let n be the total number of genes under analysis and K be the total number of genes annotated for that class. Is the observed number untypical, or does it rather express a random distribution of the specific functional class? This problem can be translated into an urn model (cf. Example 3.15). If the m genes were randomly drawn from the total of n genes, then the probability of having exactly k out of K genes from the functional class would be given by the hypergeometric distribution

$$P(k) = \frac{\binom{K}{k}\binom{n-K}{m-k}}{\binom{n}{m}}.$$ (9-25)

The *P*-value for the cluster can then be calculated as the probability of having more than the observed number of hits of that functional group using Eq. (9-25), i.e., $p = \sum_{j \geq k} P(j)$.

9.5
Classification Methods

In this section we will introduce the basic principles of classification methods for microarray data. In Section 9.5.1 we discuss the basic concepts, in Section 9.5.2 we describe the basic idea of support vector machines as one of the most important classification methods, and in Section 9.5.3 we list some alternatives. Section 9.5.4 discusses cross-validation as a method to validate the performance of classification algorithms.

9.5.1
Basic Concepts

An important medical application of microarray analysis is the diagnosis of diseases and subtypes of a disease, e.g., cancer. Normal cells can evolve into malignant cancer cells by mutations of genes that control cell cycle, apoptosis, and other processes (Hanahan and Weinberg 2000). Determination of the exact cancer type and stage is essential for the correct medical treatment of the patient. The task of sample diagnostics cannot be undertaken by the methods discussed so far. This task defines a complementary set of mathematical algorithms for gene expression – classification procedures. Recall that the purpose of clustering is to partition genes (and possibly conditions) into co-expression groups by a suitable optimization method based on the expression matrix (Section 9.3). The purpose of classification is to assign a given condition (e.g., a patient's expression profile across a set of genes) to preexisting classes of conditions (e.g., groups of patient samples from known disease stages). The clustering methods discussed so far do not utilize any supporting tissue annotation (e.g., tumor vs. normal). This information is used only to assess the performance of the method. Such methods are often referred to as *unsupervised*. In contrast, *supervised* methods attempt to predict the classification of new tissues based on their gene expression profiles after training on examples that have been classified by an external "supervisor."

The practical problems underlying the classification of patients to disease subtypes are that (1) new/unknown disease classes have to be identified, (2) marker genes that separate the disease classes have to be found, and (3) patients have to be classified by assigning them to one of the classes. The first problem has already been discussed in Section 9.3. Clustering methods can be used to group the samples and identify subtypes of disease conditions. The identification of marker genes can be carried out using statistical tests (compare Section 9.2) or by the selection of groups of co-regulated genes that are significantly different across the disease subtypes. This program has been published previously in several large-scale studies. For example, Bittner et al. (2000) studied malignant melanoma and identified two subtypes of cutaneous melanoma with different characteristics in cell motility and invasiveness. They discovered a subset of melanomas identified by mathematical clustering of gene expression in a series of samples. Many genes underlying the classification of this subset are differentially regulated in invasive melanomas that form primitive tubular networks *in vitro*, a feature of some highly aggressive metastatic melanomas.

Golub et al. (1999) have described a generic approach to cancer classification based on gene expression profiling and applied this to human acute leukemias as a test case. A class-discovery procedure automatically discovered the distinction between acute myeloid leukemia (AML) and acute lymphoblastic leukemia (ALL) without previous knowledge of these classes. On the basis of 50 pre-selected "informative" genes (from a total of 6817 genes), they assigned 36 out 38 patients correctly to the two cancer classes.

Once the set of marker genes and the disease classes have been determined, a new patient sample can be classified according to the expression profile among the marker genes and the comparison with the training set. We focus here on the simplest classification task, i.e., the assignment to only two different classes (normal vs. disease). Here, the general classification problem can be stated as follows. Let T be a set of n training samples consisting of pairs (x_i, z_i), $T = \{(x_1, z_1), \ldots, (x_n, z_n)\}$, where x_i is a p-dimensional vector and $z_i \in \{-1, 1\}$ is a binary label (class label). Each vector consists of the expression profile of the patient sample across the p marker genes and each label assigns this vector to one of the classes. Given a new query, $x \in \Re_p$, the classification method (classifier) has to predict the group label, z, of x given the training set. Thus, each classification method can be interpreted as a function $F : \Re_p \times T \to \{-1, 1\}$.

9.5.2
Support Vector Machines

Support vector machines (SVMs) are the most widely used group of methods for classification (Vapnik 1995). Several studies have been published using SVMs in recent years, in particular for cancer diagnostics (e.g., Furey et al. 2000; Statnikov et al. 2004). A recent implementation can be found in Chang and Lin (2003).

The intuition of support vector machines is that of a linear decision rule. Consider two different groups of vectors in $\Re_p$. We want to find a hyperplane that separates these two samples by making the least possible error. The usual problem is that there are many such separating hyperplanes so that we have to define some kind of optimization criterion. Figure 9.9 illustrates the problem with the simple case of a two-di-

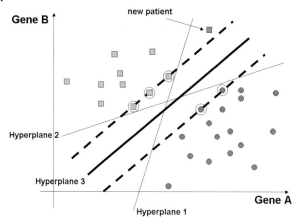

Fig. 9.9 Support vector machines. Two classes of patient data are separated in the plane that is spanned by the expression levels according to two genes. Hyperplanes 1 and 2 yield two perfect linear separations of the groups; however, when classifying a new patient, they disagree in the classification. Hyperplane 1 assigns the patient to group 1 (circles), whereas hyperplane 2 assigns the patient to group 2 (squares) due to the fact that both hyperplanes are geometrically too close to one of the subsets. The support vector machine classifier tries to maximize the margin between the two groups by defining support vectors (circled data points) and a hyperplane that maximizes the minimum distances to these support vectors (hyperplane 3).

mensional space spanned by the expression levels of the patients according to two marker genes (A and B). Hyperplanes 1 and 2 both separate the two samples perfectly. However, given a new patient profile (red square), both methods would lead to different classification results. The problem here is that both hyperplanes are geometrically too close to one of the samples and thus risk misassigning a future datum.

The idea behind SVMs is to select a hyperplane that is more likely to generalize on future data. This is achieved by finding a hyperplane that maximizes the minimum distances of the closest points and thus maximizes the width of the margin between the two classes. The hyperplane is specified by the boundary training vectors (support vectors).

Recall the classification problem from the previous section. A hyperplane can be described by $H(w, b) = \{x; wx + b = 0\}$, with a vector $w \in \Re_p$ that determines the orientation of the hyperplane and a scalar b that determines the offset of the hyperplane from the origin. Here, wx denotes the inner or dot product of the two vectors. A hyperplane in two dimensions is given by a straight line (Fig. 9.9) and in three dimensions by a plane. We say that a hyperplane supports a class if all points in that class fall on one side. Thus, we would like to find a pair w, b so that $wx_i + b \geq 1$ for the points with class label $z_i = 1$ and $wx_i + b \leq 1$ for the points with class label $z_i = -1$. To compute the hyperplane with the largest margin, we search two supporting hyperplanes for the two classes. The support planes are pushed apart until they fall into a specific number of data vectors from each class (the support vectors marked with a circle in Fig. 9.9). Thus, the solution depends only on these support vectors. The distance between the supporting hyperplanes $wx + b = 1$ and

$wx + b = -1$ is equal to $\dfrac{2}{\|w\|}$, where $\|.\|$ denotes the Euclidean norm. Thus, maximizing the margin is equivalent to the following problem:

Minimize $\|w\|^2$
subject to $z_i (x_i w + b) \geq 1$ for $i = 1, ..., n$. (9-26)

This problem can be represented by the Langrangian dual problem:

Minimize α values $\dfrac{1}{2} \sum_{i,j} z_i z_j \alpha_i \alpha_j x_i x_j - \sum_i \alpha_i$
subject to $\sum_i z_i \alpha_i = 0$ and $\alpha_i \geq 0$. (9-27)

Both problems lead to the same solution, i.e., a solution with the property that $w = \sum_i z_i \alpha_i x_i$. The classification rule found by the algorithm then reads for any new datum

$$F_T(x) = sign\left(\sum_i z_i \alpha_i x_i x + b\right).$$ (9-28)

It should be noted that this classification rule depends only on the support vectors since the dual problem assigns values $\alpha_i = 0$ to all other data vectors.

In practice, it might be that in the original dimension, p, no linear separation can be performed on the training data. SVMs then map the data to a higher-dimensional space where a linear separation is possible, using a map $\Phi : \Re_p \rightarrow \Re_m, m > p$. Since the optimization problem involves only inner products of the vectors, an optimal separating hyperplane in the projected space can be found by solving the problem for the inner products $\Phi(x_i) \Phi(x_j)$. Fortunately (due to Mercer's theorem, which is beyond the scope of this book), it is known that for certain mappings and any two vectors the inner product in the projected dimension can be calculated using a kernel function $K : \Re_p \times \Re_p \rightarrow \Re$ such that

$$K(x_i, x_j) = \Phi(x_i) \Phi(x_j).$$ (9-29)

Two kernels are widely used:

- linear kernel: $K(x_i, x_j) = x_i x_j$ and
- polynomial kernel: $K(x_i, x_j) = (\gamma x_i x_j + \varepsilon)^d$.

A further modification resulting from the fact that, in practice, misclassifications will occur is the introduction of an error parameter, C, in the optimization problem (Eq. (9-24)) and the dual problem (Eq. (9-25)). This error parameter represents the tradeoff between the training set misclassification error and the size of the margin. The optimization problem involving the kernel and this parameter reads

Minimize α values $\dfrac{1}{2}\sum_{i,j} z_i z_j \alpha_i \alpha_j K(x_i x_j) - \sum_i \alpha_i$

subject to $\sum_i z_i \alpha_i = 0$ and $C \geq \alpha_i \geq 0$, $\qquad\qquad$ (9-30)

and the classification is based on

$$F_T(x) = sign\left(\sum_i z_i \alpha_i K(x_i x) + b\right). \qquad\qquad (9\text{-}31)$$

Further reading on SVMs can be found in Cristianini and Shawe-Taylor (2000). SVMs seem to be the method of choice for classifying samples according to gene expression profiles. They have been proven to outperform other procedures, in particular in cancer diagnosis, by several independent studies (e.g., Furey et al. 2000; Statnikov et al. 2004).

9.5.3
Other Approaches

A very simple classification approach is the k-nearest neighbor classification method (Duda and Hart 1973). Consider a training dataset of n pairs, (x_i, z_i), $i = 1, ..., n$, of p-dimensional expression profiles and group labels. If a query, x, is to be classified, then it is likely that the group label of x equals the group label of the most similar training datum. Thus, the classification rule is given by

$$F_T(x) = z_{i_0} \quad \text{where} \quad i_0 \in \arg\max\{S(x, x_i); x_i \in T\}, \qquad (9\text{-}32)$$

where S is a suitable similarity function between the expression profiles, for example, the Pearson correlation coefficient. Taking into account the high error rates in microarray experiments, it is not reasonable to base the classification on just the nearest neighbor of the query in the training set but rather on the k-nearest neighbors. Thus, the result of the classification of the query is defined as the majority vote of these k data vectors. Further refinements are performed by weighting the group labels of the data vectors according to their similarity to the query. K-nearest neighbor methods yield surprisingly good results in many classification procedures and can be used as a borderline test for more sophisticated algorithms.

Classification can also be combined with clustering methods using clustering-based classification (Alon et al. 1999; Ben-Dor et al. 2000). If we consider the n training samples (tumor subtypes, cell lines etc.) as expression vectors whose coordinates are the expression levels of some genes, i.e., essentially transposing the expression matrix discussed in Section 9.3, then we can perform a clustering of the training sample in two or more clusters. This yields groups of samples that are similar to each other based on the selected set of genes. Clustering-based classification methods simply cluster the query sample together with the training samples and assign the label of the highest confidence calculated from all training labels in the same cluster to the query.

A third group of algorithms is based on *boosting* (Freund and Shapire 1996). The idea of boosting is to construct a good classifier by repeated calls of weak learning procedures. An example for a boosting algorithm is the AdaBoost algorithm by Freund and Shapire.

9.5.4
Cross-validation

Methods of classification rely heavily on the use of the specific training set. It is, however, important to get an idea of how well the learning procedure would perform when asking for new predictions for unknown data. A method of choice to answer this question is cross-validation. Cross-validation is a model evaluation method. The basic idea of cross-validation is to divide the entire dataset in a training and a test set. Some of the data is removed before training begins. Then, the data that was removed can be used to test the performance of the classification method on potentially "new" data. Several strategies involving this basic idea are detailed below.

9.5.4.1 The Holdout Method
In this method, the dataset is separated into two sets, called the training set and the test set. A classifier is computed using the training set only. Then the classifier is asked to predict the output values for the data in the test set. The errors are accumulated as before to give the mean absolute test set error, which is used to evaluate the method. It should be noted that holdout methods are very dependent on the holdout test set and thus that evaluation can have a high variance.

9.5.4.2 *k*-fold Cross-validation
Here, the dataset is divided into k subsets, and the holdout method is repeated k times. Each time, one of the k subsets is used as the test set and the other k–1 subsets are put together to form a training set. Then the average error across all k trials is computed. The advantage of this method is that it matters less how the data gets divided. Every data point gets to be in a test set exactly once and gets to be in a training set k–1 times. The variance of the resulting estimate is reduced as k is increased. A variant of this method is to randomly divide the data into a test and training set k different times. The advantage of doing this is that you can independently choose how large each test set is and how many trials you average over.

9.5.4.3 Leave-one-out Cross-validation
This method is k-fold cross-validation, with k equal to n, the number of data points in the set. That means that n separate times, the function approximator is trained on all the data except for one point and a prediction is made for that point. As before, the average error is computed and used to evaluate the model. The evaluation given by leave-one-out cross-validation error is very expensive to compute, but it has been applied as a standard cross-validation method to classification studies.

9.6
Reverse Engineering Genetic Networks

The methods discussed so far analyze the transcriptome level of genes in an explorative way. Co-expressed genes might have similar regulatory characteristics, but it is not possible to get information about the nature of the regulation. This task is tackled by the analysis of genetic networks.

Genetic networks are composed of a set of molecular entities (genes, proteins, compounds) and interactions between those entities. The purpose of these interactions is to carry out some cellular functions. The dynamics of a genetic network describe functional pathways of a cell (or tissue) such as metabolism, gene regulation, and signaling.

The task of reverse engineering of a genetic network is the reconstruction of the interactions in a qualitative way from experimental data using algorithms that weight the nature of the possible interactions with numerical values (cf. Section 3.5). In contrast to the forward modeling of networks with known interactions, which tries to determine network behavior by topological and dynamical characteristics (cf. Chapter 8), reverse engineering is data-based and tries to estimate regulatory interactions from the experimental data. Once determined, these networks can be used to make predictions on the gene expression of the corresponding genes. *In silico* predictions can be used to characterize vital functions of this network, e.g., predicting the behavior of the network when knocking down a certain gene by a suitable model system. In Section 9.6.1 we describe the simplest gene regulatory network model, the Boolean network. Here, algorithms exist that can infer the Boolean rules from the state transitions, which is exemplified with the REVEAL algorithm (Liang et al. 1999). In Section 9.6.2 we review alternative approaches, and in Section 9.6.3 we report on recent findings that support the occurrence of specific modules in gene regulation – the identification of common network motifs.

9.6.1
Reconstructing Boolean Networks

Consider a set of experimental conditions. An interesting question is whether we can reconstruct the qualitative interactions of the corresponding genes. Obviously, the general answer is no, because the set of experimental conditions might be too general. However, there are two setups where we might succeed: time-dependent measurements and knockout experiments. In time-dependent measurements, the conditions are dependent on each other in the sense that (theoretically) a strong expression of a transcription factor at a certain time point will lead to activation (or repression) of the gene expression of its targets at the next time point. Similarly, knocking out the transcription factor should point to expression changes of its targets.

The simplest models of gene regulatory networks are Boolean models (see Section 3.5 and Section 8.2). Here, genes have only discrete states and the regulatory interactions are described by Boolean functions (Kauffman 1993). Quite a number of reverse engineering algorithms for Boolean networks have been proposed (Akutsu et al. 1999, 2000; Liang et al. 1999). Recall that in a Boolean network, genes are represented as nodes, some of which are connected by edges with weights equal to 1 or −1 depending on whether the nature of regulation is activation or repression, respectively.

Reverse engineering methods are based on the following principle idea. Consider a pair of consecutive time-dependent conditions (time t and $t + 1$) on n gene probes. Binarize the expression values and define a set of rules that allows the computation of binarized expression levels at time $t + 1$ from those at time t. These rules represent the expression changes occurring from the consecutive time points. A second pair of consecutive time points will generate a second set of rules that may overlap with those rules reconstructed from the first pair. This procedure iterates over all pairs of consecutive time points, and the resulting set of rules are those that are consistent to explain the whole dataset.

One of the first algorithms to reconstruct a Boolean network was REVEAL (Liang et al. 1999). The basic idea of REVEAL is to use mutual information measurement from the state transition tables to extract the regulatory Boolean rules (for definitions of the concepts of entropy and mutual information, see Section 11.3). Recall the state transition table (Tab. 8.1) for the four-gene network described in Fig. 8.2. Denote by a_t, b_t, c_t, d_t the state vector of the genes across the 16 possible system states at time t. Figure 9.10 describes the individual steps of the algorithm. A critical parameter of the algorithm is the connectivity, k, i.e., the number of inputs for each gene.

input abcd	output abcd
0000	0001
0001	0101
0010	0000
0011	0000
0100	0001
0101	0101
0110	0000
0111	0000
1000	1001
1001	1101
1010	1000
1011	1000
1100	1011
1101	1111
1110	1010
1111	1010

gene state vectors

Step 1 ($k=1$):

a_{t+1} = (0000000011111111)
=> $H(a_{t+1}; a_t)=H(a_{t+1})$
a_t = (0000000011111111)

Rule table for a

input	output
0	0
1	1

d_{t+1} = (1100110011001100)
=> $H(d_{t+1}; c_t)=H(d_{t+1})$
c_t = (0011001100110011)

Rule table for d

input	output
0	1
1	0

Step 2 ($k=2$):

b_{t+1} = (0100010001000100)
=> $H(b_{t+1}; c_t,d_t)=H(b_{t+1})$
c_t = (0011001100110011)
d_t = (0101010101010101)

Rule table for b

input	output
00	0
10	0
01	1
11	0

c_{t+1} = (0000000000001111)
=> $H(c_{t+1}; a_t,b_t)=H(c_{t+1})$
a_t = (0000000011111111)
b_t = (0000111100001111)

Rule table for c (AND rule)

input	output
00	0
10	0
01	0
11	1

Fig. 9.10 Analysis of a Boolean gene regulatory network with the REVEAL algorithm.

The different steps of the algorithm iterate between the identification of perfect input-output state pairs and the determination of the Boolean rule. Note that for a perfect input-output state pair, the relation

$$H(x;y) = H(x) \tag{9-33}$$

holds for binary vectors x and y.

1. Identification of perfect input-output state pairs of connectivity $k=1$: Compute the mutual information of all input-output state vector pairs. The calculation of the mutual information values reveals that $H(a_{t+1};a_t) = H(a_{t+1})$, i.e., a_t uniquely determines a_{t+1}. Likewise, $H(d_{t+1};c_t) = H(d_{t+1})$, i.e., c_t uniquely determines d_{t+1}. For all other genes there is no perfect match.
2. Determination of the rules for the identified pairs at $k = 1$: We retrieve the rules $a(t + 1) = a(t)$ and $d(t + 1) = \text{not } c(t)$ by the respective rule tables.
3. Identification of perfect input-output state pairs of connectivity $k = 2$: If not all rules can be retrieved by $k = 1$, we consider $k = 2$ by comparing the output state vectors of the remaining genes with all possible pairs of input state vectors. The calculation gives $H(b_{t+1};c_t,d_t) = H(b_{t+1})$, i.e., the pair c_t, d_t determines b_{t+1}. Likewise, $H(c_{t+1};a_t,b_t) = H(c_{t+1})$, i.e., the pair a_t, b_t determines c_{t+1}.
4. Determination of the rules for the identified pairs at $k = 2$: We retrieve the rules $b(t + 1) = (\text{not } c(t))$ and $d(t)$ and likewise $c(t + 1) = a(t)$ and $b(t)$.
5. Identification of perfect input-output state pairs of connectivity $k = p$.
6. Determination of the rules for the identified pairs at $k = p$. Stop if all genes have been assigned a rule; otherwise, increment p and go to 5.

The REVEAL algorithm has the advantage of calculating simple networks (as in our example) very quickly. Essentially two steps are needed to retrieve the network. The disadvantage is that higher connectivity involves the calculation of the joint entropy of many state vectors, which can be difficult. For example, for $k = 2$ we have

$$H\left(x_{t+1};y_t,z_t\right) = H(x_{t+1}) + H\left(y_t,z_t\right) - H\left(x_{t+1},y_t,z_t\right) \tag{9-34}$$

and likewise for higher k. Furthermore, experimental data needs to be transformed into binary values, which might lead to imperfect and "noisy" state vectors so that no exact match can be calculated in steps 1 and 3. Despite these drawbacks, mostly implied by the model's simplicity, Boolean models currently represent the only tractable result on larger networks, i.e., with a number of nodes >100.

9.6.2
Other Approaches

Several other models have been described for reverse engineering genetic networks. The linear model approach (compare Section 3.4.4) of D'Haeseleer et al. (1999) assumes that the expression level of a gene in a network depends on a linear combination of the expression levels of other genes, according to a model similar to Eq. (3-100) in Chapter 3. The authors applied this model to the study of 65 genes at 28 time points (concerning cervical spinal cord and hippocampus development of rats). They interpolated the time courses of the genes covering an interval of seven months of development by a cubic interpolation and estimated the weights of the regulatory interactions by least-squares estimation.

A linear model is a very simple approach for determining the weights of the regulatory network. Therefore, extensions have been proposed to nonlinear approaches, i.e., with the nonlinear activation function of Eq. (3-100) in Chapter 3. One such example is the backpropagation through time (BPTT) algorithm described in Werbos (1990). This algorithm essentially is an iterated gradient learning method that incorporates a time-ordered derivation operator that measures the effect of weight changes propagated through time.

Friedman et al. (2000) and Pe'er et al. (2001) pioneered the analysis of gene regulatory networks with Bayesian networks (cf. Section 3.5.2 and Section 8.3). They applied their methodology to time course data on the yeast cell cycle (Spellman et al. 1998) as well as yeast perturbation experiments described in Hughes et al. (2000). They investigated data identifying lower complex properties of the network, such as Markov relations. A Markov relation between a pair of genes holds if the relation of the genes is not separated by other genes, e.g., a parent-child relationship. If there is a Markov relation between two genes, this indicates that both are related in some biological interaction. Pe'er et al. (2001) showed that 30% of these pairs could not be recovered by simple pairwise correlation measurements and thus that the context-related network analysis improved. They were able to identify known transcriptional interactions as well as previously uncharacterized genes participating in those interactions.

A new approach based on dynamic Bayesian networks has been proposed recently (Kim et al. 2003). These approaches overcome the disadvantage that a Bayesian network does not allow regulatory circles by introducing time delays.

9.6.3
Network Motifs

The dimensionality of the gene regulatory network is the major problem of reverse engineering methods. Thus, modularity has become a major concept in recent years. The strategy is to break down this network into smaller components, called modules or network motifs, and connect them loosely to so-called ensemble networks. Extremely exiting and encouraging findings for such a bottom-up strategy have been published recently – the detection of regulatory motifs.

Davidson et al. (2002) investigated the gene regulatory network, involving nearly 50 genes, controlling the specification of the endoderm and mesoderm in the sea urchin embryo. Experimental techniques include perturbation experiments with QPCR, subtractive hybridizations on macroarray filters, whole-mount *in situ* hybridizations, and computational analysis of *cis*-regulatory elements. The result is a complex network representing a logic map of the genetic regulatory interactions that define the inputs and outputs to each *cis*-regulatory element resulting from the expression of other genes.

Whereas this map for development is rather large, two other groups were able to define smaller common regulatory motifs employing different techniques and tested on different organisms. Shen-Orr et al. (2002) analyzed the transcriptional regulation network of *Escherichia coli*. They used the RegulonDB database information for transcriptional regulation (Salgado et al. 2001) and performed additional literature mining and were able to identify three highly significant network motifs by comparisons with random networks. Furthermore, they were able to characterize general motif functionalities, e.g., time-dependent gene expression in the reaction to external stimuli.

Lee et al. (2002) performed an experimentally driven study on *Saccharomyces cerevisiae*. They performed chromatin immunoprecipitation (ChIP) on 106 different yeast regulators and identified ChIP-enriched promoter regions of genes by hybridization to microarrays that contained a genome-wide set of yeast promoters. They identified approximately 4000 highly significant interactions of regulators to promoter regions, with an average of 38 promoter regions per regulator. Their analysis revealed six different network motifs in the yeast interaction network, entailing the three motifs found in the other study. The network motifs according to Lee et al. (2002) are:

1. Autoregulation motif: a regulator that binds to the promoter region of its own gene.
2. Multicomponent loop: a circuit involving two or more factors.
3. Feed-forward loop: a regulator controls a regulator and additionally both bind to the promoter of a target gene.
4. Single-input motif: a regulator binds a set of promoters of different genes.
5. Multi-input motifs (dense overlapping regulons): a set of regulators binds commonly to a set of promoter regions.
6. Regulatory chain: a chain of regulators where the nth regulator binds to the promoter of the $n + 1$th regulator.

Motifs can be assigned to characteristic biological functions. For example, particularly interesting motifs are feed-forward loops. They have the potential to provide temporal control of a process because expression of the target gene may depend on persistent accumulation of activation signals for the regulators (Shen-Orr et al. 2002). For example, modeling a feed-forward loop with the Boolean AND rule (compare Section 8.3) will reject gene activation of the target gene caused by rapid variations in the first regulator and respond only on persistent activation. Here, the second regulator functions as a control for the length of activation. Both studies characterize single-input motifs as a functional element for coordinating a specific biological function, such as the regulation of enzymes.

The classification of network motifs and the construction and integration of such motifs in larger networks is a new research component of systems biology. The future goal will be to construct a kind of lexicon of motifs for higher-order functioning that gives insights into the fundamental gene regulatory design principles of living organisms. Driven by the tremendous challenges of new experimental techniques such as the above combination of chromatin immunoprecipitation and DNA microarrays, it is now possible to measure protein-DNA interactions and thus to combine gene regulation with gene expression.

References

AKUTSU, T., MIYANO, S. and KUHARA, S. Identification of genetic networks from a small number of gene expression patterns under the Boolean network model (1999) In: R.B. Altman et al., ed. Proceedings of the Pacific Symposium on Biocomputing 99. Singapore, pp 17–28.

AKUTSU, T., MIYANO, S. and KUHARA, S. Inferring qualitative relations in genetic networks and metabolic pathways (2000) Bioinformatics *16*, 727–734.

ALON, U., BARKAI, N., NOTTERMAN, D.A., GISH, G., YBARRA, S., MACK, D. and LEVINE, A.J. Broad patterns of gene expression revealed by clustering analysis of tumor and normal colon tissues probed by oligonucleotide arrays (1999) Proc. Natl. Acad. Sci. USA *96*, 6745–6750.

BEN-DOR, A., SHAMIR, R. and YAKHINI, Z. Clustering gene expression patterns (1999) J. Comput. Biol. *6*, 281–297.

BEN-DOR, A., BRUHN, L., FRIEDMAN, N., NACHMAN, I., SCHUMMER, M. and YAKHINI, Z. Tissue classification with gene expression profiles (2000) J. Comput. Biol. *7*, 559–584.

BENJAMINI, Y. and HOCHBERG, Y. Controlling the false discovery rate: a practical and powerful approach to multiple testing (1995) J Royal Statist Soc B *57*, 289–300.

BITTNER, M., MELTZER, P. and CHEN, Y., et al. Molecular classification of cutaneous malignant melanoma by gene expression profiling (2000) Nature *406*, 536–540.

BROWN, M., GRUNDY, W. and LIN, D., et al. Knowledge-based analysis of microarray gene expression data using support vector machines (1999) PNAS *97*, 262–267.

CHANG, C.C. and LIN, C.J. LIBSVM: a library for support vector machines (2003) http://www.csie.ntu.edu.tw/~cjlin/libsvm.

CHRISTENSEN, R. Plane answers to complex questions (1996) 2nd Edition Springer, New York.

CHUDIN, E., WALKER, R., KOSAKA, A., WU, S.X., RABERT, D., CHANG, T.K. and KREDER, D.E. Assessment of the relationship between signal intensities and transcript concentration for Affymetrix GeneChip arrays (2001) Genome Biol *3*, RESEARCH0005.

CLEVELAND, W.S. Robust locally weighted regression and smoothing scatterplots (1979) J. Am. Stat. Assoc. *74*, 829–836.

CLEVELAND, W.S. and DEVLIN, S.J. Locally weighted regression: an approach to regression analysis by local fitting (1983) J. Am. Stat. Assoc. *83*, 596–610.

CRISTIANINI, N. and SHAWE-TAYLOR, J. An introduction to support vector machines (2000) Cambridge University Press, Cambridge.

DAVIDSON, E.H., RAST, J.P., OLIVERI, P., RANSICK, A., CALESTANI, C., YUH, C.H., MINOKAWA, T., AMORE, G., HINMAN, V., ARENAS-MENA, C., OTIM, O., BROWN, C.T., LIVI, C.B., LEE, P.Y., REVILLA, R., RUST, A.G., PAN, Z., SCHILSTRA, M.J., CLARKE, P.J., ARNONE, M.I., ROWEN, L., CAMERON, R.A., McCLAY, D.R., HOOD, L. and BOLOURI, H. A genomic regulatory network for development (2002) Science *295*, 1669–78.

DeRISI, J., PENLAND, L., BROWN, P.O., BITTNER, M.L., MELTZER, P.S., RAY, M., CHEN, Y., SU, Y.A. and TRENT, J.M. Use of cDNA microarray to analyse gene expression patterns in human cancer (1996) Nature Genetics *14*, 457–460.

DeRISI, J., IYER, V.R. and BROWN, P.O. Exploring the metabolic and genetic control of gene expression on a genomic scale (1997) Science *278*, 680–686.

D'HAESELEER, P., WEN, X., FUHRMAN, S. and SOMOGYI, R. (1999) Linear modeling of mRNA expression levels during CNS development and injury. Pacific Symposium on Biocomputing. R. Altman, ed., World Scientific, Singapore, pp. 41–52.

DICKMEIS, T., AANSTAD, P., CLARK, M., FISCHER, N., HERWIG, R., MOURRAIN, P.,

BLADER, P., ROSA, F., LEHRACH, H. and STRAHLE, U. Identification of nodal signaling targets by array analysis of induced complex probes (2001) Dev. Dyn. *222*, 571–80.

DRAGHICI, S. Data analysis tools for DNA microarrays (2003) Chapman & Hall/CRC Press, Boca Raton.

DUDA, R.O. and HART, P.E. Pattern classification and scene analysis (1973). J. Wiley & Sons, New York.

DURBIN, B.P., HARDIN, J.S., HAWKINS, D.M. and ROCKE, D.M. A variance-stabilizing transformation for gene-expression microarray data (2002) Bioinformatics *18 Suppl 1*, S105-S110.

EISEN, M.B., SPELLMAN, P.T., BROWN, P.O. and BOTSTEIN, D. Cluster analysis and display of genome-wide expression patterns (1998) Proceedings of the Natl. Acad. Sci. USA *95*, 14853–14868.

FREUND, Y. and SHAPIRE, R. (1996) Experiments with a new boosting algorithm. In: Machine Learning: Proceedings of the 13th International Conference, Saitta, L., ed., Morgan Kauffman, San Francisco, pp. 148–156.

FRIEDMAN, N., LINIAL, M., NACHMAN, I. and PE'ER, D. Using Bayesian networks to analyze expression data (2000) J. Comput. Biol. *7*, 601–620.

FUREY, T.S., CRISTIANINI, N., DUFFY, N., BEDNARSKI, D.W., SCHUMMER, M. and HAUSSLER, D. Support vector machine classification and validation of cancer tissue samples usng microarray expression data (2000) Bioinformatics *16*, 906–914.

Gene Ontology Consortium. The gene ontology (GO) database and information resource (2003) Nucleic Acids Res. *32*, D258-D261.

GOLUB, J., et al. Molecular classification of cancer: Class discovery and class prediction by gene expression monitoring (1999) Science *286*, 531–537.

GRANJEAUD, S., NGUYEN, C., ROCHA, D., LUTON, R. and JORDAN, B. From hybridisation image to numerical values: a practical high-throughput quantification system for high density filter hybridisations. (1996) Genet. Anal. *12*, 151–162.

GRESS, T., HOHEISEL, J., LENNON, G., ZEHETNER, G. and LEHRACH, H. Hybridization fingerprinting of high-density cDNA library arrays with cDNA pools derived from whole tissues. (1992) Mamm. Genome *3*, 609–619.

GRESS, T., MULLER-PILLASCH, F. and GREG, T.,

et al. A pancreatic cancer-specific expression profile (1996) Oncogene *13*, 1819–1830.

HANAHAN, D. and WEINBERG, R.A. The hallmarks of cancer (2000) Cell *100*, 57–70.

HASTIE, T., TIBSHIRANI, R., EISEN, M.B., ALIZADEH, A., LEVY, R., STAUDT, L. and CHAN, W., et al. Gene shaving as a method for identifying distinct sets of genes with similar expression patterns (2000) Genome Biology *1*, research0003.1–0003.21.

HERWIG, R., POUSTKA, A.J., MÜLLER, C., LEHRACH, H. and O'BRIEN, J. Large-scale Clustering of cDNA Fingerprinting Data (1999) Genome Research 9, 1093–1105.

HERWIG, R., AANSTAD, P., CLARK, M. and LEHRACH, H. Statistical evaluation of differential expression on cDNA nylon arrays with replicated experiments (2001) Nucleic Acids Res. *29*, E117.

HUBER, W., VON HEYDEBRECK, A., SÜLTMANN, H., POUSTKA, A. and VINGRON, M. Variance stabilisation applied to microarray data calibration and to the quantification of differential expression (2002) Bioinformatics *18 Suppl 1*, S96-S104.

HUGHES, T., MARTON, M. and JONES, A., et al. Functional discovery via a compendium of expression profiles (2000) Cell *102*, 109–126.

HUGHES, T., MAO, M. and JONES, A., et al. Expression profiling using microarrays fabricated by an ink-jet oligonucleotide synthesizer (2001) Nat. Biotechnol. *19*, 342–347.

IRIZARRY, R.A., BOLSTAD, B.M., COLLINS, F., COPE, L.M., HOBBS, B. and SPEED, T.P. Summaries of Affymetrix GeneChip probe level data (2003) Nucleic Acids Res. *31*, e15.

IYER, V.R., EISEN, M.B., ROSS, D.T., SCHULER, G., MOORE, T., LEE, J., TRENT, J., STAUDT, L.M., HUDSON, J., BOGUSKI, M., LASHKARI, D., SHALON, D., BOTSTEIN, D. and BROWN, P.O. The transcriptional program in the response of human fibroblasts to serum (1999) Science *283*, 83–87.

JAIN, A.K. and DUBES, R.C. Algorithms for clustering data (1988) Prentice Hall, Englewood Cliffs, NJ.

JAIN, A.N., TOKUYASU, T.A., SNIJDERS, A.M., SEGRAVES, R., ALBERTSON, D.G. and PINKEL, D. Fully automated quantification of microarray image data (2002) Genome Res. *12*, 325–332.

JOLLIFFE, I.T. Principal Component Analysis (1986) Springer, New York.

KAHLEM, P., SULTAN, M., HERWIG, R., STEINFATH, M., BALZEREIT, D., EPPENS, B., SARAN,

N.G., Pletcher, M.T., South, S.T., Stetten, G., Lehrach, H., Reeves, R.H. and Yaspo, M.L. Transcript level alterations reflect gene dosage effects across multiple tissues in a mouse model of down syndrome (2004) Genome Res. *14*, 1258–67.

Kauffman, S.A. The origins of order: Self-organization and selection in evolution (1993) Oxford University Press, New York.

Kerr, M.K., Martin, M. and Churchill, G.A. Analysis of variance for gene expression microarray data (2000) J. Comput. Biol. *7*, 819–837.

Kim, S.Y., Imoto, S. and Miyano, S. Inferring gene networks from time series microarray data using dynamic Bayesian networks (2003) Briefings Bioinf. *4*, 228–235.

Kohonen, T. Self-organizing maps (1997) Springer, Berlin.

Kuo, W.P., Jenssen, T.K., Butte, A.J., Ohno-Machado, L. and Kohane, I.S. Analysis of matched mRNA measurements from two different microarray technologies (2002) Bioinformatics *18*, 405–12.

Lee, T.I., Rinaldi, N.J., Robert, F., Odom, D.T., Bar-Joseph, Z., Gerber, G.K., Hannett, N.M., Harbison, C.T., Thompson, C.M., Simon, I., Zeitlinger, J., Jennings, E.G., Murray, H.L., Gordon, D.B., Ren, B., Wyrick, J.J., Tagne, J.B., Volkert, T.L., Fraenkel, E., Gifford, D.K. and Young, R.A. Transcriptional regulatory networks in Saccharomyces cerevisiae (2002) Science *298*, 799–804.

Lehmann, E.L. Nonparametrics: Statistical methods based on ranks (1979) Holden-Day, San Francisco.

Lehrach, H., Drmanac, R., Hoheisel, J., Larin, Z., Lennon, G., Monaco, A.P., Nizetic, D., Zehetner, G. and Poustka, A. Hybridization fingerprinting in Genome Mapping and Sequencing (1990) In: K. E. D. a. S. Tilghman, ed. Genome analysis. Cold Spring Harbor, New York, pp 39–81.

Lennon, G. and Lehrach, H. Hybridization analyses of arrayed cDNA libraries (1991) Trends in Genetics *7*, 314–317.

Li, C. and Wong, W.H. Model-based analysis of oligonucleotide arrays: Expression index computation and outlier detection (2001) Proc. Natl. Acad. Sci. USA *98*, 31–36.

Liang, S., Fuhrman, S. and Somogyi, R. REVEAL, a general reverse engineering algorithm for inference of genetic network architecture (1999) In: R. Altman et al., ed. Proceed-

ings of the Pacific Symposium on Biocomputing 98. Singapore, pp 18–28.

Lipshutz, R.J., Fodor, S.P., Gingeras, T.R. and Lockhart, D.J. High density synthetic oligonucleotide arrays (1999) Nature Genetics *21*, 20–24.

Lockhart, D.J., Dong, H., Byrne, M.C., Follettie, M.T., Gallo, M.S.C.M.V., Mittmann, M., Wang, C., Kobayashi, M., Horton, H. and Brown, E.L. Expression monitoring by hybridizaion to high-density oligonucleotide arrays (1996) Nature Biotechnology *14*, 1675–1680.

MacQueen, J.B. Some methods for classification and analysis of multivariate observations (1967) In: L. M. LeCam and J. Neymann, eds. Proceedings of the 5th Berkeley Symposium on Mathematical Statistics and Probability. UCLA Press, Los Angeles.

Mirkin, B. Mathematical Classification and Clustering (1996) Elsevier, Dordrecht.

Nguyen, C., Rocha, D., Granjeaud, S., Baldit, M., Bernard, K., Naquet, P. and Jordan, B.R. Differential gene expression in the murine thymus assayed by quantitative hybridization of arrayed cDNA clones (1996) Genomics *29*, 207–216.

Pe'er, D., Regev, A., Elidan, G. and Friedman, N. Inferring subnetworks from perturbed expression profiles (2001) Bioinformatics *17 Suppl 1*, S215-S224.

Poustka, A., Pohl, T., Barlow, D.P., Zehetner, G., Craig, A., Michiels, F., Ehrich, E., Frischauf, A.M.A.M. and Lehrach, H. Molecular approaches to mammalian genetics (1986) Cold Spring Harbor Symposia on Quant. Biol., Cold Spring Harbor, New York, pp 131–139.

Quakenbush, J. Microarray data normalization and transformation (2002) Nature Genetics, 496–501.

Ross, D.T., Scherf, U., Eisen, M.B., Perou, C.M., Rees, C., Spellman, P., Iyer, V., Jeffrey, S., de~Rijn, M.V., Waltham, M., Pergamenschikov, A., Lee, J., Lashkari, D., Shalon, D., Myers, T., Weinstein, J., Botstein, D. and Brown, P. Systematic variation in gene expression patterns in human cancer cell lines (2000) Nature Genetics *24*, 227–235.

Rousseeuw, P.J. Least median of squares regression (1984) J. Am. Stat. Assoc. *79*, 871–880.

Salgado, H., et al. RegulonDB (version 3.2): transcriptional regulation and operon organization in Escherichia coli K-12. (2001) Nucleic Acids Res. *29*, 72–74.

SCHENA, M., SHALON, D., DAVIS, R. and BROWN, P. Quantitative monitoring of gene expression patterns with a complementary DNA microarray (1995) Science *270*, 467–470.

SCHENA, M., SHALON, D., HELLER, R., CHAI, A., BROWN, P. and DAVIS, R. Parallel human genome analysis: microarray-based expression monitoring of 1000 genes (1996) Proc. Natl. Acad. Sci. USA *93*, 10614–10619.

SHARAN, R. and SHAMIR, R. CLICK: a clustering algorithm with applications to gene expression analysis (2000) In: P. Bourne. et al., ed. Proceedings of the 8th International Conference on Intelligent Systems for Molecular Biology (ISMB). Menlo Park, pp. 307–316.

SHEN-ORR, S.S., MILO, R., MANGAN, S. and ALON, U. Network motifs in the transcriptional regulation network of Escherichia coli (2002) Nat. Genet. *31*, 64–8.

SPELLMAN, P., SHERLOCK, G. AND ZHANG, M., et al. Comprehensive identification of cell cycle-regulated genes of the yeast saccharomyces cerevisiae by microarray hybridisation (1998) Mol. Biol. Cell. *9*, 3273–3297.

STATNIKOV, A., ALIFERIS, C.F., TSAMARDINOS, I., HARDIN, D. and LEVY, S. A comprehensive evaluation of multicategory classification methods for microarray gene expression cancer diagnosis (2004) Bioinformatics *Epub ahead of print*.

STEINFATH, M., WRUCK, W., SEIDEL, H., LEHRACH, H., RADELOF, U. and O'BRIEN, J. Automated image analysis for array hybridization experiments (2001) Bioinformatics *17*, 634–41.

STOREY, J.D. and TIBSHIRANI, R. Statistical significance for genome-wide studies (2003) PNAS *100*, 9440–9445.

TAMAYO, P., SLONIM, D., MESIROV, J., ZHU, Q., KITAREEWAN, S., DIMITROVSKY, E., LANDER, E.S. and GOLUB, T.R. Interpreting patterns of gene expression with self-organizing maps: Methods and application to hematopoietic differentiation (1999) Proc. Natl. Acad. Sci. USA *96*, 2907–2912.

TAN, P.K., DOWNEY, T.J., SPITZNAGEL, E.L., JR., XU, P., FU, D., DIMITROV, D.S., LEMPICKI, R.A., RAAKA, B.M. and CAM, M.C. Evaluation of gene expression measurements from commercial microarray platforms (2003) Nucleic Acids Res. *31*, 5676–84.

TAVAZOIE, S., HUGHES, J.D., CAMPBELL, M.J., CHO, R.J. and CHURCH, G.M. Systematic determination of genetic network architecture (1999) Nat. Genet. *22*, 281–5.

TÖRÖNEN, P., KOLEHMAINEN, M., WONG, G. and CASTREN, E. Analysis of gene expression data using self-organizing maps (1999) FEBS Lett. *451*, 142–146.

TUSHER, V.G., et al. Significance analysis of microarrays applied to the ionizing radiation response (2001) PNAS *98*, 5116–5121.

VAPNIK, V.N. The Nature of Statistical Learning Theory (1995) Springer, New York.

WEN, X., FUHRMAN, S., MICHAELS, G.S., CARR, D.B., SMITH, S., BARKER, J.L. and SOMOGYI, R. Large-scale temporal gene expression mapping of central nervous system development (1998) Proc. Natl. Acad. Sci. USA *95*, 334–339.

WERBOS, P.J. Backpropagation through time: what it does and how to do it (1990) Proc IEEE *78*, 1550–1560.

WESTFALL, P.H. and YOUNG, S.S. Resampling-based multiple testing: examples and methods for p-value adjustment (1993) Wiley, New York.

WHITFIELD, M.L., SHERLOCK, G. and SALDANHA, A.J., et al. Identification of genes periodically expressed in the human cell cycle and their expression in tumors (2002) Mol. Biol. Cell *13* 1977–2000.

WIERLING, C.K., STEINFATH, M., ELGE, T., SCHULZE-KREMER, S., AANSTAD, P., CLARK, M., LEHRACH, H. and HERWIG, R. Simulation of DNA array hybridization experiments and evaluation of critical parameters during subsequent image and data analysis (2002) BMC Bioinformatics *3*, 29.

WODICKA, L., DONG, H., MITTMANN, M. and LOCKHART, D.J. Genome-wide expression monitoring in Saccharomyces cerevisiae (1997) Nature Biotechnology *15*, 1359–1367.

YANG, Y. and SPEED, T.P. Design issues for cDNA microarray experiments (2002) Nature Rev. Genet. *3*, 579–583.

YANG, H., DUDOIT, S., LUU, P., LIN, D.M., PENG, V., NGAI, J. and SPEED, T.P. Normalization for cDNA microarray data: a robust composite method addressing single and multiple slide systematic variations (2002) Nucleic Acids Res. *30*, e15.

YEUNG, K.Y., HAYNOR, D.R. and RUZZO, W.L. Validating clustering for gene expression data (2001) Bioinformatics *17*, 309–318.

ZIEN, A., FLUCK, J., ZIMMER, R. and LENGAUER, T. Microarrays: How many do you need? (2003) J. Comput. Biol. *10*, 653–667.

10
Evolution and Self-organization

Introduction

Since Darwin's famous book *On the Origin of Species by Means of Natural Selection, or the Preservation of Favoured Races in the Struggle for Life* (1859), it has been a widely accepted view that biological species gradually developed from a few common ancestors in an iterative process of mutations and natural selection over millions of years. Throughout this evolution, new species appeared and existing species adapted themselves to changing environmental conditions.

Mutations are changes in the genetic material (genotype) of organisms. They usually cause changes in properties of the organisms (phenotype) and occur by chance. Natural selection proves fitness with respect to survival and reproduction in the actual environment with no further goal or plan. The fittest in gaining the necessary resources will win and survive, while the others become extinct. The term *natural selection* has to be distinguished from *artificial selection*. Artificial selection chooses specific features to be retained or eliminated depending on a goal or intention (e. g., the objective of a farmer to have corn that permits maximal harvest).

The view that biological systems developed during evolution can be applied not only to species but also to other units of biological consideration, such as cells, metabolic pathways, and gene expression networks. It has been questioned, however, whether the principle of development by mutation and selection can be used to understand evolution in a theoretical way, to learn how and why biological systems assumed their current state, and to predict structures of biological networks using simple analogies.

A basic assumption of theoretical considerations is that evolution is based on the trial-and-error process of variation and natural selection of systems at all levels of complexity. The development of biological systems further involves the feature of self-organization, i.e., assuming stable structures that (1) employ a global cooperation between the elements, (2) are inherent in the system, and (3) are contained independently of external pressure.

Biological evolution is a complex process. As with other subjects of systems biology, this complexity conflicts with the attempt to develop general models for evolution. Biological diversity increases the number of components to be considered in models. Therefore, it seems unrealistic to develop a detailed and fundamental de-

Systems Biology in Practice. Concepts, Implementation and Application.
E. Klipp, R. Herwig, A. Kowald, C. Wierling, H. Lehrach
Copyright © 2005 WILEY-VCH Verlag GmbH & Co. KGaA, Weinheim
ISBN: 3-527-31078-9

scription of phenomena, as is sometimes possible in theoretical physics. In general, evolutionary models can rarely be experimentally tested, since we will not survive the necessary time span. Nevertheless, steps have been undertaken to clarify features of biological phenomena such as competition and cooperativity, self-organization, and emergence of new species with mathematical modeling. Such models provide a better understanding of biological evolution; they also give generalized descriptions of biological experiments. The following types of evolutionary models have been developed.

Models of the origin of self-replicating systems have been constructed in connection with the origin-of-life problem. M. Eigen and P. Schuster introduced the concepts of quasispecies and hypercycles (Eigen 1971b; Eigen and Schuster 1977–1979, 1982). These models describe mathematically some hypothetical evolutionary stages of prebiological self-reproducing macromolecular systems. General models of evolution describe some informational and cybernetic aspects of evolution, such as the neutral evolution theory by M. Kimura (Kimura and Ota 1971, 1974; Kimura 1979, 1983) and S. Kauffman's automata (Kauffman and Weinberger 1989; Kauffman 1991, 1993; Kauffman and Macready 1995). Models of artificial life are aimed at understanding the formal laws of life and evolution. These models analyze the evolution of artificial "organisms," living in computer-program worlds.

Computer algorithms that use evolutionary methods of optimization to solve practical problems have been developed. The genetic algorithm by J. H. Holland (Holland 1975, 1992; Domingo and Holland 1997) and the evolutionary programming initiated by Fogel et al. (1966), the evolution strategies by Rechenberg (1994), and the genetic programming propagated by Koza et al. (2001) are well-known examples of this research. Evolutionary optimization has been applied to models of biological systems. The idea is to predict features of a biological system from the requirement that it function optimally in order to be the fittest that survives.

These models are usually very abstract and much simpler than biological processes. But the abstractness is necessary to find a general representation of the investigated features despite their real complexity and diversity. Furthermore, the concepts must be simple enough to be perceived and to be applicable.

10.1
Quasispecies and Hypercycles

In the 1970s, Eigen and Schuster and others studied the origin-of-life problem (Eigen and Schuster 1977, 1979; Eigen et al. 1980b; Swetina and Schuster 1982). They wanted to understand the behavior of simple self-reproducing systems and therefore developed several mathematical concepts, including the quasispecies model and the hypercycle model. The quasispecies model is a description of the process of the Darwinian evolution of self-replicating entities within the framework of physical chemistry. It is useful mainly in providing a qualitative understanding of the evolutionary processes of self-replicating macromolecules such as RNA or DNA or simple asexual organisms such as bacteria or viruses. Quantitative predictions based on this model are difficult because the parameters that serve as its input are hard to obtain from actual biological systems.

The model relies on four assumptions:

1. The self-replicating entities can be represented as sequences composed of letters from an alphabet, e.g., sequences of DNA consisting of the four bases A, C, G, and T.
2. New sequences enter the system solely as either correct or erroneous copies of other sequences that are already present.
3. The substrates, or raw materials, necessary for ongoing replication are always present in sufficient quantity in the considered volume. Excess sequences are washed away in an outgoing flux.
4. Sequences may decay into their building blocks.

In the quasispecies model, mutations occur by errors made during copying of already-existing sequences. Further, selection arises because different types of sequences tend to replicate at different rates, which leads to the suppression of sequences that replicate more slowly in favor of sequences that replicate faster. In the following sections, we will show how to put this into equations.

10.1.1
Selection Equations for Biological Macromolecules

The dynamics of selection processes in early evolution may be described with equations of the type used in population dynamics. Instead of species, here we consider the macromolecules that are able to self-replicate as a model. For example, DNA molecules are replicated by complementary base pairing ($A = T$ and $C \equiv G$):

$$DNA \rightarrow 2\,DNA \tag{10-1}$$

A population is defined as a set $\{S_1, S_2, ..., S_n\}$ of n sequences. Each sequence is a string of N symbols, s_{ik}, with $k = 1, ..., N$ and $i = 1, ..., n$. The symbols are taken from an alphabet containing λ letters. Using DNA as an example, we consider a four-letter alphabet ($\lambda = 4$, $s_{ik} = A, C, G, T$). Thus, the space of possible sequences covers λ^N different sequences. The sequence length N and the population size n are assumed to be large: $N, n \gg 1$. The concentration of molecules with identical sequences S_i is x_i. We assume that the DNA molecules have some selective value f_i that depends on the sequence of nucleotides. During propagation of the replication process, the molecules with higher selective value will have an advantage over those with a lower value. The evolution character depends strongly on the population size n. If n is very large ($n \gg \lambda^N$), the number of all sequences in a population is large and evolution can be considered a deterministic process. In this case, the population dynamics can be described in terms of the ordinary differential equations. In the opposite case ($n \ll \lambda^N$), the evolution process should be handled as stochastic (not done here).

Example 10-1

Consider a "soup" containing a million molecules. For a sequence of length $N = 5$ from an alphabet with $\lambda = 4$ letters, there are $4^5 = 1024$ possibilities for different sequences S_i, and the mean abundance per sequence is about 1000. The number of possibilities in the case of a string length $N = 20$ is about 10^{12}, meaning that on average only one of a million possible sequences is present in the soup. In the latter case, a mutation would (most probably) result in a new sequence that was not present before. In the first case, a mutation of one molecule would result in an increase of the abundance of another already-present sequence.

A basic assumption of this concept is that there is a master sequence S_m, having the maximal selective value f_m. The selective value f_i of any other sequence S_i depends on the Hamming distance h (the number of different symbols at corresponding places in sequences) between S_i and the master sequence S_m: $f_i = f_i(h(S_i, S_m))$ – the smaller the distance h, the greater the selective value f_i.

10.1.1.1 Self-replication Without Interaction

Assume that DNA molecules perform identical replication and are also subject to decay. The time course of their concentration x_i is determined by the ordinary differential equation (ODE)

$$\frac{dx_i}{dt} = a_i x_i - d_i x_i = (a_i - d_i) x_i ,$$ (10-2)

where a_i and d_i are the rate constants for the replication and the decay. For constant values of a_i and d_i and an initial concentration x_i^0 for $t = 0$, the solution of Eq. (10-2) is given by

$$x_i(t) = x_i^0\, e^{(a_i - d_i)t} .$$ (10-3)

Depending on the difference $f_i = a_i - d_i$, Eq. (10-3) describes a monotonous increase $(a_i > d_i)$, a decrease $(a_i < d_i)$, or a constant concentration $(a_i = d_i)$, respectively. Therefore, the difference f_i can be considered as the selective value (also called excess productivity).

10.1.1.2 Selection at Constant Total Concentration of Self-replicating Molecules

In Eq. (10-3) the dynamics of species S_i is independent of the behavior of the other species. However, selection will happen only if there is interaction between the species, leading to selective pressure. This is given if, e.g., the number of building blocks (mononucleotides) is limited or if the concentration may not exceed a certain maximum. In the latter case, the total concentration of species can be kept constant by introducing a term describing elimination of supernumerary individuals or dilution by flow-out of the considered volume. This is called selection at constant organization (Schuster et al. 1978). Assuming that the dilution rate is proportional to the actual concentration of the species, it follows that

$$\frac{dx_i}{dt} = f_i \cdot x_i - \varphi \cdot x_i . \tag{10-4}$$

Under the condition of constant total concentration $\left(\sum_i x_i = x_{total} = const.\right.$ or $\left.\sum_i \frac{dx_i}{dt} = 0\right)$ it follows that

$$\varphi = \frac{\sum_i f_i x_i}{\sum_k x_k} = \bar{f} . \tag{10-5}$$

Since f_i denotes the excess productivity of species S_i, $\varphi = \bar{f}(x)$ is the mean excess productivity. Introducing Eq. (10-5) into Eq. (10-4) yields the selection equation

$$\frac{dx_i}{dt} = \left(f_i - \bar{f}\right) x_i . \tag{10-6}$$

This is a system of coupled nonlinear ODE. Nevertheless, it is easy to see that the concentrations increase over time for all species with $f_i > \bar{f}$ and that the concentrations decrease for all species with $f_i < \bar{f}$. The mean excess productivity $\bar{f}$ is, therefore, a selection threshold. Equation (10-6) shows that the concentrations of species with high selective value increase with time. Hence, the mean excess productivity also increases according to Eq. (10-5). Successively, the selective values of more and more species become lower than $\bar{f}$, their concentrations start to decrease, and eventually they die out. Finally, only the species with the highest initial selective value survives, the so-called master species.

The explicit solution of Eq. (10-6) reads

$$x_i(t) = \frac{x_{total} \cdot x_i^0 e^{f_i t}}{\sum_j x_j^0 e^{f_j t}} . \tag{10-7}$$

The species with the highest excess productivity is the master sequence S_m. In the current scenario, it will survive and the other species will die out.

Example 10-2

Consider $n = 4$ competing sequences with equal initial concentrations $x_i^0 = n/4$ and different selective values $f_1 < f_2 < f_3 < f_4$. This results in the temporal behavior depicted in Fig. 10.1.
For $t = 0$, $f_1 < \bar{f} < f_2 < f_3 < f_4$ holds; hence, the concentration x_1 decreases, while the other concentrations increase. With time progression, f_2 and f_3 fall one after the other under the rising threshold $\bar{f}$, and the respective concentrations x_2 and x_3 eventually decrease. Concentration x_4 always moves up until it asymptotically reaches the total concentration. Species 4 is the master species, since it has the highest selective value.

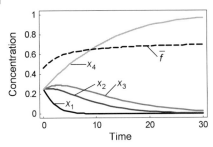

Fig. 10.1 Time course of concentration of four competing sequences performing identical replication as described in Eq. (10-7). Initial concentrations are $x_i^0 = n/4$; the selective values are $f_1 = 0.01, f_2 = 0.52, f_3 = 0.58, f_4 = 0.7$. The dashed line shows the mean excess productivity $\bar{f}$ that increases with time.

10.1.1.3 Self-replication with Mutations: The Quasispecies Model

Up to now we considered only the case of identical self-replication. However, mutations are an important feature of evolution. In the case of erroneous replication of sequence S_i, a molecule of sequence S_j is produced that also belongs to the space of possible sequences. The right-hand side of Eq. (10-4) can be extended in the following way:

$$\frac{dx_i}{dt} = a_i\, q_i\, x_i - d_i\, x_i + \sum_{j \neq i} m_{ij}\, x_j - \varphi x_i .\qquad(10\text{-}8)$$

The expression $a_i\, q_i\, x_i$ denotes the rate of identical self-replication, where $q_i \leq 1$ is the ratio of correctly replicated sequences. The quantity q_i characterizes the quality of replication. The term $d_i\, x_i$ denotes again the decay rate of sequence S_i, and φx_i is the dilution term ensuring constant total concentration. The expression $\sum_{j \neq i} m_{ij} x_j$ characterizes the synthesis rate of sequence S_i from other sequences S_j by mutation.

Since every replication results in the production of a sequence from the possible sequence space, the rate of erroneous replication of all sequences must be equal to the synthesis rate of sequences by mutation. Therefore, it holds that

$$\sum_i a_i \left(1 - q_i\right) x_i = \sum_i \sum_{j \neq i} m_{ij}\, x_j .\qquad(10\text{-}9)$$

Taking again into account the constant total concentration and Eq. (10-9) yields

$$0 = \sum_i \frac{dx_i}{dt} = \sum_i a_i\, x_i - \sum_i d_i\, x_i - \varphi \sum_i x_i .\qquad(10\text{-}10)$$

This way, for φ Eq. (10-5) holds again. The selection equation for self-replication with mutation reads

$$\frac{dx_i}{dt} = \left(a_i\, q_i - d_i - \bar{f}\right) x_i + \sum_{j \neq i} m_{ij}\, x_j .\qquad(10\text{-}11)$$

Equation (10-11) differs from Eq. (10-6) by an additional coupling term that is due to the mutations. A high precision of replication requires small coupling constants

(m_{ij}). For small m_{ij} one may expect behavior similar to that in the case without muta-tion: the sequences with the high selective value will accumulate, sequences with low selective value die out. But the existing sequences always produce erroneous se-quences that are closely related to them and differ only in a small number of muta-tions. A species and its close relatives that appeared by mutation are referred to as quasispecies. Therefore, there is not selection of a single master species, but rather of a set of species. The species with the highest selective value and its close relatives form the master quasispecies distribution.

In conclusion, the quasispecies model does not predict the ultimate extinction of all but the fastest replicating sequence. Although the sequences that replicate more slowly cannot sustain their abundance level by themselves, they are constantly re-plenished as sequences that replicate faster mutate into them. At equilibrium, re-moval of slowly replicating sequences due to decay or outflow is balanced by replen-ishing, so that even relatively slowly replicating sequences can remain present in fi-nite abundance.

Due to the ongoing production of mutant sequences, selection acts not on single sequences but rather on so-called mutational clouds of closely related sequences, the quasispecies. In other words, the evolutionary success of a particular sequence de-pends not only on its own replication rate but also on the replication rates of the mu-tant sequences it produces and on the replication rates of the sequences of which it is a mutant. As a consequence, the sequence that replicates fastest may even disap-pear completely in selection-mutation equilibrium, in favor of more slowly replicat-ing sequences that are part of a quasispecies with a higher average growth rate (Swe-tina and Schuster 1982). Mutational clouds as predicted by the quasispecies model have been observed in RNA viruses and in *in vitro* RNA replication (Domingo and Holland 1997; Burch and Chao 2000).

10.1.1.4 The Genetic Algorithm

The evolution process in the quasispecies concept can also be viewed as a stochastic algorithm. This can be used as a strategy for a computer search algorithm. The evo-lution process produces consequent generations. We start with an initial population $S(0) = \{S_1(0), ..., S_n(0)\}$ at time $t = 0$. A new generation $S(t + 1)$ is obtained from the old one $S(t)$ by random selection and mutation of sequences $S_i(t)$, where t corre-sponds to the generation number. Assume that all $f_i \leq 1$, which can be ensured by normalization. The model evolution process can be described formally in the follow-ing computer program–like manner.

1. Initialization. Form an initial population $S(0) = \{S_1(0), ..., S_n(0)\}$ by choosing ran-domly for every sequence $i = 1, ..., n$ and for every position $k = 1, ..., N$ in the se-quence a symbol from the given alphabet (e.g., A, T, C, G or "0" and "1").
2. Sequence selection for the new generation. Select sequences by choosing ran-domly numbers i' with the probability $f_{i'}$ and add a copy of the old sequence $S_{i'}(t)$ to the new population as $S_{i'}(t + 1)$.
3. Control of population size. Repeat step 2 until the new population has reached size n of the initial population.

4. Mutation. Change with a certain probability for every sequence $S_i(t)$ with $i = 1, ..., n$ and for every position $s_{ik}(t)$ with $k = 1, ..., N$ the current symbol to another symbol of the alphabet.
5. Iteration. Repeat steps 2–4 for successive time points.

The application of this algorithm allows for a visualization of the emergence of quasispecies and the master quasispecies distribution from an initial set of sequences during time.

10.1.1.5 Assessment of Sequence Length for Stable Passing-on of Sequence Information

The number of possible mutants of a certain sequence depends on its length N. Since the alphabet for DNA molecules has four letters, each sequence has $3N$ neighboring sequences (mutants) with a Hamming distance of $h = 1$. For mutants with arbitrary distance h, there are $N_h = 3^h \binom{N}{h}$ possibilities. Therefore, the number of sequences belonging to a quasispecies can be very high.

The quality measure q entering Eq. (10-8) for a sequence of length N can be expressed by the probability p_q of correct replication of the individual nucleotides. Assuming that this probability is independent of position and type of the nucleotide, the quality measure reads

$$q = p_q^N. \tag{10-12}$$

Mathematical investigation confirms that stable passing-on of information is possible only if the value of the quality measure is above a certain threshold $q > 1/s$. The parameter s is the relative growth rate of the master sequence, which is referred to as superiority. The generation of new species and, therefore, development during evolution, is possible only with mutations. But too-large mutation rates lead to destruction of information already accumulated. The closer q is to 1, the longer sequences may replicate in a stable manner. For the maximal length of a sequence, Eigen and coworkers (Eigen 1971 a) determined the relation

$$N(1 - p_q) < \ln s. \tag{10-13}$$

During evolution self-reproducing systems became more and more complex and the respective sequences became longer. Hence, the accuracy of replication also had to increase. Since the number of nucleotides in mammalian cells is about $N \approx 10^9$, Eq. (10-13) implies that the error rate per nucleotide is on the order of 10^{-9} or lower. This is in good agreement with the accuracy of the replication in mammalian cells. Such a level of accuracy cannot be reached by simple self-replication based on chemical base pairing; it necessitates help from polymerases that catalyze the replication. For uncatalyzed replication of nucleic acids, the error rate is at least 10^{-2}, which implies a maximal sequence length of $N \approx 10^2$.

10.1.1.6 Coexistence of Self-replicating Sequences: Complementary Replication of RNA

As we have seen, only mutation and selection cannot explain the complexity of currently existing sequences and replication mechanisms. Their stable existence necessitates cooperation between different types of molecules in addition to their competition.

Consider the replication of RNA molecules, a mechanism used by RNA phages. The RNA replicates by complementary base pairing. There are two complementary strands, R_i^+ and R_i^-. The synthesis of one strand always requires the presence of the complementary strand, i.e., R_i^+ derives from R_i^- and vice versa. Thus, both strands have to cooperate for replication.

For a single pair of complementary strands we have the following scheme:

$$\xleftarrow{d^+} R_i^+ \underset{a^-}{\overset{a^+}{\rightleftharpoons}} R_i^- \xrightarrow{d} , \qquad (10\text{-}14)$$

with the kinetic constants a^+ and a^- for replication and the kinetic constants d^+ and d^- for degradation. Denoting the concentrations of R_i^+ and R_i^- with x^+ and x^-, respectively, the corresponding ODE system reads

$$\frac{dx^+}{dt} = a^- x^- - d^+ x^+$$

$$\frac{dx^-}{dt} = a^+ x^+ - d^- x^- \qquad (10\text{-}15)$$

and in matrix notation holds

$$\frac{d}{dt}\begin{pmatrix} x^+ \\ x^- \end{pmatrix} = \begin{pmatrix} -d^+ & a^- \\ a^+ & -d^- \end{pmatrix}\begin{pmatrix} x^+ \\ x^- \end{pmatrix}. \qquad (10\text{-}16)$$

The eigenvalues of the Jacobian matrix in Eq. (10-16) are

$$\lambda_{1/2} = -\frac{d^+ + d^-}{2} \pm \sqrt{\left(\frac{d^+ - d^-}{2}\right)^2 + a^+ a^-} . \qquad (10\text{-}17)$$

They are always real, since the kinetic constants have nonnegative values. While λ_2 (the "–" solution) is negative, λ_1 (the "+" solution) may assume positive or negative values depending on the parameters:

$$\lambda_1 < 0 \quad \text{for} \quad a^+ a^- < d^+ d^-$$
$$\lambda_1 > 0 \quad \text{for} \quad a^+ a^- > d^+ d^- . \qquad (10\text{-}18)$$

The solution of Eq. (10-16) reads

$$x(t) = b^{(1)} e^{\lambda_1 t} + b^{(2)} e^{\lambda_2 t} , \qquad (10\text{-}19)$$

with concentration vector $x = (x^+, x^-)^T$ and eigenvectors $b^{(1)}, b^{(2)}$ of the Jacobian.

According to Eq. (10-19) a negative eigenvalue λ_1 indicates the extinction of both strands R_i^+ and R_i^-. For a positive eigenvalue λ_1, the right site of Eq. (10-19) comprises an exponentially increasing and an exponentially decreasing term, the first of which dominates for progressing time. Thus, the concentrations of both strands rise exponentially. Furthermore, the growth of each strand depends not only on its own kinetic constants but also on the kinetic constants of the other strand.

Example 10-3

For the simple case that both strands have the same kinetic properties ($a^+ = a^- = a$ and $d^+ = d^- = d$), the temporal behavior is shown in Fig. 10.2.
If $a > d$, the exponential increase dominates and both strands accumulate. If $a < d$, both strands become extinct. In both cases, the initial concentration differences eventually become negligible and both strands behave identically.

10.1.2
The Hypercycle

The hypercycle model describes a self-reproducing macromolecular system in which RNAs and enzymes cooperate in the following manner. There are n RNA species; the i-th RNA codes for the i-th enzyme ($i = 1, 2, ..., n$). The enzymes cyclically increase the replication rates of the RNAs, i.e., the first enzyme increases the replication rate of the second RNA, the second enzyme increases the replication rate of the third RNA, ..., and eventually the n-th enzyme increases the replication rate of the first RNA. In addition, the described system possesses primitive translation abilities, in that the information stored in RNA sequences is translated into enzymes, analogous to the usual translation processes in contemporary cells. M. Eigen and P. Schuster consider hypercycles to be predecessors of protocells (primitive unicellular biological organisms). The action of the enzymes accelerates the replication of the RNA species and enhances the accuracy. Although the hypercycle concept may explain the advantages of the cooperation of RNA and enzymes, it cannot explain how it arose during evolution. A special problem in this regard is the emergence of a genetic code.

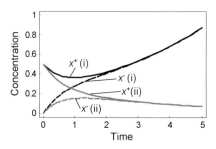

Fig. 10.2 Concentration time courses for complementary replication of RNA molecules according to Eq. (10-15). Both strands have the same kinetic properties. Parameters in case (i) are $a = 1$ and $d = 0.75$ (black lines, solid: +strand, dashed: –strand); both strands accumulate. In case (ii) it holds that $a = 0.75$ and $d = 1$ (gray lines, solid: +strand, dashed: –strand); both strands become extinct with time.

The simplest cooperation between enzymes and nucleotide sequences is given when (1) the enzyme E_i is the translation product of the nucleic acid I_i and (2) the enzyme E_i primarily catalyzes the identical replication of I_i as depicted below

$$a^R \, \text{(} \, I_i \, \xrightarrow{a^T} \, E_i \, \text{)} \, . \tag{10-20}$$

a^T and a^R are the kinetic constants of translation and replication.

In general, a hypercycle involves several enzymes and RNA molecules. In addition, the mentioned macromolecules cooperate to provide primitive translation abilities so that the information, coded in RNA sequences, is translated into enzymes, analogous to the usual translation processes in biological objects. The cyclic organization of the hypercycle (Fig. 10.3) ensures its structure stability.

In the following, we will consider the dynamics for the competition of two hypercycles of the type depicted in Eq. (10-20). Under the conditions of constant total concentration and negligible decay of compounds, the ODE system for RNAs with concentrations I_1 and I_2 and enzymes E_1 and E_2 reads

$$\frac{dE_1}{dt} = a_1^T I_1 - \varphi_E E_1$$

$$\frac{dI_1}{dt} = a_1^R I_1 E_1 - \varphi_I I_1$$

$$\frac{dE_2}{dt} = a_2^T I_2 - \varphi_E E_2$$

$$\frac{dI_2}{dt} = a_2^R I_2 E_2 - \varphi_I I_2 \, . \tag{10-21}$$

For the ODE system in Eq. (10-21) it is assumed that all reactions follow simple mass action kinetics. Since the total concentrations of RNAs and enzymes are constant ($I_1 + I_2 = c_I$ and $E_1 + E_2 = c_E$), it follows for the dilution terms that

$$\varphi_E = \frac{a_1^T I_1 + a_2^T I_2}{c_E} \quad \text{and} \quad \varphi_I = \frac{a_1^R I_1 E_1 + a_2^R I_2 E_2}{c_I} \, . \tag{10-22}$$

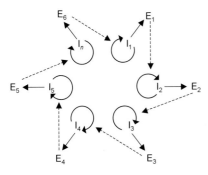

Fig. 10.3 Schematic representation of the hypercycle consisting of RNA molecules I_i and enzymes E_i ($i = 1, ..., n$). The i-th RNA codes for the i-th enzyme E_i. The enzymes cyclically increase RNA's replication rates, namely, E_1 increases the replication rate of I_2, E_2 increases the replication rate of I_3, ..., and, eventually, E_n increases the replication rate of I_1.

There are three steady-state solutions to Eq. (10-21) under consideration of Eq. (10-22) with nonnegative concentration values. The following two steady states are stable:

(i) $E_1^{(i)} = 0,$ $I_1^{(i)} = 0,$ $E_2^{(i)} = c_E,$ $I_2^{(i)} = c_I$

(ii) $E_1^{(i)} = c_E,$ $I_1^{(i)} = c_I,$ $E_2^{(i)} = 0,$ $I_2^{(i)} = 0,$ (10-23)

and the third steady state is not stable (a saddle). In both stable steady states, one of the hypercycle survives and the other one becomes extinct.

Example 10-4

Let's consider the dynamics of two competing hypercycles as described in Eq. (10-21). Here, the chosen parameters allow for better growth of the first hypercycle ($a_1^T > a_2^T$, $a_1^R > a_2^R$). Nevertheless, it is not always the case that the first hypercycle survives and the second hypercycle dies out. The final steady state depends strongly on the initial conditions. The temporal behavior can be illustrated as a time course and in the phase plane as shown in Fig. 10.4.

For competing hypercycles the dynamics depends on both the individual kinetic parameters of the hypercycles and the initial conditions. Both steady states are attrac-

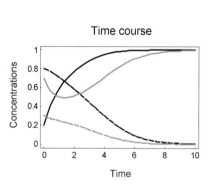

Time course

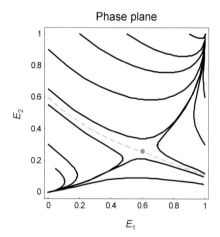

Phase plane

Fig. 10.4 Dynamics of competing two-component hypercycles as given in Eq. (10-21). Parameters: $a_1^T = 1$, $a_1^R = 1$, $a_2^T = 0.75$, $a_2^R = 0.75$, $c_I = 1$, $c_E = 1$. Left panel: time course of RNA and enzymes for the initial conditions $I_1(0) = 0.7$, $E_1(0) = 0.2$. The solid and dashed lines represent quantities of the first and second cycles, while the black and gray lines stand for enzyme and RNA concentrations, respectively. For the given parameters and initial conditions, the first hypercycle succeeds, while the second hypercycle dies out. Right panel: phase plane representation for the first hypercycle (values for the second hypercycle are determined by the condition of constant total concentrations for enzymes and RNAs). Depending on the initial conditions, the system evolves towards one of the stable steady states (Eq. (10-23)). The gray dot at point (0.6, 0.257) marks the saddle point, and the dotted gray line separates the basin of attraction of both stable steady states.

tive for a certain region of the concentration space. If the initial state belongs to the basin of attraction of a steady state, the system will always move towards this state. The hypercycle with less favorable parameters and a lower growth rate may survive if it is present with high initial concentration. Nevertheless, the steady state that ensures the survival of the hypercycle with higher growth rates has a larger basin of attraction, and this hypercycle may also win with a lower initial concentration.

The dependence on initial conditions in the selection of hypercycles is a new property compared to the identical or complementary self-replication without catalysts. If a new hypercycle would emerge due to mutation, the initial concentrations of its compounds are very low. It can only win against the other hypercycles if its growth rate is much larger. Even then it may happen that it becomes extinct – depending on the actual basins of attraction for the different steady states. This dependence leads to the possibility that during evolution even non-optimal systems may succeed if they are present in sufficiently high initial concentrations. This is called once forever selection, favoring the survival of systems that had good conditions by chance, independent of their actual quality. This behavior is quite different from the classical Darwinian selection process.

Even the non-optimal hypercycles advantageously combine the properties of polynucleotides (self-reproduction) with the properties of enzymes (enhancement of speed and accuracy of polynucleotide replication). The cyclic organization of the hypercycle ensures its structural stability. This stability is enhanced even if hypercycles are organized into compartments (Eigen et al. 1980a). This way, external perturbations by parasites can be limited and functionally advantageous mutations can be selected for.

In conclusion, one may state that the considered models cannot explain the real life-origin process, because these models are based on various plausible assumptions rather than on strong experimental evidence. Nevertheless, quasispecies and hypercycles provide a well-defined mathematical background for understanding the first molecular-genetic systems evolution. These models can be considered a step towards the development of more realistic models.

10.2
Other Mathematical Models of Evolution

10.2.1
Spin-glass Model of Evolution

The quasispecies concept as model of evolution (Section 10.2.1) implies a strong assumption, i.e., that the Hamming distance between the particular and unique master sequences determines the selective value. Only one maximum of the selective value exists. Using the physical spin-glass concept, we can construct a similar model wherein the fitness function can have many local maxima.

D. Sherrington and S. Kirkpatrick (1975, 1978) proposed a simple spin-glass model to interpret the physical properties of the systems, consisting of randomly interacting spins. This well-known model can be described briefly as follows:

1. There is a system s of spins s_k with $k = 1, ..., N$, where N is large $(N \gg 1)$. Each spin has the value of either 1 or -1.
2. Spins can exchange their values by random interactions, which lead to spin reversals.
3. The energy $E(s)$ of the spin system is

$$E(s) = -\sum_{k<l} J_{kl}\, s_k\, s_l \,.\tag{10-24}$$

The values J_{kl} are elements of the exchange interaction matrix with normally distributed random values and a probability density P_D of

$$P_D\left(J_{kl}\right) = (2\pi)^{-\frac{1}{2}} (N-1)^{\frac{1}{2}} \exp\left[-J_{kl}^2 \frac{(N-1)}{2}\right].\tag{10-25}$$

According to Eqs. (10-24) and (10-25), the mean spin-glass energy is zero, $\langle E \rangle = 0$, and for one-spin reversal the mean square root of energy variation is equal to 2.

The interesting feature of the spin-glass concept is the large number of local energy minima M, where a local energy minimum is defined as a state s_L at which any one-spin reversal would increase the energy E. Furthermore, there is a global energy minimum E_0 with $E_0 \approx 0.8\,N$.

A spin-glass model of evolution represents a model sequence as a vector S_i of spins and a population as a set $S = \{S_1, ..., S_n\}$ of n sequences. Each sequence has a selective value that depends on its energy:

$$f(S_i) = \exp\left[-\beta E(S_i)\right]\tag{10-26}$$

for a choice of J_{kl}. β is a parameter for the selection intensity.

Spins s_{ik} and s_{il} interact according to the interaction matrix J_{kl}. The selective value of a sequence becomes maximal and its energy minimal when the combinations of spins in the sequences provide maximally cooperative interactions for a given matrix J_{kl}.

To this end we again consider an evolutionary process with subsequent generations (compare Section 10.2.1.4). The initial population is generated by chance. New generations are obtained by selection and mutation. Selection occurs with respect to the selective value defined in Eq. (10-26). Mutation is a sign reversal of a spin $s_{ik} \rightarrow -s_{ik}$ with certain probability P.

The evolutionary process can be followed by considering for successive generations the number of sequences possessing certain energy $n(E)$, as illustrated in Fig. 10.5.

In the spin-glass-type of evolution, the system converges to one of the local energy minima E_L, which can be different for different runs of simulation. One may compare this evolutionary method with the sequential method of energy minimization, i.e., consequent changes of symbols $(s_{ik} \rightarrow -s_{ik})$ of one sequence and fixation of only successful reversals. The sequential search is computationally simpler than the evolution search. Nevertheless, the evolution search results on average in a deeper local energy minimum E_L, because different valleys in the energy landscape that are never reached

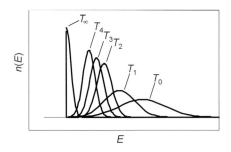

Fig. 10.5 Schematic representation of sequence distributions $n(E)$ for subsequent generations $T_0 < T_1 < ... < T_4$. For T_∞ the system is trapped into a local energy minimum E_L. The global energy minimum is E_0.

in the sequential method are simultaneously examined in the evolution process. Thus, in the spin-glass case, the evolutionary search has a certain advantage with respect to the sequential search: it results on average in the greater selective value.

10.2.2
Neutral Theory of Molecular Evolution

The neutral theory of molecular evolution introduced by Kimura (1983) states that mutations are mostly neutral or only slightly disadvantageous. The historical background for this statement was the deciphering of the genetic code and the structure of DNA by Watson and Crick (1953a–c) and the understanding of the principle of protein synthesis. In addition, the evolutionary rate of amino acid substitutions and protein polymorphism was estimated. The assumption of neutrality of mutations agrees both with the mutational molecular substitution rate observed experimentally and with the fact that the rate of the substitutions for the less biologically important part of macromolecules is greater than for the active centers of macromolecules.

The mathematical models of the neutral theory are essentially stochastic, i.e., a relatively small population size plays an important role in the fixation of the neutral mutations. The features of neutral selection can easily be explained using the game of neutral evolution.

Consider populations (of sequences or organisms or, in the following example, of balls) with a finite population size n. The rules describing the evolutionary process are as follows. (1) The population contains black and white balls with a total population size n. (2) The next generation is created in two steps. First, all balls are duplicated preserving their color. A black ball has a black offspring, a white ball a white one. Secondly, half of the population is removed irrespective of the "age" of a ball (i.e., whether it is an offspring or a parent ball) and with equal probability for black and white balls.

The state of the population is given by the number l of black balls. Consequently, there are $n - l$ white balls. The evolution is characterized by the probability P_{lm} for the transition from a state with l black balls to a state with m black balls in the next generation. P_{lm} can be calculated by applying combinatorial considerations:

$$P_{lm} = \begin{cases} \dfrac{\dbinom{2l}{m} \cdot \dbinom{2n-2l}{n-m}}{\dbinom{2n}{n}}, & \text{if } 2l-n \le m \le 2l \\ \\ 0, & \text{if } 2l < m \text{ or } m < 2l-n \end{cases} \tag{10-27}$$

with $\dbinom{a}{b} = \dfrac{a!}{(a-b)!\,b!}$.

Possible evolutionary processes for a population of size 10 with initially five black and five white balls are illustrated in Fig. 10.6.

The matrix P_{lm} determines the random Markovian process, which can be considered as an example of a simple stochastic genetic process. Concerning the behavior of this process, the following can be stated. (1) The process always converges to one of two states, $l = 0$ (only white balls) or $l = n$ (only black balls). (2) For a large population size n, the characteristic number of generations needed to converge to either of these states is equal to $2n$. Thus, although this evolution is purely neutral (black and white balls have equal chances of survival), only one species is selected.

It can be questioned how progressive evolution is possible if molecular substitutions are neutral. To answer this question, M. Kimura uses the concept of gene duplication developed by Ohno (1970). According to Kimura, gene duplications create unnecessary, surplus DNA sequences, which in turn drift further because of random mutations, providing the raw material for creation of new, biologically useful genes.

The evolutionary concepts of the neutral theory came from interpretations of biological experiments; this theory was strongly empirically inspired. The other type of theory, a more abstract one, was proposed by Stuart A. Kauffman: *NK* automata or Boolean networks.

10.2.3
Boolean Network Models

Boolean models are based on proposition logic founded by George Boole (1815–1864). This type of logic entails the principle of bivalence: any statement is either true or false. A third possibility or contradictions are excluded. Statements can be

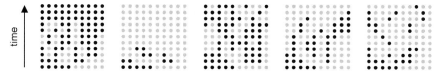

Fig. 10.6 Representative runs for the game of neutral evolution. Starting with five black balls and five white balls at generation T_0 (bottom line), the system converges within several generations to a state with either only black balls (left panel) or only white balls (second and forth panel from left). For the third and fifth panels, the final state is not yet decided at generation T_{10}.

combined using the operators "and," "or," or "not" and combinations thereof. The truth-value of combined statements depends only on the truth-value of the individual statements and their connection.

Boolean logic is applied to biological processes such as regulation of gene expression in the framework of Kauffman's NK Boolean networks (Kauffman and Weinberger 1989; Kauffman and Johnsen 1991; Kauffman 1993; Kauffman and Macready 1995). Genes are the elements of the network. Levels of gene expression are approximated by only two states: each gene is either expressed (is assigned the value "1") or not expressed ("0"). The network has N elements or nodes. Each element has K inputs (regulatory interactions) and one output. Input and output have binary values (1 or 0). The values are updated in discrete time steps.

Boolean networks always have a finite (although possibly large) number of possible states and hence only a finite number of possible state changes. The state changes of an individual element are specified by rules that relate the output to the inputs. There are 2^{2^K} possible rules for a node with K inputs. The labeling of the rules corresponds to numbers representing the respective binary numbers of output or to their meaning in normal life (*and, or*) (see Tabs. 10.1 and 10.2).

Tab. 10.1 Boolean rules for $K = 1$. The rules represent a functional dependence of the output of an element from the input. The second row indicates verbal notions for the rules, and the last row presents the numbering of the rules according to the decimal value of the binary number corresponding to the output values.

Input	Output			
A	0	A	not A	1
0	0	0	1	1
1	0	1	0	1
Rule	0	1	2	3

Tab. 10.2 Boolean rules for $K = 2$. The rules represent a functional dependence of the output of an element from the input (e. g., "xor" = "exclusive or," "nor" = "not or," "nand" = "not and"). The second row indicates verbal notions for the rules, and the last row presents the numbering of the rules according to the decimal value of the binary number corresponding to the output values.

Input		Output															
A	B	0	and		A		B	xor	or	nor		not B		not A		nand	1
0	0	0	0	0	0	0	0	0	0	1	1	1	1	1	1	1	1
0	1	0	0	0	0	1	1	1	1	0	0	0	0	1	1	1	1
1	0	0	0	1	1	0	0	1	1	0	0	1	1	0	0	1	1
1	1	0	1	0	1	0	1	0	1	0	1	0	1	0	1	0	1
Rule		0	1	2	3	4	5	6	7	8	9	10	11	12	13	14	15

Example 10-5

The network

$$A \longrightarrow B \longrightarrow C \longrightarrow D \qquad (10\text{-}28)$$

has the connectivity $K = 1$. Let $A = const.$, $B = f(A) = \text{not } A$, $C = f(B) = \text{not } B$, and $D = f(C) = C$, with the initial state $(A,B,C,D)(t_0) = (1,0,0,0)$. The following states are

$$(A,B,C,D)(t_1) = (1,0,0,1)$$

$$(A,B,C,D)(t_2) = (1,0,1,1)$$

...

$$(A,B,C,D)(t_i) = (1,0,1,1) \quad \text{for} \quad i = 2, ..., \infty.$$

After two steps the system has attained a fix point.

Example 10-6

$$\begin{array}{c} A \longrightarrow B \\ \nearrow \qquad \searrow \\ E \qquad \qquad C \\ \nwarrow_{D}\nearrow \end{array} \qquad (10\text{-}29)$$

Another typical structure of a Boolean network with $K = 1$ is the closed loop, where the input of the first element is the output of the last element.
Periodic behavior is possible if all elements obey rules 1 or 2. Assume, for example, that all elements follow rule 1 and the initial state is $(ABCDE) = (10000)$. The states for the following time steps will be (01000), (00100), (00010), (00001), and again (10000), which closes the cycle. Rules 0 or 3 break the periodic behavior, since the output of the respective element is no longer dependent on the input.

Example 10-7

The network

$$\qquad (10\text{-}30)$$

has $N = 3$ elements and may assume $2^N = 8$ different states. Let the rules be as follows:

$$A(t+1) = A(t) \text{ and } B(t)$$
$$B(t+1) = A(t) \text{ or } \quad B(t)$$
$$C(t+1) = A(t) \text{ or } \quad (\text{not } B(t) \text{ and } C(t))$$

The following table lists the possible actual states and the respective following states for (ABC).

Actual state	000	001	010	011	100	101	110	111
Next state	000	001	010	010	011	011	111	111

It can be seen that the states (000), (001), (010), and (111) are fix points, since they will not be left. The states (000), (001), (100), (101), and (110) cannot be reached from other states (see also Fig. 10.7).

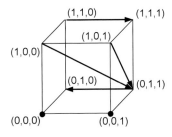

Fig. 10.7 The eight possible states for a network of $N = 3$ elements are represented as corners of a cube. The possible transitions are symbolized by arrows.

An NK automaton is an autonomous random network of N elements with K inputs and one output per element. The Boolean elements of the network and the connections between elements are chosen randomly. There are no external inputs to the network. The number of elements N is assumed to be large. Since N and K are finite, the number of possible states is also finite – although possibly too large to be inspected in reasonable time.

In reverse engineering of gene expression networks, it is of interest how many gene expression states have to be measured independently to find out the network connections. It has been estimated that this number is about 2^N for fully connected Boolean networks, about $K \cdot 2^K \log(N)$ for networks with connectivity K, and about $\log(N)$ in the case of pairwise correlation of gene expression values.

10.3
Prediction of Biological Systems from Optimality Principles

Biological systems developed through evolution by mutation and selection. Evolution can be considered as an optimization process that took place over millions of years. It seems that present-day systems show properties that are optimal with respect to certain selective conditions. Hence, system properties may be predicted from mathematical models based on optimality criteria.

Evolution is considered to be without aim or direction, but it forces development of species towards maximizing fitness. The formulation of a function that measures fitness is not straightforward. Several optimality criteria have been proposed. For cellular reaction systems, they involve, e.g., (1) maximization of steady-state fluxes, (2) minimization of the concentrations of metabolic intermediates, (3) minimization of transition times, (4) maximization of sensitivity to an external signal, and (5) optimization of thermodynamic efficiencies (Heinrich and Schuster 1998).

Evolution and optimization of cellular systems are subject to physical constraints. Such constraints include, for example, differences in free energy for participants of a reaction expressed by the equilibrium constant, diffusion limitations in the movement of compounds through the cell, structural requirements in the composition of macromolecules, or the stoichiometry of metabolic systems.

In order to take into account biological constraints, the concept of a cost function has been introduced (Reich 1983). The following have been suggested as cost functions: the total amount of enzyme in a cell or the pathway under consideration (Reich 1983), the total energy utilization (Stucki 1980), or the evolutionary effort (Heinrich and Holzhutter 1985) counting the number of mutations or events necessary to attain a certain state.

In the following three sections we will study how metabolic networks should be designed if they were designed according to optimality principles. We investigate the consequences of the demand for rapid conversion of substrate into product on the catalytic properties of single enzymes and on the appropriate amount of enzymes in a metabolic pathway. In the first two sections, we determine conditions that yield maximal steady-state fluxes. In the third section, an example for temporal regulation of pathway properties is studied.

10.3.1
Optimization of Catalytic Properties of Single Enzymes

An important function of enzymes is to increase the rate of a reaction. Therefore, evolutionary pressure should lead towards a maximization of the reaction rate $v \to \max$ (Pettersson 1989, 1992; Heinrich and Hoffmann 1991; Wilhelm et al. 1994). High reaction rates may be achieved only if the kinetic properties of the enzymes are suitably adapted. We identify the optimal kinetic parameters that maximize rates for the reversible conversion of substrate S into product P (Klipp and Heinrich 1994).

There are two constraints to be considered. First, the action of an enzyme cannot alter the thermodynamic equilibrium constant for the conversion of S to P (Eq. (5-13)). Changes of kinetic properties must obey the thermodynamic constraint. Second, the values of the kinetic parameters are limited by physical constraints even for the best enzymes. Their maximal possible values are denoted by k^{max}, and we consider all rate constants to be normalized by their respective k^{max}, such that the maximal values of the normalized kinetic constants are one.

For a reaction that can be described with linear kinetics

$$E+S \underset{k_{-1}}{\overset{k_1}{\rightleftarrows}} E+P \tag{10-31}$$

with the thermodynamic equilibrium constant

$$q = k_1/k_{-1}, \tag{10-32}$$

the rate equation reads

$$v = E_{total} \cdot (S \cdot k_1 - P \cdot k_{-1}) = E_{total} \cdot k_{-1} \cdot (S \cdot q - P) = E_{total} \cdot k_1 \cdot \left(S - \frac{P}{q} \right). \tag{10-33}$$

It is easy to see that v becomes maximal for fixed values of E, S, P, and q, if k_1 and k_{-1} become maximal. Note that usually only one of the two rate constants may attain its maximal value. The value of the other, submaximal constant is given by Eq. (10-32).

For the reversible reaction obeying the Michaelis-Menten kinetics (Eq. (5-34)) with the reaction rate given in Eq. (5-36), the optimal result depends on the value of P. For $P \le 1/q$ the rate becomes maximal if k_1, k_2, and k_{-2} assume maximal values and k_{-1} is submaximal (R_1 in Fig. 10.8). For $P \ge q$ we obtain submaximal values of only k_{-2} (R_2). For $1/q < P < q$ the optimal solution is characterized by submaximal values of k_{-1} and k_{-2}, with $k_{-1} = \sqrt{P/q}$ and $k_{-2} = \sqrt{1/(Pq)}$ (R_3).

Comparison of the optimal state with a reference state can assess the effect of the optimization. One choice for a reference state is $k_1 = k_2 = 1$ and $k_{-1} = k_{-2} = 1/\sqrt{q}$, i.e., equal distribution of the free energy difference represented by the equilibrium constant on the first and the second step. The respective reference rate reads

$$v^{ref} = \frac{Sq - P}{(S+1)q + (P+1)\sqrt{q}}$$ and the optimal rate in regions R_1, R_2, and R_3 read

$$v^{opt, R_1} = \frac{Sq - P}{(S+1)q + 1 + Pq}, \quad v^{opt, R_2} = \frac{Sq - P}{(S+1)q + q + P}, \quad \text{and } v^{opt, R_3} = \frac{Sq - P}{(S+1)q + 2\sqrt{Pq}}.$$

For example, in the case $P = q$ and $q = 100$, the maximal rate for optimal kinetic constants is $v^{max} = \frac{S-1}{S+3}$ and the reference rate calculates as $v^{ref} = \frac{S-1}{S+11.1}$, which is lower than the maximal rate.

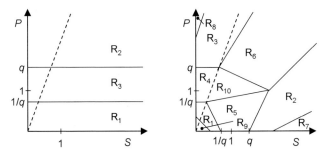

Fig. 10.8 Subdivision of the plane of substrate and product concentrations (S, P) into regions of different solutions for the optimal microscopic rate constants (schematic representation). The dashed lines indicate the function $Sq = P$. (a) Solution regions for the two-step mechanism. (b) Solution regions for the three-step mechanism.

For the reversible three-step mechanism involving the binding of the substrate to the enzyme, the isomerization of the ES complex to an EP complex, and the release of product from the enzyme

$$E+S \underset{k_{-1}}{\overset{k_1}{\rightleftharpoons}} ES \underset{k_{-2}}{\overset{k_2}{\rightleftharpoons}} EP \underset{k_{-2}}{\overset{k_3}{\rightleftharpoons}} E+P \tag{10-34}$$

the reaction rate is given as

$$v = E_{total} \cdot \frac{S \cdot k_1 k_2 k_3 - P \cdot k_{-1}k_{-2}k_{-3}}{k_2 k_3 + k_{-1}k_3 + k_{-1}k_{-2} + S \cdot k_1 (k_2 + k_3 + k_{-2}) + P \cdot k_{-3}(k_2 + k_{-1} + k_{-2})} \tag{10-35}$$

It turns out that the optimal solution for this mechanism depends on the values of both S and P; there are 10 different solutions (see Tab. 10.3 and Fig. 10.8).

There are three solutions with a submaximal value of one backward rate constant, three solutions with submaximal values of two backward rate constants, three solutions with submaximal values of one backward and one forward rate constant, and one solution with submaximal values of all three backward rate constants. The con-

Tab. 10.3 Optimal solutions for the rate constants of the three-step enzymatic reaction as functions of the concentrations of substrate and product for $q \geq 1$.

Solution	k_1	k_{-1}	k_2	k_{-2}	k_3	k_{-3}
R_1	1	$1/q$	1	1	1	1
R_2	1	1	1	$1/q$	1	1
R_3	1	1	1	1	1	$1/q$
R_4	1	$\sqrt{P/q}$	1	1	1	$\sqrt{1/Pq}$
R_5	1	$\sqrt{\dfrac{S+P}{q(1+P)}}$	1	$\sqrt{\dfrac{1+P}{q(S+P)}}$	1	1
R_6	1	1	1	$\sqrt{\dfrac{2P}{q(1+S)}}$	1	$\sqrt{\dfrac{1+S}{2Pq}}$
R_7	$\sqrt{\dfrac{2q(1+P)}{S}}$	1	1	$\sqrt{\dfrac{2(1+P)}{qS}}$	1	1
R_8	1	1	$\sqrt{\dfrac{2q(1+S)}{P}}$	1	1	$\sqrt{\dfrac{2(1+S)}{qP}}$
R_9	1	$\sqrt{\dfrac{2(S+P)}{q}}$	1	1	$\sqrt{2q(S+P)}$	1
R_{10}	1	*	1	$\dfrac{P}{qk_{-1}^2}$	1	$\dfrac{1}{qk_{-1}k_{-2}}$

* k_{-1} is the solution to the equation $k_{-1}^4 + k_{-1}^3 - k_{-1}\dfrac{P}{q} - \dfrac{SP}{q} = 0$

straint imposed by the thermodynamic equilibrium constant leads to the following effects. At very low substrate and product concentrations, maximal rate is achieved by improving the binding of S and P to the enzyme (the so-called high (S,P)-affinity solution). If S or P is present in very high concentrations, they are weakly bound (low S- or P-affinity solutions). For intermediate values of S and P, only backward constants assume submaximal values. For concentrations of S and P equal to unity, the optimal solution reads

$$k_{-1} = k_{-2} = k_{-3} = q^{-1/3} \quad \text{and} \quad k_1 = k_2 = k_3 = 1. \tag{10-36}$$

This case represents an equal distribution of the drop in free energy on all three elementary steps.

10.3.2
Optimal Distribution of Enzyme Concentrations in a Metabolic Pathway

By means of regulated gene expression and protein degradation, cells can adjust the amount of enzyme allocated to the reactions of a metabolic pathway according to the current metabolic supply and demand. In many cases the individual amounts of enzymes should be regulated such that the metabolic fluxes necessary for the maintenance of cell functions can be achieved while the total enzyme amount is low. One reason for this is that enzymes are osmotically active substances. One strategy to achieve osmotic balance is, therefore, to keep the total amount of enzyme constrained. Furthermore, enzyme synthesis is expensive for the cell, with respect to both energy and material. It is therefore reasonable to assume that various pathways or even individual reactions compete for the available resources.

In theoretical terms we can study how a maximal steady-state flux through a pathway is achieved with a given fixed total amount of enzyme (Klipp and Heinrich 1999). The optimization problem is to distribute the total protein concentration $E_{total} = \sum_{i=1}^{r} E_i$ optimally among the r reactions. We will exemplify this for the simple unbranched pathway presented in Eq. (5-180). To assess the effect of optimization we will compare the optimal state to a reference state where the given total concentration of enzymes is distributed uniformly such that $E_i = E_{total}/r$.

The optimal enzyme concentrations E_i^{opt} in states of maximal steady-state flux J can be determined by the variational equation

$$\frac{\partial}{\partial E_i}\left(J - \lambda\left(\sum_{i=1}^{r} E_i - E_{total}\right)\right) = 0 \quad (i = 1, .., r), \tag{10-37}$$

where λ denotes the Lagrange multiplier. From this equation it follows that

$$\frac{\partial J}{\partial E_i} = \lambda, \tag{10-38}$$

and by multiplication with E_i^{opt}/J we find that

$$\frac{E_i^{opt}}{J}\left(\frac{\partial J}{\partial E_i}\right)_{E_j=E_j^{opt}} = \frac{E_i^{opt}}{J}\lambda . \tag{10-39}$$

The left-hand term of Eq. (10-39) represents the flux-control coefficient $(C_i)_{E_j=E_j^{opt}} = C_i^{opt}$ of reaction i over steady-state flux J in optimal states. Since the sum of the flux-control coefficients over all reactions equals unity (summation theorem, Eq. (5-143)), it follows that

$$1 = \sum_{i=1}^{r} \frac{E_i^{opt}}{J}\lambda = \frac{E_{total}}{J}\lambda . \tag{10-40}$$

Therefore, it holds that

$$C_i^{opt} = \frac{E_i^{opt}}{E_{total}} . \tag{10-41}$$

This means that the allocation of the flux-control coefficient in optimal states (here: states of maximal steady-state fluxes), C_i^{opt}, is equal to the allocation of the relative enzyme concentrations along the pathway.

Example 10-8

For the special case that every reaction of the pathway obeys mass action kinetics $v_i = E_i(k_i S_{i-1} - k_{-i} S_i)$ with the equilibrium constant $q_i = k_i/k_{-i}$, the expression for the steady-state flux reads

$$J = \frac{P_0 \prod\limits_{j=1}^{r} q_j - P_r}{\sum\limits_{l=1}^{r} \frac{1}{E_l k_l} \prod\limits_{m=l}^{r} q_m} . \tag{10-42}$$

Introducing Eq. (10-42) into Eq. (10-38) leads to

$$E_i^{opt} = \frac{E_{total}}{r} \frac{\sqrt{Y_i}\sum\limits_{h=1}^{r}\sqrt{Y_h}}{\sum\limits_{l=1}^{r} Y_l} \quad \text{with} \quad Y_m = \frac{1}{k_m}\prod\limits_{n=m}^{r} q_n . \tag{10-43}$$

And for the flux-control coefficients it holds that

$$C_i^{opt} = \frac{\sqrt{Y_i}}{\sum\limits_{h=1}^{r}\sqrt{Y_h}} . \tag{10-44}$$

The distribution of flux-control coefficients in the reference state is given in Eq. (5-182).

The effect of optimization for a chain of four consecutive reactions is discussed in Example 5-27 and is shown in Fig. 5.9. The larger the deviation of the value of equilibrium constant q from 1, the stronger the effect of the optimization is, i.e., the larger the difference between maximal flux and reference flux is.

The problem of maximizing the steady-state flux at a given total amount of enzyme is related to the problem of minimizing the total enzyme concentration that allows for a given steady-state flux. For an unbranched reaction pathway (Eq. (5-180)), obeying the flux equation (Eq. (10-42)), the minimization of E_{total} results in the same optimal allocation of relative enzyme concentrations and flux-control coefficients as maximization of J.

The principle of minimizing the total enzyme concentration at fixed steady-state fluxes is in some respect more general since it may also be applied to branched reaction networks. Application of the principle of maximal steady-state flux to branched networks either could lead to conflicting interests between different fluxes in different branches or necessitate determination of an objective function that balances the weight of the different fluxes.

Special conditions hold for the flux-control coefficients in states of minimal total enzyme concentration at fixed steady-state fluxes. Since the reaction rates v_i are proportional to the enzyme concentrations, a fixation of the steady-state fluxes J^0 leads to the following relation between enzyme concentrations and substrate concentrations:

$$E_i = E_i(S_1, S_2, .., S_{r-1}) = \frac{v_i^0}{f_i}, \tag{10-45}$$

where the function f_i expresses the thermodynamic part of the reaction rate that is independent of the enzyme concentration. The principle of minimal total enzyme concentration implies that

$$\frac{\partial E_{total}}{\partial S_j} = -\sum_{i=1}^{r} \frac{v_i^0}{f_i^2} \frac{\partial f_i}{\partial S_j} = 0, \tag{10-46}$$

which determines the metabolite concentrations in the optimal state. Since $f_i = v_i^0 / E_i$, it follows that

$$\frac{E_i^{opt}}{v_i^0} \frac{\partial v_i^0}{\partial S_j} = 0, \tag{10-47}$$

and in matrix representation

$$\left(\frac{d\mathbf{v}}{d\mathbf{S}}\right)^T (dg\,\mathbf{J})^{-1} \mathbf{E}^{opt} = \mathbf{0}, \tag{10-48}$$

where $\boldsymbol{E}^{opt}$ is the vector containing the optimal enzyme concentrations. An expression for the flux-control coefficients in matrix representation has been given in Eq. (5-163). Its transposed matrix reads

$$\left(\boldsymbol{C}^{J}\right)^{T} = \boldsymbol{I} - \left(dg\,\boldsymbol{J}\right)\boldsymbol{N}^{T}\left(\left(\boldsymbol{N}\frac{\partial\boldsymbol{v}}{\partial\boldsymbol{S}}\right)^{-1}\right)^{T}\left(\frac{\partial\boldsymbol{v}}{\partial\boldsymbol{S}}\right)^{T}\left(dg\,\boldsymbol{J}\right)^{-1}. \tag{10-49}$$

Post-multiplication with the vector $\boldsymbol{E}^{opt}$ leads to

$$\left(\boldsymbol{C}^{J}\right)^{T}\boldsymbol{E}^{opt} = \boldsymbol{E}^{opt} \tag{10-50}$$

under consideration of Eq. (10-48). Equation (10-50) represents a functional relation between enzyme concentrations and flux-control coefficients for enzymatic networks in states of minimal total enzyme concentration.

10.3.3
Temporal Transcription Programs

In this section, temporal adaptation of enzyme concentration is studied (Klipp et al. 2002) rather than steady-state solutions. Consider a pathway that can be switched on or off by the cell depending on actual requirements. The product P of the pathway is important but is not essential for the reproduction of the cell. The faster the initial substrate S_0 can be converted into P, the more efficiently the cell may reproduce and outcompete other individuals. If S_0 is available, then the cell produces the enzymes of the pathway to make use of the substrate. If the substrate is not available, then for economical reasons the cell does not synthesize the respective enzymes. Bacterial amino acid synthesis is organized this way. This scenario shall be studied theoretically by starting with a resting pathway (i.e., although the genes for the enzymes are present, they are not expressed due to lack of the substrate). Suddenly, S_0 appears in the environment (by feeding or change of place). How can the cell make use of S_0 as soon as possible?

The system of ODEs describing the dynamics of the pathway reads

$$\frac{dS_0}{dt} = -k_1 \cdot E_1 \cdot S_0$$

$$\frac{dS_i}{dt} = k_i \cdot E_i \cdot S_{i-1} - k_{i+1} \cdot E_{i+1} \cdot S_i \quad (i = 1, .., n-1)$$

$$\frac{dP}{dt} = k_n \cdot E_n \cdot S_{n-1}. \tag{10-51}$$

For simplicity's sake, we assume that the cell can make the enzymes instantaneously when necessary (neglecting the time necessary for transcription and translation) but that the total amount of enzyme is limited due to limited capacity of the cell to produce and store proteins. The time necessary to produce P from S_0 is measured as transition time

$$\tau = \frac{1}{S_0(0)} \int\limits_{t=0}^{\infty} (S_0(0) - P(t))\, dt.$$ (10-52)

The optimization problem to be solved is to find a temporal profile of enzyme concentrations that allows for $\tau = \min$ at $E_{tot} = \sum_{i=1}^{n} E_i(t) = const.$

Example 10-9

For a pathway consisting of only $n = 2$ reactions with $k_i = k\,(i = 1, ..., n)$, there is an explicit solution (Klipp et al. 2002). The optimal enzyme profile consists of two phases and an abrupt switch at time T_1. In the first interval for $0 \le t \le T_1$, only the first enzyme is present. In the second interval for $T_1 < t < \infty$, both enzymes are present with a constant concentration. The switching time is $T_1 = \textit{ln}\,(2/(3 - \sqrt{5}))$. In the first interval it holds that $E_1 = E_{total}$, $E_2 = 0$, and in the second interval it holds that $E_1 = E_{total} \cdot (3 - \sqrt{5})/2$, $E_2 = E_{total} \cdot (\sqrt{5} - 1)/2$. Note, for curiosity, that here the ratio E_2/E_1 equals the Golden Ratio (i.e., $(1 + \sqrt{5})/2:1$). The minimal transition time for these optimal concentrations is $\tau_{min} = 1 + T_1 + (1 - e^{-T_1})^{-1} = 3.58$ in units of $(k \cdot E_{total})^{-1}$. This means that in the first phase all available enzymes are used to catabolize the initial substrate; product is made only in the second phase. The fastest possible conversion of S_0 to P employs a delayed onset in formation of P that favors an accelerated decay of S_0 in the initial phase and pays off in the second phase. The temporal profiles of enzyme and metabolite concentrations are shown in Fig. 10.9.

To solve the optimization problem for pathways with n enzymes, the time axis can be divided into m intervals in which the enzyme concentrations are constant. The quantities to be optimized are the switching times T_1, T_2, ... defining the time intervals and the enzyme concentrations during these intervals. In the reference case with only one interval ($m = 0$ switches), the optimal enzyme concentrations are all equal ($E_i = E_{total}/n\ (i = 1, ..., n)$). The optimal transition time for this case reads $\tau = n^2$ in units of $(k \cdot E_{total})^{-1}$. Permitting one switch ($m = 1$) between intervals of constant enzyme concentrations allows for a considerably lower transition time. An increasing number of possible switches ($m > 1$) leads to a decrease in the transition time un-

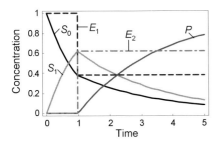

Fig. 10.9 Optimal enzyme and metabolite concentration time profiles for a linear metabolic pathway as explained in Example 10-9.

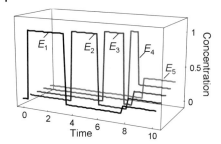

Fig. 10.10 Optimal temporal enzyme profiles yielding the minimal transition time for a pathway of five reactions. The switching times are $T_1 = 3.08$, $T_2 = 5.28$, $T_3 = 6.77$, and $T_4 = 7.58$.

til the number of switches reaches $m = n - 1$. The corresponding optimal enzyme profiles have the following characteristics. Within any time interval, except for the last one, only a single enzyme is fully active, whereas all others are shut off. At the beginning of the process, the whole amount of available protein is spent exclusively to the first enzyme of the chain. Each of the following switches turns off the active enzyme and allocates the total amount of protein to the enzyme that catalyzes the following reaction. The last switch allocates a finite fraction of protein to all enzymes with increasing amounts from the first one to the last one (Fig. 10.10).

If one compares the case of no switch (the reference case) with the case of $m = n - 1$ switches, the drop in transition time (gain in turnover speed) amplifies with increasing length n of the reaction chain. This simple example shows that temporal adjustment of enzyme activities, e. g., by regulation of gene expression, may lead to a considerable improvement in metabolic efficiency. Bacterial amino acid production pathways are possibly regulated in the described manner: Zaslaver and colleagues (2004) experimentally investigated the amino acid biosynthesis systems of *Escherichia coli*, identified the temporal expression pattern, and showed a hierarchy of expression that matches the enzyme order in the unbranched pathways.

References

BURCH, C.L. and CHAO, L. Evolvability of an RNA virus is determined by its mutational neighbourhood (2000) Nature *406*, 625–8.

DARWIN, C. The Origin of Species (1859).

DOMINGO, E. and HOLLAND, J.H. RNA virus mutations and fitness for survival (1997) Annu. Rev. Microbiol. *51*, 151–178.

EIGEN, M. Molecular self-organization and the early stages of evolution (1971a) Q Rev Biophys *4*, 149–212.

EIGEN, M. Molekulare Selbstorganisation und Evolution (Self organization of matter and the evolution of biological macro molecules) (1971b) Naturwissenschaften *58*, 465–523.

EIGEN, M. and SCHUSTER, P. The hypercycle. A principle of natural self-organization.

Part A: Emergence of the hypercycle (1977) Naturwissenschaften *64*, 541–65.

EIGEN, M. and SCHUSTER, P. The hyper cycle. A principle of natural self organization. Part B. The abstract hypercycle. (1978) Naturwissenschaften *65*, 7–41.

EIGEN, M. and SCHUSTER, P. The hypercycle – A principle of natural self-organization (1979) Springer-Verlag, Berlin.

EIGEN, M. and SCHUSTER, P. Stages of emerging life–five principles of early organization (1982) J. Mol. Evol. *19*, 47–61.

EIGEN, M., GARDINER, W.C., JR. and SCHUSTER, P. Hypercycles and compartments. Compartments assist – but do not replace – hypercyclic organization of early genetic information (1980a) J. Theor. Biol. *85*, 407–11.

EIGEN, M., SCHUSTER, P., SIGMUND, K. and WOLFF, R. Elementary step dynamics of catalytic hypercycles (1980 b) Biosystems *13*, 1–22.

FOGEL, L.J., OWENS, A.J. and WALSH, M.J. Artificial intelligence through simulated evolution (1966) Wiley, New York.

HEINRICH, R. and HOFFMANN, E. Kinetic parameters of enzymatic reactions in states of maximal activity; an evolutionary approach (1991) J. Theor. Biol. *151*, 249–83.

HEINRICH, R. and HOLZHUTTER, H.G. Efficiency and design of simple metabolic systems (1985) Biomed. Biochim. Acta *44*, 959–69.

HEINRICH, R. and SCHUSTER, S. The modelling of metabolic systems. Structure, control and optimality (1998) Biosystems *47*, 61–77.

HOLLAND, J.H. Adaptation in natural and artificial systems (1975) MIT Press, Boston.

HOLLAND, J.H. Adaptation in natural and artifical systems (1992) MIT Press, Cambridge, MA.

KAUFFMAN, S.A. Antichaos and adaptation (1991) Sci. Am. *265*, 78–84.

KAUFFMAN, S.A. The origins of order: Self-organization and selection in evolution (1993) Oxford University Press, New York.

KAUFFMAN, S.A. and JOHNSEN, S. Coevolution to the edge of chaos: coupled fitness landscapes, poised states, and coevolutionary avalanches (1991) J. Theor. Biol. *149*, 467–505.

KAUFFMAN, S.A. and MACREADY, W.G. Search strategies for applied molecular evolution (1995) J. Theor. Biol. *173*, 427–40.

KAUFFMAN, S.A. and WEINBERGER, E.D. The NK model of rugged fitness landscapes and its application to maturation of the immune response (1989) J. Theor. Biol. *141*, 211–45.

KIMURA, M. The neutral theory of molecular evolution (1979) Sci. Am. *241*, 98–100, 102, 108 passim.

KIMURA, M. The neutral theory of molecular evolution (1983) Cambridge University Press, Cambridge.

KIMURA, M. and OTA, T. On the rate of molecular evolution (1971) J. Mol. Evol. *1*, 1–17.

KIMURA, M. and OTA, T. On some principles governing molecular evolution (1974) Proc. Natl. Acad. Sci. USA *71*, 2848–52.

KLIPP, E. and HEINRICH, R. Evolutionary optimization of enzyme kinetic parameters; effect of constraints (1994) J. Theor. Biol. *171*, 309–23.

KLIPP, E. and HEINRICH, R. Competition for enzymes in metabolic pathways: implications for optimal distributions of enzyme concentrations and for the distribution of flux control (1999) Biosystems *54*, 1–14.

KLIPP, E., HEINRICH, R. and HOLZHUTTER, H.G. Prediction of temporal gene expression. Metabolic opimization by re-distribution of enzyme activities (2002) Eur. J. Biochem. *269*, 5406–13.

KOZA, J.R., MYDLOWEC, W., LANZA, G., YU, J. and KEANE, M.A. Reverse engineering of metabolic pathways from observed data using genetic programming (2001) Pac. Symp. Biocomput. 434–45.

OHNO, S. Evolution by gene duplication (1970) Springer-Verlag, Berlin.

PETTERSSON, G. Effect of evolution on the kinetic properties of enzymes (1989) Eur. J. Biochem. *184*, 561–6.

PETTERSSON, G. Evolutionary optimization of the catalytic efficiency of enzymes (1992) Eur. J. Biochem. *206*, 289–95.

RECHENBERG, I. Evolutionsstragie 94 (1994) Friedrich Frommann Verlag.

REICH, J.G. The economy of protein maintenance in the living cell (1983) Biomed. Biochim. Acta *42*, 839–48.

SCHUSTER, P., SIGMUND, K. and WOLFF, R. Dynamical systems under constant organization I. Topological analysis of a family of nonlinear differential equations–a model for catalytic hypercycles (1978) Bull. Math. Biol. *40*, 743–69.

SHERRINGTON, D. and KIRKPATRICK, S. Solvable model of a spin glass (1975) Phys. Rev. Lett. *35*, 1792–1796.

SHERRINGTON, D. and KIRKPATRICK, S. Infiniteranged models of spin-glasses (1978) Phys. Rev. B *17*, 4384.

STUCKI, J.W. The optimal efficiency and the economic degrees of coupling of oxidative phosphorylation (1980) Eur. J. Biochem. *109*, 269–83.

SWETINA, J. and SCHUSTER, P. Self-replication with errors. A model for polynucleotide replication (1982) Biophys. Chem. *16*, 329–45.

WATSON, J.D. and CRICK, F.H. Genetical implications of the structure of deoxyribonucleic acid (1953 a) Nature *171*, 964–7.

WATSON, J.D. and CRICK, F.H. Molecular structure of nucleic acids; a structure for deoxyribose nucleic acid (1953 b) Nature *171*, 737–8.

WATSON, J.D. and CRICK, F.H. The structure of

DNA (1953 c) Cold Spring Harb. Symp. Quant. Biol. *18*, 123–31.

WILHELM, T., HOFFMANN-KLIPP, E. and HEINRICH, R. An evolutionary approach to enzyme kinetics; optimization of ordered mechanisms. (1994) Bull. Math. Biol. *56*, 65–106.

ZASLAVER, A., MAYO, A.E., ROSENBERG, R., BASHKIN, P., SBERRO, H., TSALYUK, M., SURETTE, M.G. and ALON, U. Just-in-time transcription program in metabolic pathways (2004) Nat. Genet. *36*, 486–91.

11
Data Integration

Introduction

In this chapter we follow our data integration schema outlined in Section 1.3. Data integration is a central part of systems biology. The typical data integration problems arising in practical research can be described on three levels of complexity.

The first level of data integration consists of the integration of heterogeneous data resources and databases with the aim to parse data between these databases and to query for information. There are multiple databases available today covering DNA and protein sequences of various organisms, experimental data, interaction data, pathway data, databases of chemical compounds, etc. (for a review of important databases, see Chapter 13). Technically, database integration requires the definition of data exchange protocols and languages as well as the development of parsers that interconnect the databases to a data layer that is able to display the heterogeneous data sources in a unified way.

The second level of data integration consists of the identification of correlative associations across different datasets with the aim to gain a more comprehensive and coherent view of the same objects in light of the diverse data sources. For example, transcription factor–binding sites are correlated with gene expression profiles (cf. Section 8.2) and protein and gene expression are analyzed simultaneously to derive cellular networks (Ideker et al. 2002). To identify such correlative associations across heterogeneous data is mainly a task of defining adequate statistical procedures that are robust enough to cope with the diversity of the data. Furthermore, conflicts in data measurements have to be handled.

The third level is focused on mapping of the information gained for interactions of the objects into networks and pathways that may be used as basic models for the underlying cellular systems. The task here is to define common sets of objects that show a similar behavior through subsets of experimental conditions. In contrast to the analysis of data from a single source, as described with DNA arrays in Chapter 9, data integration methods allow the joint analysis of experimental conditions from various sources.

In this chapter we discuss solutions and some practical applications for each of these three data integration levels. Section 11.1 discusses the main concepts and problems of database integration. This has been a major research topic in recent years and several practical solutions exist, based mainly on two concepts: database federa-

Systems Biology in Practice. Concepts, Implementation and Application.
E. Klipp, R. Herwig, A. Kowald, C. Wierling, H. Lehrach
Copyright © 2005 WILEY-VCH Verlag GmbH & Co. KGaA, Weinheim
ISBN: 3-527-31078-9

tion and data warehouse. As an example of a federated system, we describe the SRS tool, while the EnsMart tool illustrates an application of a data warehouse system. Furthermore, we discuss XML, the most prominent data-exchange format. We list several XML-based languages for the storage and exchange of data that are relevant in systems biology. In Section 11.2 we introduce a specific concept of defining correlative associations across different datasets – information measurement based on the entropy concept. This concept is widely used in electrical engineering and mathematics and has also recently found some applications in bioinformatics. Section 11.3 describes the integration of different data sources and the identification of groups of objects and groups of conditions using the biclustering framework, which is an extension of the general clustering concept (cf. Section 9.3).

11.1
Database Networks

There are many autonomous databases for functional genomics and systems biology research, some of which are described in Chapter 13. In practical research the user typically needs a number of these databases in parallel for conducting research. Most of the public biological databases were originally stored in plain text files. As the size and complexity of data increased, these databases incorporated database management systems. Users can access them by submitting queries via Web interfaces or by downloading the entire database, in text format, to a local machine. Direct access to the database through the database management system is often not allowed. Some of the most popular databases are sequence databases such as GenBank at NCBI, EMBL at EBI, and the DNA Databank of Japan (DDBJ); protein-related databases such as SWISS-PROT, PDB, and Pfam; and bibliographic databases such as PubMed. These databases include a broad range of information that is specific neither to a given organism nor to a given subject matter. Another group of databases includes information related to a specific subject such as the study of a given organism or the study of a given biological process (e.g., metabolic pathways). Subject-specific databases include, e.g., MGD (mouse genome database); SGD (*Saccharomyces* genome database); FlyBase; BRENDA, a database on enzyme-related information; and MetaCyc, a metabolic pathway database that integrates pathway information from various literature databases. A comprehensive recent list of available databases can be found in Baxevanis (2003).

Most of these databases have connections to each other and allow browsing queries among each other. However, this browsing process allows just screening one database after another. Consideration of the heterogeneity and complexity of the data available for the same object (gene, protein) has identified the need for tools that enable simultaneous queries across whole networks of databases. In this section we introduce the basic concepts of such database connections and describe some of the currently available tools for database integration, in particular SRS and EnsMart. Furthermore, we will describe data-exchange formats based on XML.

11.1.1
Basic Concepts of Database Integration

A database integration system connects distributed databases and involves several of the following steps:

1. integration of the schemas of the individual databases to a common data model,
2. establishment of the relationship between the objects in different databases,
3. decomposing of multi-database queries into database-specific sub-queries,
4. accessing the component databases to retrieve the data, and
5. combining the results of the sub-queries.

Database integration has to cope with severe practical problems. Biological data are highly complex. In addition, data vary between sequences, numerical values (e.g., gene expression values), and entire pathways so that the development of a common data schema is difficult. Furthermore, data are extremely heterogeneous, in particular considering the semantic aspect. For example, the term "gene" has different meanings in different database schemas. Semantic data integration attempts to resolve this problem and to enhance the quality and the completeness of integrated data from multiple sources through the use of ontologies, i.e., formal descriptions of the concepts and entities for a specific part of knowledge and the relations among them. Ontologies typically carry synonyms and lexical variants of terms (thesaurus) and apply them in the query process. An important challenge arises because data models for the different databases can vary. A data model is an abstraction of the entities (objects) and their relations in the database. It describes the constraints imposed on the data, how the attributes of an entity are structured, and how the entities (objects) are related to each other. There are two widely used data models: the relational model and the object-oriented model. Under the relational data model, the data are organized into a table format, where each column of the table represents an attribute of an object and each row (record) of the table represents a single entity. In each table, one or more attributes are designated as the primary key that is used to uniquely identify each record. To reduce redundancy and a data overhead, the entity-related information is often distributed among several tables that are linked via different keys. The object-oriented model is based on concepts that are similar to ones used in object-oriented programming languages. For example, encapsulation, inheritance, and polymorphism are also applicable to the object-oriented data model. Each data object is defined as a class that has multiple attributes. These attributes can describe features of the object or can be a reference to other classes. Usually, common attributes of several specific classes are subsumed into a more general class of which the specific classes can inherit. A further difficulty is the fact that data in different databases can be redundant and conflicting. Thus an important and yet partially unsolved problem in database integration is how to handle such data conflicts.

Different approaches to the database integration of biological databases have been proposed. Extendable data integration techniques follow two main approaches, database federation systems and data warehouses (data marts). One of the main advan-

A   B

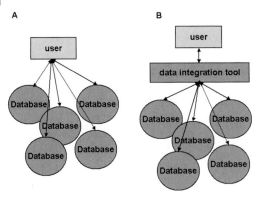

Fig. 11.1 Basic schema illustrating the concept of database integration. The common situation is that the user works with different heterogeneous and autonomous databases (a). This requires the interaction with each database, and each query has to be inserted into each database separately. (b) In a database integration setup the user interacts with the integration tool. Queries will then be translated by the integration tool and sent to the individual database and a consistent output will be provided.

tages of federated databases is that they do not require that component databases be physically combined into one database. A database federation system does not modify the primary data resources. The databases are connected through a specialized network service shared by applications (databases and tools) and users to create a virtual integrated database (Fig. 11.1).

In the data warehouse approach, the component databases are mapped to a single database called the data warehouse. Creating a data warehouse is a process that consists of two steps (Karp 1995). First the schemas of the component databases are mapped onto the global schema (i.e., the schema of the data warehouse). Second, data is extracted from the component databases and used to populate the data warehouse. A data warehouse stores the core data (a set of relational databases) in a central store. The warehouse is connected to other relational databases from which a subset of the data can be selectively extracted and loaded for analysis. Slightly different are data marts, which store specialized data derived from a data warehouse. The emphasis here is on content, presentation, and ease of use in formats familiar to the specialized user.

11.1.2
SRS

One of the first database integration platforms developed was SRS (Sequence Retrieval System). SRS was originally developed as a tool for providing easy access to biological sequence databases (Etzold and Argos 1993; Etzold et al. 1996) and has been extended to other data sources as well. SRS was acquired by LION Bioscience AG in 1998 and further developed as a commercial product. SRS version 6 is freely available for academic research. Currently, there are more than 100 servers worldwide (http://downloads.lionbio.co.uk/publicsrs.html). The EBI SRS server contains wrappers for more than 400 databases and 20 applications connected to the system. Applications include, for example, sequence-matching tools such as BLAST and FASTA.

The federated databases are stored locally with a query integration engine acting as middleware. SRS is based on the indexing of flat files. Text files are still the *de facto* standard for biological databases such as EMBL, SWISS-PROT, etc. XML files have a more structured format but are still considered as text files. In this system, each database record in any component database is processed separately as a collection of data fields. An index is created for each data field (data field index). This index classifies each record in the database according to a set of keywords from a controlled vocabulary. Each database will have one index per data field. A different type of index (link index) is used to link individual databases. A link index is created for each pair of databases that includes cross-references to each other and these links are bidirectional. Databases that do not directly reference each other can still be connected by traversing links through intermediate databases. SRS has a unique approach to addressing syntactic and semantic heterogeneities.

SRS has an object-oriented design. It uses metadata to define a class for a database entry object and rules for text-parsing methods, coupled with the entry attributes. SRS incorporates a proprietary parsing language (Icarus) for generating the database wrappers and another language (SRS query language) for the formulation of queries (Zdobnov et al. 2002). Data in SRS can be subdivided into sections that correspond to the main contents of the integrated databases such as DNA sequences, protein sequences, mapping data, SNPs, and metabolic processes.

SRS is a keyword-based system. Queries can be combined using logical operators such as "&" (AND), "|" (OR) and "!" (BUT NOT). An HTML interface is available for the formulation of queries and for viewing the results of the data retrieval. Thus, SRS can be used as a front end to independently query multiple data sources.

There are some APIs of SRS version 6 to most widely used programming languages such as C++ and Java. This allows the development of customized interfaces to proprietary analysis tools.

11.1.3
EnsMart

EnsMart (http://www.ensembl.org/EnsMart) provides a generic data warehouse system (Kasprzyk et al. 2004). The system organizes data from individual databases into one query-optimized system by the incorporation of the data-warehousing technique for descriptive data. Currently, it is focused on Ensembl and thus primarily entails data with genomic annotation such as genes and SNPs, functional annotation, and expression data. Data are available for nine different species annotated in Ensembl (*Homo sapiens, Mus musculus, Rattus norvegicus, Danio rerio, Fugu rubripes, Anopheles gambiae, Drosophila melanogaster, Caenorhabditis briggsae,* and *Caenorhabditis elegans*) (Birney et al. 2004).

EnsMart data are organized around central objects, so-called foci, and additional satellite data. Currently, two foci exist, gene and SNP, and all additional data are presented in relation to these foci. EnsMart comes up with three different user interfaces. The MartView is an Internet user interface in the "wizard" style. It allows navigating through pages to specify user input. Furthermore, it is used to specify the output format and to handle data export. The MartExplorer is a local database. It is installed as a program and has a graphical user interface that allows displaying the query as a tree in an interactive manner. The MartShell is a command line shell that uses a query language specifically designed for mart queries.

EnsMart has powerful querying facilities. The querying process is organized into three steps: start, filter, and output. The start stage specifies the organism and the focus for the query. The filter step offers the possibility of narrowing the search according to several criteria. For example, chromosomes and specific regions on the chromosome can be specified as an attribute using the region filter. Other filters restrict the search to specific gene classes ("novel genes," "disease genes," etc.) or genes that are mapped to a particular identifier (e.g., HUGO gene symbols). The output stage defines the attributes that are used for exporting the data. This is dependent on the focus that has been selected previously. Queries can be chained, i.e., the file output from previous queries can be used as filters for the current query.

11.1.4
DiscoveryLink

DiscoveryLink was developed by IBM and is another example of a federated database approach. It has been the result of the fusion of two products: IBM's Garlic federated database prototype for multimedia information and DataJoiner, a federated database management product based on the DATABASE 2 (DB2) relational database product. It supports SQL (standard query language) for queries and comes up with wrappers in C++. DiscoveryLink requires a DB2 instance. Wrappers are available for most relational database management engines, e.g., ORACLE. The system consists of a logical data model for the federated data resources in the DB2 instance and a series of "nicknames." A nickname in IBM's terminology is a reference to a relational table that belongs to one of the federated data resources. For example, the nickname "protein" associated with a set of attributes would correspond to a "protein" table in a relational database specifically designed to store protein-associated information. Queries can be sent containing any combination of nicknames in the DB2 instance as if they were relational tables. The set of nicknames defined for the federated data sources forms a global schema. This schema determines the types of searches that can be formulated, similar to a relational data model. DiscoveryLink is essentially a middleware engine and applications and user interfaces must be developed externally.

11.1.5
Data Exchange

eXtensible Markup Language (XML) is a widespread standard for formatting text files in a hierarchical order. XML consists of key words (or tags) and attributes associated with these key words (cf. Section 14.2). The set of key words can be defined flexibly, which distinguishes XML from, for example, HTML. This feature has given rise to multiple XML conform data-exchange languages for specific purposes so that XML is now the working standard for storing and exchanging information with an inherent hierarchical structure (Achard et al. 2001). Most databases are available in

Tab. 11.1 Some available XML conform markup languages.

Language	Description	Use
BSML	Bioinformatic Sequence Markup Language	Genomic sequences and biological function
MATHML	Mathematical Markup Language	Mathematical formulas
BioML	Biopolymer Markup Language	Complex annotation for protein and DNA sequences
MAGEML	Microarray and Gene Expression Markup Language	Microarray data exchange
SBML	Systems Biology Markup Language	Biochemical networks and models
CML	Chemical Markup Language	Managing chemical information
CellML	Cell Markup Language	Mathematical models

XML-compatible format and come up with tools to parse the information. Table 11.1 gives an overview of several relevant XML conform markup languages.

The recent advent of high-throughput technologies in genomics and proteomics has given rise to large consortia that attempt to define common schemas for data storage and data exchange mostly based on XML. One example is the MIAME consortium, which attempts to unify descriptions of microarray experiments (Brazma et al. 2001). MIAME requires detailed annotation about experimental conditions, materials, and procedures to be captured. The MIAME-required information can be encoded in MAGE-ML.

MAGE-ML is a formal XML language designed to describe and communicate information about microarray-based experiments such as microarray designs, microarray manufacturing information, microarray experiment setup and execution information, gene expression data, and data analysis results.

A similar approach has been attempted in proteomics for sophisticated algorithms and methods on data standardization, data integration, and data exchange in order to gain improvements in data reproducibility and data quality control. This attempt has been targeted in recent publications (Taylor et al. 2003; Hermjakob et al. 2004). Proteomics technologies (MS, 2D gels, protein-protein interactions etc.) generate large and diverse datasets that require standardized schemas for interchanging data. For example, different MS manufacturers store data in different proprietary formats, which limits to a large extent data analysis, exchange of raw datasets, and software development. Furthermore, many strategies exist for assigning peptides to mass spectra that end up in partly conflicting results. Protein-protein interactions and the construction of networks suffer from high false-positive and false-negative rates (incorrect folding, inadequate subcellular localization, etc.), which tremendously downgrade the reproducibility and comparability of these approaches. The exchange, storage, and standardization of proteomics data based on XML-like schemas are a central goal of the above-mentioned projects and consortia (PEDRo, HUPO).

11.2
Information Measurement in Heterogeneous Data

Chapter 9 introduced the main analysis tools for DNA array data, basically targeting measurements of the transcriptome. System-wide approaches will measure data on several levels of cellular information, e.g., adding textual data in the form of gene annotation, gene regulation, interaction data, etc. A particularly interesting question is whether heterogeneous data can be integrated by analytical concepts in order to give a coherent view of the objects under analysis across these data. Essentially, this is a problem of suitable similarity functions that allow the measurement of correlation in the different data sources. Commonly used similarity measures are mathematical functions based on the feature matrices of two datasets that are based on geometric considerations such as distances and correlations. Such measures are less appropriate since datasets are heterogeneous and it is not straightforward to add a topological meaning to some data sources, e.g., to categorical data or data derived from binary classifications. In contrast, measures based on information concepts can be applied here. In this section we will introduce such concepts, namely, entropy and mutual information. Entropy and mutual information have been applied in the analysis of DNA sequences and gene expression (Herwig et al. 1999). Furthermore, in Section 9.6 we showed the application of mutual information to derive interaction rules in the reverse engineering of Boolean networks (Liang et al. 1999). We will highlight a recent example from the literature where this concept was used to combine gene expression data with functional annotations.

11.2.1
Information and Entropy

The concept of information was originally introduced by Shannon (1948) in the context of communication theory. Given a source of information that sends discrete symbols from an alphabet $A = \{a_1, ..., a_K\}$ with probabilities $p_1, ..., p_K$, i.e., $\sum_{i=1}^{K} p_i = 1$, the information content of a single letter of the alphabet, a_i, is defined as $I(a_i) = -\log_2(p_i)$. This definition is motivated through the following considerations:

- Non-negativity: The information content of a single letter is nonnegative since we have $p_i \in [0,1]$ and thus $-\log_2(p_i) \geq 0$.
- Monotony: The idea here is that rare letters should have a high information content since they are unexpected because of their low probability. Conversely, frequent symbols should have a low information content since they correspond to highly probable events. Thus, the information content of single letters should increase reciprocally to their probability.
- Additivity: The amount of information of K independent letters $a_1, ..., a_K$ with the same probability, p, should scale linearly with the amount of information of single symbols. This is implied by the functional characteristics of the log function

$$I(a_1, ..., a_K) = -\log_2(p(a_1, ..., a_K)) = -K\log_2(p) = KI(a_1). \tag{11-1}$$

This concept extends straightforwardly if more than one information source is used independently. Consider A and B to be two alphabets, $A = \{a_1, ..., a_K\}$ and $B = \{b_1, ..., b_L\}$. The composed alphabet, $A \times B$, consists of KL letter pairs (a_k, b_l). Intuitively, since the sources are independent of each other, the information content of a letter pair should be the sum of the information content of the individual letters. This is assured by the functional characteristic of the log function:

$$I((a_k, b_l)) = -\log_2 (p_{kl}) = -\log_2 (p_k\, p_l) = -\log_2 (p_k) - \log_2 (p_l) = I(a_k) + I(b_l).$$

The base of the logarithm is equal to two, which is motivated by information theory where information is stored in bits. The more bits that are stored in a memory unit, the higher the information content is. For example, a unit of n bits can store 2^n binary-coded digits, which have an information content of $-\log_2 \left(\dfrac{1}{2^n} \right) = n$.

To characterize the source completely, the information content of single letters is not sufficient. Therefore, the entropy concept has been introduced. Entropy is defined as the average (or expected) information content of the source with respect to all letters, i.e.,

$$H(A) = -\sum_{i=1}^{K} p_i \log (p_i). \tag{11-2}$$

Entropy is commonly denoted by the symbol H. This points back to early concepts of entropy in thermodynamics in the 19th century introduced by Boltzmann (defining the H function) to characterize systems in high-dimensional phase spaces in order to locate these systems between order and chaos.

Alternatively to the motivation from information theory, entropy is sometimes introduced in statistics in order to describe the grade of uncertainty of a probability distribution (compare Section 3.4). Let $P = \{p_1, ..., p_n\}$ be a finite probability distribution, i.e., a set of n nonnegative numbers that sum up to one, $\sum_{i=1}^{n} p_i = 1$. The entropy of P is defined, similarly to Eq. (11-2), as

$$H(P) = -\sum_{i=1}^{n} p_i \log (p_i). \tag{11-3}$$

Figure 11.2 displays the entropy as a function of the individual probabilities in the case of $n = 2$ and $n = 3$. If all probability weights are concentrated on a single event, then entropy is zero. If the events have equal weights, then entropy is maximal. Entropy is a measure of the mean information inherent in the probability distribution and can be considered as the expectation of the probability distribution under a log transformation of the data.

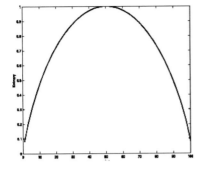

Number of events: 2

p   probability of event 1
1-p   probability of event 2

$H = -p*log_2(p)-(1-p)*log_2(1-p)$

Number events: 3

p   probability of event 1
q   probability of event 2
1-p-q   probability of event 3

$H = -p*log_2(p)-q*log_2(q)-(1-p-q)*log_2(1-p-q)$

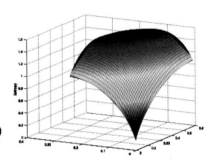

Fig. 11.2 Entropy as a function of the individual probabilities of the probability distribution for the case of distributions of size two (upper part) and three (lower part).

11.2.2
Mutual Information

Mutual information is a concept introduced by Shannon (1948) in order to measure information coherence in two datasets. Consider an alphabet $A \times B$ composed of two discrete alphabets, $A = \{a_1, ..., a_K\}$ and $B = \{b_1, ..., b_L\}$, that are not necessarily independent of each other. The mutual information of A and B is defined as

$$H(A; B) = \sum_{k,l} p_{kl} \log_2 \left(\frac{p_{kl}}{p_k \, p_l} \right). \tag{11-4}$$

Here, p_{kl} is the probability of the letter pair (a_k, b_l) and p_k and p_l are the probabilities of the letters a_k and b_l, respectively.

Similarly, mutual information can be defined with respect to two random variables, x and y, with corresponding probability distributions. If we denote by $\{p_{kl}\}$ the set of probabilities of the joint probability distribution of x and y, then mutual information is defined, similarly to Eq. (11-4), by

$$H(x; y) = \sum_{k,l} p_{kl} \log_2 \left(\frac{p_{kl}}{p_k \, p_l} \right). \tag{11-5}$$

Mutual information measures the amount of information of x inherent in y. Using the characteristic of the log function, it can be shown that

$$H\left(x;y\right) = H\left(x\right) + H\left(y\right) - H\left(x,y\right),\tag{11-6}$$

where $H(x,y)$ is the entropy of the joint probability distribution of x and y.

Several properties of mutual information can be derived (Cover and Thomas 1991):

$$0 \leq H\left(x;y\right) \leq \min\left\{H\left(x\right), H\left(y\right)\right\}\tag{11-7}$$

$$H\left(x;y\right) = H\left(y;x\right)\tag{11-8}$$

$$H\left(x;x\right) \geq H\left(x;y\right)\tag{11-9}$$

$$H\left(x;y\right) = 0, \text{ if and only if } x \text{ and } y \text{ are stochastically independent.}\tag{11-10}$$

The first inequality states that mutual information cannot be higher than the entropy of individual sources. This follows intuition because we cannot gain information from x through y that is not inherent in either x or y. Furthermore, if both variables are independent of each other, we cannot gain any information from x about y and *vice versa* (Eq. (11-10)).

Practically, mutual information is used to evaluate contingency tables. Suppose that we have two data measurements that partition the data in K and L groups, respectively. The coherence of the measurements can be described by a $K \times L$ contingency table of the following form:

x/y	1	2	...	L	Total
1	n_{11}	n_{12}	...	n_{1L}	$n_{1.}$
2	n_{21}	n_{22}	...	n_{2L}	$n_{2.}$
...	...	...	...	...	...
K	n_{K1}	n_{K2}	...	n_{KL}	$n_{K.}$
Total	$n_{.1}$	$n_{.2}$	...	$n_{.L}$	n

Here, $n_{k.}$ and $n_{.l}$ refer to the kth and lth marginal of the row and column classes, respectively, and n is the overall number of measured features. Mutual information is calculated according to the frequency of the cell entries:

$$H\left(x;y\right) = \sum_{k,l} \frac{n_{kl}}{n} \log_2 \left(\frac{n_{kl}\, n}{n_{k.}\, n_{.l}}\right).\tag{11-11}$$

Mutual information is an indicator of the coherence of information in the two datasets. It should be noted that mutual information does not distinguish between correlation (high agreement in the diagonal of the contingency table) and anti-correlation (high agreement in the anti-diagonal of the table [see Example 11-1]).

Example 11-1

Consider the binary data vectors $x = (0000011111)$, $y = (0000011111)$, and $z = (1111100000)$. Mutual information will result in similar values when judging the pairwise similarities, i.e., $H(x; y) = H(x; z)$, although the former two vectors are identical and the latter two vectors are completely diverse. This might be a desired effect. For example, if the vectors describe the state vectors of two components of a Boolean network, y and z, in relation to a third, x, then an immediate interaction rule would retrieve that x is an activator of y and an inhibitor of z. However, sometimes this is an undesired effect that identifies the need for correcting mutual information for anti-correlation. By applying the correction below, we will get a negative result for the latter pair, i.e., $H(x; z) = -H(x; y)$, which takes into account anti-correlation.

For simplicity we will assume a binary categorization of the data. Thus the above contingency table reduces to the following table:

x/y	1	2	Total
1	n_{11}	n_{12}	$n_{1.}$
2	n_{21}	n_{22}	$n_{2.}$
Total	$n_{.1}$	$n_{.2}$	n

Intuitively, one would assign results that have more weights in the anti-diagonal than in the diagonal a negative result, similar to the Pearson correlation coefficient, where anti-correlation is measured with negative values close to -1. Thus, the exact threshold should be a function of the diagonal elements and should take into account the marginals of the table. A reasonable indicator for anti-correlation is the occurrence of fewer weights in the diagonal than one would get from a random assignment of class attributes. Consider two n-dimensional vectors that carry information for two categories. Let $n_{.2}$ and $n_{2.}$ be the marginals of the occurrences of the second category (we have to consider only one category since the other values are then uniquely determined). We can ask for the probability that we will observe k times an agreement of that category by chance in the two vectors. This probability is given by the hypergeometric distribution, i.e.,

$$P(k) = \frac{\binom{n_{2.}}{k}\binom{n - n_{2.}}{n_{.2} - k}}{\binom{n}{n_{.2}}} . \tag{11-12}$$

The expectation of this distribution in dependence on the marginals is

$$E = \frac{n_{2.}\, n_{.2}}{n} . \tag{11-13}$$

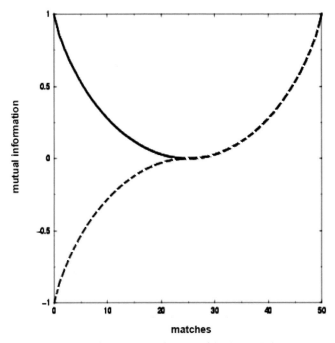

Fig. 11.3 Mutual information as a function of the diagonal element in a 2 × 2 contingency table derived from a binary classification from two different measurements (solid line). In this example, $n = 100$ and $n_2. = n_{.2} = 50$. Mutual information is minimal if n_{22} equals its expectation, i.e., $n_{22} = \frac{n_2.n_{.2}}{n}$. This quantity can be used to adjust the measure for anti-correlation (dashed line).

The expectation value is a natural indicator for anti-correlation of the two measurements, in the sense that any observed agreement should have significantly more matches. Thus, in the binary case a correction of mutual information would read

$$H\left(x;y\right) = sign\left(n_{22} - \frac{n_2.n_{.2}}{n}\right) \sum_{k,l=1}^{2} \frac{n_{kl}}{n} \log_2\left(\frac{n_{kl}\,n}{n_{k.}n_{.l}}\right). \tag{11-14}$$

Figure 11.3 displays the effect of correction for anti-correlation of mutual information. It should be pointed out that this correction cannot be straightforwardly extended to the case of more than two classes.

11.2.3
Information Correlation: Example

In this subsection we discuss the application of mutual information as a method for validating the results of clustering gene expression profiles with functional annotation (Gibbons and Roth 2002). These authors addressed the question of how clustering results can be validated using external information, i.e., information that is not given by the gene expression measurements. They used several datasets and performed different clustering algorithms with different parameter sets (compare Section 9.3). These methods were evaluated based on the assumption that good clustering solutions will agglomerate genes of similar function. They defined a figure of merit that is based on mutual information between the clustering result and gene annotation data. Clustering was done for publicly available sets of yeast expression data (Tavazoie et al. 1999) and GO annotations from the SGD database. The figure of merit is essentially a Z-score derived from comparison of observed results with random sets and indicates global relationships between a clustering and functional annotation.

The score was derived from a binary table displaying genes as rows and GO attributes as columns:

GO attributes Genes	1	2	...	P	Total
1	n_{11}	n_{12}	...	n_{1P}	$n_{1.}$
2	n_{21}	n_{22}	...	n_{2P}	$n_{2.}$
...	...	...	...	...	...
N	n_{N1}	n_{N2}	...	n_{NP}	$n_{N.}$
Total	$n_{.1}$	$n_{.2}$	...	$n_{.P}$	n

Here, n_{kl} are binary features indicating whether the gene has a specific functional attribute ("1") or not ("0").

From this table they evaluated entropies for cluster-attribute pairs (cf. Section 11.2) and computed mutual information according to

$$H(C;A) = \sum_i H(C;A_i) = nH(C) + \sum_i H(A_i) - \sum_i H(C, A_i),$$

where C refers to the clustering result determining the groups of similar genes and A_i refers to the ith attribute. The score is derived by the following procedure:

1. Compute $H(C; A)$ for the observed clustering result.
2. Randomly assign genes to clusters of equal size and compute $H(\bar{C}, A)$ for this random partition $\bar{C}$.
3. Repeat step 2a number of times and compute the mean and the standard deviation of the observed scores, μ and σ.
4. Return the score as $Z = \dfrac{H(C;A) - \mu}{\sigma}$.

Using this score, the authors were able to identify clustering procedures that perform better than others. A particularly striking result was that hierarchical clustering using single-linkage analysis led to results that perform worse than random. This bad performance of the single-linkage method has been reported before in independent studies.

11.3
Biclustering

The third level of data integration aims to derive interactions and structures of the biological objects combining data from heterogeneous sources. Concepts that define such tasks are rather rare. One popular method to organize the objects into groups is biclustering. In this section we introduce the problem of biclustering originally developed for improving clustering of expression profiles. We describe the first of these algorithms introduced by Cheng and Church (2000). Recently, this technique was successfully applied for integrating data from heterogeneous sources (Tanay et al. 2004); this will be described in the final subsection.

11.3.1
The Problem

Given an *nxp* data matrix X, where n is the number of objects (e.g., genes) and p is the number of conditions (e.g., DNA array experiments), a bicluster is defined as a submatrix, X_{IJ}, of X that is composed of a subset of objects, I, and a subset of conditions, J, whereby the objects in X_{IJ} express similar behavior across the subset of conditions. Different algorithms define different ways of judging this kind of similarity. Typical elements of a bicluster algorithm are a preprocessing step to equalize the data from heterogeneous sources and a post-processing step to eliminate redundancies. In contrast to the clustering procedures described in Section 9.3, biclustering assigns objects (and conditions) to several biclusters that might be highly similar.

In contrast to clustering algorithms, where the similarity is computed for pairs of objects across all conditions in an equally weighted manner, the similarity computed in a biclustering procedure measures the coherence of specific objects under specific conditions. This is a more adequate procedure when using biologically diverse experimental conditions where, for example, groups of genes behave similarly within the first group and are uncorrelated in the second group of conditions (e.g., using different knockout experiments). Thus, biclustering allows the joining of many types of experimental conditions.

The biclustering situation can be visualized with a bipartite graph (Fig. 11.4). Experimental conditions are listed on top and objects (e.g., genes) at the bottom. Whenever an object is associated with a condition, there is an edge connecting the object-condition pair. Dense regions of edges define object-condition modules. If a dense region is significant with respect to some criterion, it is called a bicluster.

The art of a biclustering procedure is to define reasonable frameworks that assign weights to the edges according to the specific types of object-condition relationships, to define a scoring scheme that allows one to judge the significance of the observed bicluster, and to develop efficient algorithms to identify the biclusters in the entire bipartite graph.

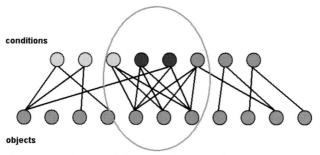

conditions

objects

Fig. 11.4 Conditions and objects can be organized in a bipartite graph. If a data object is associated with a condition (e. g., through expression strength or a binary classification), an edge is drawn between the condition and the object. Biclusters are defined as regions of densely connected groups of objects and conditions.

11.3.2
Algorithmic Example

The first biclustering algorithm was published by Cheng and Church (2000) in order to identify better clusters in gene expression profiling, although the strategy itself had been proposed before (Mirkin 1996). The algorithm is a node-deletion/-addition algorithm for identifying submatrices in the gene expression matrix that have low mean squared residue scores. In their study the authors compared the performance of the biclustering procedure with standard clustering procedures on several datasets and showed that they improved the cluster quality.

Let X be the *nxp* data matrix and let X_{IJ} be a submatrix. Here, I and J are subsets of row and columns, respectively. Denote the submatrix's ith row average by $x_{iJ} = \frac{1}{|J|} \sum_{j \in J} x_{ij}$, the submatrix's jth column average by $x_{Ij} = \frac{1}{|I|} \sum_{i \in I} x_{ij}$, and the total submatrix average by $x_{IJ} = \frac{1}{|I||J|} \sum_{i \in I, j \in J} x_{ij}$. The residue score of an element, $x_{ij} \in X_{IJ}$, is defined as $RS_{IJ}(x_{ij}) = x_{ij} - x_{Ij} - x_{iJ} + x_{IJ}$. The mean squared residue is the variance of the set of all elements in the bicluster plus the mean row and column variances, respectively, and is defined as $S(X_{IJ}) = \frac{1}{|I||J|} \sum_{i \in I, j \in J} RS_{IJ}^2(x_{ij})$.

If the submatrix is totally uniform, i.e., there are no differences in expression of the genes across the selected conditions, this would lead to a score equal to zero. Despite this trivial case, if all gene profiles are coherently changing across the selected conditions, and thus the bicluster has a highly specific profile, this will lead to small scores as well. Conversely, if the values in the submatrix were randomly drawn (e. g., from a Gaussian distribution), then the expected score would be equal to the variance of the distribution. Thus, good biclusters can be defined as subsets of objects/conditions with low residue scores. If the score is not zero, then it is always possible to remove a row or column to lower the score until the bicluster becomes constant.

In their algorithm, the authors define a biclusters as submatrices X_{IJ} of X with a score below δ, i.e., $S(X_{IJ}) \leq \delta$. The parameter δ is an algorithmic parameter that can be specified by the user. For example, δ could be the minimum score for clusters computed with a standard clustering algorithm. The goal of the algorithm is to find the largest δ bicluster in the data. This optimization problem cannot be solved by brute computer power since it is NP-hard (for proof, see Cheng and Church [2000]). Thus, heuristics must be implied that find a large δ bicluster. A naïve approach would start with the entire matrix and consider stepwise single-row and column addition and deletion. If the best operation improves the score, it will be applied; otherwise, the procedure stops. This approach, however, is computationally unfeasible for the commonly large data matrices.

Consider a specific row $i \in I$ of the submatrix X_{IJ}. If the average contribution to the total score is greater than the row's relative share, i.e., $\frac{1}{|J|} \sum_j RS_{IJ}^2(x_{ij}) > S(X_{IJ})$, then it can be shown that the removal of the row from the submatrix will decrease the score. A similar argument holds for a specific column $j \in J$. This leads to the following node-deletion algorithm:

1. Start with the entire matrix, $X_{IJ} = X$.
2. If $S(X_{IJ}) \leq \delta$, stop.
3. For each row, i, and column, j, of the bicluster, compute $d_i = \frac{1}{|J|} \sum_{j \in J} RS_{IJ}^2(x_{ij})$ and $d_j = \frac{1}{|I|} \sum_{i \in I} RS_{IJ}^2(x_{ij})$.
4. Delete the row or column giving the highest average residue if this residue is above the threshold. This defines a smaller modified bicluster, X_{IJ}. Go to step 2.

Now consider a specific row $i \in I$. If the average contribution to the total score is lower than the row's relative share, i.e., $\frac{1}{|J|} \sum_{j \in J} RS_{IJ}^2(x_{ij}) \leq S(X_{IJ})$, then the addition of the row to the submatrix will decrease the score as well. Again, a similar argument holds for additional columns. This leads to the following node-addition algorithm:

1. Start with a given bicluster X_{IJ}. Compute all values x_{iJ}, x_{Ij}, x_{IJ} and $S(X_{IJ})$.
2. Add columns, $j \notin J$, with $\frac{1}{|I|} \sum_{i \in I} RS_{IJ}^2(x_{ij}) \leq S(X_{IJ})$ to the bicluster.
3. Recompute all values x_{iJ}, x_{Ij}, x_{IJ} and $S(X_{IJ})$.
4. Add rows, $i \notin I$, with $\frac{1}{|J|} \sum_{j \in J} RS_{IJ}^2(x_{ij}) \leq S(X_{IJ})$.
5. If nothing is added, stop.

The final algorithm iterates between deletion and addition of rows and columns until no improvement of the score can be achieved. The result is a bicluster. After the first bicluster is found, the entries in the respective rows and columns of the initial data matrix are masked using random data and the iteration is started again. The whole loop is iterated until a pre-fixed number of biclusters is found or until no more submatrices are available.

Several other algorithms for biclustering have been published. Coupled two-way clustering (CTWC) (Getz et al. 2000) defines a generic scheme for transforming a one-dimensional clustering algorithm into a biclustering algorithm. The iterative signature algorithm (ISA) (Bergmann et al. 2003) validates biclusters according to the row and column averages through the selected set of objects and conditions using a simple linear model approach. The statistical algorithmic method for bicluster analysis (SAMBA) (Tanay et al. 2002) uses a sophisticated scoring scheme for biclusters based on a probabilistic concept. The latter algorithm has been shown to work efficiently for data integration, as will be discussed below.

11.3.3
Biclustering and Data Integration

A practical example illustrating the powerful biclustering approach for data integration has been recently published by Tanay et al. (2004). The authors have used heterogeneous, genome-wide data from yeast experiments such as DNA arrays, protein interactions, transcription factor binding data, and phenotype data to reveal functional modules. These modules (essentially biclusters) are defined as the maximal group of genes that express common features across a subset of experiments. The clusters were identified with the SAMBA algorithm. The computation was done using a statistical representation of the data sources. The authors were able to derive global architectural properties by the identified modular organization of gene expression. This modular organization has been postulated before (Ihmels et al. 2002; Segal et al. 2003). The analysis provides evidence for a global hierarchical organization of the yeast system in the sense that small modules could be clustered to higher modules that characterize common behavior under specific conditions.

Data integration was performed with expression profiles from 70 different conditions (~1000 different profiles), 110 transcription factor binding location profiles (Lee et al. 2002), and more than 6000 protein-protein interactions and complex interactions. Using this data the authors were able to identify 665 significant modules with maximal overlap. Overlap was defined according to gene-condition vertex pairs of the modules. The statistical significance of the module was judged according to a randomized control set, and the biological function of the module was assigned according to overrepresentation of GO categories of the corresponding gene set of the module using the strategy described in Chapter 9 (Section 9.4.3). The authors used the identified modules for the study of the transcriptional network and predicted the function of more than 800 uncharacterized genes.

References

ACHARD, F., VAYSSEIX, G. and BARILLOT, E.
XML, bioinformatics and data integration
(2001) Bioinformatics *17*, 115–25.

BAXEVANIS, A.D. The Molecular Biology Database Collection: 2003 update (2003) Nucleic
Acids Res. *31*, 1–12.

BERGMANN, S., IHMELS, J. and BARKAI, N.
Iterative signature algorithm for the analysis
of large-scale gene expression data (2003)
Phys. Rev. E. Stat. Nonlin. Soft. Matter Phys.
67, 1–18.

BIRNEY, E., ANDREWS, T.D., BEVAN, P., CACCAMO,
M., CHEN, Y., CLARKE, L., COATES, G., CUFF, J.,
CURWEN, V., CUTTS, T., DOWN, T., EYRAS, E.,
FERNANDEZ-SUAREZ, X.M., GANE, P.,
GIBBINS, B., GILBERT, J., HAMMOND, M.,
HOTZ, H.R., IYER, V., JEKOSCH, K., KAHARI, A.,
KASPRZYK, A., KEEFE, D., KEENAN, S.,
LEHVASLAIHO, H., McVICKER, G., MELSOPP, C.,
MEIDL, P., MONGIN, E., PETTETT, R., POTTER, S.,
PROCTOR, G., RAE, M., SEARLE, S., SLATER, G.,
SMEDLEY, D., SMITH, J., SPOONER, W.,
STABENAU, A., STALKER, J., STOREY, R.,
URETA-VIDAL, A., WOODWARK, K.C., CAMERON,
G., DURBIN, R., COX, A., HUBBARD, T. and
CLAMP, M. An overview of Ensembl (2004)
Genome Res. *14*, 925–8.

BRAZMA, A., HINGAMP, P., QUACKENBUSH, J.,
SHERLOCK, G., SPELLMAN, P., STOECKERT, C.,
AACH, J., ANSORGE, W., BALL, C.A., CAUSTON,
H.C., GAASTERLAND, T., GLENISSON, P.,
HOLSTEGE, F.C., KIM, I.F., MARKOWITZ, V.,
MATESE, J.C., PARKINSON, H., ROBINSON, A.,
SARKANS, U., SCHULZE-KREMER, S., STEWART, J.,
TAYLOR, R., VILO, J. and VINGRON, M. Minimum information about a microarray experiment (MIAME)-toward standards for microarray data (2001) Nat. Genet. *29*, 365–71.

CHENG, Y. and CHURCH, G.M. (2000) Biclustering of expression data. In: Proceedings of the
8th International Conference on Intelligent
Systems for Molecular Biology, eds. P. Bourne
et al., AAAI Press, Menlo Park, pp. 93–103.

COVER, T.M. and THOMAS, J.A. Elements of
information theory (1991). J. Wiley & Sons,
New York.

ETZOLD, T. and ARGOS, P. SRS – an indexing and
retrieval tool for flat file data libraries (1993)
Comp. Appl. Biosc. *9*, 49–57.

ETZOLD, T., ULYANOV, A. and ARGOS, P.
SRS: information retrieval system for molecular biology data banks (1996) Methods
Enzymol. *266*, 114–28.

GETZ, G., LEVINE, E. and DOMANY, E. Coupled
two-way clustering analysis of gene microarray
data (2000) PNAS *97*, 12079–12084.

GIBBONS, F.D. and ROTH, F.P. Judging the
quality of gene expression-based clustering
methods using gene annotation (2002)
Genome Res. *12*, 1574–1581.

HERMJAKOB, H., MONTECCHI-PALAZZI, L.,
BADER, G., WOJCIK, J., SALWINSKI, L., CEOL, A.,
MOORE, S., ORCHARD, S., SARKANS, U.,
VON MERING, C., ROECHERT, B., POUX, S.,
JUNG, E., MERSCH, H., KERSEY, P., LAPPE, M.,
LI, Y., ZENG, R., RANA, D., NIKOLSKI, M.,
HUSI, H., BRUN, C., SHANKER, K., GRANT, S.G.,
SANDER, C., BORK, P., ZHU, W., PANDEY, A.,
BRAZMA, A., JACQ, B., VIDAL, M., SHERMAN, D.,
LEGRAIN, P., CESARENI, G., XENARIOS, I.,
EISENBERG, D., STEIPE, B., HOGUE, C. and
APWEILER, R. The HUPO PSI's molecular
interaction format – a community standard for
the representation of protein interaction data
(2004) Nat. Biotechnol. *22*, 177–83.

HERWIG, R., POUSTKA, A.J., MULLER, C., BULL, C.,
LEHRACH, H. and O'BRIEN, J. Large-scale
clustering of cDNA-fingerprinting data (1999)
Genome Res. *9*, 1093–105.

IDEKER, T., OZIER, O., SCHWIKOWSKI, B. and
SIEGEL, A.F. Discovering regulatory and signalling circuits in molecular interaction networks
(2002) Bioinformatics *18 Suppl 1*, S233–40.

IHMELS, J., FRIEDLANDER, G., BERGMANN, S.,
SARIG, O., ZIV, Y. and BARKAI, N. Revealing
modular organization in the yeast transcriptional network (2002) Nat. Genet. *31*, 370–7.

KARP, P.D. A strategy for database interoperation
(1995) J. Comput. Biol. *2*, 573–86.

KASPRZYK, A., KEEFE, D., SMEDLEY, D.,
LONDON, D., SPOONER, W., MELSOPP, C.,
HAMMOND, M., ROCCA-SERRA, P., COX, T. and
BIRNEY, E. EnsMart: a generic system for fast
and flexible access to biological data (2004)
Genome Res. *14*, 160–9.

LEE, T.I., RINALDI, N.J., ROBERT, F., ODOM, D.T.,
BAR-JOSEPH, Z., GERBER, G.K., HANNETT, N.M.,
HARBISON, C.T., THOMPSON, C.M., SIMON, I.,
ZEITLINGER, J., JENNINGS, E.G., MURRAY, H.L.,
GORDON, D.B., REN, B., WYRICK, J.J.,
TAGNE, J.B., VOLKERT, T.L., FRAENKEL, E.,
GIFFORD, D.K. and YOUNG, R.A. Transcrip-

tional regulatory networks in Saccharomyces cerevisiae (2002) Science *298*, 799–804.

LIANG, S., FUHRMAN, S. and SOMOGYI, R. REVEAL, a general reverse engineering algorithm for inference of genetic network architecture (1999) in R. Altman et al., ed. Proceedings of the Pacific Symposium on Biocomputing 98. Singapore, pp 18–28.

MIRKIN, B. Mathematical classification and clustering (1996) Elsevier, Dordrecht.

SEGAL, E., SHAPIRA, M., REGEV, A., PE'ER, D., BOTSTEIN, D., KOLLER, D. and FRIEDMAN, N. Module networks: identifying regulatory modules and their condition-specific regulators from gene expression data (2003) Nat. Genet. *34*, 166–76.

SHANNON, C. A mathematical theory of communication (1948) Bell Systems Technology Journal *27*, 379–423.

TANAY, A., SHARAN, R. and SHAMIR, R. Discovering statistically significant biclusters in gene expression data (2002) Bioinformatics *18*, S136-S144.

TANAY, A., SHARAN, R., KUPIEC, M. and SHAMIR, R. Revealing modularity and organization in the yeast molecular network by integrated analysis of highly heterogeneous genomewide data (2004) PNAS *101*, 2981–2986.

TAVAZOIE, S., HUGHES, J.D., CAMPBELL, M.J., CHO, R.J. and CHURCH, G.M. Systematic determination of genetic network architecture (1999) Nat. Genet. *22*, 281–285.

TAYLOR, C.F., PATON, N.W., GARWOOD, K.L., KIRBY, P.D., STEAD, D.A., YIN, Z., DEUTSCH, E.W., SELWAY, L., WALKER, J., RIBA-GARCIA, I., MOHAMMED, S., DEERY, M.J., HOWARD, J.A., DUNKLEY, T., AEBERSOLD, R., KELL, D.B., LILLEY, K.S., ROEPSTORFF, P., YATES, J.R., 3rd, BRASS, A., BROWN, A.J., CASH, P., GASKELL, S.J., HUBBARD, S.J. and OLIVER, S.G. A systematic approach to modeling, capturing, and disseminating proteomics experimental data (2003) Nat. Biotechnol. *21*, 247–54.

ZDOBNOV, E.M., LOPEZ, R., APWEILER, R. and ETZOLD, T. The EBI SRS server – recent developments (2002) Bioinformatics *18*, 368–373.

12
What's Next?

12.1
Systems Biology: The Core of Biological Research and Medical Practice of the Future?

Biological research is at a crossroad. We have, on the one hand, a very successful tradition of research by the now "classical" paradigm (complex processes are studied in small sections, which can be analyzed in isolation; experiments are at least supposed to be designed to test hypotheses, etc.; results are typically published in the free-text format of a journal article and are designed to be read and understood by other researchers). On the other hand, we have started a new tradition in genomic research, based on the systematic analysis of all components of complex processes (data are generated systematically and are primarily made available online in databases). To interpret the data generated in this "genomic" phase, we have two main strategies available. We can use systematically generated data as part of the normal research as well as data-interpretation process. But in addition, we are also able to employ a number of statistical tools to identify patterns in large amounts of data, which would be very hard to find using the classical, hypothesis-driven paradigm.

We see the possibility of modeling complex networks as the centerpiece of a new, third wave of biological research, likely to be associated with a dramatic improvement in our capability to analyze complex systems.

For this, we need a new systems biology phase of biological research, based on a combination of automated high-throughput data generation and sophisticated programs comparing the predictions made by different models with the available data. We can expect further dramatic changes in the rate, accuracy, and resolution of the data we generate. The thousand-dollar genome has become an official goal of funding by the National Institutes of Health. It is highly likely that the patterns of gene expression at the RNA level and even the protein level will be used routinely in tumor diagnosis in the not-too-distant future.

Large amounts of information can even now be generated from sequence variants of genes, which govern rates of uptake and metabolism of many drugs that are commonly being used in medicine. The results of decades of research on the effects of variants of single genes on cellular processes (e.g., single-nucleotide polymorphism analysis) fill the current literature.

Systems Biology in Practice. Concepts, Implementation and Application.
E. Klipp, R. Herwig, A. Kowald, C. Wierling, H. Lehrach
Copyright © 2005 WILEY-VCH Verlag GmbH & Co. KGaA, Weinheim
ISBN: 3-527-31078-9

The development of quantitative models, based on all general (information from the literature, systematic data generation) and individual (patient-specific) data available, to predict, e.g., treatment outcomes would be an enormously powerful model to make large amounts of information available to the treating physician. Pragmatically, systems biology might very well be our only hope to make these tremendous amounts of information useful for achieving our goals in medicine, food production, or biotechnology.

The problem might, however, be much deeper than this. The classical approach to biology is based, to a large extent, on subdividing complex problems into simple parts, e.g., the function of a single gene or a small group of genes. Individual groups generate data on these systems, and attempt to understand them, with the ultimate hope of being able to reconstitute all of these results into a global understanding of the entire problem. We do, however, have to keep in mind that there is really no proof that this strategy will work for many of the problems that are most important to people outside the narrow scientific community. In mathematics, for example, a number of problems exist that cannot be subdivided in this form. It is, for instance, not possible to identify the shortest path connecting a large number of places (the "traveling salesman" problem) by such a strategy. In this case, the only solution would be to use techniques that are able to probe in parallel most or all components of the complex networks under investigation and to combine this with modeling approaches that are also able to treat components that cannot be analyzed experimentally. This way, we might be able to predict the future behavior of a system such as a patient who is receiving personalized treatment for a specific tumor (a question of major importance to the large number of people likely to undergo cancer treatment in the future).

12.2
Experimental Planning in the Systems Biology Phase of Biological Research

The systems biology phase of biological and medical research will change the way we plan and carry out experiments to probe the complex networks of processes; our ability to predict must be greatly improved in order to help to solve these types of problems.

Experimental planning and data generation in the recent, pre-genomic phase of biological research has, at least in principle, been guided by hypotheses (hypothesis-driven research, a principle that has, however, been mitigated by the many unexpected observations that often contribute more to our understanding of biology than the hypothesis-driven research originally planned). In the genomic phase, this has been replaced largely by the systematic analysis of all components of a process and, ideally, of all components that an organism has or is able to produce (all genes, all transcripts, all proteins, all protein complexes, all metabolites, etc.). The systems biology phase of biological research might represent a synthesis of both principles. Since our knowledge (or hypothesis) about a process is defined by the model or models we can formulate about the process as well as the exact parameters we use in this modeling (initial concentrations, kinetic constants etc.), we can use computational and mathematical techniques to compare these models, to identify key experiments, and to program robotic systems to carry out these experiments. Such a strategy has, for example, been used recently to carry out an analysis of yeast mutations (*The Robot Scientist*; King et al. 2004), in which the experimental planning and control of the robots actually carrying out the experiments were performed by a computer program.

12.3
Publication in the Era of Systems Biology

Before the genome sequencing project, information was transmitted between different scientists and different groups predominantly in the form of text (although nowadays, this text is transmitted more and more often in electronic form). In contrast, genomic data has been predominantly shared electronically via databases or as supplemental material linked to publications. Since the best description of a complex biological process is likely to be its computational and mathematical model, the information can be exchanged by exchanging functional models, which can be compared to alternative models and can even be plugged into robot scientist systems to guide the production of new data needed to develop the models further. For this, it will be essential to standardize interfaces between the modeling tools and to standardize model description, a process that has started with, for example, the development of the Systems Biology Workbench (SBW) (see Section 14.1.5) and Systems Biology Markup Language (SBML) (see Section 14.2.2).

12.4
Systems Biology and Text Mining

Despite the growing importance of databases for research in molecular biology and medicine, most knowledge is still published in scientific papers rather than in structured database entries. This knowledge is essentially incomprehensible for computer programs and is difficult to find even for humans. The task of finding and understanding relevant publications in any specific area takes a major and increasing fraction of a researcher's time. However, there is a high potential that computational methods from machine learning and natural language processing can help to alleviate this situation (Raychaudhuri et al. 2003; Chang et al. 2004; Hakenberg et al. 2004).

Systems biology studies predominantly gene expression networks, signal transduction pathways, metabolic networks, or combinations of these. Information about proteins, their interactions, their correlation with phenotypes, and their role in complex networks is of high importance. Such information is available only in the form of scientific publications that have to be found, read, and understood by researchers.

Development of algorithms and software tools for text mining will support literature research and will help to combine data from multiple articles into new scientific findings. Given a set of documents, tasks such as the following can be tackled: (1) recognizing biological entities including genes, gene products, pathways, and diseases; (2) extracting all protein-protein relationships and showing the network of interactions graphically; (3) extracting the interaction network of a specific pathway in a specific cell type and, as far as possible, the kinetic parameters that are required to run a computer simulation of these reactions; and (4) building a database storing the extracted information.

12.5
Systems Biology in Medicine

One of the most important applications of systems biology in the short and medium term will be in guiding the treatment of patients. There is an enormous amount of information on the role of single genes or single mutations in these genes in different diseases – information that is typically not used to optimize the treatment of patients. In addition, as mentioned before, it is not at all clear whether anything short of a computational model of patients and their diseases will ever be sufficiently predictive to allow the optimal treatment of each patient. It is very likely that significant progress in this direction is possible for using such an approach in the treatment of cancer (if sufficient resources are made available). Similarly, other diseases that manifest themselves at the level of the cell (metabolic diseases) could be relatively straightforward to model. In the case of infectious diseases, modeling both the host and the infecting bacterium could similarly lead to significant progress. However, modeling can be based only on a fairly detailed molecular understanding of the basic processes behind the disease. Any diseases for which we have little understanding of the molecular causes (e. g., schizophrenia) will not be amenable to this approach.

12.6
Systems Biology in Drug Development

The development of new drugs has become increasingly difficult. Rising sums of money for research have resulted in the development of fewer and fewer new therapeutic substances. It is quite likely that the development of accurate models of the complex biological processes affected by a specific disease will provide a completely new platform for drug development. The effect of drugs can be modeled and predictions from the model can be tested against experimental data. After the effects of different drugs are incorporated into the model, predictions can be made on, e. g., the effects of combinations of drugs, allowing the development of new combination therapies, identifying potential toxic side effects, and possibly even guiding the medicinal chemists in optimizing the drug.

Systems biology could also become a key technique in reducing the number of animal tests, while at the same time increasing the information gained from the remaining tests and therefore increasing the safety of the drugs or other compounds developed. This could be particularly important for predicting side effects in vulnerable populations or in stages difficult to cover in the normal toxicity tests (e. g., the developing embryo).

12.7
Systems Biology in Food Production and Biotechnology

Plants (or animals) used in food production are extremely complex systems. The process of optimizing specific important aspects is therefore difficult, slow, error prone, and fraught with the danger of unintended side effects. This is partly because simple breeding schemes, or even the construction of transgenic plants, will typically optimize only a single parameter and will tend to ignore side effects due to the limited number of *in vivo* tests that can typically be carried out in such an optimization experiment, as well as to the large number of parameters that control the behavior of each individual. Because of the lower cost of modeling and the easy access to all parameters of such a model, combinations of large-scale modeling runs with a limited number of experiments could improve the results dramatically.

Such an approach could also be used to optimize the production of energy from renewable sources (plants or microorganisms). It could improve biotechnological techniques and help to reduce the environmental problems and energy consumption associated with many of the current chemical procedures. It could lead to the production of new compound classes, which could, for example, be used as antibacterial agents in medicine and could even help to predict the outcome of the complex processes used, e. g., in the production of many types of food (rice etc.).

12.8
Systems Biology in Ecology

Ecological systems are based on the interaction of many organisms. These interactions can be modeled and predictions can be made on the development of an ecological system, as well as on the effect (positive or negative) of any external influence (Westerhoff et al. 2002). Simulations therefore could be an essential step in trying to understand such systems and improving the ecology of areas that have been damaged by human intervention. Similar problems arise in trying to understand infectious diseases, since here too the ultimate outcome depends on the interaction between the pathogen and the host (often modulated by the presence of other organisms, e. g., natural symbionts).

12.9
Systems Biology and Nanotechnology

Both establishment and application of models will require the routine generation of very large amounts of data on genes, proteins, metabolites, and many other aspects of the complex processes we are studying. In addition, many of these processes might very well differ from cell to cell. In many cases we will not be able to identify and pool cells of identical type and state, in order to carry out the measurements on larger aggregates, without losing information about the cell-to-cell differences, which could be critical for the models and their interpretation.

Many of the current techniques are costly (resequencing the genome of a patient would be feasible in principle, but would, with current technologies, cost tens of millions of dollars, clearly not feasible as a routine medical diagnostic procedure). They are also very often rather insensitive, requiring the analysis of pools of materials, usually containing many cell types, and often also material from a number of individuals. To be able to routinely analyze the material from single patients, we might very well want to carry out the equivalent of the entire human genome project on each patient. In fact, we might want to carry the analysis much further down to the level of regions of similar cells or, where necessary, to the level of single cells.

Progress in these directions might come from new developments in nanotechnologies and a number of other areas, which might allow us to dramatically increase throughput, to reduce cost, and to increase the sensitivity of our measurements (Heath et al. 2003). Nanosensors based on carbon nanotubes (Kong et al. 2000; Star et al. 2001) or semiconductor nanowires (Cui and Lieber 2001; Cui et al. 2001) could, for example, allow us to analyze expression patterns on unamplified samples from very few or even single cells, to score changes in the genome of a cancer cell on minute amounts of material, and to measure minute amounts of proteins. In addition, the very small scale of such devices might allow more rapid measurements of dynamic changes taking place in cells, an additional important source of information in developing and testing models of the many complex processes taking place in the cell.

Another important area of development is that of nanofluidic devices (nanolab). New techniques allowing highly integrated fluidic systems (Thorsen et al. 2002) might, within the foreseeable future, be able to automate and miniaturize many of the analyses that we are currently carrying out on a much larger scale (and therefore also with less sensitivity and at much higher cost). Development of such nanofluidic devices could help to transfer many of the operations currently dependent on highly trained experimenters using complex machinery into routine applications, enabling us to carry out a "genome project" on the genome (and the genome of the tumor) of any individual patient.

12.10
Guiding the Design of New Organisms

There are a number of reasons to try to design new (micro-) organisms from scratch. Such organisms could carry out new chemical transformations, degrade components in the environment that have proven indigestible to all available organisms, and compete with pathogenic strains to eliminate specific diseases. In contrast to natural selection, which has come up with a wide range of organisms (including many surviving under some of the most extreme conditions imaginable), computer models have the advantage of being able to evolve through stages that would not be viable in nature, or even in the laboratory, and can select for phenotypes, for which it is hard to develop a selection system for organisms. (On the other hand, natural selection is able to carry out many more trials than will be feasible by computational techniques for a long time.) It can, however, also simply be the ultimate test that our models are correct. If we can design a new organism and predict all of its features correctly, we have come as close to the truth as we will ever be able to get.

The design of a new organism could in principle be carried out in a single step, i.e., designing all the components and assembling them in one single step. However, more promising is a stepwise approach that starts from an existing organism and adds (or eliminates) genes until, in a process similar to natural evolution, all the components of the new cells are encoded by the new genome or are produced by components encoded by this genome.

Using such strategies to design new bacterial strains seems quite feasible in the medium term. The design of eukaryotic microorganisms could prove considerably more difficult, due to the larger number of cellular compartments needed there. The design of completely novel organisms of high complexity, with complex nervous systems, is far outside the range we can imagine being feasible in the foreseeable future.

12.11
Computational Limitations

The computational complexity of systems biology approaches is tremendous, simply because of the size of the networks under analysis. For example, describing a gene interaction network with n genes with a simple Boolean network results in 2^n different possible states, a number that is beyond the computation power for large n. Likely, the parameter space of kinetic models described by differential equation systems is theoretically unlimited. An important focus of future research will thus be the reduction of the parameter space of such models. Here, approaches can proceed in several directions.

Investigation of the topology of networks can lead to robust solutions that are fairly invariant against changes of the kinetic parameters (von Dassow et al. 2000). These authors investigated the segment polarity network in *Drosophila* using a simple continuous dynamical model, and their results suggested that once the correct topology of the network was determined, the model predicted the correct behavior with different sets of kinetic parameters quite stably. This is a good argument against the usual criticism of large-scale modeling that we will never measure enough kinetic parameters with sufficient accuracy to develop a sensible model.

Parallelization of computation using multiprocessor machines will enable us to apply detailed simulations on large models. Here, simple brute force methods in analogy to chess computers will be developed, varying parameter sets and evaluating the results, for example, by sensitivity analysis. This will go in turn with parameter reduction methods that take into account the fact that most matrices representing the biological object are sparse and that the full complexity of the problem is not valid for biological problems.

Hybrid methods will be an option for future computational approaches. The combination of model predictions with different granularity (e. g., qualitative and quantitative prediction, deterministic and probabilistic predictions) will lead to new computational approaches.

12.12
Potential Dangers

As with every other development of major importance that increases our knowledge and capabilities, there is the potential for dangerous developments arising out of our new powers. The release of new organisms may result in unintended consequences for the environment or human health. Much more worrying, however, is the possible use of these new developments in research on biological weapons. In its long history, mankind has unfortunately developed many ways to kill each other. It is therefore important to be aware of the possible misuse of new developments. But, as with other powerful and dangerous developments (nuclear physics, organic chemistry), controlling bodies can be instituted to monitor and contain possible risks, while allowing us to profit from the positive potential of the new techniques.

References

CHANG, J.T., SCHUTZE, H. and ALTMAN, R.B. GAPSCORE: finding gene and protein names one word at a time (2004) Bioinformatics *20*, 216–25

CUI, Y. and LIEBER, C.M. Functional nanoscale electronic devices assembled using silicon nanowire building blocks (2001) Science *291*, 851–3

CUI, Y., WEI, Q., PARK, H. and LIEBER, C.M. Nanowire nanosensors for highly sensitive and selective detection of biological and chemical species (2001) Science *293*, 1289–92

HAKENBERG, J., SCHMEIER, S., KOWALD, A., KLIPP, E. and LESER, U. Finding kinetic parameters using text mining (2004) Omics *8*, 131–52

HEATH, J.R., PHELPS, M.E. and HOOD, L. Nano-Systems biology (2003) Mol. Imaging Biol. *5*, 312–25

KING, R.D., WHELAN, K.E., JONES, F.M., REISER, P.G., BRYANT, C.H., MUGGLETON, S.H., KELL, D.B. and OLIVER, S.G. Functional genomic hypothesis generation and experimentation by a robot scientist (2004) Nature *427*, 247–52

KONG, J., FRANKLIN, N.R., ZHOU, C., CHAPLINE, M.G., PENG, S., CHO, K. and DAI, H. Nanotube molecular wires as chemical sensors (2000) Science *287*, 622–5

RAYCHAUDHURI, S., CHANG, J.T., IMAM, F. and ALTMAN, R.B. The computational analysis of scientific literature to define and recognize gene expression clusters (2003) Nucleic Acids Res. *31*, 4553–60

STAR, A., STODDART, J.F., STEUERMAN, D., DIEHL, M., BOUKAI, A., WONG, E.W., YANG, X., CHUNG, S.W., CHOI, H. and HEATH, J.R. Preparation and Properties of Polymer-Wrapped Single-Walled Carbon Nanotubes We would like to acknowledge the following agencies and foundations for supporting various aspects of this work: the polymer synthesis and spectroscopic characterization of the nanotube-polymer complex was funded by ONR; the chemical preparation and AFM analysis of these materials was supported by the NSF; device fabrication and charge-transport measurements were funded by DARPA and ONR; and the nonlinear microscopy experiments were supported by DARPA and the Keck Foundation (2001) Angew Chem. Int. Ed. Engl. *40*, 1721–1725

THORSEN, T., MAERKL, S.J. and QUAKE, S.R. Microfluidic large-scale integration (2002) Science *298*, 580–4

VON DASSOW, G., MEIR, E., MUNRO, E.M. and ODELL, G.M. The segment polarity network is a robust developmental module (2000) Nature *406*, 188–192

WESTERHOFF, H.V., GETZ, W.M., BRUGGEMAN, F., HOFMEYR, J.H., ROHWER, J.M. and SNOEP, J.L. ECA: control in ecosystems (2002) Mol. Biol. Rep. *29*, 113–7

Part III
Computer-based Information Retrieval and Examination

Systems Biology in Practice. Concepts, Implementation and Application.
E. Klipp, R. Herwig, A. Kowald, C. Wierling, H. Lehrach
Copyright © 2005 WILEY-VCH Verlag GmbH & Co. KGaA, Weinheim
ISBN: 3-527-31078-9

13
Databases and Tools on the Internet

Introduction

With the rapid increase of biological data, it has become even more important to organize and structure the data in a way that information can easily be retrieved. As a result,
the number of databases has also increased rapidly over the past few years. Most of
these databases have a Web interface and can be accessed from everywhere in the
world, which is an enormously important service for the scientific community. Again
we have to emphasize that we can give only a very brief summary of a small number of
databases. An extensive list of databases can be found at http://www.mpiem.gwdg.de/
Forschung/Biol/biol_index_en.html. Furthermore, the journal *Nucleic Acids Research*
offers a databases issue each year in January that is dedicated to factual biological databases and, additionally, a Web server issue in July presenting Web-based services such
as tools for sequence comparison or prediction of 3-D protein structure.

13.1
Gene Ontology

The accumulation of scientific knowledge is a decentralized, parallel process. Consequently, the naming and description of new genes and gene products is not necessarily systematic. Often, gene products with identical functions are given different
names in different organisms or the verbal description of the location and function
might be quite different (e.g., protein degradation vs. proteolysis). This, of course,
makes it very difficult to perform efficient searching across databases and organisms.

This problem has been recognized, and in 1998 the Gene Ontology (GO) project
(http://www.geneontology.org) was initiated as a collaborative effort of the Saccharomyces Genome Database (SGD), the Mouse Genome Database (MGD), and FlyBase.
The aim of the Gene Ontology is to provide a consistent, species-independent, functional description of gene products. Since 1998 the GO project has grown considerably and now includes databases for plant, animal, and prokaryotic genomes. Effectively, GO consists of a controlled vocabulary (the GO terms) used to describe the
biological function of a gene product in any organism. The GO terms have a defined
parent-child relationship and form a directed acyclic graph (DAG) (cf. Section 3.5.1).

Systems Biology in Practice. Concepts, Implementation and Application.
E. Klipp, R. Herwig, A. Kowald, C. Wierling, H. Lehrach
Copyright © 2005 WILEY-VCH Verlag GmbH & Co. KGaA, Weinheim
ISBN: 3-527-31078-9

In a DAG, each node can have multiple child nodes, as well as multiple parent nodes. Cyclic references, however, are forbidden. The combination of vocabulary and relationship between nodes is referred to as ontology. At the root of the GO are the three top-level categories, molecular function, biological process, and cellular component, which contain many levels of child nodes (GO terms) that describe a gene product with increasing specificity. The GO consortium, in collaboration with other databases, develops and maintains the three top-level ontologies (the set of GO terms and their relationship) themselves, creates associations between the ontologies and the gene products in the participating databases, and develops tools for the creation, maintenance, and use of the ontologies.

Let's look at a practical example to see how the concept works. The enzyme superoxide dismutase, for instance, is annotated in FlyBase (the *Drosophila melanogaster* database) with the GO term "cytoplasm" in the cellular component ontology, with the GO terms "defense response" and "determination of adult lifespan" in the biological process ontology, and with the terms "antioxidant activity" and "copper, zinc superoxide dismutase activity" in the molecular function ontology. The GO term cytoplasm itself has the single parent "intracellular," which has the single parent "cell," which is finally connected to the cellular component. The other GO terms for superoxide dismutase are connected in a similarly hierarchical way to the three top categories.

The following table gives the number of gene products that have been annotated to the top-level categories of the GO for several popular databases. The table dates from January 2004 and excludes annotations that are based exclusively on electronic inferences.

Database	Biological process	Molecular function	Cellular component
SGD *Saccharomyces cerevisiae*	6455	6438	6441
FlyBase *Drosophila melanogaster*	4974	7084	4291
MGI *Mus musculus*	6634	7127	8175
TAIR *Arabidopsis thaliana*	13,962	6449	11746
WormBase *Caenorhabditis elegans*	3903	410	756
RGD *Rattus norvegicus*	1436	1833	745
Gramene *Oryza sativa*	5459	2770	16,628
ZFIN *Danio rerio*	413	315	296
DictyBase *Dictyostelium discoideum*	410	426	5383
GO Annotations@EBI Human	8109	7585	7037

To use the Gene Ontology effectively, many different tools have been developed that are listed on the GO Web site (http://www.geneontology.org/GO.tools.html). The repertoire encompasses Web-based and standalone GO browsers and editors, microarray-related tools, and programs for many specialized tasks. In the remainder of this section, we will have only a quick look at three such tools. Our first candidate is AmiGO (http://godatabase.org/), which is a Web-based GO browser maintained by the GO consortium (Fig. 13.1a). First of all, AmiGO can be used to browse the terms of the ontologies. The numbers in parenthesis behind the GO terms show how many gene products in the currently selected database are annotated to this term. The seven-digit number behind GO is the GO-ID that links each GO term to a unique identifier. One or more species and one or more data sources can be selected to restrict the results of the search. A click on a leaf of the GO hierarchy (such as biological_processes unknown) brings up a window that lists the genes in the selected databases that have been annotated to this term. Instead of browsing the GO tree, one can also search for specific GO terms and get to the gene products associated with these terms or search for gene products and find the connected GO terms. Finally, it is also possible to get a graphical view, which shows where the selected term is located within the ontology tree.

AmiGO's search options are quite limited since it is only possible to search for several terms that are connected via the OR function (under advanced query). The Java applet GoFish v1.11 (http://llama.med.harvard.edu/~berriz/GoFishWelcome.html) is a good alternative for such cases (Fig. 13.1b). Different GO terms can be selected from a GO tree (left side), which can then be combined into complex Boolean expressions (window in the middle). In the case shown here, we are searching for gene products in the FlyBase that are antioxidants or are involved in defense/immunity but are not concerned with programmed cell death. When the user selects a specific database, the applet downloads the GO terms and associations for this database, and therefore the response time of GoFish is normally faster than for AmiGO.

Recently developed high-throughput techniques such as DNA chips enable researchers to measure the expression profile of thousands of genes in parallel. Often, one is interested in whether the genes that are over- or underexpressed share biological functions. The Web-based program GOstat (http://gostat.wehi.edu.au/) makes use of the Gene Ontology to test whether certain GO terms are statistically over- or underrepresented in a group of genes of interest. GOstat can compare the list of genes either against a user-supplied control list or against the complete list of genes in a selected database. It then uses Fisher's exact test or the Chi-square test to determine whether the observed differences of the frequencies of GO terms are significant or not (cf. Section 9.4). The output is a list of *P*-values that state how specific the associated GO terms are for the list of genes provided. The list can then be obtained as text or as an HTML file.

This was only a brief introduction of three of the many available programs that make use of GO annotations. Furthermore, it is always possible to develop one's own programs, since all GO-related files such as lists of GO definitions or database annotations can be downloaded at http://www.geneontology.org.

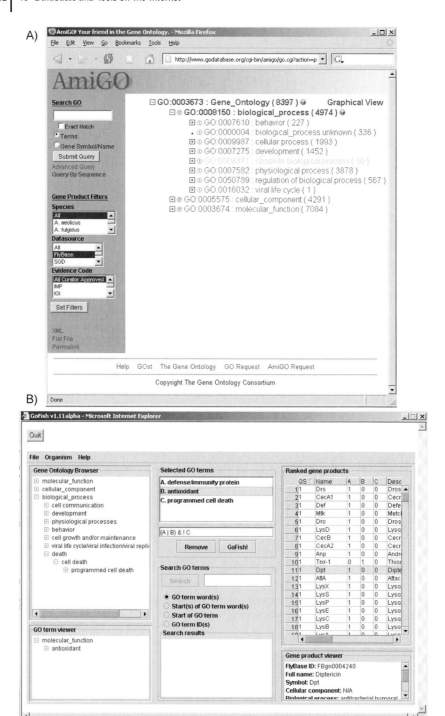

13.2
KEGG

KEGG (Kyoto Encyclopedia of Genes and Genomes; http://www.genome.ad.jp/ kegg/) is a reference knowledgebase offering information about genes and proteins, biochemical compounds, reactions, and pathways. The data are organized in three parts: the gene universe (consisting of the GENES, SSDB, and KO databases), the chemical universe (with the COMPOUND, GLYCAN, REACTION, and ENZYME databases which are merged as the LIGAND database), and the protein network consisting of the PATHWAY database (Kanehisa et al. 2004). In addition, the KEGG database is hierarchically classified into categories and subcategories at four levels. The five topmost categories are metabolism, genetic information processing, environmental information processing, cellular processes, and human diseases. Subcategories of metabolism are, e.g., carbohydrate, energy, lipid, nucleotide, or amino acid metabolism. These are subdivided into the different pathways, such as glycolysis, citrate cycle, purine metabolism, etc. Finally, the fourth level corresponds to the KO (KEGG Orthology) entries. A KO entry (internally identified by a K number, e.g., K00001 for the alcohol dehydrogenase) corresponds to a group of orthologous genes that have identical functions.

The gene universe offers information about genes and proteins generated by genome sequencing projects. Information about individual genes is stored in the GENES database, which is semiautomatically generated from submissions to GenBank, the NCBI RefSeq database, the EMBL database, and other publicly available organism-specific databases. K numbers are further assigned to entries of the GENES database. The SSDB database contains information about amino acid sequence similarities between protein-coding genes computationally generated from the GENES database. This is carried out for many complete genomes and results in a huge graph depicting protein similarities with clusters of orthologous and paralogous genes.

The chemical universe offers information about chemical compounds and reactions relevant to cellular processes. It includes more than 11,000 compounds (internally represented by C numbers, e.g., C00001 denotes water), a separate database for carbohydrates (nearly 11,000 entries; represented by a number preceded by G, e.g., G10481 for cellulose), more than 6000 reactions (with R numbers, e.g., R00275 for the reaction of the superoxide radical into hydrogen peroxide), and more than 4000 enzymes (denoted by EC numbers as well as K numbers for orthologous entries). All these data are merged as the LIGAND database (Goto et al. 2002). Thus, the chemical universe offers comprehensive information about metabolites with their respective chemical structures and biochemical reactions.

◀ **Fig. 13.1** (a) AmiGO, a Web-based GO browser developed by the GO consortium. It allows browsing the GO hierarchy and searching for specific GO terms or gene products in different databases. The numbers in brackets behind the GO terms indicate how many gene products have been annotated to this term in the selected database. (b) GoFish, a Java applet, can also connect to several databases and allows the user to search for gene products using complex Boolean expressions of GO terms.

KEGG's protein network provides information about protein interactions comprising pathways and protein complexes. The 235 KEGG reference pathway diagrams (maps) offered on the Web site give clear overviews of important pathways. Organism-specific pathway maps are automatically generated by coloring of organism-specific genes in the reference pathways.

The KEGG database can be queried via the Web interface, e. g., for genes, proteins, compounds, etc. Access to the data via FTP (http://www.genome.ad.jp/anonftp) as well via a SOAP server (http://www.genome.ad.jp/kegg/soap) is possible for academic users, too (SOAP is a protocol for the exchange of messages between computer software based on XML; see Section 14.2.1).

13.3
BRENDA

High-throughput projects, such as the international genome sequencing efforts, accumulate large amounts of data at an amazing rate. These data are essential for the reconstruction of phylogenetic trees and gene-finding projects. However, for kinetic modeling, which is at the heart of systems biology, kinetic data of proteins and enzymes are needed. Unfortunately, this type of data is notoriously difficult and time-consuming to obtain, since proteins often need individually tuned purification and reaction conditions. Furthermore, the results of such studies are published in a large variety of journals from different fields.

In this situation, BRENDA aims to be a comprehensive enzyme information system (http://www.brenda.uni-koeln.de). Basically, BRENDA is a curated database that contains a large amount of functional data for individual enzymes. These data are gathered from the literature and made available via a Web interface. The table on the next page gives an overview of the types of information that is collected and the number of entries for the different information fields (as of June 2004). For instance, enzymes representing 4379 different EC numbers and over 50,000 different K_m values are contained in the database.

One of BRENDA's strengths is the multitude of ways the database can be searched. It is easy to find all enzymes that are above a specific molecular weight, belong to *C. elegans*, or have a temperature optimum above 30°C. If desired, the list of results can then be downloaded as a tab-separated text file for later inspection. Using the Advanced Search feature, it is possible to construct arbitrarily complex search queries involving the information field shown in the table.

Sometimes one wants to search for all enzymes that are glycosylases without knowing the corresponding EC number or to find all enzymes that are found in horses without knowing the exact scientific name. In this situation, the ECTree browser and the TaxTree search are helpful by providing a browser-like interface to search down the hierarchy of EC number descriptions or taxonomic names. A similar browser is also available for Gene Ontology terms, which were discussed in Section 13.1.

BRENDA is also very well connected to other databases that can provide further information about an enzyme in question. Associated GO terms are directly linked

Information Field	Entries	Information Field	Entries
Enzyme nomenclature		*Functional parameters*	
EC number	4379	K_m value	52,343
Recommended name	4376	Turnover number	9035
Systematic name	3469	Specific activity	22,108
Synonyms	30,475	pH range and optimum	5063/18,866
CAS registry number	4005	Temperature range and optimum	1396/8014
Reaction	3864	*Molecular properties*	
Reaction type	6326	pH stability	3899
Enzyme structure		Temperature stability	9124
Molecular weight	18,725	General stability	5847
Subunits	11,666	Organic solvent stability	468
Sequence links	65,249	Oxidation stability	487
Post-translational modifications	2069	Storage stability	8249
Crystallization	1741	Purification	15,102
3D structure, PDB links	11,236	Cloned	6666
Enzyme-ligand interactions		Engineering	6190
Substrates/products	82,194	Renatured	346
Natural substrates	33,619	Application	1641
Cofactor	9967	*Organism-related information*	
Activating compound	11,780	Organism	99,502
Metals/ions	16,162	Source-tissue, organ	28,181
Inhibitors	75,584	Localization	11,711
Bibliographic data			
References	73,406		

to the AmiGO browser; substrates and products of the catalyzed reactions can be displayed as chemical structures; links to the taxonomic database NEWT (http://www.e-bi.ac.uk/newt) exist for information of the organism; sequence data can be obtained from Swiss-Prot; and if crystallographic data exist, a link to PDB (see Section 13.8) is provided. Finally, literature references (including PubMed IDs) from where the protein data originated are provided.

13.4
Databases of the National Center for Biotechnology

The National Center for Biotechnology (NCBI) (http://www.ncbi.nlm.nih.gov/) provides several databases that are widely used in biological research. Most important are the molecular databases, offering information about nucleotide sequences, proteins, genes, molecular structures, and gene expression. Besides this, several databases comprising scientific literature are available. The NCBI also provides a taxonomy database that contains names and lineages of more than 130,000 organisms. For more than 1000 organisms, whole genomes (either already completely sequenced or for which sequencing is still in progress) and corresponding gene maps are available, as well as tools for their inspection. A full overview of the databases provided by the NCBI can be found under http://www.ncbi.nlm.nih.gov/sitemap/index.html. All these databases are searchable via the Entrez search engine accessible through the NCBI homepage.

Among the nucleotide sequence databases, the Genetic Sequence database (GenBank), the Reference Sequences database (RefSeq), and UniGene can be found. GenBank (Release 143.0, from August 2004) comprises 41.8 billion nucleotide bases from more than 37 million reported sequences. The RefSeq database (Maglott et al. 2000; Pruitt et al. 2000; Pruitt and Maglott 2001) is a curated, non-redundant set of sequences including genomic DNA, mRNA, and protein products for important model organisms. In UniGene, expressed sequence tags (ESTs) and full-length mRNA sequences are organized into clusters, each representing a unique known or putative gene of a specific organism. (For molecular biological analyses, e.g., sequencing or expression profiling, the mRNA of expressed genes is usually translated into a complementary DNA [cDNA, copy DNA], since this is more stable and feasible for standard biotechnological methods. An EST is a short, approximately 200–600 bp long, sequence from either side of a cDNA clone that is useful for identifying the full-length gene, e.g., for locating the gene in the genome.)

In addition to nucleotide sequences, protein sequences can also be searched for at the NCBI site via Entrez-Proteins. Searches are performed across several databases, including RefSeq, Swiss-Prot, and PDB.

Finally, the LocusLink database (http://www.ncbi.nlm.nih.gov/LocusLink) offers diverse information about specific genetic loci (the location of a specific gene). Thus, LocusLink provides a central hub for accessing gene-specific information for a number of species, such as human, mouse, rat, zebrafish, nematode, fruit fly, cow, and sea urchin.

Among the literature databases are PubMed and OMIM (Online Mendelian Inheritance in Man). PubMed is a database of citations and abstracts for biomedical literature. Citations are from MEDLINE (http://medline.cos.com) and additional life science journals. OMIM is a catalog of human genes and genetic disorders with textual information and copious links to the scientific literature.

Thus, the databases at the NCBI are one of the major resources for sequence data, annotations, and literature references. They can be used to determine what is known about a specific gene or its protein or to get information about the sequences and their variants or polymorphisms. In addition to this, the NCBI also offers a database on gene expression data (Gene Expression Omnibus, GEO).

Besides all these databases, the NCBI also provides tools mostly operating on sequence data. These include programs comparing one or more sequences with the provided sequence databases.

13.5
Databases of the European Bioinformatics Institute

The European Bioinformatics Institute (EMBL-EBI) also offers several biologically relevant databases (http://www.ebi.ac.uk/Databases). These include databases on nucleotide sequences, genes, and genomes (EMBL Nucleotide Database, Ensembl automatic genome annotation database), a database on alternative splicing sites (ASD), a database of protein modifications (RESID), a database on protein families and protein domains (InterPro), a database on macromolecular structures (E-MSD), and a database on gene expression data (ArrayExpress). The protein databases Swiss-Prot, TrEMBL, and UniProt as well as the Reactome database on pathways and processes relevant for humans will be discussed in separate sections below.

13.5.1
EMBL Nucleotide Sequence Database

The EMBL Nucleotide Sequence Database (http://www.ebi.ac.uk/embl) incorporates, organizes, and distributes nucleotide sequences from public sources and synchronizes its data in a daily manner with the DNA Database of Japan (DDBJ) and GenBank, which are the two other most important nucleotide sequence databases worldwide (Kulikova et al. 2004).

13.5.2
Ensembl

The Ensembl project (http://www.ensembl.org/) is developing and maintaining a system for the management and presentation of genomic sequences and annotation for eukaryotic genomes (Hubbard et al. 2002; Birney et al. 2004a, 2004b; Hammond and Birney 2004). What does annotation mean in this context? Annotation is the characterization of features of the genome using computational and experimental methods. In the first place, this is the prediction of genes, including structural elements like introns and exons, from the assembled genome sequence and the characterization of genomic features, like repeated sequence motifs, conserved regions, or single-nucleotide polymorphisms (SNPs). SNPs (pronounced „snips") are common DNA sequence variations among individuals, where a single nucleotide is altered. Furthermore, annotation includes information about functional domains of the proteins encoded by the genes and the roles that the gene products fulfill in the organism.

The central component of Ensembl is a relational database storing the genome sequence assemblies and annotations produced by Ensembl's automated sequence-annotation pipeline, which utilizes the genome assemblies and data from external resources for this purpose. In September 2004, Ensembl provided genomic annotations for several vertebrates (human, chimp, mouse, rat, puffer fish, zebrafish, and chicken), arthropods (mosquito, honeybee, and fruit fly), and nematodes (*Caenorhabditis elegans* and *Caenorhabditis briggsae*). Annotations, such as genes with their intron/exon structure, SNPs, etc., can be viewed along the assembled sequence contigs using the Ensembl ContigView, which is accessible via the organism-specific Web pages (e.g., for humans, http://www.ensembl.org/Homo_sapiens/).

13.5.3
InterPro

InterPro (http://www.ebi.ac.uk/interpro/) is a protein signature database comprising information about protein families, domains, and functional groups (Biswas et al. 2002; Mulder et al. 2003). It combines many commonly used protein signature databases and is a very powerful tool for the automatic and manual annotation of new or predicted proteins from sequencing projects. In addition, InterPro entries are mapped to the Gene Ontology (GO, see Section 13.1) and are linked to protein entries in UniProt (see Section 13.6).

13.6
Swiss-Prot, TrEMBL, and UniProt

In addition to several nucleotide sequence databases, a variety of protein sequence databases also exist, ranging from simple sequence repositories to expertly curated universal databases that cover many species and provide a great deal of additional information. One of the leading protein databases is Swiss-Prot (http://www.ebi.ac.uk/swissprot/). As of August 2004 (release 44.4), it contains 158,010 protein sequence entries. Swiss-Prot is maintained by the Swiss Institute of Bioinformatics (SIB) and the European Bioinformatics Institute (EBI) and offers a high level of annotation comprising information about the protein origin (gene name and species), amino acid sequence, protein function and location, protein domains and sites, quaternary structure, references to the literature, protein-associated disease(s), and many other details. In addition, Swiss-Prot provides cross-references to several external data collections such as nucleotide sequence databases (DDBJ/EMBL/GenBank), protein structure databases, databases providing protein domain and family characterizations, disease-related databases, etc. (Boeckmann et al. 2003).

Since the creation of fully curated Swiss-Prot entries is a highly laborious task, another database called TrEMBL (Translation from EMBL), which uses an automated annotation approach, was introduced. TrEMBL (http://www.ebi.ac.uk/trembl/) contains computer-annotated entries generated by *in silico* translation of all coding sequences (CDS) available in the nucleotide databases (DDBJ, EMBL, GenBank). The entries offered at TrEMBL do not overlap with those found in Swiss-Prot.

The world's most comprehensive catalog providing protein-related information is the UniProt database (http://www.uniprot.org). UniProt is composed of information of Swiss-Prot, TrEMBL, and PIR (http://pir.georgetown.edu). One part of UniProt, UniParc, is the most comprehensive, publicly accessible, non-redundant protein sequence collection available (Apweiler et al. 2004).

13.7
Reactome

Sequence and annotation databases such as RefSeq (Pruitt et al. 2000; Pruitt and Maglott 2001), GeneCards (Safran et al. 2002), or YPD (Costanzo et al. 2000), provide a gene-by-gene view of the genome. These databases present all the information known about the structure and function of a gene and its protein(s) in a single record. However, important for biology – especially systems biology – is information about the complex interactions among proteins, nucleic acids, and other molecules, e. g., metabolites that carry out complex biological processes. Such data about biological processes and pathways are not covered by the above-mentioned gene-centric databases but often are found in the scientific literature. Reactome (formerly known as Genome Knowledgebase, Joshi-Tope et al. 2003), is an open, online database of fundamental human biological processes that tries to narrow this gap. The Reactome project is managed as a collaboration of the Cold Spring Harbor Laboratory, the European Bioinformatics Institute (EBI), and the Gene Ontology Consortium.

A screenshot of the Reactome homepage (http://www.reactome.org) is shown in Fig. 13.2. The database is divided into several modules of fundamental biological processes that are thought to operate in humans. Each module of the database has one or more primary authors and is further peer reviewed by experts in the specific fields. Each module can also be referenced by its revision date and thus can be cited like a publication.

On one hand the Reactome database is intended to offer valuable information for wet-lab scientists who want to know, e. g., more about a specific gene product they are unfamiliar with. On the other hand the Reactome database can be used by computational biologists to draw conclusions from large datasets such as expression data gained by cDNA chip experiments. For the latter purpose, the database can be downloaded and locally installed as a MySQL database (DuBois 2002). Due to its clear, hierarchical, object-oriented design, it can be queried very flexibly by Structured Query Language (SQL) statements. (SQL is a popular computer language used to create, modify, and query databases.)

The data model of Reactome consists of three fundamental data types: physical entity, reaction, and pathway. A physical entity is any kind of molecule or complex that participates in a biological process. A reaction consumes one or more physical entities as input and produces one or more physical entities as output. Reactions can be further grouped into pathways. With the help of these data types, the topology of a reaction network can be described. Kinetic data (e. g., rate constants or concentration gradients) that are required for true physiological modeling are not accounted for by the database. Gene products mentioned in the database are linked to the gene-specific databases SwissProt, Ensembl, and RefSeq.

Another tool offered by Reactome is the "Pathfinder." This utility enables the user to find the shortest path between two physical entities, e. g., the shortest path between the metabolites D-fructose and pyruvate, or the steps from the primary mRNA to its processed form. The computed path can be shown graphically. The pathfinder also offers the possibility to exclude specific entities, such as the metabolites ATP or

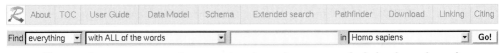

Reactome – a knowledgebase of biological processes

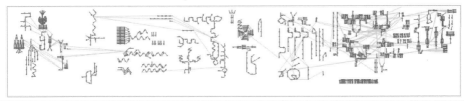

Cell Cycle, Mitotic	Cell Cycle Checkpoints	DNA Repair	DNA Replication
Hsa | Mmu | Rno | Fru | Dre | Gga	Hsa | Mmu | Rno | Fru | Dre | Gga	Hsa | Mmu | Rno | Fru | Dre | Gga	Hsa | Mmu | Rno | Fru | Dre | Gga
Gene Expression	Lipid metabolism	Insulin receptor mediated signalling	Metabolism of amino acids and related nitrogen–containing molecules
Hsa | Mmu | Rno | Fru | Dre | Gga	Hsa | Mmu | Rno | Fru | Dre | Gga	Hsa | Mmu | Rno | Fru | Dre	Hsa | Mmu | Rno | Fru | Dre | Gga
Metabolism of glucose, other sugars, and ethanol	mRNA Processing	Nucleotide metabolism	Oxidative decarboxylation of pyruvate and TCA cycle
Hsa | Mmu | Rno | Fru | Dre | Gga	Hsa | Mmu | Rno | Fru | Dre | Gga	Hsa | Mmu | Rno | Fru | Dre | Gga	Hsa | Mmu | Rno | Fru | Dre | Gga
Transcription	Translation		
Hsa | Mmu | Rno | Fru | Dre | Gga	Hsa | Mmu | Rno | Fru | Dre | Gga		

Fig. 13.2 Reactome (http://www.reactome.org) is a database of fundamental human biological processes. The homepage offers a graphical representation of the human reaction network. Each arrow in the diagram represents a single event, which is a biological process during which input entries are converted into output entries by one or more steps. The separate modules covered by the Reactome database are listed below the diagram. Pointing with the mouse to one of the module names highlights all events assigned to it. Furthermore, for each module, orthologous events occurring in other organisms can be highlighted. Clicking on either a module or a single event in the diagram offers more details about it. The link "TOC" at the top of the page refers to a table reporting the review state of each module. The header line also has a reference to the "Pathfinder" tool.

NADH, which show high connectivity and whose input thus might lead to a path that is not the one intended to be found.

A further add-on currently under construction is an export facility of the models as SBML code. SBML is a language designed for the exchange of biological models in systems biology, which is discussed in more detail in Section 14.2.2.

13.8
PDB

Biological macromolecules, i.e. proteins and nucleic acids, fold into specific three-dimensional structures. Using techniques such as X-ray crystallography or nuclear magnetic resonance (NMR), these structures can be solved and the three-dimen-

Year	Deposited structures per year	Deposited structures in total
1990	236	568
1991	412	756
1992	554	964
1992	782	1673
1994	1025	2995
1995	1188	3932
1996	1429	5098
1997	1836	6669
1998	2150	8740
1999	2570	11110
2000	2937	13755
2001	3209	16612
2002	3381	19624
2003	4684	23793
2004	3078	26485

sional coordinates of the atoms can be determined. Obviously, such information is extremely valuable for understanding the biological activity of the molecules and their interaction with possible reaction partners. The Protein Data Bank, PDB, is the main repository for 3D structures of biological macromolecules (Berman et al. 2000). As of August 2004 the databank holds more than 26,000 structures and, as the previous table shows, the number is growing exponentially.

Currently the PDB Web site (http://www.pdb.org) is undergoing a major restructuring. Although the new site (http://pdbbeta.rcsb.org) is still under construction and is not yet free of bugs, we will concentrate on the new site, since it is foreseeable that it will soon replace the old Web site. The new site is based on the Data Uniformity Project (Westbrook et al. 2002), the aim of which is to improve the consistency of data formats and content across the PDB archive. One way to achieve this was the introduction of a new data format, mmCIF (macromolecular Crystallographic Information File), which is superior to the old PDB format.

The new, overhauled Web site offers extensive search and browse capabilities, similar to the features found at the BRENDA Web site (see Section 13.3). In the simplest case, one can enter a PDB ID, a four-character alphanumeric identifier, to get straight to a specific structure (Fig. 13.3). 1B06, for instance, brings up the information for the superoxide dismutase of *Sulfolobus acidocaldarius*, a thermophilic archaebacterium. The resulting page gives essential information about the protein such as literature references, quality parameters for the crystal structure, and GO terms. Via the available pull-down menus, further functions can be reached. Probably the most important functions are downloading structure (PDB or mmCIF format) or sequence (FASTA format) files and accessing different 3D viewers. Some viewers, such as KiNG or WebMol, require only a Java-enabled Web browser, while others, such as Rasmol or the Swiss-PDB viewer, need a special browser plug-in.

If a PDB ID is not available, the database can be browsed, for instance, according to GO terms (see Section 13.1). Under "Browse Database/Molecular Function" we

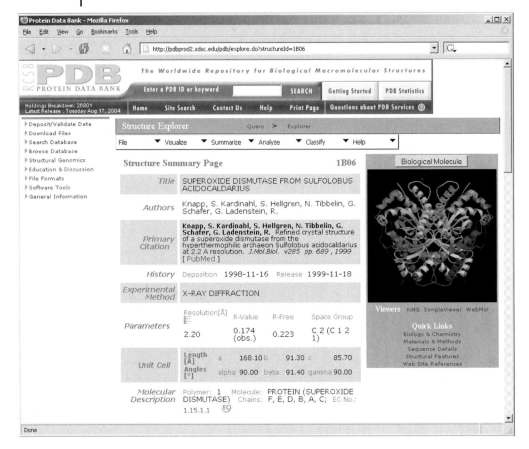

Fig. 13.3 PDB, the Protein Data Bank, is the major repository for 3D structures of biological macromolecules (http://pdbbeta.rcs-b.org). The Web interface allows browsing and searching the database in a multitude of different ways. This screenshot shows the entry for the superoxide dismutase of *Sulfolobus acidocaldarius*, a thermophilic archaebacterium.

can drill down the GO terms to find "catalytic activity/oxidoreductase activity/oxidoreductase activity, acting on superoxide radicals as acceptor/superoxide dismutase activity." This GO term is linked to 129 PDB structures, one of which is shown in Fig. 13.3. And, as for BRENDA, there is also the option of browsing according to EC number or species. Finally, the database can also be browsed for SCOP (http://scop.mrc-lmb.cam.ac.uk/scop) and CATH (http://www.biochem.ucl.ac.uk/bsm/cath) classifiers, hierarchical classification schemes for protein domain structures, and structural similarities.

The two most important methods for searching PDB are SearchLite and SearchFields. SearchLite is quite powerful, since it allows one to combine search terms using "and," "or," and "not." The search phrase "superoxide dismutase and sulfolobus," for instance, results in two hits, one of which is 1B06, shown in Fig. 13.3. For more complex search tasks, SearchFields can be used. There it is possible to search specific database fields (e.g., GO terms, resolution, organism) and combine them using Boolean operators. If the search query results in more than one hit, it is possible to download structure or sequence files for some or all of the results.

If one is interested in much larger datasets, structure files (PDB and mmCIF format) can be directly downloaded from the anonymous FTP server at ftp:// ftp.rcsb.org/pub/pdb/data/structures/divided. Entries are grouped by the middle characters of the PDB-ID. For example, entry file 1B06 can be found in pub/pdb/ data/structures/divided/pdb/B0 or pub/pdb/data/structures/divided/mmCIF/B0. Additionally, PDB releases data on CD-ROM four times a year. The January release contains all structures, while the other three releases are update releases.

13.9
TRANSFAC and EPD

The transcriptional activity of genes, and thus their biological function, is controlled by the interaction of transcription factors with promoter regions on the DNA. Thus, a better understanding of this interaction would be very valuable for a systems biological description of cellular processes. Promoter databases such as TRANSFAC or EPD provide important information for the modeler and the experimentalist.

13.9.1
TRANSFAC

TRANSFAC can be reached at http://www.gene-regulation.com. It contains information about eukaryotic transcription factors (TF) and their DNA-binding sites (cf. Section 8.2). The database requires a registration, but a public version is free of charge for academic users. TRANSFAC consists of six different ASCII flat file tables called SITE, GENE, FACTOR, CELL, CLASS, and MATRIX. SITE contains information about the transcription factor–binding site on the DNA, GENE gives a short description of the gene the site belongs to, FACTOR describes the transcription factors binding to this site, CELL holds information about the cell types in which the transcription factors have been found that bind to a given site, CLASS provides information about the class the transcription factor belongs to, and the MATRIX table gives nucleotide distribution matrices for the binding sites of transcription factors.

The contents of the tables are described by different fields. The following list provides an overview of the field names of the SITE table together with a short description.

Each of the different sets of tables can be searched for either globally or restricted to a specific field. Wildcards ("*" and "?") can be used, so that a global search for "*" finds all entries for the selected table. The public version of TRANSFAC currently

Field	Field description
AC	Accession number
ID	Identifier
DT	Date and author
TY	Sequence type
DE	Description (gene or gene product), GENE accession number
RE	Gene region like promoter or enhancer
SQ	Sequence of the regulatory element
EL	Denomination of the element
SF	First position of factor-binding site
ST	Last position of factor-binding site
S1	Definition of first position if it is not the transcription start site
BF	Binding factor with FACTOR accession number, name, and biological species
MX	MATRIX accession number for deduced matrix
OS	Organism or species
OC	Organism classification
SO	CELL accession number for FACTOR source
MM	Method
CC	Comments
DR	Link to external databases
RX	Medline ID
RN	Reference number
RA	Reference authors
RT	Reference title
RL	Reference data

contains 6627 SITE entries, 4219 FACTOR entries, 1755 GENE entries, 1432 CELL entries, 44 CLASS entries, and 336 MATRIX entries. The MATRIX tables are probably the most interesting for modeling, since they contain information about the frequencies of the different nucleotides at the transcription factor-binding site.

13.9.2
EPD

The Eukaryotic Promoter Database (EPD) is hosted at the Swiss Institute for Bioinformatics (SIB) and contains a collection of eukaryotic polymerase II promoters, for which the transcription start site has been determined experimentally and whose sequence is available in the EMBL Data Library (http://www.epd.isb-sib.ch). As of August 2004, EPD is based on EMBL release 79 and contains 4810 entries. Up to release 72, promoters were classified according to a hierarchically numbered system, not unlike the EC numbering system for enzymes. Top levels of this system are (1) plant promoters, (2) nematode promoters, (3) arthropod promoters, (4) mollusk promoters, (5) echinoderm promoters, and (6) vertebrate promoters. Unfortunately, this system has been discontinued since it is often difficult to determine how a new promoter should be classified, especially if the gene product is a multifunctional protein.

Like TRANSFAC, EPD is based on ASCII flat files containing different fields, indicated by field identifiers in the first two columns. Also, the search capabilities are similar in that search queries can be performed on all fields or a selected subset of fields. An example search for "superoxide dismutase" on all fields results in three hits. For each hit, further information can then be displayed: either the content of the flat file entry or the promoter sequence (plus upstream/downstream nucleotides) in FASTA or EMBL format.

It is also possible to download larger lists of promoter sequences (http://www.epd.isb-sib.ch/seq_download.html) by selecting groups of promoters from a hierarchical list that is based on the mentioned classification scheme. This makes it easy to retrieve all promoter sequences of *Mus musculus* or even for all vertebrates. Finally, using the EPD FTP server (ftp://ftp.epd.unil.ch/pub/databases/epd/views), it is possible to download the complete database.

13.10
Genome Matrix

The integration of information from functional genomics approaches represents a major challenge to bioinformatics and computational biology (cf. Chapter 11). In contrast to sequence databases, which are restricted to a single data class, data from functional genomics experiments can be extremely complex and are typically useful only if a large amount of information on the experiment, the materials used, the exact experimental conditions, etc., is provided. In addition, many experiments are technically possible (or at least available) only with genes of one species. It is therefore essential to combine functional genomics information from many experimental sources and across many organisms, based on the orthology between the genes in the different species.

A number of relevant databases have been developed. Expression data, for example, have dedicated databases (ArrayExpress at the EBI, http://www.ebi.ac.uk/arrayexpress/; Gene Expression Omnibus, GEO, at the NCBI, http://www.ncbi.nlm.nih.gov/geo/; Stanford Microarray Database, SMD, http://genome-www.stanford.edu/microarray/) in which expression data following the MIAME standard can be deposited. There are a number of databases for protein interactions (DIP, http://dip.doe-mbi.ucla.edu/; BIND, http://www.bind.ca), protein structure (PDB, see Section 13.8), gene traps (German Genetrap Consortium, http://www.genetrap.de/), and many other aspects of functional genomics. In addition to these databases centered around the type of information they store, there are many curated databases gathering all available information on the genes of a specific organism, e.g., for mouse (the Jackson Laboratory, http://www.jax.org/), rat (Rat Genome Database, http://rgd.mcw.edu/; Ratmap, http://ratmap.gen.gu.se/), the nematode *Caenorhabditis elegans* (WormBase, http://www.wormbase.org/), the fruit fly *Drosophila melanogaster* (FlyBase, http://flybase.bio.indiana.edu/), the zebrafish *Danio rerio* (Zebrafish Information Network, ZFIN, http://zfin.org/), or the budding yeast *Saccharomyces cerevisiae* (Saccharomyces Genome Database, SGD, http://www.yeastgenome.org/).

Access to this information is, however, typically focused on gene-by-gene queries and therefore is not optimal for the display of information on thousands of genes at a time.

This has been the main driving force behind the development of Genome-Matrix (http://www.genome-matrix.org), a database/database interface system developed by the Max Planck Institute for Molecular Genetics and the German Resource Center for Genome Research (RZPD). This system displays information on different genes of different organisms in the form of a matrix of colored rectangles, with each column representing one gene (and its orthologs in the other organisms displayed), while each row corresponds to one particular type of information relevant for the comprehension of the function of the genes (Fig. 13.4). Thus, for each gene (or groups of genes) the system allows the display of the available information in a com-

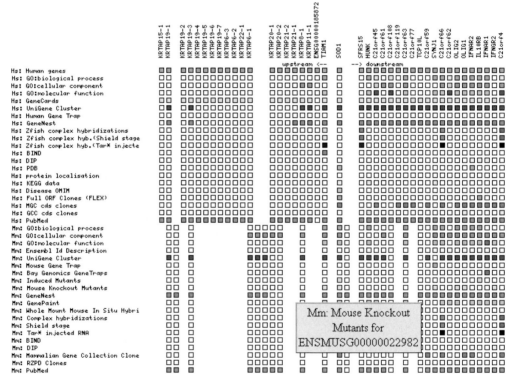

Fig. 13.4 Genome matrix (http://www.genome-matrix.org) is a database/database interface system providing genomic information as a matrix. Each column of the matrix corresponds to a particular gene of an organism (or its ortholog(s), if displayed) and each row represents one particular type of information relevant for the comprehension of the function of the genes. As far as possible, the information of one particular data type is coded by the color of the boxes in a row. The screenshot shows the information available for the gene superoxide dismutase (SOD1) in human (Hs) and mouse (Mm) as well as its neighboring genes on chromosome 21. By pointing to one particular box, a pop-up menu is produced that provides a short description of the information that is linked to that particular box.

prehensive way. The display can either output groups of genes (e.g., sharing the term "kinase") or view a single gene in its chromosomal neighborhood (i.e., genes downstream or upstream in the DNA sequence).

As far as possible, the information of one particular data type for one particular gene is represented by the color of the box (usually possible for scalar information). The color of the box can, for example, identify the function of the gene (GO annotation), represent a quantitative measure (normalized expression levels for a gene displayed on a red-green or yellow-blue scale), or simply indicate that there is information of one particular type for this particular gene available (e.g., an X-ray structure of a protein, a picture showing a developmental phenotype of a mouse knockout strain, an RNAi phenotype in *C. elegans*, etc.). Clicking on the boxes then displays the information available, stored either locally or in a database or Web site anywhere in the world. Since this system has a very low overhead, it is easy to adapt to changes in the many databases holding the primary information, a feature required for any realistic system attempting to keep track of the multitude of relevant data produced worldwide.

References

APWEILER, R., BAIROCH, A., WU, C.H., BARKER, W.C., BOECKMANN, B., FERRO, S., GASTEIGER, E., HUANG, H., LOPEZ, R., MAGRANE, M., MARTIN, M.J., NATALE, D.A., O'DONOVAN, C., REDASCHI, N. and YEH, L.S. UniProt: the Universal Protein knowledgebase (2004) Nucleic Acids Res. *32 Database issue*, D115–9

BERMAN, H.M., WESTBROOK, J., FENG, Z., GILLILAND, G., BHAT, T.N., WEISSIG, H., SHINDYALOV, I.N. and BOURNE, P.E. The Protein Data Bank (2000) Nucleic Acids Res. *28*, 235–42

BIRNEY, E., ANDREWS, D., BEVAN, P., CACCAMO, M., CAMERON, G., CHEN, Y., CLARKE, L., COATES, G., COX, T., CUFF, J., CURWEN, V., CUTTS, T., DOWN, T., DURBIN, R., EYRAS, E., FERNANDEZ-SUAREZ, X.M., GANE, P., GIBBINS, B., GILBERT, J., HAMMOND, M., HOTZ, H., IYER, V., KAHARI, A., JEKOSCH, K., KASPRZYK, A., KEEFE, D., KEENAN, S., LEHVASLAIHO, H., McVICKER, G., MELSOPP, C., MEIDL, P., MONGIN, E., PETTETT, R., POTTER, S., PROCTOR, G., RAE, M., SEARLE, S., SLATER, G., SMEDLEY, D., SMITH, J., SPOONER, W., STABENAU, A., STALKER, J., STOREY, R., URETA-VIDAL, A., WOODWARK, C., CLAMP, M. and HUBBARD, T. Ensembl 2004 (2004a) Nucleic Acids Res. *32 Database issue*, D468–70

BIRNEY, E., ANDREWS, T.D., BEVAN, P., CACCAMO, M., CHEN, Y., CLARKE, L., COATES, G., CUFF, J., CURWEN, V., CUTTS, T., DOWN, T.,

EYRAS, E., FERNANDEZ-SUAREZ, X.M., GANE, P., GIBBINS, B., GILBERT, J., HAMMOND, M., HOTZ, H.R., IYER, V., JEKOSCH, K., KAHARI, A., KASPRZYK, A., KEEFE, D., KEENAN, S., LEHVASLAIHO, H., McVICKER, G., MELSOPP, C., MEIDL, P., MONGIN, E., PETTETT, R., POTTER, S., PROCTOR, G., RAE, M., SEARLE, S., SLATER, G., SMEDLEY, D., SMITH, J., SPOONER, W., STABENAU, A., STALKER, J., STOREY, R., URETA-VIDAL, A., WOODWARK, K.C., CAMERON, G., DURBIN, R., COX, A., HUBBARD, T. and CLAMP, M. An overview of Ensembl (2004b) Genome Res. *14*, 925–8

BISWAS, M., O'ROURKE, J.F., CAMON, E., FRASER, G., KANAPIN, A., KARAVIDOPOULOU, Y., KERSEY, P., KRIVENTSEVA, E., MITTARD, V., MULDER, N., PHAN, I., SERVANT, F. and APWEILER, R. Applications of InterPro in protein annotation and genome analysis (2002) Brief Bioinform. *3*, 285–95

BOECKMANN, B., BAIROCH, A., APWEILER, R., BLATTER, M.C., ESTREICHER, A., GASTEIGER, E., MARTIN, M.J., MICHOUD, K., O'DONOVAN, C., PHAN, I., PILBOUT, S. and SCHNEIDER, M. The SWISS-PROT protein knowledgebase and its supplement TrEMBL in 2003 (2003) Nucleic Acids Res. *31*, 365–70

COSTANZO, M.C., HOGAN, J.D., CUSICK, M.E., DAVIS, B.P., FANCHER, A.M., HODGES, P.E., KONDU, P., LENGIEZA, C., LEW-SMITH, J.E.,

LINGNER, C., ROBERG-PEREZ, K.J., TILLBERG, M., BROOKS, J.E. and GARRELS, J.I. The yeast proteome database (YPD) and Caenorhabditis elegans proteome database (WormPD): comprehensive resources for the organization and comparison of model organism protein information (2000) Nucleic Acids Res. *28*, 73–6

DUBOIS, P. MySQL cookbook (2002) O'Reilly and Associates, Sebastopol, California

GOTO, S., OKUNO, Y., HATTORI, M., NISHIOKA, T. and KANEHISA, M. LIGAND: database of chemical compounds and reactions in biological pathways (2002) Nucleic Acids Res. *30*, 402–4

HAMMOND, M.P. and BIRNEY, E. Genome information resources – developments at Ensembl (2004) Trends Genet. *20*, 268–72

HUBBARD, T., BARKER, D., BIRNEY, E., CAMERON, G., CHEN, Y., CLARK, L., COX, T., CUFF, J., CURWEN, V., DOWN, T., DURBIN, R., EYRAS, E., GILBERT, J., HAMMOND, M., HUMINIECKI, L., KASPRZYK, A., LEHVASLAIHO, H., LIJNZAAD, P., MELSOPP, C., MONGIN, E., PETTETT, R., POCOCK, M., POTTER, S., RUST, A., SCHMIDT, E., SEARLE, S., SLATER, G., SMITH, J., SPOONER, W., STABENAU, A., STALKER, J., STUPKA, E., URETA-VIDAL, A., VASTRIK, I. and CLAMP, M. The Ensembl genome database project (2002) Nucleic Acids Res. *30*, 38–41

JOSHI-TOPE, G., VASTRIK, I., GOPINATH, G.R., MATTHEWS, L., SCHMIDT, E., GILLESPIE, M., D'EUSTACHIO, P., JASSAL, B., WU, G., BIRNEY, E., STEIN, L. The genome knowledgebase: a resource for biologists and bioinformaticists (2003) Cold Spring Harb. Symp. Quant. Biol. *68*: 237–43

KANEHISA, M., GOTO, S., KAWASHIMA, S., OKUNO, Y. and HATTORI, M. The KEGG resource for deciphering the genome (2004) Nucleic Acids Res. *32 Database issue*, D277–80

KULIKOVA, T., ALDEBERT, P., ALTHORPE, N., BAKER, W., BATES, K., BROWNE, P., VAN DEN BROEK, A., COCHRANE, G., DUGGAN, K., EBERHARDT, R., FARUQUE, N., GARCIA-PASTOR, M., HARTE, N., KANZ, C., LEINONEN, R., LIN, Q.,

LOMBARD, V., LOPEZ, R., MANCUSO, R., MCHALE, M., NARDONE, F., SILVENTOINEN, V., STOEHR, P., STOESSER, G., TULI, M.A., TZOUVARA, K., VAUGHAN, R., WU, D., ZHU, W. and APWEILER, R. The EMBL Nucleotide Sequence Database (2004) Nucleic Acids Res. *32 Database issue*, D27–30

MAGLOTT, D.R., KATZ, K.S., SICOTTE, H. and PRUITT, K.D. NCBI's LocusLink and RefSeq (2000) Nucleic Acids Res. *28*, 126–8

MULDER, N.J., APWEILER, R., ATTWOOD, T.K., BAIROCH, A., BARRELL, D., BATEMAN, A., BINNS, D., BISWAS, M., BRADLEY, P., BORK, P., BUCHER, P., COPLEY, R.R., COURCELLE, E., DAS, U., DURBIN, R., FALQUET, L., FLEISCHMANN, W., GRIFFITHS-JONES, S., HAFT, D., HARTE, N., HULO, N., KAHN, D., KANAPIN, A., KRESTYANINOVA, M., LOPEZ, R., LETUNIC, I., LONSDALE, D., SILVENTOINEN, V., ORCHARD, S.E., PAGNI, M., PEYRUC, D., PONTING, C.P., SELENGUT, J.D., SERVANT, F., SIGRIST, C.J., VAUGHAN, R. and ZDOBNOV, E.M. The InterPro Database 2003 brings increased coverage and new features (2003) Nucleic Acids Res. *31*, 315–8

PRUITT, K.D. and MAGLOTT, D.R. RefSeq and LocusLink: NCBI gene-centered resources (2001) Nucleic Acids Res. *29*, 137–40

PRUITT, K.D., KATZ, K.S., SICOTTE, H. and MAGLOTT, D.R. Introducing RefSeq and LocusLink: curated human genome resources at the NCBI (2000) Trends Genet. *16*, 44–7

SAFRAN, M., SOLOMON, I., SHMUELI, O., LAPIDOT, M., SHEN-ORR, S., ADATO, A., BEN-DOR, U., ESTERMAN, N., ROSEN, N., PETER, I., OLENDER, T., CHALIFA-CASPI, V. and LANCET, D. GeneCards 2002: towards a complete, object-oriented, human gene compendium (2002) Bioinformatics *18*, 1542–3

WESTBROOK, J., FENG, Z., JAIN, S., BHAT, T.N., THANKI, N., RAVICHANDRAN, V., GILLILAND, G.L., BLUHM, W., WEISSIG, H., GREER, D.S., BOURNE, P.E. and BERMAN, H.M. The Protein Data Bank: unifying the archive (2002) Nucleic Acids Res. *30*, 245–8

14
Modeling Tools

Introduction

The databases described in the previous chapter are huge repositories for the biological data that have been gathered by various techniques. The information in the databases represents raw material for most types of modeling efforts. Modeling tools help to formulate theoretical ideas and hypotheses and to extract information relevant to these hypotheses from the raw material stored in the databases. Mathematica and Matlab are general-purpose tools for solving mathematical problems analytically or numerically and for visualizing the results by using different kinds of graphics. Another general-purpose tool that will not be described because of space limitations is the freely available software package R (http://www.r-project.org). Although enormously powerful and flexible, general-purpose tools have a steep learning curve and require some effort to get used to. Consequently, many specialized tools have been developed, some of which are described in the different subsections of Section 14.1. As we will see, these tools are normally easier to master and often concentrate on a certain method or technique.

Irrespective of the tool used, however, it has become clear that it is essential to be able to exchange systems biological models developed by different pieces of software. Section 14.2 describes some of the available exchange formats with special emphasis on the Systems Biology Markup Language (SBML), which is emerging as common standard.

14.1
Modeling and Visualization

14.1.1
Mathematica and Matlab

Mathematica and Matlab are two extensive general-purpose tools for the computation and visualization of any type of mathematical model.

Mathematica is produced by Wolfram Research (http://www.wolfram.com) and exists currently as version 5 for the operating systems Microsoft Windows, Macintosh, Linux, and several Unix variants. The Mathematica system consists of two com-

Systems Biology in Practice. Concepts, Implementation and Application.
E. Klipp, R. Herwig, A. Kowald, C. Wierling, H. Lehrach
Copyright © 2005 WILEY-VCH Verlag GmbH & Co. KGaA, Weinheim
ISBN: 3-527-31078-9

ponents: the kernel that runs in the background performing the calculations and the graphical user interface (GUI) that communicates with the kernel. The GUI has the form of a so-called notebook that contains all the input, output, and graphics. Apart from its numerical calculation and graphics abilities, Mathematica is renowned for its capability to perform advanced symbolic calculations. Mathematica can be used either by interactively invoking the available functions or by using the built-in programming language to write larger routines and programs, which are also stored as or within notebooks. For many specialized topics, Mathematica packages (a special kind of notebook) that provide additional functionality are available. Two products that ship with Mathematica, J/Link and MathLink, enable the two-way communication with Java or C/C++ code. This means that Mathematica can access external code written in one of these languages and that the Mathematica kernel can actually be called from other applications. The former is useful if an algorithm has already been implemented in one of these languages or to speed up time-critical calculations that would take too long if implemented in Mathematica itself. In the latter case other programs can use the Mathematica kernel to perform high-level calculations or render graphics objects. Besides an excellent Help utility, there are also many sites on the Internet that provide additional help and resources. The site http://mathworld. wolfram.com contains a large repository of contributions from Mathematica users all over the world. If a function or algorithm does not exist in Mathematica, it is worthwhile to check this site before implementing it yourself. If questions and problems arise during the use of Mathematica, a valuable source of help is also the newsgroup news://comp.soft-sys.math.mathematica.

The major rival of Mathematica is Matlab 6.5, produced by MathWorks (http://www.mathworks.com). In many respects both products are very similar and it is up to the taste of the user which one he prefers. Matlab is available for the same platforms as Mathematica, has very strong numerical capabilities, and can also produce many different forms of graphics. It also has its own programming language and functions are stored in so-called M-files. Toolboxes (special M-files) add additional functionality to the core Matlab distribution, and, like Mathematica, Matlab can be called by external programs to perform high-level computations. A repository exists for user-contributed files (http://www.mathworks.com/matlabcentral/fileexchange and http://www.mathtools.net/MATLAB/toolboxes.html) as well as a newsgroup (news://comp.soft-sys.matlab) for getting help. Despite these similarities, there are also differences between the two programs. The table on the next page gives a very short, superficial, and subjective list of important differences. The available space is unfortunately not sufficient to go into more detail or describe finer differences.

Let's have a look at Mathematica and Matlab using a practical example. The superoxide radical, $O_2^{\cdot-}$, is a side product of the electron transport chain of mitochondria and contributes to the oxidative stress a cell is exposed to. Different forms of the enzyme superoxide dismutase (SOD) exist that convert this harmful radical into hydrogen peroxide, H_2O_2. This itself causes oxidative stress, and again different enzymes, such as catalase (cat) or glutathione peroxidase, exist to convert it into water. If we want to describe this system, we can write down the following reaction scheme and set of differential equations.

Topic	Mathematica	Matlab
Debugging	Cumbersome and difficult. No dedicated debugging facility.	Dedicated debugger allows one to single-step through M-files using breakpoints.
Add-ons	Many standard packages ship with Mathematica and are included in the price.	Many important toolboxes have to be bought separately. See http://www.mathworks.com/products/product_listing.
Deployment	User needs Mathematica to perform the calculations specified in notebooks.	Separately available compiler allows one to produce standalone applications.
Symbolic computation	Excellent built-in capabilities.	Possible with commercial toolbox.
Storage	All input, output, and graphics are stored in a single notebook.	Functions are stored in individual M-files. A large project can have hundreds of M-files.
Graphics	Graphics are embedded in a notebook and cannot be changed after their creation.	Graphics appear in a separate window and can be manipulated as long as the window exists.
ODE model building	Differential equations are specified explicitly.	Dynamical processes can be graphically constructed with Simulink, a companion product of Matlab.

$$\xrightarrow{c1} O_2^{\cdot-} \xrightarrow[\text{SOD}]{c2} H_2O_2 \xrightarrow[\text{cat}]{c3} H_2O$$

$$\frac{dO_2^{\cdot-}}{dt} = c_1 - c_2 \cdot SOD \cdot O_2^{\cdot-}$$

$$\frac{dH_2O_2}{dt} = c_2 \cdot SOD \cdot O_2^{\cdot-} - c_3 \cdot cat \cdot H_2O_2$$

14.1.1.1 Mathematica Example

First we define the differential equations (and assign them to the variables eq1 and eq2) and specify the numerical values for the constants.

```
eq1 = O2'[t] == c1-c2*SOD*O2[t];
eq2 = H2O2'[t] == c2*SOD*O2[t]-c3*cat*H2O2[t];
par = {c1→6.6*10⁻⁷, c2→1.6*10⁹, c3→3.4*10⁷, SOD→10⁻⁵, cat→10⁻⁵}
```

Now we can solve the equations numerically with the function NDSolve and assign the result to the variable "sol." As boundary conditions we specify that the initial concentrations of superoxide and hydrogen peroxide are zero and instruct NDSolve to find a solution for the first 0.01 seconds. NDSolve returns an interpolating function object, which can be used to obtain numerical values of the solution for any time point between 0 and 0.01. We see that at 0.01 seconds the concentrations are in the nanomolar range and the level of H_2O_2 is approximately 50-fold higher than the concentration of superoxide. Finally, we use Plot to produce a graphic showing the time course of the variable concentrations. We specify several options such as axes labels and colors to make the plot more informative.

```
sol = NDSolve[{eq1, eq2, O2[0]==0, H2O2[0]==0}/.par, {O2, H2O2}, {t,0,0.01}]
{O2[0.01], H2O2[0.01]}/.sol   ⇒     {{4.125*10⁻¹¹, 1.84552*10⁻⁹}}
Plot[Evaluate[{O2[t], H2O2[t]/50}/.sol], {t,0,0.01}, PlotRange->All,
    PlotStyle->{Hue[0.9],Hue[0.6]}, AxesLabel->{"time","concentration"}];
```

14.1.1.2   Matlab Example
In Matlab the routine that solves the ODE systems requires as one of its arguments a function that evaluates the right-hand side of the ODE system for given times and variable values. Because the example system is so small, we can define this function as an inline function and avoid writing a separate M-file. Next the options for the ODE solver are defined. The absolute values of the solution are very small, and therefore the absolute tolerance has to be adjusted accordingly.

```
dydt = inline('[c1-c2*SOD*y(1);c2*SOD*y(1)-c3*cat*y(2)]','t','y','tmp','
    SOD','cat','c1','c2','c3');
options = odeset('OutputFcn',[ ], 'AbsTol', 1e-30, 'RelTol', 1e-6);
```

Now ode45 is called, which solves the ODE system for the specified time span. In addition to dydt, which evaluates the derivatives, we also supply the starting concentrations of the variables and the numerical values for the constants that were used in dydt. ode45 is only one of a whole set (ode45, ode23, ode113, ode15s, ode23s, ode23t, and ode23tb) of possible solvers with different properties (differing in accuracy or suitability for stiff problems). The function returns a vector, *t*, holding time points for which a solution is returned and a matrix, *y*, that contains the variable values at these time points. To find out which concentration exists at a given time, the function "interp1" can be used, which also interpolates between existing time points if necessary. Finally, the resulting time course is plotted and the axes are labeled appropriately.

```
[t, y] = ode45(dydt, [0,0.01], [0;0], options, 1e-5, 1e-5, 6.6e-7, 1.6e9, 3.4e7);
interp1(t,y,0.01)      ⇒      4.125*10⁻¹¹, 1.84552*10⁻⁹
plot(t, y(:,1), t, y(:,2)/50)
xlabel('time')
ylabel('concentration')
```

14.1.2
Gepasi

Matlab and Mathematica are huge and expensive general-purpose tools for mathematical modeling. They can be used to model anything that can be modeled, but at the cost of a steep learning curve. The opposite approach is used by specialized tools that are designed for a certain task. Gepasi is one of these tools that have been developed for the modeling of biochemical reaction systems. It was written by Pedro Mendes (Mendes 1993, 1997) and is available free of charge (http://www.gepasi.org). It runs native under Microsoft Windows but can also be used under Unix/Linux in connection with the Wine emulator (http://www.winehq.com).

In Gepasi, reactions are entered not as differential equations but rather in a notation similar to chemical reactions (Fig. 14.1). Each reaction has to be assigned to a specific kinetics, and Gepasi allows the user to select from a large range of predefined kinetics types (Michaelis-Menten, Hill Kinetics, Uni-Uni, etc.). In addition it is also possible to create user-defined kinetics types. Once a system is defined, the program allows one to perform several tasks such as plotting a time course, scanning the parameter space, fitting models to data, optimizing any function of the model, and performing metabolic control analysis and linear stability analysis.

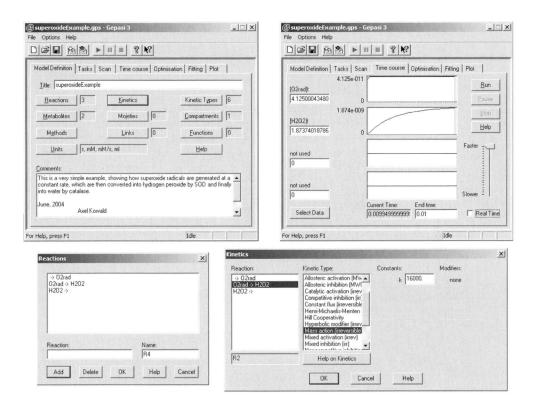

Fig. 14.1 The simulation tool Gepasi. Top left: The main window, which contains tabs for activities such as input of the reaction system, calculating a time course, fitting the system to experimental data or scanning the parameter space. Bottom left: Reactions are entered in a chemical notation, not as ODEs. Irreversible reactions are entered with the symbol -> and reversible reactions with an equal sign (=). Bottom right: A kinetics has to be assigned to each reaction and the necessary numerical constants have to be specified. Top right: If the system has been defined, Gepasi can calculate the time course of selected variables.

It is also possible to create multi-compartment models with Gepasi to model reactions that take place, for instance, in the cytoplasm and the nucleus. If a metabolite crosses a boundary between two compartments of different volume, the change of concentration in the originating compartment is not equal to that in the destination compartment. Gepasi automatically takes care of the conversions between concentrations into absolute amounts and back, which is necessary for the calculations. Apart from its own format, Gepasi can also save and load models that are described in the Systems Biology Markup Language (SBML) level 1 (see Section 14.2.2).

Gepasi is a handy tool that is designed to perform many of the standard tasks for studying a system of biochemical reactions. It is easy to handle, except that one has to get used to the strange fact that all windows are of a fixed size and rather small. Graphical simulation results, however, can also be redirected to a companion program, gnuplot, which does not have these restrictions.

14.1.3
E-Cell

The E-Cell system, initially developed in 1996 at Keio University (Japan), is designed for the simulation of cellular processes. Its first version (E-Cell 1) was used for the construction of a hypothetical cell model with 127 genes, which proved to be sufficient for the modeling of transcription, translation, energy production, and phospholipid synthesis. For this model, a gene collection of *Mycoplasma genitalium* was employed as template (Tomita et al. 1999), as this microorganism is equipped with one of the smallest genomes known. A further model developed for use with E-Cell deals with the mitochondrial metabolism and describes several pathways and processes such as the respiratory chain, the TCA cycle, the fatty acid β-oxidation, and the metabolite transport system (Yugi and Tomita 2004).

The latest version of E-Cell (E-Cell 3, http://www.e-cell.org/) – as well as E-Cell 2 – runs under Microsoft Windows and Linux. E-Cell 3 allows the user to perform multialgorithm calculations, e.g., deterministic models described by ODEs can coexist with stochastic models. Since different cellular processes take place on different timescales – e.g., enzymatic reactions occur on the order of milliseconds and gene regulatory events happen on the order of minutes or hours – E-Cell 3 also includes an algorithm that handles the multiple timescales associated with different cellular processes (Takahashi et al. 2004).

E-Cell models are constructed by employing three fundamental object classes: substance, reactor, and system. Substances represent state variables. Reactors are processes that operate on the state variables. Systems can contain other objects and represent logical and/or physical compartments that can be used for the development of hierarchical models for cellular systems.

Figure 14.2a shows the Session Monitor of E-Cell. Via the Session Monitor, simulations of previously loaded models can be performed. Simulation results can be plotted in a diagram using the TracerWindow (Fig. 14.2b), which is created via the EntityList window. The EntityList window (Fig. 14.2c) further presents the model hierarchy given by the nested structure of systems and a list of the variables (or pro-

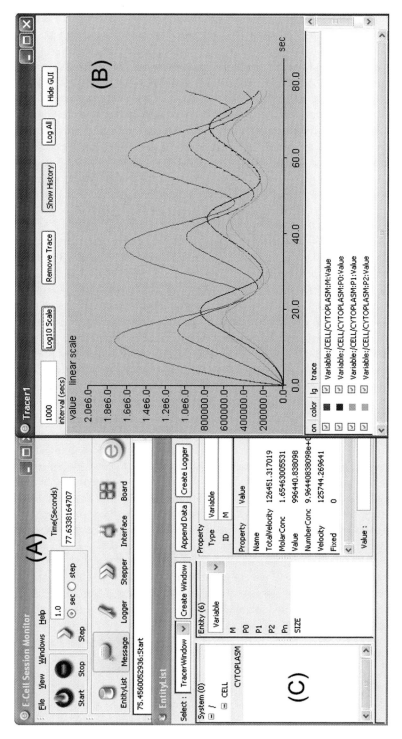

Fig. 14.2 The E-Cell system. (a) The Session Monitor is used to load models and perform simulations. Simulation results can be viewed, e.g., via the TracerWindow (b). The EntityList (c) offers functionalities to browse the model or to edit properties of the variables and processes.

cesses) contained in the selected system. Furthermore, it is used to edit variable or process properties such as the values of the initial concentrations or kinetic constants.

A model file (with the file extension *.eml) can be created either from a separate script file (with the file extension *.em) or directly via a separate application, the Model Editor. In addition to this a further system called GEM (Genome-based E-Cell Modeling) has been developed. The purpose of this system is to automate the generation of E-Cell models. GEM implements a powerful annotation system that utilizes public databases. Via GEM, E-Cell models can be generated simply from genome sequences (Ishii et al. 2004).

14.1.4
PyBioS

PyBioS is designed for applications in systems biology and supports modeling and simulation. In contrast to e.g., Gepasi or E-Cell, which are installed locally, PyBioS is a Web-based environment running on a server that is accessible via http://pybios. molgen.mpg.de/. The purpose of PyBioS is to provide a framework for the conduction of kinetic models of various sizes and levels of granularity. The tool can be used as a standalone modeling platform for ediding and analyzing biochemical models in order to predict the time-dependent behavior of the models. Alternatively, the platform offers the possibility of database interfaces (e.g., KEGG, Reactome) where models can automatically be populated from database information. In particular, the high level of automation enables the analysis of large models.

Figure 14.3 shows screenshots of the PyBioS modeling and simulation environment. Predefined models can be selected from a model repository. Alternatively, users can also create their own models. Using the "View" tab, the user can inspect the hierarchical model. A list of all reactions of the model and a diagram of the whole reaction network are available via the "Reactions" and "Network" tabs, respectively. Model simulations performed by numerical integration of ordinary differential equation systems (ODEs) are possible via the "Simulation" tab. The "Population" tab offers functions for the creation and modification of a model, e.g., forms to edit kinetic parameters and initial concentrations of model components representing state variables. One question a systems biologist might be interested in is how the steady-state behavior of a system might change if one parameter (e.g., the rate of glucose uptake of a cell) is varied. PyBioS provides functionalities to scan the steady-state behavior (via successive simulations or root finding) given a varying parameter. This function, which also includes basic stability analysis, as well as other functions such as the computation of conservation relations are provided via the "Analysis" tab. Finally, via the "Export/Import" tab users can exchange models with other modeling systems, e.g., via SBML language Level 1 (see Section 14.2.2). One important feature of PyBioS is the possibility of using information of public databases directly for the creation of models. It offers, e.g., an interface to the metabolic data of KEGG (see Section 13.2) or an interface to the Reactome database (see Section 13.7), the latter still being under development.

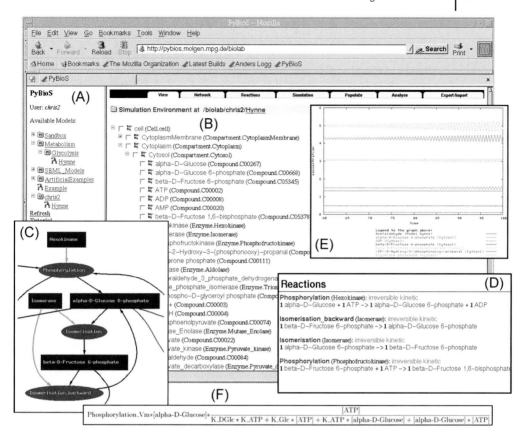

Fig. 14.3 The PyBioS simulation environment. A particular model can be selected from the model repository (a) and its hierarchical model structure can be inspected via the "View" tab at the top of the browser window (b). A graphical representation of the model is provided by an automatically generated network diagram (accessible via the "Network" tab), e.g., (c) shows the forward and reverse reaction of the isomeri- zation of glucose-phosphate to fructose-phosphate of a glycolysis model. The "Reactions" tab offers an overview of all reactions of the model (d). Simulations can be performed via the "Si- mulation" tab (e). A simulation is based on an automatically generated mathematical model derived from the corresponding object-oriented model that comprises the network of all reactions and their respective kinetics (f).

The underlying object-oriented structure of PyBioS entails a set of predefined object classes for biological entities (in the following, referred to as BioObjects). Available BioObjects are Cell, Compartment, Compound, Chromosome, Polypeptide, Protein, Enzyme, Complex, Gene, etc. All of these BioObjects correspond to their respective biological counterpart and can be used for the creation of computational models that are hierarchically ordered according to fundamental cytological, and molecular structures (e.g., compartments or molecule complexes). Object-specific information is stored as properties of the BioObjects; for instance, each BioObject has an identifier and a concentration, and a Chromosome or Polypeptide can have a nucleotide or amino acid sequence, respectively. Furthermore, each BioObject can have one or more actions. For example, an action can be a chemical reaction or a transport process of molecules between different compartments. Actions describe the stoichiometry of the reactions and their kinetics. PyBioS provides a list of several predefined kinetic laws from which an appropriate one can be chosen for a specific reaction. Moreover, users can define their own kinetic laws. The hierarchical object-oriented model composed of several BioObjects is internally stored in an object-oriented database and is used for further applications provided by PyBioS. For instance, for a time course simulation, the object-oriented model is used for the automatic generation of a system of ODEs.

14.1.5
Systems Biology Workbench

So far we have discussed quite a few different modeling tools, and more will be described in the next sections. One reason for this multitude of simulation tools is that no single tool can provide all the possible simulation methods and ideas that are available. This is especially true since new experimental techniques and theoretical insights constantly stimulate the development of new ways to simulate and analyze biological systems. Consequently, different researchers have written different tools in different languages running on different platforms. A serious problem with this development is that most tools save models in their own format, which is not compatible with the other tools. Accordingly, models cannot easily be exchanged between tools but have to be re-implemented by hand. Another problem is the overhead involved with programming parts of the tool that are not part of the actual core function. This means that although a program might be specialized in analyzing the topology of a reaction network, it also has to provide means for the input and output of the reaction details.

Two closely related projects aim at tackling these problems. One is the development of a common format for describing models. This resulted in the development of the Systems Biology Markup Language (SBML), which is described in detail in Section 14.2.2. The other project is the Systems Biology Workbench (SBW) (Hucka et al. 2002), which is a software system that enables different tools to communicate with each other (http://www.sys-bio.org). Thus, SBW-enabled tools can use services provided by other modules and in turn advertise their own specialized services. Figure 14.4 gives an overview of SBW and some of the currently available SBW-enabled programs. At the center of the system is the SBW broker that receives messages from one module and relays them to other modules. Let's have a quick look at this mechanism using JDesigner and Jarnac, two modules that come with the SBW standard installation. JDesigner is a program for the graphical creation of reaction networks, and Jarnac is a tool for the numerical simulation of such networks (time course and steady state). Jarnac runs in the background and advertises its services to the SBW broker. JDesigner contacts the broker to find out which services are available and displays the found services in a special pull-down menu called SBW. A reaction model that has been created in JDesigner can now be sent to the simulation ser-

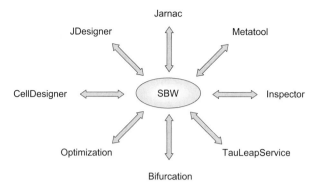

Fig. 14.4 The systems biology workbench (SBW) and SBW-enabled programs. The SBW broker module (in the center) forms the heart of the SBW and provides message passing and remote procedure invocation for SBW-enabled programs. The programs can concentrate on a specialized task such as graphical model building (JDesigner, CellDesigner) or simulation and analysis (Jarnac, TauLeapService, Metatool, Optimization, Bifurcation) and otherwise use the capabilities of already-existing modules.

vice of Jarnac. A dialog box opens to enter the necessary details for the simulation, and then the broker calls the simulation service of Jarnac. After a time course simulation finishes, the result is transmitted back to JDesigner (via the broker) and can be displayed. Further technical details of the SBW system are given in Sauro et al. (2003).

The representative list of SBW-enabled programs shown in Fig. 14.4 contains programs specialized in the graphical creation of reaction networks (JDesigner and CellDesigner), simulation tools (Jarnac and TauLeapService), analysis and optimization tools (Metatool, Bifurcation and Optimization), and utilities such as the Inspector module, which provides information about other modules.

SBW and SBML are very interesting developments that hopefully will help to facilitate the exchange of biological models and thus stimulate the discussion and cooperation among modelers. The more tool-writers adopt the SBML format and render their applications SBW aware, the more powerful this approach will be. Steps are under way to integrate BioSPICE (http://www.biospice.org) into the SBW framework (Sauro et al. 2003), which will strengthen SBW's data handling capabilities and support its status as the *de facto* standard for modeling in systems biology. To give readers an idea of what working with SBW is like, we will now describe the programs JDesigner and CellDesigner in more detail.

14.1.5.1 JDesigner

JDesigner is a Microsoft Windows program that is included with the SBW installation. It can be used in combination with SBW or as standalone application. If used alone, it is a graphical network designer. In this mode only the graphics canvas, which can be seen in the top right part of Fig. 14.5, is available. An icon bar allows the easy construction of networks consisting of compartments, molecular species, and reactions between the species. In the example shown, the network consists of

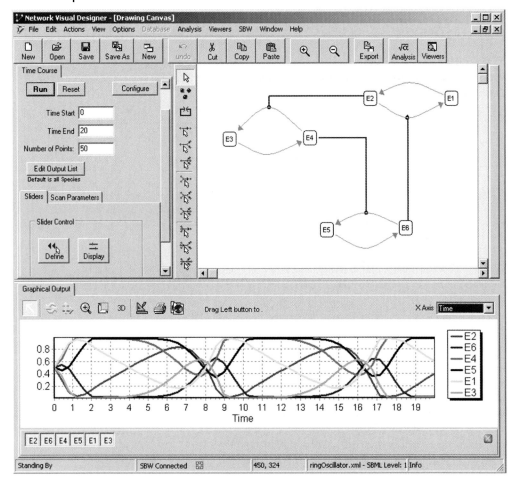

Fig. 14.5 JDesigner is an SBW-enabled application that allows the visual construction of reaction networks. The upper right part of the screenshot shows a network of six species cyclically connected by six reactions. Connection to the time course service of the Jarnac module brings up the control panel on the upper left part. After Jarnac has finished the simulation, the results are passed back to JDesigner, where they are displayed in the bottom part of the window.

six species (E1 to E6) that are connected via six reactions. JDesigner allows changing the shape, color, and position of the graphical elements to achieve a visually pleasing result. But if we are actually interested in the dynamics of the system, we have to define initial concentrations for the species and kinetic laws for the reactions. JDesigner has a list of predefined kinetic laws that can be assigned to a reaction, but it also allows defining arbitrary custom kinetics. The model can then be saved in SBML Level 1 or 2. However, the current version of JDesigner, 1.934, seems to have subtle problems with the produced SBML. Unfortunately, none of the supplied

SBML example models passes the online syntax validation that is available at http://sbml.org/tools/htdocs/sbmltools.php, which prevents, for instance, the transfer of models from JDesigner to CellDesigner.

Like all SBW-enabled programs, JDesigner has a special menu called SBW that lists the services provided by other SBW modules. Services provided with the standard distribution are stochastic time course simulations, deterministic time course and steady-state calculations, and the generation of a Matlab ODE function file of the current model. However, JDesigner also offers another, tighter, integration with Jarnac, a network simulation module. The menu entry "Actions/Connect Simulator" establishes a direct connection to Jarnac, which in turn enables several entries in the Analysis menu. The left side of Fig. 14.5 shows the control panel that appears if the Time Course Simulation is chosen from this menu. After the simulation is finished, a graphical representation of the solution can be examined (bottom of Fig. 14.5). The graphical output is very flexible and allows selection of the variables to be plotted, of the axes labels and scaling, and of titles and legends. Furthermore, the result can be saved in different graphic formats and the numerical values can be exported as text, XML, or Excel format. Finally, a good tutorial on how to use JDesigner is available from http://public.kgi.edu/~hsauro/sysbio/papers/JDBooklet.pdf.

14.1.5.2 CellDesigner

CellDesigner, another network creation tool, might be an alternative to JDesigner for people who do not use Microsoft Windows (Funahashi et al. 2003). The application is written in Java and therefore also runs under MacOS X and Linux. The current version is 2.0 and can be downloaded from http://systems-biology.org. As with JDesigner, networks can be constructed from compartments, species, and reactions. However, CellDesigner comes with a large number of predefined shapes that can be used for different types of molecules such as proteins, receptors, ion channels, small metabolites, etc. It is also possible to modify the symbols to indicate phosphorylations or other modifications (Fig. 14.6, center). The program also provides several icons for special reaction types such as catalysis, transport, inhibition, and activation.

Reading and writing of the models is SBML-based (Level 1 and 2), and the models written by CellDesigner pass the online validation at http://sbml.org/tools/htdocs/sbmltools.php and thus conform to the SBML standard. A nice feature in this respect is the ability to display the SBML model structure as a tree (Fig. 14.6, left side). A click on a species or reaction in this tree highlights the corresponding elements in the graphics canvas and in the matching tab on the right side showing further details. This tab is also the place where initial concentrations and reaction details are entered. Like JDesigner, CellDesigner allows entering arbitrary kinetic equations, but unfortunately it has no list of standard kinetics (mass action or Michaelis-Menten) that can be applied. For each reaction, the rate law has to be typed in by hand. A connection to SBW is realized via the standard SBW menu and provides the services described together with JDesigner. For a further introduction to CellDesigner, a startup guide can be obtained from the download page at http://systems-biology.org.

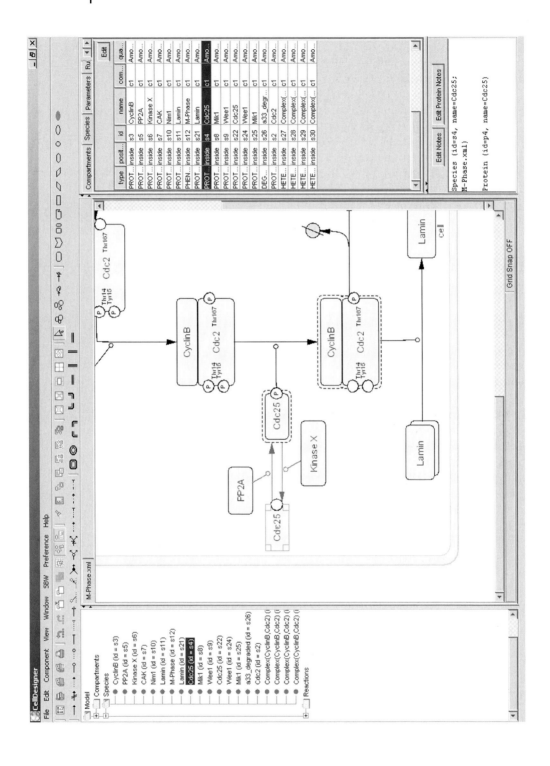

14.1.6
Petri Nets

A Petri Net is a graphical and mathematical modeling tool for discrete and parallel systems. The mathematical concept was developed in the early 1960s by Adam Petri. The basic elements of a Petri Net are places, transitions, and arcs that connect places and transitions. When represented graphically, places are shown as circles and transitions as rectangular bars (see Fig. 14.7). Places represent objects (molecules, cars, machine parts), and transitions describe whether and how individual objects are inter-converted. Places can contain zero or more tokens, indicating the number of objects that currently exist. The tokens are shown as dots in Fig. 14.7a (one in place P1 and two in place P3). Whether a transition can take place (can fire) or not depends on the places that are connected to the transition by incoming arcs to contain enough tokens. If this condition is fulfilled, the transition fires and changes the state of the system by removing tokens from the input places and adding tokens to the output places. The number of tokens that are removed and added depends on the weight of the arcs. The movement of tokens during successive firing events is called the token game.

Petri Nets are not only an optically pleasing representation of a system but they can also be described mathematically in terms of integer arithmetic. For simple types of Petri Nets, certain properties can thus be calculated analytically, but often the net has to be run to study the long-term system properties. Over the years many extensions to the basic Petri Net model have been developed for different simulation purposes (Bernardinello and de Cindio 1992):

1. Hybrid Petri Nets that add the possibility to have places that contain a continuous token number instead of discrete values.
2. Timed Petri Nets that extend transitions to allow for a specific time delay between the moment when a transition is enabled and the actual firing.
3. Stochastic Petri Nets that go one step further and allow a random time delay drawn from a probability distribution.
4. Hierarchical Petri Nets, in which modularity is introduced by representing whole nets as a single place or transition of a larger net.
5. Colored Petri Nets that introduce different types (colors) or tokens and more complicated firing rules for transitions.

With these extensions Petri Nets are powerful enough to be used for models in systems biology. Biochemical pathways can be modeled with places representing me-

---

◀ Fig. 14.6 CellDesigner 2.0 is another program that is SBW aware and can be used to construct reaction networks that can be analyzed by other SBW modules or saved in SBML format. The special strength of CellDesigner is its advanced graphical representation skills. Different shapes are available for different types of molecules, such as ions, proteins, receptors, genes, DNA, or RNA. Another highlight is the model tree (left side) that provides a convenient overview of the SBML structure and components.

A)

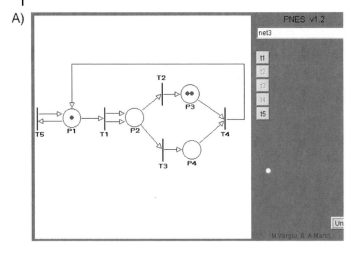

B)

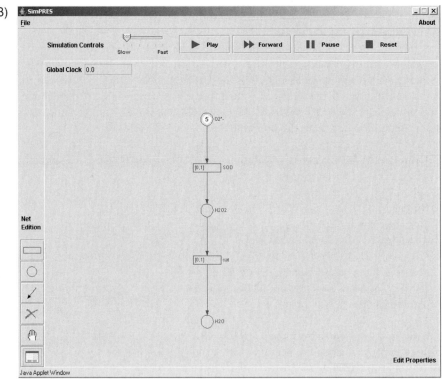

Fig. 14.7 Several Java applets exist to get started with Petri Nets. (a) For a very first contact, PNES at http://web.tiscali.it/marconthe-net/Pnes.Pnes.html is a good choice. It contains numerous predefined nets, and by firing enabled transitions manually, the network behavior can be studied. (b) A simple applet that also allows users to construct and run their own Petri Nets can be found at http://www.ida.liu.se/~luico/ SimPRES. It allows one to specify different time delays for transitions, and thus simple Timed Petri Nets can be created.

tabolites and transitions representing reactions, and stoichiometric coefficients are encoded as different weights of input and output arcs. Consequently, Petri Nets have been used to model metabolic networks (Reddy et al. 1996; Küffner et al. 2000) and signal transduction pathways (Matsuno et al. 2003). Many free and commercial tools are available to explore the behavior of Petri Nets. The Petri Nets World homepage (http://www.daimi.au.dk/PetriNets) is an excellent starting point for this purpose. It contains a large amount of information about tutorials, software, and conferences as well as a large bibliography regarding Petri Nets. In addition to comprehensive standalone packages, there are also a number of Petri Nets available that have been implemented as Java applets. The Petri Net Educational Simulator (PNES) at http://web.tiscali.it/marconthenet/Pnes.Pnes.html is very limited because it displays only a collection of predefined nets, but by stepping through the net (playing the token game) one can get a first impression. Figure 14.7a shows the user interface of PNES. A more advanced applet (can also be installed as application) that also allows the creation and modification of Petri Nets is SimPRES (http://www.ida.liu.se/~luico/SimPRES). Figure 14.7b shows the applet with our well-known reaction system from superoxide to water (see Section 14.1.1) implemented as Petri Net.

However, these applets can run only simple Petri Nets, which are restricted in their computational capabilities. Consequently, the radical detoxification reactions shown in Fig. 14.7b lack realism. The number of superoxide radicals that is converted into hydrogen peroxide is constant per unit time. A more realistic assumption is that the reaction follows the mass action (as done in Sections 14.1.1 and 14.1.2). But for such calculations larger packages are needed, e.g., CPN Tools (http://wiki.daimi.au.dk/cpntools), which is an actively developed Colored Petri Net tool developed at the university of Aarhus, Denmark, or the commercially available Cell Illustrator (http://www.gene-networks.com/ci), which is based on a Hybrid Petri Net.

14.1.7
STOCKS 2

The stochastic simulation tool STOCKS 2 was developed by Andrzej Kierzek and Jacek Puchalka and is available free of charge under the GNU GPL license (http://www.sysbio.pl/stocks/). Versions are available for Microsoft Windows and Linux.

Simulations using differential equations assume that the number of molecules in the described system is so large that it can be treated as a continuous variable. A second assumption of ODE modeling is that the system is completely deterministic. Random fluctuations do not occur. The smaller the number of molecules, the more unrealistic those assumptions become. Most molecules in a cell exist in large numbers, but some are very rare. Transcription factors, for example, exist in notoriously low numbers in cells. There are only approximately 10 molecules of the Lac repressor in an *E. coli* cell (Levin 1999). Proteins involved in signal transduction pathways are also very rare, as are defective mitochondria that might be relevant for the aging process (see Section 7.3.2). Under those circumstances it becomes important that four or five molecules might be in a cell, but not fractional amounts like 4.325 (as assumed by ODEs). Of special importance can be the difference between zero and one items if this item is a self-reproducing object like a defective mitochondrion. If modeled with ODEs it is practically impossible to obtain zero defective mitochondria; a small amount (well below one) will always remain. Because of their self-reproducing property, a population of defective mitochondria could always regrow from this artifact. If modeled stochastically, all defective organelles disappear (zero concentration) if the last one is destroyed, and thus they cannot regrow. If the simulated system has more than one possible steady state, there can also be qualitative differences between a deterministic simulation with differential equations and a stochastic simulation that takes random effects into account. In an ODE model the system will settle into one of the possible steady states and remain there forever. If modeled stochastically, however, the system can jump from one steady state to the other if they are close enough together.

As discussed in Section 3.6, the basic algorithms used for stochastic simulations are Gillespie's first reaction method and direct method (Gillespie 1977) or the more efficient, recently developed, next reaction method (Gibson and Bruck 2000). However, all these methods have problems to model systems that contain both intensive reactions involving molecule species present in large numbers and reactions involving rare molecules. The majority of computation time is used for the intensive reactions, which occur in very short time intervals and thus are called fast reactions. It therefore often requires an unacceptably long computation time before the interesting slow reactions are simulated.

STOCKS 2 (Puchalka and Kierzek 2004) is based on the idea of modeling fast reactions with an approximate method (Gillespie 2001) and the slow reactions with the exact next reaction method. The assignment of reactions into slow and fast is done automatically and dynamically. This means that if a molecular species increases in number during the course of a simulation, which in turn increases the reaction rate, STOCKS 2 automatically moves it from the list of slow reactions to the group of fast reactions. The program uses as input a model description in SBML (Section 14.2.2) and generates as output text files containing the molecule numbers of the different variables at user-specified time points. SBML is a very bulky and verbose format, and hence writing an SBML model description by hand is a painful process. Luckily an input editor is provided to create the model and the SBML file (Fig. 14.8a). The documentation is, at the time of this writing, rather sparse, but the buttons and associated dialog boxes roughly have to be processed from top to bottom. "Model Parameters" allows one to enter several details relevant for the actual simulation, such as the simulation time, the number of repetitions of an experiment (to get a feeling for the spread of individual trajectories), the time interval for saving output, and whether to save debug information (very handy during model development). "Parameters" leads to the definition of constants for the model, the next button allows one to define compartments of different sizes, and in "Species" the used variables have to be declared. The most important part is finally the definition of the reactions. It is possible to choose from a variety of different kinetics types or to define an arbitrary kinetics. However, this has to be entered in MathML format, which is discussed in Section 14.2.3. The last two buttons are for advanced topics and will not be discussed here.

The output of STOCKS 2 is a plain text file, but for illustrative purposes Fig. 14.8b compares the processed stochastic results of an example model (accumulation of de-

A)

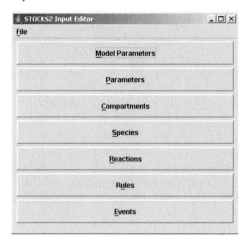

B)

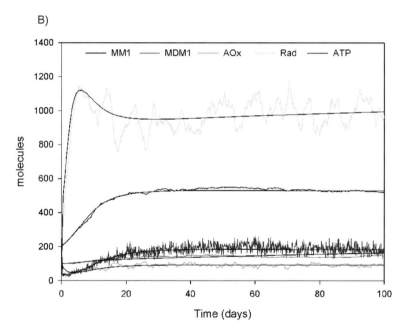

Fig. 14.8 STOCKS 2 is a simulation tool for stochastic models. (a) Models can be constructed with the Input Editor, which generates the SBML format used by STOCKS 2. Each of the seven buttons opens dialog boxes that allow one to enter simulation parameters, variables, reactions, compartments, etc. (b) Comparison of the stochastic trajectories generated by STOCKS 2 and the corresponding ODEs of an example model describing the population dynamics of mitochondria.

fective mitochondria, similar to Section 7.3.2) with the solutions of a corresponding differential equations model. In this case there is excellent agreement between the two types of simulation. We would like to recommend this dual modeling approach since the ODEs can be used to derive the stochastic reactions, a simulation of the ODE system can give a quick and rough feeling for the model behavior, and disagreement between the two approaches can often be used to spot implementation errors of the stochastic model. If there are differences they have to be understandable by the special above-mentioned differences between the deterministic and stochastic approaches.

14.1.8
Genetic Programming

Genetic programming (Koza 1992) is a variation of genetic algorithms (Holland 1975). This means that it uses techniques borrowed from evolution. A solution to a problem is obtained by letting many different versions of a program compete against each other. From one generation to the next, they can undergo mutations and recombination and propagate according to their fitness. The better a variant solves the problem at hand, the higher its fitness is. The main difference between genetic programming (GP) and genetic algorithms lies in the way the solution is presented. GP produces a ready-to-use program in a Lisp-like presentation, while genetic algorithms create a string of numbers that represents the solution.

As an example, assume that the problem at hand is to find the mathematical function that most accurately approximates the data points shown in Fig. 14.9a. The critical point is to find a way to represent the solution (a mathematical function) as a tree-like structure as seen in Fig. 14.9b. Such a tree consists of internal nodes, consisting of problem-specific functions (here mathematical operators), and terminal nodes, consisting of the input for the functions. Each tree represents one individual of the competing population. An appropriate measure of fitness is another important point for successfully applying GP. In this case the sum of squares of the distance between the data points and the corresponding function values could be used. New individuals can be generated by mutating nodes (replacement of one operator by another or modification of a numerical constant) or by recombination between two individuals (exchange of sub-branches). If those modifications follow certain syntactical constraints, it can be guaranteed that syntactically correct mutants are always generated.

Genetic programming has been used successfully in such diverse areas as the automatic creation of the topology and sizing of analogue electrical circuits (Koza et al. 1999), the design of antennas according to high-level specifications (Comisky et al. 2000), and the reverse engineering of metabolic pathways (Koza et al. 2000, 2001). The last example is especially interesting because it relates directly to systems

---

Fig. 14.9 (a) Function to data fitting as simple example of Genetic Programming (GP). (b) Possible solutions to the problem (mathematical functions) are represented as a tree. (c) The structure and numerical constants of this meta- bolic reaction network are to be reverse engi- neered by GP using only concentration values of diacyl-glycerol for different enzyme concentra- tions. (d) Tree-like representation of two of the four enzyme reactions seen in (c). ▶

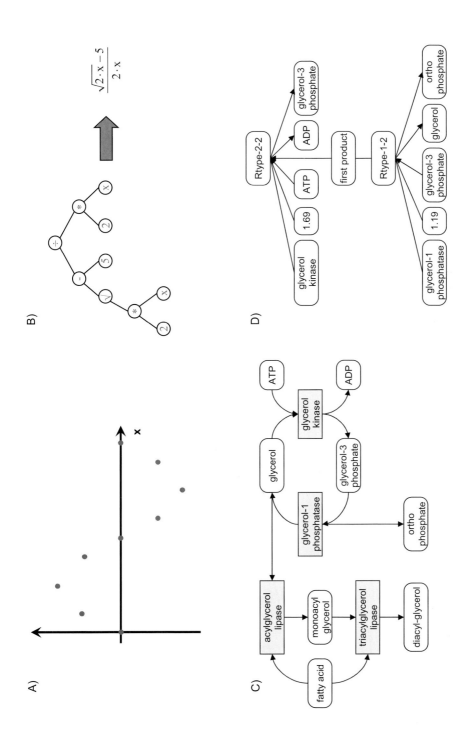

biology and its implementation is not trivial. The task is to re-create the topology as well as the numerical values of the involved rate constants of the network shown in Fig. 14.9 c, purely from the measured time course of the diacyl-glycerol concentration for different amounts of the involved enzymes. The first challenge is to represent enzyme reactions as a tree structure suitable for genetic programming. For this purpose four different chemical reaction functions and two selector functions are defined. The reaction functions work on reactions with one or two substrates and products. Assuming simple mass action kinetics, the reaction of glycerol-1 phosphatase is described by a one-substrate, two-products reaction type (Fig. 14.9 d). The function node takes two further arguments specifying the enzyme and the value of the rate constant. Glycerol kinase takes two substrates, one of which is the first product of the reaction catalyzed by glycerol-1 phosphatase. The first product selector function takes the first product of a chemical reaction function and feeds it as input into another reaction function.

The second important task is to calculate the fitness of a reaction network that is represented through a tree structure. This is done by converting the tree into a set of differential equations and solving them numerically for 270 different enzyme concentrations. Then the diacyl-glycerol concentration produced under those conditions by the evolved tree is compared with the simulation of the correct network (sum of squares), giving the required fitness measure. Koza et al. (2000) have used a population of 100,000 individuals to tackle this problem, and after 225 generations an individual evolved with the correct topology and all rate constants within 2% of the true value.

Several programs are available that facilitate the use of genetic programming. Most packages are designed in such a way that the user has to supply routines that define problem-specific functions and evaluate the fitness of an individual, while the software takes care of mutating and breeding the population of genetic programs. Examples of such software are ECJ (http://cs.gmu.edu/~eclab/projects/ecj/), jrgp (http://www.sourceforge.net/projects/jrgp), JGProg (http://jgprog.sourceforge.net/), or the commercial program Discipulus (http://www.aimlearning.com/Prod-Discipulus.htm). The most comprehensive and flexible package is probably ECJ-11, a Java-based evolutionary computation and genetic programming research system. A detailed description of this large package is unfortunately not possible in the available space. However, depending on the Java skills of the user, several days to weeks might be necessary to fully master this excellent package.

14.2
Model Exchange Languages, Data Formats

14.2.1
Introduction to XML

The easiest way to store and exchange data for the computer is a plain text that is readable by humans. Since data represented by such files are compatible with almost all computational operating systems, plain text files are also widely used in biological research, e. g., for the storage of sequence information and its annotations. The type of information (e. g., sequence identifier, origin, preparation method, and the sequence data itself) is indicated by special tags and/or is defined in a separate description. A similar but more flexible tool for the storage of data in a well-defined way is the Extensible Markup Language (XML). XML is recommended by the World Wide Web Consortium (W3C) for the definition of special-purpose markup languages (http://www.w3.org/TR/2004/REC-xml-20040204/). XML is a lightweight adaptation of the even more general Standard Generalized Markup Language (SGML). Documents using an XML conform markup language are written as plain text and have a very clear and simple syntax that can easily be read by both humans and computer programs; however, it is generally intended to be written and read by computers, not by humans. The following example of some cellular components illustrates XML's major characteristics:

Example

```
<?xml version="1.0"?>
<cell id="yeast cell">
  <compartment id="cytoplasm">
    <compartment id="cytosol">
      <enzyme id="SOD1" name="Cu,Zn-superoxide dismutase"
             reaction="2 O2*- + 2 H+ = O2 + H2O2"/>
      <molecule> H2O2 </molecule>
    </compartment>
  </compartment>
  <compartment id="nucleus">
    <chromosome id="chromsosome 1" length="230209 bp"/>
  </compartment>
</cell>
```

In XML, information is associated with tags indicating the type or formatting of the information. Tags are enclosed in sharp brackets and have a tag name (<tag name>, e. g., <molecule>). They are used to delimit and denote parts of the document or to add further information to the document structure. Text blocks delimited by a start tag and a corresponding end tag (in an end tag the tag name is preceded by a slash, "/") are called nonempty elements. A nonempty element contains simple text and/or further tags. Thus, XML documents are usually hierarchically organized. Elements that do not embrace further information (empty elements) are defined by an empty-element tag – a tag that ends with a slash in front of the closing sharp bracket (<tag name/>). In the example above <cell>, <compartment>, and <molecule> are nonempty tags and <enzyme> and <chromosome> are empty tags. The hierarchical structure becomes clear by the <cell> tag that embraces <compartment> tags, which again directly or indirectly embrace other elements (e. g., <compartment>, <enzyme>, or <chromosome>) and text data (e. g., "H2O2" in the example above). Tag names are case sensitive and have to start with a letter or underscore followed by any number of letters, numbers, hyphens, dots, or underscores. Furthermore, start tags or empty-element tags can have attributes that offer additional information. Attributes follow the tag name delimited by spaces and have a name and a value that are connected by an equal sign ("="), e.g., in the example above, the <cell> tag has an attribute id carrying the value "yeast cell". A well-formatted document expects quotation marks around the value. XML documents are preceded by a prolog (the first line in the example above) that identifies the document as an XML document and can contain further information about the used version.

We have described the basic components of XML; for further reading, please consult, e.g., Ray (2003). In the following subsections we will describe two markup languages that conform to XML and are used in systems biology: Systems Biology Markup Language (SBML) and MathML. Besides these, other XML conform languages for representing data in biology have been defined, such as Chemical Markup Language (CML) for the representation of molecule structures (Liao and Ghanadan 2002), MAGE-ML for the exchange of microarray and expression data (Spellman et al. 2002), ProML for the representation of essential features of proteins (Hanisch et al. 2002), and others.

14.2.2
Systems Biology Markup Language

Many different tools for modeling and simulation of biological systems have already been developed (cf. Section 14.1). All of them offer functionalities to enter the model data and to make the model persistent by storing it, e.g., in an application-specific file. Since all of these tools offer different strength and capabilities (e.g., one offers a good graphical representation of models and the other provides very accurate methods for numerical simulations), a systems biologist is often interested in using several of these tools. But this typically requires the re-encoding of a model in a new tool, which is usually a time-consuming and error-prone process. Therefore, software-independent common standards for the representation of qualitative and quantitative models of biochemical reaction networks are required. CellML (Lloyd et al. 2004, http://www.cellml.org) and SBML (Hucka et al. 2003, 2004) are two XML-based formats facing up to this problem. Since SBML is the most prominent, we will describe it in more detail below.

SBML (http://www.sbml.org) is a free and open format for "describing models common to research in many areas of computational biology, including cell signaling pathways, metabolic pathways, gene regulation, and others" (Hucka et al. 2003). It is already supported by many software tools (Hucka et al. 2004); in September 2004 the SBML homepage listed more than 60 software systems supporting SBML.

The following SBML Level 2 code (differences to Level 1 will be discussed below) shows the general structural elements of an SBML document:

Example

```
<?xml version="1.0"?>
<sbml xmlns="http://www.sbml.org/sbml/level2" level="2"
        version="1">
  <model id="My_model">
    <listOfFunctionDefinitions>
      ...
    </listOfFunctionDefinitions>
    <listOfUnitDefinitions>
      ...
    </listOfUnitDefinitions>
    <listOfCompartments>
      ...
    </listOfCompartments>
    <listOfSpecies>
      ...
    </listOfSpecies>
    <listOfParameters>
      ...
    </listOfParameters>
    <listOfRules>
      ...
    </listOfRules>
    <listOfReactions>
      ...
    </listOfReactions>
    <listOfEvents>
      ...
    </listOfEvents>
  </model>
</sbml>
```

The <sbml> element with a single included <model> element indicates an SBML model. The optional attribute id of <model> defines a model name. This model name has to begin with a letter or underscore followed by zero or more characters of letters, numbers, or the underscore. Model definitions and model data are subdivided into several lists. The <listOfFunctionDefinitions> element contains user-defined functions that can be used throughout the model. User-defined unit names that are not in a list of predefined units (including several names of SI units defined by the International System of Units and derivatives of these units) can be defined in the <listOfUnitDefinitions> element. The declaration of compartment names, <listOfCompartments>, enables the definition of the spatial organization of the species involved in the model. It also supports the definition of nested compartments.

Basic components of a model are declared in the three elements <listOfSpecies>, <listOfParameters>, and <listOfReactions>. The <listOfSpecies> element declares all species of the model, where the term species refers to any kind of molecule relevant for the model. Species can represent either variables that change during time or external variables with constant values. For instance, a list of species can look like this:

Example

```
<listOfSpecies>
  <species id="Glucose_cytosol" name="Glucose (Cytosol)"
          compartment="cytosol" initialConcentration="4"/>
  <species id="Glucose_6_P" name="Glucose-6-phosphate"
          compartment="cytosol" initialConcentration="0.75"/>
  <species id="Glucose_external" name="Glucose (extracellular)"
          compartment="medium" initialConcentration="9.35"/>
</listOfSpecies>
```

The id has to be a unique identifier with the same character restrictions as for the model id; the name attribute is a more readable, non-unique character string.

Parameters, such as kinetic constants, can be defined either in a global namespace, if listed in the <listOfParameters> element, or in a local namespace, if declared in a reaction listed in <listOfReactions>. In the following example of the superoxide dismutase (SOD) reaction (cf. Section 14.1.1), the declaration of a reaction in SBML is illustrated.

Example

```
<?xml version="1.0"?>
<sbml xmlns="http://www.sbml.org/sbml/level2"
          level="2" version="1">
  <model id="SOD model">
    <listOfCompartments>
        <compartment id="cytosol"/>
    </listOfCompartments>

    <listOfSpecies>
      <species id="O2radical" name="O2 radical"
          compartment="cytosol" initialConcentration="0.0"/>
      <species id="H2O2" name="hydrogen peroxide"
          compartment="cytosol" initialConcentration="0.0"/>
      <species id="SOD" name="superoxide dismutase"
          compartment="cytosol" initialConcentration="1.0e-5"/>
    </listOfSpecies>
```

```
<listOfReactions>
  <reaction id="SOD_reaction">
    <listOfReactants>
      <speciesReference species="O2radical"/>
    </listOfReactants>
    <listOfProducts>
      <speciesReference species="H2O2"/>
    </listOfProducts>
    <listOfModifiers>
      <modifierSpeciesReference species="SOD"/>
    </listOfModifiers>
    <kineticLaw>
      <math xmlns="http://www.w3.org/1998/Math/MathML">
        <apply>
          <times/>
          <ci> c2 /ci>
          <ci> SOD /ci>
          <ci> O2radical /ci>
        </apply>
      </math>
      <listOfParameters>
        <parameter id="c2" value="1.6e9"/>
      </listOfParameters>
    </kineticLaw>
  </reaction>
</listOfReactions>
</model>
</sbml>
```

The <reaction> element describes the reactants (substrates), products, and modifiers of a reaction. Modifiers are species that are neither created nor destroyed in the particular reaction, like the catalyzing enzyme SOD in this example. The <kineticLaw> element describes the rate at which the reaction takes place. The expression of the mathematical formula is done by the use of MathML, which is described in the next subsection. In SBML the kinetic law is not equivalent to a traditional rate law, since it is expressed in terms of substance/time rather than concentration/time. This is because of the support for multi-compartment models. For example, suppose two species S and P of the reaction $S \rightarrow P$ are located in different compartments that differ in volume. The rate of change in concentration by time can readily be calculated via dividing the rate of change in substance by time by the respective volumes.

Rules, defined in the <listOfRules> element, provide a way to create constraints on parameters and variables that cannot be expressed using reactions. Events, defined in the <listOfEvents> element, describe explicit instantaneous discontinuous state changes in the model, e. g., that a species concentration is halved when another species exceeds a given threshold concentration.

A full overview and description of the SBML syntax is given in the SBML specification "Systems Biology Markup Language (SBML) Level 2: Structures and Facilities for Model Definitions", which can be downloaded from http://sbml.org/documents/.

SBML is being developed in levels, wherein each new level extends the language by new features. Currently, Level 1 and Level 2 are defined. The main differences between both levels are (Finney and Hucka 2003):

- Level 2 uses MathML (see next section) instead of text strings (used in Level 1) for the expression of mathematical formula.
- Level 2 enables the addition of metadata. Metadata is supportive information (e. g., the model's literature reference or an alternative name of a biological entity) that provides context to a resource (e. g., to the model or its components).
- Level 1 provides only a limited set of predefined mathematical functions. In Level 2 additional named functions can be defined and used in mathematical expressions throughout the model.
- Occasionally, some biological processes of a model have a delayed response that should not be modeled in detail. Level 2 also provides a construct for the definition of such delay functions.
- Level 2 also supports the definition of discrete events that can occur at defined transitions and thus affect the values of model variables.

Interfaces for the use of SBML with the popular mathematical environments Matlab and Mathematica (cf. Section 14.1.1) are also available:

- MathSBML (Shapiro et al. 2004, http://www.sbml.org/mathsbml.html) is an open-source package that provides facilities for Mathematica to read SBML models and convert them into ODE systems that can be used for simulations and plotting. It supports SBML Levels 1 and 2.
- SBMLToolbox (http://sbml.org/software/sbmltoolbox) provides an interface for reading, writing, and manipulating of SBML models within the Matlab environment.

The current SBML Level 2 specification does still have some limitations regarding the needs of some software tools. Therefore, the following extensions for SBML Level 3 are proposed:

- support for the inclusion of diagrammatic renditions of a model;
- support for the composition of models from instances of submodels;
- support for multicomponent species such as molecule complexes;
- support for index collections of objects of the same type, as it would be helpful for the construction of, e. g., tissues of almost identical cells; and
- support for spatial features such as the geometry of compartments, diffusion properties of species, and different species concentrations across different regions of a cell, as well as support for partial differential calculus.

14.2.3
MathML

SBML is designed to describe models in systems biology but is not intended to represent complicated mathematical expressions. MathML is an XML-based markup language especially created for this task (http://www.w3.org/Math). At places in SBML that require a mathematical expression, e. g., a user-defined kinetic law, MathML can be inserted. MathML comes in two flavors, as markup language for presenting the layout of mathematical expressions and as markup language for conveying the mathematical content of a formula. The major use of the presentation markup is to enable Internet browsers to directly display equations, something that is not possible with normal HTML tags. However, it is the content markup variant of MathML that is of greater interest for modeling. It can be used to exchange mathematical expressions in a common low-level format between software packages that need to evaluate these expressions (instead of displaying them). The following table contains MathML for the Michaelis-Menten expression $\frac{E \cdot S}{Km+S}$.

MathML presentation markup	MathML content markup

`<math xmlns='http://www.w3.org/`
`          1998/Math/MathML'>`
` <mfrac>`
`  <mrow>`
`   <mi>E/mi>`
`   <mo>*/mo>`
`   <mi>S/mi>`
`  </mrow>`
`  <mrow>`
`   <mi>Km/mi>`
`   <mo>+/mo>`
`   <mi>S/mi>`
`  </mrow>`
` </mfrac>`
`</math>`
	`<math xmlns='http://www.w3.org/`
	`          1998/Math/MathML'>`
	` <apply>`
	`  <divide/>`
	`  <apply>`
	`   <times/>`
	`    <ci>E/ci>`
	`    <ci>S/ci>`
	`  </apply>`
	`  <apply>`
	`   <plus/>`
	`    <ci>Km/ci>`
	`    <ci>S/ci>`
	`  </apply>`
	` </apply>`
	`</math>`

MathML is a very verbose format and is not intended to be generated or edited by hand. Specialized authoring tools should be used to import or export MathML expressions. Many different programs are available to make Web browsers MathML aware, to generate PDF or DVI from MathML, to save equations in MS Word in MathML format, or to create mathematical expressions interactively and save them in both types of MathML (http://www.w3.org/Math/implementations.html). One reason to look closer at the content markup MathML is STOCKS2 (see Section 14.1.7), which needs MathML input if the user wants to define a new kinetic type. The required MathML format could be generated with a commercial editor like WebEQ from Design Science (http://www.dessci.com) or by using a free service offered at http://www.mathmlcentral.com, a Web site of Wolfram Research (the company that produces Mathematica). This site offers three valuable Web services for free: validating whether a given MathML expression is syntactically correct, rendering of presentation markup MathML into different graphics formats, and conversion of a mathematical expression that is given in Mathematica syntax into the different types of MathML. With this wealth of resources available on the Net, it should be no problem to master MathML.

References

BERNARDINELLO, L. and DE CINDIO, F. A survey of basic net models and modular net classes (1992) Springer Verlag, Berlin.

CAMPBELL, N.A. and REECE, J.B. Biology (2001) 6th Edition, Benjamin Cummings.

COMISKY, W., YU, J. and KOZA, J.R. Automatic synthesis of a wire antenna using genetic programming (2000) Genetic and Evolutionary Computation Conference.

FINNEY, A. and HUCKA, M. Systems biology markup language: Level 2 and beyond (2003) Biochem. Soc. Trans. *31*, 1472–3.

FUNAHASHI, A., TANIMURA, N., MOROHASHI, M. and KITANO, H. CellDesigner: a process diagram editor for gene-regulatory and biochemical networks (2003) Biosilico *1*, 159–162.

GIBSON, M.A. and BRUCK, J. Efficient exact stochastic simulation of chemical systems with many species and many channels (2000) J. Phys. Chem. *104*, 1876–1889.

GILLESPIE, D.T. Exact stochastic simulation of coupled chemical reactions (1977) J. Phys. Chem. *81*, 2340–2361.

GILLESPIE, D.T. Approximate accelerated stochastic simulation of chemically reacting systems (2001) J. Chem. Phys. *115*, 1716–1733.

HANISCH, D., ZIMMER, R. and LENGAUER, T. ProML–the protein markup language for specification of protein sequences, structures and families (2002) In Silico Biol. *2*, 313–24.

HOLLAND, J.H. Adaptation in natural and artificial systems: An introductory analysis with applications to biology, control, and artificial intelligence (1975) University of Michigan Press, Ann Arbor, MI.

HUCKA, M., FINNEY, A., SAURO, H.M., BOLOURI, H., DOYLE, J. and KITANO, H. The ERATO Systems Biology Workbench: enabling interaction and exchange between software tools for computational biology (2002) Pac. Symp. Biocomput. 450–61.

HUCKA, M., FINNEY, A., SAURO, H.M., BOLOURI, H., DOYLE, J.C., KITANO, H., ARKIN, A.P., BORNSTEIN, B.J., BRAY, D., CORNISH-BOWDEN, A., CUELLAR, A.A., DRONOV, S., GILLES, E.D., GINKEL, M., GOR, V., GORYANIN, II, HEDLEY, W.J., HODGMAN, T.C., HOFMEYR, J.H., HUNTER, P.J., JUTY, N.S., KASBERGER, J.L., KREMLING, A., KUMMER, U., LE NOVERE, N., LOEW, L.M., LUCIO, D., MENDES, P., MINCH, E., MJOLSNESS, E.D., NAKAYAMA, Y., NELSON, M.R., NIELSEN, P.F., SAKURADA, T., SCHAFF, J.C., SHAPIRO, B.E., SHIMIZU, T.S., SPENCE, H.D., STELLING, J., TAKAHASHI, K., TOMITA, M., WAGNER, J. and WANG, J. The systems biology markup language (SBML): a medium for representation and exchange of biochemical network models (2003) Bioinformatics *19*, 524–31.

HUCKA, M., FINNEY, A., BORNSTEIN, B.J., KEATING, S.M., SHAPIRO, B.E., MATTHEWS, J., KOVITZ, B.L., SCHILSTRA, M.J., FUNAHASHI, A., DOYLE, J.C. and KITANO, H. Evolving a lingua franca and associated software infrastructure for computational systems biology: the Systems Biology Markup Language (SBML) project (2004) Syst. Biol. *1*, 41–53.

ISHII, N., ROBERT, M., NAKAYAMA, Y., KANAI, A. and TOMITA, M. Toward large-scale modeling of the microbial cell for computer simulation (2004) J. Biotechnol. *113*, 281–94.

KOZA, J.R. Genetic programming: On the programming of computers by means of natural selection (1992) MIT Press, Cambridge, MA.

KOZA, J.R., BENNETT, I.F.H., ANDRE, D. and KEANE, M.A. Genetic programming III: Darwinian invention and problem solving (1999) Morgan Kaufmann, San Francisco, CA.

KOZA, J.R., MYDLOWEC, W., LANZA, G., YU, J. and KEANE, M.A. Reverse engineering and automatic synthesis of metabolic pathways from observed data using genetic programming

(2000) Stanford Medical Informatics Technical Report *SMI-2000–0851*.

KOZA, J.R., MYDLOWEC, W., LANZA, G., YU, J. and KEANE, M.A. Reverse engineering of metabolic pathways from observed data using genetic programming (2001) Pac. Symp. Biocomput. 6, 446–458.

KÜFFNER, R., ZIMMER, R. and LENGAUER, T. Pathway analysis in metabolic databases via differential metabolic display (DMD) (2000) Bioinformatics 16, 825–36.

LEVIN, B. Genes VII (1999) Oxford University Press, Oxford.

LIAO, Y.M. and GHANADAN, H. The chemical markup language (2002) Anal. Chem. 74, 389A-390A.

LLOYD, C.M., HALSTEAD, M.D. and NIELSEN, P.F. CellML: its future, present and past (2004) Prog. Biophys. Mol. Biol. 85, 433–50.

MATSUNO, H., TANAKA, Y., AOSHIMA, H., DOI, A., MATSUI, M. and MIYANO, S. Biopathways representation and simulation on hybrid functional Petri net (2003) In Silico Biol. 3, 389–404.

MENDES, P. GEPASI: a software package for modelling the dynamics, steady states and control of biochemical and other systems (1993) Comput Appl Biosci 9, 563–71.

MENDES, P. Biochemistry by numbers: Simulation of biochemical pathways with Gepasi 3 (1997) Trends Biochem. Sci. 22, 361–363.

PUCHALKA, J. and KIERZEK, A.M. Bridging the gap between stochastic and deterministic regimes in the kinetic simulations of the biochemical reaction networks (2004) Biophys. J. 86, 1357–1372.

RAY, E.T. Learning XML (2003) 2nd Edition O'Reilly.

REDDY, V.N., LIEBMAN, M.N. and MAVROVOUNIOTIS, M.L. Qualitative analysis of biochemical reaction systems (1996) Comput. Biol. Med. 26, 9–24.

SAURO, H.M., HUCKA, M., FINNEY, A., WELLOCK, C., BOLOURI, H., DOYLE, J. and KITANO, H. Next generation simulation tools: the Systems Biology Workbench and BioSPICE integration (2003) Omics 7, 355–72.

SHAPIRO, B.E., HUCKA, M., FINNEY, A. and DOYLE, J. MathSBML: a package for manipulating SBML-based biological models (2004) Bioinformatics 20, 2829–31.

SPELLMAN, P.T., MILLER, M., STEWART, J., TROUP, C., SARKANS, U., CHERVITZ, S., BERNHART, D., SHERLOCK, G., BALL, C., LEPAGE, M., SWIATEK, M., MARKS, W.L., GONCALVES, J., MARKEL, S., IORDAN, D., SHOJATALAB, M., PIZARRO, A., WHITE, J., HUBLEY, R., DEUTSCH, E., SENGER, M., ARONOW, B.J., ROBINSON, A., BASSETT, D., STOECKERT, C.J., JR. and BRAZMA, A. Design and implementation of microarray gene expression markup language (MAGE-ML) (2002) Genome Biol. 3, RESEARCH0046.

TAKAHASHI, K., KAIZU, K., HU, B. and TOMITA, M. A multi-algorithm, multi-timescale method for cell simulation (2004) Bioinformatics 20, 538–46.

TOMITA, M., HASHIMOTO, K., TAKAHASHI, K., SHIMIZU, T.S., MATSUZAKI, Y., MIYOSHI, F., SAITO, K., TANIDA, S., YUGI, K., VENTER, J.C. and HUTCHISON, C.A., 3rd E-CELL: software environment for whole-cell simulation (1999) Bioinformatics 15, 72–84.

YUGI, K. and TOMITA, M. A general computational model of mitochondrial metabolism in a whole organelle scale (2004) Bioinformatics 20, 1795–6.

Subject Index

Systems Biology in Practice. Concepts, Implementation and Application.
E. Klipp, R. Herwig, A. Kowald, C. Wierling, H. Lehrach
Copyright © 2005 WILEY-VCH Verlag GmbH & Co. KGaA, Weinheim
ISBN: 3-527-31078-9

mitosis 54, 235, 239
model 6, 8, 424
– continuous model 8
– discrete model 8
– mitochondrial metabolism 424
– *Mycoplasma genitalium* 424
model development 9
modeling tools 419 ff.
modules 10
– modularity 10
moiety conservation 149
molecular biology 23 ff.
molecular tags 124
molecularity 141
Monod-Wyman-Changeux rate expression
  155
monolayer 29, 39
monosaccharide 27
mortality 240
morula 21
motif 217
M-phase 52 ff.
mRNA *see* messenger RNA
MS *see* mass spectrometry
multi-compartment models 424
multiple testing 128, 303 ff.
– Bonferroni correction 304
– false discovery rate 305
– family-wise error rate 304
– Holm's stepwise correction 305
– Westfall and Young step-down correction
  305
mutation 50, 337, 339, 342
mutation-accumulation theory 241
mutational clouds 343
mutation-selection balance 241
mutual information 329, 376 ff.
myosin 41

n
nanofluidic devices 392
nanosensors 392
nanotechnology 391
National Center for Biotechnology (NCBI)
  405
natural selection 337
NCBI *see* National Center for Biotechnology
negative feedback 220, 232, 236, 278
network 10, 174
network motifs 331 ff.
– autoregulation motif 332
– feed-forward loop 332
– multicomponent loop 332
– multi-input motif 332

– regulatory chain 332
– single-input motif 332
neurula 21
neutral theory of molecular evolution 351
NEWT 405
NF-κB 275
nitrocellulose filter 120
NK automaton 352, 355
NLS *see* nuclear localization sequence
noncompetitive inhibition 150
normalization 176, 296 ff.
– d-chip 297
– global measures 296
– iterative regression 296
– linear model approaches 297
– LOWESS 297
– variance stabilization 298
normalization factor 175
northern blotting 121
NP-hard 383
nuclear envelope 43
nuclear localization sequence 50
nuclear pore 40
nucleic acid 35
nucleoid 40
nucleolus 40
nucleoside 35 f.
nucleosome 41
nucleus 37, 40 f., 46
null hypothesis 91
null space 65
nullclines 228
nylon membrane 120

o
objective function 165
object-oriented model 428
ODE *see* ordinary differential equation
oligomer proteins 153
OMIM 406
once forever selection 349
oncogenes 235
ontology 369, 400
operator 51, 283, 353
operon 278
optimal state 357, 359
optimality principles 355 ff.
optimization 355 ff., 363
ordinary differential equations 66 f., 266, 286
– explicit ODE 67
– implicit ODE 67
– linear systems of ODEs 68
– solution 67
– solution of linear ODE systems 70